Central Service
Technical Manual

Seventh Edition

www. evole. com

Disclaimer

This publication is designed to provide accurate and authoritative information in regard to the subject matter covered. It is sold with the understanding that the publisher is not engaged in rendering legal, accounting, or other professional service. If legal advice or other expert assistance is required, the services of a competent professional person should be sought.

From the Declaration of Principles jointly adopted by the American Bar Association and a Committee of Publishers and Associations.

The authors are solely responsible for the contents of this publication. All views expressed herein are solely those of the authors and do not necessarily reflect the views of the International Association of Healthcare Central Service Materiel Management.

Nothing contained in this publication shall constitute a standard, an endorsement, or a recommendation of the International Association of Healthcare Central Service Materiel Management. The International Association of Healthcare Central Service Materiel Management also disclaims any liability with respect to the use of any information, procedure, or product, or reliance thereon by any member of the healthcare industry.

FOREWORD

CENTRAL SERVICE TECHNICAL MANUAL
Seventh Edition

This seventh edition of the Central Service Technical Manual has evolved from the first edition which was published by the International Association of Healthcare Central Service Materiel Management (IAHCSMM) in 1969. The intervening editions during these (almost) 40 years have detailed successive improvements in the discipline to help keep Central Service Technicians and other professionals current in an industry where the term, "fast- paced," is a conservative description. This new seventh edition reflects the latest in technology, innovations, and protocols which impact "how things are done" in contemporary Central Service departments.

How has this new Central Service Technical Manual changed from the previous edition? It's easy to start with the obvious: the extensive use of color, photographs, and graphics that help make it easy to read and to learn. Probing just a little deeper, you will notice the format of each chapter:

- Objectives that introduce each chapter, and then begin each section of the chapter.

- Extensive use of "key terms" that are introduced and defined throughout the chapter to help assure that readers understand the basic language of the Central Service discipline.

- An organization that is simplified with use of headings and lists that focus on specific topics.

An extensive end-of-manual glossary is provided to continue the emphasis on basic language comprehension as a critical on-the-job communication tool.

As you begin to read this new edition of the Central Service Technical Manual, you'll quickly discover that it is not just attractive and easy-to-comprehend. Its completely revised content explores the world of Central Service for new readers, and brings experienced professionals up-to-date on the latest industry standards. Authors have made extensive use of the new American National Standard ST 79 developed by the Association for the Advancement of Medical Instrumentation (AAMI) which combines previously separate technical standards applicable to the Central Service profession. The result: the Central Service Technical Manual is an indispensable resource in the working library of every Central Service director, manager, supervisor, and employee.

This new edition was, like no previous edition, written "by the industry for the industry." The development process began 14 months before the Central Service Technical Manual was published. Volunteer members of IAHCSMM's Professional Development Resource Council:

- Reviewed content of the sixth edition text.

- Compiled data from several inputs (member surveys, instructor surveys, student surveys, and changes in standards and technologies).

- Determined additional subject-matter that was needed.

- Suggested the appropriate organization for the manual and its chapters.

- Reviewed first, edited, and final drafts of every chapter.

Members of the PDRC who served as the development team for this seventh edition manual deserve special recognition:

Tracy Johnson*

Patti Koncur

Cheron Rojo

Jean Sargent

Richard Schule

BJ Schuler

The old saying, "If you want to get something done, assign the task to the persons who are the busiest!" is certainly true, and you'll note that PDRC committee members were also actively involved writing chapters and developing workbook and instructor materials.

The Central Service Technical Manual, Seventh Edition, will, more than ever before, help Central Service professionals to learn the "why's" behind the "how's" applicable to the knowledge and skills needed for their profession. As with previous editions, it was written with the following constituencies at the forefront:

• Central Service Technicians studying to complement their skills as they prepare for certification programs sponsored by IAHCSMM.

• Central Service and Materiel Management staff members looking for solutions to daily operating problems, and answers to questions about ways to improve their products and services.

• Today's students—members of tomorrow's healthcare team—who are enrolled in courses leading to positions within the profession.

The greatest influence of this new edition of the Central Service Technical Manual may stem from its continued use as a study guide in IAHCSMM's certification program for Central Service Technicians. Thousands of healthcare professionals have used previous editions to help them become certified: recognized for their knowledge of and dedication to the ever-expanding role of Central Service in healthcare facilities.

In many respects, the earlier editions of the Central Service Technical Manual have been a basic "primer" for the profession. They have literally shaped and influenced the careers of certified professionals—many of whom have gone on to distinguish themselves in their chosen field, and who now hold the highest positions in their facilities and with affiliated associations. It is expected that this new edition will continue this tradition. It will be used as a study guide today, and tomorrow it will be on the bookshelves of those who will most influence the Central Service profession as it evolves.

It is testimony to the experts who have contributed to this manual that such a wide variety of needs can be met by a single text. This new edition draws upon the contributions made by authors of earlier editions, and our thanks are extended to them.

ACKNOWLEDGEMENTS AND FINAL THOUGHTS

Many association members and others assisted PDRC members and chapter contributors with the development of this Central Service Technical Manual. They devoted their time, knowledge, and energies to help assure that this manual was absolutely as good as it could be. Special recognition goes to, Patti Koncur and Jean Sargent who provided the final technical review of the entire manual. We also wish to thank Mr. Stan Burkat, Burkat Design, for his assistance in developing this first-ever format and production process used for the Central Service Technical Manual.

The concluding paragraph in the Foreword to the sixth edition of the Central Service Technical Manual is worth repeating:

It is the past, present, and future members of the International Association of Healthcare Central Service Materiel Management to whom this Central Service Technical Manual is dedicated. It truly was written by them and for them. They, along with the patients being cared for, will be better served as the contents of this manual are implemented in the day-to-day operations of our nation's healthcare facilities.

It has been an honor, pleasure, and rewarding learning experience to serve as co-editors of this important healthcare resource.

Natalie Lind, CRCST, CHL
IAHCSMM Education Director
Ada, Minnesota

Jack D. Ninemeier, Ph.D.
The Eli Broad Graduate School of Management
Michigan State University
East Lansing, Michigan

A Special Thank You to the Author/Contributors who generously shared their time and expertise to develop this text and its corresponding materials. They are (alphabetically):

Bruce T. Bird
Director, Central Processing
Surgical Services Clinical Program
Urban Central Region
Intermountain Healthcare
Salt Lake City, UT

Joyce Burris, CRCST, ACE
Sterile Processing Manager
Swedish Medical Center
Seattle, WA

Dr. Mauro da Fonte
Faculty
Health Science and Math & Science Divisions
Gateway Community College
Phoenix, AZ

Scott A. Davis
Director, Technical Operations
IMS Sterile Processing Management

Sharon Greene-Golden, CRCST
Manager of Sterile Processing
BON SECOURS-Mary Immaculate Hospital
Newport News, VA

Marcia Hardick, RN, BS, CGRN, CSPDT
Clinical Education Specialist
STERIS Corporation

Gale Havrilla
Senior Microbiologist (Retired)
3M Healthcare Sterilization

Lisa Huber, BA, CRCST, ACE, FCS
Sterile Processing Director
Anderson Hospital
Maryville, IL

Lory Hunter, ST, CRCST
Vice President, SPD Educator
Best Practice Professionals, Inc.
Milwaukee, WI

Tracy Johnson*
Chief, PAD
West Palm Beach, VAMC

Victor Kennedy, M.P.H, C.I.H.
Director, Safety Department
UCLA Healthcare System

Sue Klacik, BA, FCS, ACE, CRCST, CHL
Corporate Director of Sterile Processing
Forum Health
Youngstown, OH

Patti Koncur
Director of Clinical Operations
IMS S-3
Surgeon's Support Solutions

Stephen Kovach
Director of Education
Healthmark Industries

Natalie Lind
Educational Director
IAHCSMM

Bob Marrs, BA, CRCST, CHL
Director, Sterile Processing
St. David's Medical Center
Austin, TX

David A. Narance, RN, BSN, CRCST
Manager/Clinical Specialist Sterile Reprocessing
MedCentral Health System
Mansfield, OH

Jack Ninemeier, Ph. D.
The Eli Broad Graduate School of Management
Michigan State University

Harriet Pitts, MS, CIC, RN
Long Beach Memorial Hospital
Long Beach, CA

Cheron Rojo
Educator
St. Agnes Medical Center
Fresno, CA

Jean Sargent, FCS, FAHRMM, CMRP, ACE, CRCST, CHL
Vice President Supply Chain Management
University of Kentucky Chandler Medical Center

Rick Schultz
President and Chief Executive Officer
Spectrum Surgical Instruments Corporation
Stow, OH

Linda L. Wilson, RN, BSN, Med, CNOR, BC
Staff Development Coordinator
Poudre Valley Hospital
Fort Collins, CO

We would like to thank the following Vendors, Institutions, and Organizations for their contributions to the Seventh Edition and its corresponding materials:

(Alphabetically)

3M Healthcare

Aesculap

Advanced Sterilization Products (ASP)

Case Medical

Gettinge

Healthmark Industries

Integrated Medical Services (IMS)

KEM Medical

Lighthouse Imaging Corporation

Medline Industries

Spectrum Surgical

SPS Medical

Steris Corporation

We would also like to thank the following individuals for their work reviewing the text:

Bruce Bird	Stephen Kovach
Joyce Burris	Bob Marrs
David Craig	Carla McDermott
Mauro da Fonte	David Narance
Don Gordon	Mary Olivera
Sharon Greene-Golden	Carol Petro
Larry Guittard	Cheron Rojo
Gale Havrilla	Jean Sargent
Lisa Huber	Richard Schule
Tracy Johnson*	Rick Schultz
Sue Klacik	Angela Snowden
Bob Kline	Paula Vandiver
Patti Koncur	Linda Wilson

Numerous Central Service Departments and healthcare facilities opened their doors and allowed us to take many photos for the text and corresponding materials. IAHCSMM would like to express its sincere appreciation to those individuals and departments that were so instrumental in giving the Seventh Edition a decidedly Central Service look.

In Memory of Tracy Johnson (1960 – 2007)

Nothing great was ever achieved without enthusiasm
- Ralph Waldo Emerson

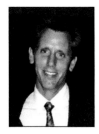

*As an advocate for the student, Tracy assured they were given every opportunity to succeed. Equally important, Tracy was also an advocate for the patient and was passionate toward all staff becoming trained/educated/certified and understanding what they were doing to assure appropriate patient care. As an active participant for the Professional Development Resource Council (PDRC), Tracy dedicated hundreds of hours toward teaching, writing chapters, proof-reading, and providing the attention to detail required of our technicians in the Central Service profession. Tracy will remain in our hearts and in our departments through Central Service education.

Contents

Chapter 5

Regulations and Standards 77

Chapter 6

Chapter 7

Chapter 8

Chapter 9

Chapter 10

Disinfection

Chapter 11

Chapter 12

Chapter 13

Chapter 14

Chapter 15

Chapter 16

Chapter 17

Chapter 18

Chapter 19

Tracking Systems 371

Chapter 20

Quality Assurance 377

Chapter 21
Safety 397

Chapter 22

Chapter 23

The International Association of Healthcare Central Service Materiel Management

The International Association of Healthcare Central Service Materiel Management (IAHCSMM) is the premier organization for professionals working in the discipline of Central Service Material Management (CS/MM). Established in 1958, it is a non-profit corporation headquartered in Chicago, Illinois, with more than 9000 members working throughout the healthcare industry in hospitals, ambulatory surgery centers, dental offices, and for medical supply manufacturers and third party reprocessors. Its members represent all 50 states and several foreign countries, and allow IAHCSMM to be a true international representative for its membership and the profession.

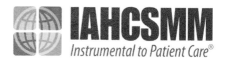

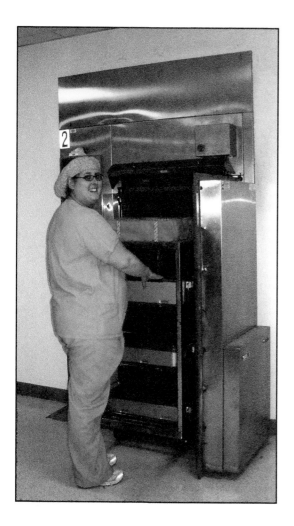

IAHCSMM AND EDUCATION

One of IAHCSMM's primary roles is to provide education and certification services to CS/MM professionals. Prior to the mid-1940's, sterilization services for all hospital departments were performed by Surgical Nurses in the surgery department. The American College of Surgeons then began a movement to standardize and centralize the preparation, sterilization, handling, and storage of all surgical supplies into one unit. The result: Central Service Departments were developed.

Today, many medical devices and supplies tend to be disposable rather than reusable. Surgical procedures and instrumentation have become more complex, and require changes in sterilization processes. Total joint replacements are performed in hospitals of every size, everyday. Physicians are performing minimally invasive procedures using endoscopes, cameras and other instruments that cost thousands of dollars (or more), and this new technology requires sterilization with methods other than saturated steam under pressure in an autoclave.

Training for physicians has evolved from apprentice-type programs to those requiring several years of specialized training after post-secondary and medical schools. Training for nurses is now university-based rather than hospital-based. By necessity, Central Service training has also changed from an on-the job ("tag along") model to a textbook-based course-of-study of which this Central Service Technical Manual, Seventh Edition, is an integral part. It is designed to provide Central Service Technicians with the latest, most current information needed to handle the changing requirements of surgical instrument sterilization, equipment management, and supply distribution.

IAHCSMM ORGANIZATIONAL STRUCTURE

Active membership in IAHCSMM is open to anyone employed in healthcare Central Service or Materiel Management departments, in a related field, or to anyone with an interest in promoting the purpose or objectives of the Association. Associate membership is open to anyone who, by virtue of their occupation, has an allied relationship with Central Service Materiel Management departments.

Although it is not required for membership, many IAHCSMM members form local chapters that offer independent meetings and provide educational offerings that follow guidelines established in IAHCSMM by-laws. The elected local chapter Presidents serve as chapter representatives, and comprise the IAHCSMM Board of Directors. This Board convenes during the annual meeting, and elects two representatives to the Executive Board from among its members.

The Executive Board is comprised of the Association's President, President-Elect, Secretary-Treasurer, and Executive Director, as well as the

IAHCSMM MISSION STATEMENT

The IAHCSMM mission shall be to provide the members of the Association and healthcare facilities with organized educational opportunities, professional development, a forum for information exchange, member services in response to member identified needs and priorities; and to represent Central Service Materiel Management in the professional community.

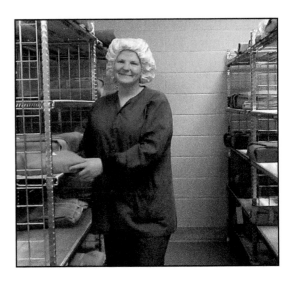

two representatives from the Board of Directors. Responsibilities of the Executive Board include transacting all administrative and financial business of the Association, planning the annual meeting, up-dating all educational materials as required, maintaining working relationships with allied associations, and interacting with IAHCSMM committees.

An Educational Director is responsible for developing and monitoring all IAHCSMM educational programs to ensure that all materials are timely, consistent, and accurate. The Executive Board, the Educational Director, and the association's Professional Development Resource Council (PDRC) work together to:

• Provide education for IAHCSMM-approved instructors.

• Develop the educational program for the Association's annual meeting.

• Develop and update all of the Association's educational resources.

Two other committees are important to IAHCSMM members: the Corporate Advisory Committee (CAC), and the Educational Advisory Committee (EAC). Along with representatives from IAHCSMM's corporate sponsors, the association's elected officers and Executive Director meet with the CAC to plan annual vendor exhibits

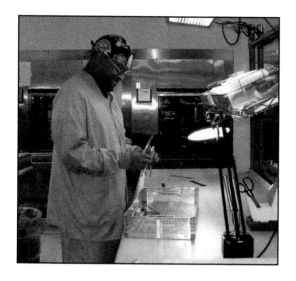

IAHCSMM PROFESSIONAL DEVELOPMENT

Completing this Central Service Technician Training Course and attaining certification is a positive first step in one's personal professional development efforts. Those pursuing a career in Central Service continually strive for recognition as professionals. It is important to understand the meaning of the term, "professional," and the requirements and responsibilities needed to earn that title. A professional is a person working in an occupation that requires extensive knowledge and skills. A profession involves membership limited to individuals with formal education in a specialized body of knowledge. Membership in a profession is usually controlled by licensing, registration, and/or certification, and is governed by a universal code of ethics. Persons working in the field of Central Service/Materiel Management certainly meet those requirements.

and education, and to consider other issues relating to corporate sponsors. The EAC members are corporate technical experts in Central Service who provide expertise to assist the Association in its program development activities.

IAHCSMM EDUCATIONAL OPPORTUNITIES

The Association's mission statement emphasizes that the provision of educational opportunities for its membership is a high priority. Held in the spring of each year, its annual meeting combines the annual membership meeting with four days of educational offerings for technicians and managers, education for IAHCSMM-approved course instructors, and the opportunity to learn about the latest products from vendors.

IAHCSMM also sponsors two day regional meetings throughout the United States that offer educational opportunities. IAHCSMM chapters also provide educational seminars to reach as many Central Service Technicians as possible. Together these educational offerings help technicians and managers keep up-to-date on the latest trends, regulations, and recommended practices, and provide an opportunity for them to network with other CS/MM professionals.

IAHCSMM develops, requires, and maintains high educational and certification standards. As the professional and technical requirements of the CS/MM profession have become more demanding, IAHCSMM has developed educational and certification programs to address these changing demands. IAHCSMM partners with Purdue University to develop academic and credentialing standards, and Purdue University endorses all IAHCSMM educational programs.

For many Central Service Technicians, the right combination of education and experience has led to the ultimate proof of competence: certification. Certification is a process that validates that a minimum level of knowledge and skills has been obtained. Someone who is certified has successfully completed a process to verify an understanding of key elements necessary to be successful in the position. Certification requirements usually include a specified amount of relevant experience, completion of specialized courses of study, and successful completion of a written exam. Whatever the steps in the process, the result is that those who are certified have proof that they are knowledgeable about and competent in their work.

IAHCSMM offers several certification courses that include:

- Certified Registered Central Service Technician (CRCST)—emphasis is on the subject -matter in this textbook which, along with a minimum of 400 clinical hours of hands-on experience, prepares one to take the examination required for certification.

- Certified Instrument Specialist (CIS)—emphasis is on identifying, handling, and processing surgical instrumentation. One must first have the CRCST credential before attaining this certification.

- Certification in Healthcare Leadership (CHL)—emphasis is on supervisory responsibilities including recruitment, selection, orientation and training, communication, leadership, motivation, and other related concepts. One must first have the CRCST credential before attaining this certification.

- Certification in Healthcare Materiel Management Concepts (CHMMC)—emphasis is on purchasing, financial management, storage and warehousing, waste control, personnel management, and related concepts.

Another designation—Fellowship in Central Service (FCS)—is available to senior Central Service professionals who are IAHCSMM members. By combining professional accomplishments with a research paper, members may achieve this, the highest designation, for Central Service Professionals.

Many healthcare organizations use Career Ladders to reward employees for successful professional development. Career ladders can provide financial incentives as well as recognition for accomplishments such as attaining certifications that benefit the healthcare organization. Maintaining each of these certifications requires proof of Continuing Education Units (CEUs) that must be earned, and then submitted at the time of annual membership renewal.

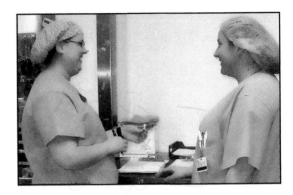

IAHCSMM INFORMATION EXCHANGE

Central Service professionals require the most current information to remain at the "top of their game." This information is vital to help keep them informed about new products and changes in recommended practices. IAHCSMM provides several methods for the sharing of information and ideas.

Communiqué is its bi-monthly publication, and an annual subscription is one of many benefits to IAHCSMM membership. With features such as

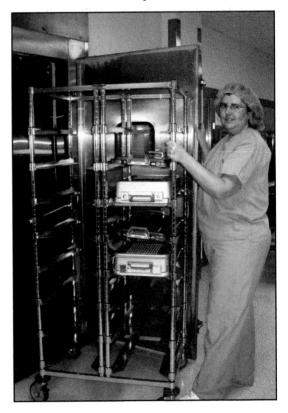

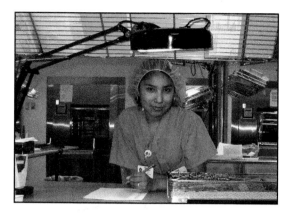

"President's Message," "Technician's Exchange," "Self-Study Lesson Plans," and "Hot Topics," and information about up-coming meetings and news from IAHCSMM chapters, Communiqué is a valuable tool for CS professionals.

IAHCSMM's website, www.iahcsmm.org, is an immediate source of a wide variety of current and helpful professional information. In addition to Communiqué Online, the website provides information about the latest available CS/MM positions, IAHCSMM certifications, links to vendor partners, and an easy way to ordering IAHCSMM products.

One of the most popular features of the website is its Discussion Forum. This real-time feature allows users to post questions about many issues Central Service professionals encounter each day. The answers are provided by other forum users, and all that is needed is internet access.

IAHCSMM MEMBER SERVICES

IAHCSMM represents the CS/MM profession and fosters relationships with several allied organizations. For example, its members serve on committees of the Association for the Advancement of Medical Instrumentation (AAMI), are in attendance at each annual congress of the Association of periOperative Nurses (AORN), and speak at the annual meetings of the Association of Surgical Technologists (AST), and the Association of Professionals in Infection Control (APIC).

Providing representation for CS/MM professionals to these allied groups helps to ensure a voice in decisions that affect IAHCSMM members.

IAHCSMM AND THE FUTURE

Healthcare organizations will continue to focus on patient safety and infection control goals. Managing costs and improving patient outcomes require that all healthcare professionals within each specialty, including sterile processing, be at the forefront of efforts to achieve these goals.

IAHCSMM leadership will always strive to improve the professional status of individuals working in the CS/MM profession. They are never content with what has been done, and are continually looking forward to changing membership needs. Current issues include:

• Advocating mandatory certification for Central Service Technicians in all 50 states.

• Continually updating and improving educational resources.

• Advocating strict regulations relating to loaner instrumentation.

• Providing opportunities for career growth and professional development.

The Central Service environment is dynamic and fast-paced, and the work is challenging and highly technical. Inefficiencies in productivity, errors, and poor quality outputs are costly to hospitals and can be life-threatening to patients. The performance of every person in every Central Service department has a direct impact on patient and employee safety. The profession is truly an evolving occupational discipline. Central Service professionals should take great satisfaction in knowing that their efforts, service, special skills, and caring are a part of every surgical procedure, each patient recovery, every birth, and each patient discharge. IAHCSMM's motto accurately reflects this: Central Service professionals are "Instrumental to Patient Care®."

Chapter 1

Introduction to Central Service

Chapter Outline

Chapter Learning Objectives

As a result of successfully completing this chapter, readers will be able to:

1. Explain the importance of the Central Service Department with an emphasis on the service provided, and its role in quality patient care.

2. Review the work flow process in an effectively organized Central Service Department.

3. Identify basic knowledge and skills required for effective Central Service Technicians.

4. Define job responsibilities of Central Service Technicians.

5. Discuss basic concerns of Central Service personnel:
   - Career growth and professional development.
   - Department organization.
   - Compensation.

The majority of medical procedures require the use of supplies, instruments, and/or equipment, some of which are used once and then discarded, and others which are used multiple times. Reusable items must be thoroughly cleaned, inspected, disinfected, and/or sterilized before they can be used to treat additional patients. The Central Service department in a health care facility performs these processes.

WHAT'S IN A NAME?

Learning Objective 1. Explain the importance of the Central Service Department with an emphasis on the service provided, and its role in quality patient care.

"Central Service" is just two words but, taken together, they appropriately describe the department that is the subject of this Technical Manual.

The "Central" in Central Service

The term, "central," suggests that services are centralized. The activities of reprocessing soiled goods and sterilizing devices to ready them for the next procedure are conducted in one centralized location under the direction and management of one individual: the Director of Central Service. (Note: The actual job title may vary by institution.) Many health care facilities find an increased demand for reprocessing services, partially as a result of a growing trend: the use of more reusable and more complex products. In addition, many facilities have expanded to clinics, surgical centers, professional offices, and other service venues that may be remote from the facility's main location.

In response to this growing demand for reprocessing services, satellite-processing units with centralized management have been established. Others have consolidated (centralized) services into an entire **integrated delivery network.** Other organizations outsource required services to specialized businesses. Regardless of where reprocessing activities are conducted, quality practices must be standardized in compliance with Central Service policies and procedures to enable standards of practice to be consistent and uniform.

Centralized management helps provide maximum utilization of human and material resources. This eliminates the costly duplication of utilities, processing equipment, space, and personnel. Educated and skilled Central Service Technicians must be knowledgeable about the complexities, precautions, and techniques required by their job. They must carry out tasks in a manner that protects the welfare and safety of patients, co-workers, themselves, and their community. Proven material handling techniques are employed to provide high levels of efficiency.

When services are centralized, when the most effective processing equipment is used, and when a better educated and prepared work force is available, fewer people can process a greater volume of materials in less time. This helps to meet the demands of increased workloads in today's health care environment.

The "Service" In Central Service

The term, "**service,**" is the key to "what Central Service is all about," and it occurs as Central Service personnel help or assist their patients and others including their health care peers. Central Service personnel must remember that they are an integral part of quality patient care. Other departments (customers) within the health care facility depend on Central Service for processed sterile supplies, instruments, equipment, and/or many products

Integrated delivery network (IDN) – A system of healthcare providers and organizations which provide (or arrange to provide) a coordinated range of services to a specific population. An IDN may be clinically and financially accountable to the population served for its health status.

Service – An activity that helps or assists one or more persons or groups of persons.

Decontamination – To make safe by removing or reducing contamination by infectious organisms or other harmful substances; the reduction of contamination to an acceptable level.

provided ready-to-use from the manufacturer. In most cases, the services provided by Central Service personnel not only "assist others," but are essential for proper patient treatment.

Central Service by Many Names

The title "Central Service" is the accepted name for this department in many health care facilities and professional organizations. In some facilities, the title "Central Service," is changed to reflect specific needs including "Central Processing," "Sterile Processing and Distribution," "Central Sterile Supply," and "Surgical Supply and Processing." Not all Central Service departments provide the same services to their customers. However, the services that are provided are always guided by the same principles and standards of operation.

CENTRAL SERVICE WORK FLOW

Learning Objective 2. Review the work flow process in an effectively organized Central Service Department.

Proper work flow in a Central Service department is important. Soiled materials must be isolated from their clean counterparts to ensure acceptable processing conditions. A one-way flow of materials from the soiled area to the clean processing area, and on to the sterile storage area is required. (See **Figure 1.1**)

To facilitate one-way flow of goods in this process, and to maintain distinction between soiled and clean work areas, physical barriers or walls segregate the functional areas of Central Service. These areas include decontamination, preparation/ packaging/sterilization, and sterile storage.

Decontamination

The decontamination area is where all soiled instruments and other items are received from using departments. **Decontamination** is the physical or chemical process that renders an inanimate object such as a medical device that may be contaminated with harmful microbes, safe for further handling. It involves a thorough cleaning process that may be accomplished with manual

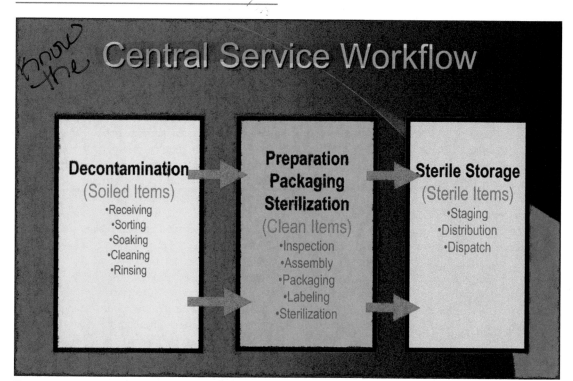

Figure 1.1 One-way Flow of Materials in a Central Service Department.

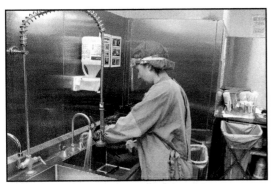

Figure 1.2 The Processing Cycle: Service Technician cleanng surgical instruments manually.

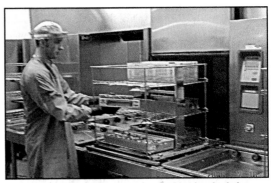

Figure 1.3 The Processing Cycle: Mechanical cleaning of surgical instruments.

cleaning (by hand, using sinks or basins) and/or with mechanical washers. Cleaning is the first step in the sterilization process. All items returned to this area are considered contaminated and potentially infectious. Central Service Technicians must have an in-depth knowledge of the items to be cleaned in this area, and incoming devices must be inspected to determine the method by which they will be decontaminated. They must then be sorted and disassembled to be cleaned properly. (See **Figure 1.2**)

Working in the decontamination area requires a thorough knowledge and understanding of microbiology and the decontamination process. Required knowledge and skills include those necessary for cleaning techniques (steps in the process and objectives of cleaning) and decontamination. Central Service staff must be able to identify and clean a wide variety of surgical instruments including syringes, needles, rubber, and specialty items. Knowledge about cleaning and disinfecting agents and their use, about the effects of the cleaning process on different metals, and about special instrument lubrication and maintenance tasks is critical. Proper disposal of all types of waste, transportation of contaminated items, and operation of equipment used in the cleaning process including washers, decontaminators, ultrasonic cleaners, cart washers, stea m guns, and scope washers further suggest the scope of their work. (See **Figure 1.3**)

Central Service Technicians working in the decontamination area must be protected from the environment. The physical layout of this area

as well as cleaning equipment used in it must meet the appropriate standards of governmental agencies, and the recommendations of professional organizations. Policies and procedures must be developed and followed to ensure that work practices minimize employee injury and exposure to pathogens. To meet the facility's and Occupational Safety and Health Administration (OSHA) safety requirements, Central Service Technicians must wear special attire called personal protective equipment (PPE). This minimizes exposure to bloodborne pathogens and other contaminates, and typically includes a facemask, eye protection, cover gown, gloves, and shoe covers or boots.

Preparation/Packaging/Sterilization

After items are safe for handling without protective attire, they are delivered to the preparation, packaging, and sterilization area of the Central Service Department. Workstations are set-up to facilitate the next steps in the processing cycle. Each item is carefully inspected for cleanliness, proper function, and possible defects. Instruments, utensils, and other devices are assembled into sets, and are then packaged and labeled in preparation for sterilization.

Central Service Technicians must be able to identify hundreds of surgical instruments. They must understand how instruments are manufactured, how they are constructed, and how to best maintain them. They must be able to inspect devices for cleanliness, proper condition, and function. Knowledge needed to care for and maintain instruments is essential, as is an understanding

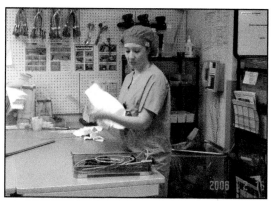

Figure 1.4 The Processing Cycle: Inspection of surgical instruments prior to set assembly.

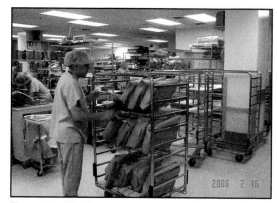

Figure 1.7 The Processing Cycle: Loading sterilizer cart and quality assurance.

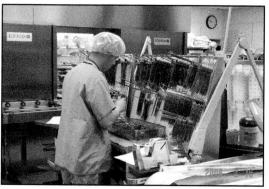

Figure 1.5 The Processing Cycle: Surgical instrument set assembly.

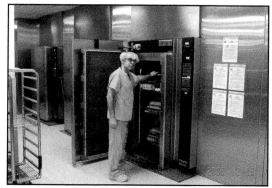

Figure 1.8 The Processing Cycle: Loading the sterilizer.

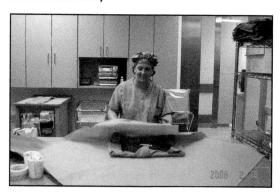

Figure 1.6 The Processing Cycle: Wrapping item prior to sterilization.

about how to prevent and solve problems such as discoloration and corrosion. (**Figures 1.4, 1.5** and **1.6** illustrate the inspection, assembly and packaging process.)

Surgical specialty instruments, equipment, and implants also require special expertise. Central Service Technicians must be able to select the

proper packaging materials, and use proper techniques for wrapping and packaging items for sterilization. Items to be sterilized must be properly identified, and the correct methods and parameters for sterilization must be followed. The principles necessary to achieve sterilization using each method of sterilization must be understood and applied. Sterilizers must be loaded and operated properly, and sterilization quality assurance measures must be followed and interpreted to ensure that items are sterile. Records must be maintained, and factors that can compromise sterile packaging must be understood, prevented, and detected. (**Figures 1.7** and **1.8** provide examples of sterilization activities.)

Personnel working in the preparation, packaging and sterilization area of Central Service normally wear facility-restricted attire such as a scrub suit and hair coverings. Dress and operating practices must protect the clean environment in this area from contamination.

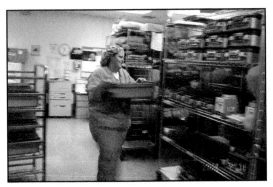

Figure 1.9 The Processing Cycle: Items sterilized in the prep & pack area are placed on shelves in the sterile storage area.

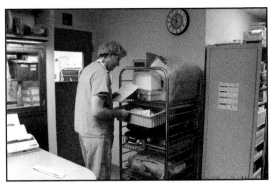

Figure 1.10 The Processing Cycle: Case cart delivered from Central Service to Surgery.

Sterile Storage

The supply area of Central Service is dedicated to the storage of sterile and clean supplies. A separate area for removing supplies from shipping cartons and containers should be provided. The major portion of the work in this area is receiving, storing, and dispensing supplies and sterile instruments. (See **Figure 1.9**)

While items may be dispensed to almost all departments within a health care facility, the major focus of this area is servicing the operating rooms. This is usually accomplished through the use of a **case cart system**. The bulk of surgical supplies is usually stored in a central location: Central Service. A dependable system must be in place to supply items to Surgery from the sterile storage area. (See **Figure 1.10**)

Surgical procedures are usually scheduled through a surgery scheduling office using a special computer program. When surgical procedures are scheduled (or at another time according to the facility's protocols), authorized personnel assign a case cart or **Doctor (Physician's) Preference Card** to each procedure. This generates a **case cart pull sheet (pick list)** that identifies items specific to the doctor and procedure. Central Service Technicians use this sheet to place supplies from the sterile storage area storage shelves onto the case carts that transport these items to the appropriate operating room. Personnel working in this area usually pull instrument sets and other required instrumentation needed for all surgical procedures for an entire day during the day or evening before they will be used.

Depending on the scope of responsibilities, other areas in the health care facility may be supplied from the sterile storage area. Also, hospital personnel from different departments frequently require items that are only available from Central Service. Those working in the sterile storage area must be familiar with all supplies within the location, because they may be required to help customers determine what is needed.

Excellent lines of communication must be maintained between those in Central Service processing and sterile storage areas to help ensure that an adequate stock of sterile items is always available. Also, the **Materiel Management Department** is an important link in the supply process. A cooperative communication and problem-solving attitude must be fostered between personnel in these two important departments.

The sterile storage area is restricted to properly attired personnel meeting facility requirements such as a scrub suit and hair coverings who are fulfilling their work requirements. Dress and work practices must protect this area's clean environment from contamination. Traffic is restricted to keep contaminates to the lowest possible level.

Personnel working in the sterile storage area must have a thorough knowledge of every item, how it is used, where it is located, and the process for obtaining it. Excellent interpersonal skills are required to interact with customers from throughout the facility. Other knowledge and skills include those needed for:

- Inventory control and supply distribution.

- Surgical specialties and procedures.

- Sterile storage.

- Sterile supply handling.

- Supply rotation.

- Computer systems relating to inventory and case carts.

- Acquisition and disposition of supplies.

- Resolution of supply problems.

All Central Service areas must exercise careful environmental control conditions. Each work area should be restricted to assigned and authorized personnel who consistently follow the facility's dress code policies. Strict traffic control patterns must regulate the movement of people and goods through the department. Air pressure levels (**negative air pressure** in decontamination areas and **positive air pressure** in the clean areas) must be maintained to control air movements. Proper air pressure control helps to prevent the flow of bacteria-laden particulates and dust from the soiled to the clean areas.

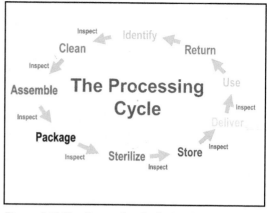

Figure 1.11 The Processing Cycle: Inspection plays an essential part of the process to ensure that a safe, quality product is provided for our patients.

The Processing Cycle

Work performed in Central Service usually follows the cycle just discussed. (See **Figure 1.11**) After use, items that can be reprocessed are returned to the decontamination area to start the process all over again. It is important to note that, at each step in the process, items are inspected to ensure that they are clean, in good repair, assembled and processed correctly, and/or that packaging materials have not been damaged to compromise sterility. **Figures 1.12** through **1.15** illustrate steps in the use cycle from the user unit (in this case Surgery) to decontamination.

Case cart system – *An inventory control system for products/equipment typically used in an operating room that involves use of an enclosed cart generally prepared for one surgical case, and not used for general supply replenishment.*

Doctor (Physician's) preference card – *A document that identifies a physician's needs (requests and preferences) for a specific medical procedure.* *Preference cards usually contain information regarding the instruments, equipment, supplies and utensils used by a specific physician. They may also include reminders for the staff of the physician's preferences regarding patient draping, etc.*

Decon air pressure (negative)

Case cart pull sheet (pick list) – *A list of specific supplies, utensils, and instruments for a specific procedure.* *Central Service Technicians use these lists to assemble the items needed for individual surgical procedures.*

Materiel Management Department – *The healthcare department responsible for researching, ordering, receiving, and managing inventory (consumable supplies).*

Negative air pressure – *The situation that occurs when air flows into a room or area because the pressure in the area is less than that of surrounding areas.* pushing air flow in.

Positive air pressure – *The situation that occurs when air flows out of a room or area because the pressure in the area is greater than that of surrounding areas.* pushing air flow out.

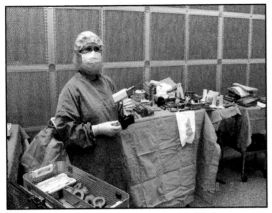

Figure 1.12 The Processing Cycle: Sterile items are used in Surgery.

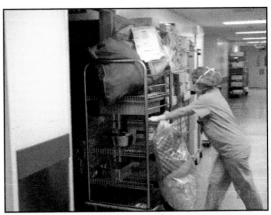

Figure 1.14 The Processing Cycle: Items are returned to Central Service for processing.

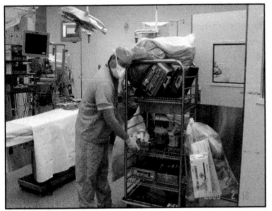

Figure 1.13 The Processing Cycle: Used items are prepared for return to Central Service after being used.

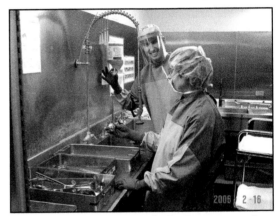

Figure 1.15 The Processing Cycle: Once returned to decontamination area of CS items are inspected to determine condition and proper method for processing.

A Basic Educational Foundation Is Needed

Numerous dimensions of knowledge and skills are required for Central Service Technicians to be effective. Taken together, they provide an overview of the breadth and depth of the discipline about which you are learning.

A basic educational foundation is necessary as a base for more specialized knowledge and skills that must be learned. Examples of this educational foundation include the ability to:

- Read and write, including the use of charts, reports, and manuals.

- Interpret technical materials used for Central Service practices and procedures.

Perform mathematical operations, including computations and weights and measures.

- Properly use healthcare and medical terminology.

- Understand basic structures, functions, and relationships between cells, tissues, organs, and systems.

- Use methods to control the spread of pathogenic microorganisms including cleaning, disinfection, and sterilization.

- Practice effective inventory and materiel management concepts and processes.

BASIC JOB KNOWLEDGE AND SKILLS

Learning Objective 3. Identify basic knowledge and skills required for effective Central Service Technicians.

Individuals employed in Central Service must have and apply significant knowledge and many skills for their department to successfully deliver quality products and services to its customers.

Let's review the knowledge and skill dimensions required to be an effective Central Service Technician.

Communication Abilities

Central Service Technicians must know alternative methods of providing and obtaining information. They must be effective oral and written communicators. To do so, they must be able to:

- Assess the ability of other people to understand what is being communicated.

- Adapt communication tactics to individual needs.

- Apply active listening skills using reflection, re-statement, and clarification techniques.

- Interact appropriately and respectfully with diverse ethnic, age, cultural, religious, and economic groups in numerous employment and social situations.

- Communicate in a straightforward, understandable, accurate, and timely manner.

- Use facility-specific guidelines and methods to send and receive information.

- Access and use electronically-produced information.

Facility Systems

Central Service Technicians must understand how their role fits into their department, their organization, and the overall health care environment. They must be able to identify how key systems affect the services they perform and

quality of care they provide. To do so requires that they:

- Are aware of the range of services offered to customers.

- Prevent unnecessary waste and duplication.

- Participate in quality improvement activities.

- Use resources including other staff members, manuals, and training opportunities.

Employability Skills

Successful Central Service Technicians practice employability skills to enhance their employment opportunities and job satisfaction, and they maintain and upgrade those skills as required. Examples arise as they:

- Maintain appropriate personal skills such as attendance and time management, and as they assume individual responsibility for their actions.

- Attain professional conduct standards.

- Use analytical skills to solve problems and make decisions.

- Formulate solutions to problems using critical thinking skills (analyze, synthesize, evaluate) independently and in teams.

- Adapt to changing situations.

- Practice personal integrity and honesty.

- Engage in continuous self-assessment and goal modification for their personal and professional improvement.

- Exhibit respectful and empathetic behavior as they interact with peers, superiors, subordinates, and customers in one-on-one and group situations.

- Listen attentively to verbal instructions, requests, and other information to verify accuracy.

- Understand various career options and the preparation required for them.

Legal Responsibilities

Central Service Technicians must understand and maintain an awareness of the legal responsibilities, limitations, and the implications of their actions within the health care delivery setting. To do so, they must:

- Solve problems relating to legal dilemmas or issues.

- Comply with established risk management factors and procedures.

- Determine when an incident must be reported.

- Maintain confidentiality.

- Operate within the required scope of practice.

- Follow mandated standards for workplace safety.

- Apply mandated standards for harassment, labor, and other employment laws.

- Comply with legal requirements for documentation.

Ethics

Ethics relates to knowing the difference between "right" and "wrong." In the health care environment, it means conforming to accepted and professional standards of conduct. Ethical behavior is "doing the right thing in the right way." Ethics should govern and guide the way Central Service Technicians act and make decisions. They must always:

- Respect patient's rights and self-determination.

- Promote justice and the equal treatment of all persons.

- Recognize the importance of patients' needs over other considerations.

- Exhibit loyalty to fellow workers and the health care facility.

- Report any activity that adversely affects the health, safety, or welfare of patients, visitors, or fellow workers.

- Comply with pertinent regulatory guidelines, including OSHA standards.

- Respect interdisciplinary differences among team members.

- Differentiate between ethical and legal issues.

- Demonstrate professionalism when interacting with co-workers and customers.

Safety Practices

Effective Central Service Technicians understand existing and potential hazards to patients, co-workers, and themselves. They prevent injury or illness through safe work practices, and consistently follow health and safety policies and procedures. They do so as they:

- Practice infection control procedures.

- Use **Standard Precautions** to control the spread of infection.

- Practice appropriate cleaning, disinfecting, and sterilizing processes.

- Apply principles of body mechanics, including use of proper lifting techniques.

- Prevent fire and electrical hazards.

Standard precautions – *Methods of using appropriate barriers to prevent transmissions of infectious organisms from contact with blood and all other body fluids, non-intact skin, and mucous membranes. Standard precautions apply to all patients, regardless of diagnosis or presumed infectious status.*

Nosocomial – *Hospital-Acquired Infection (HAI); pertaining to a hospital; applied to a disease caused in the course of being treated in a hospital.*

Job description – *A human resources tool that identifies the major tasks performed by persons in specific positions.*

- Use instruments and equipment as directed.

- Manage hazardous materials.

- Use Material Safety Data Sheets (MSDSs)

- Follow emergency procedures and protocols.

- Comply with pertinent regulatory guidelines, including OSHA standards.

Teamwork

Central Service Technicians must understand the roles and responsibilities of individual members as part of the health care team, including their ability to promote the delivery of quality health care. They must interact effectively and sensitively with all members of their team, and they do so when they:

- Practice team membership skills such as cooperation, leadership, and anticipation of their co-workers' needs.

- Respect cultural and religious differences of team members.

- Interact with others in a manner consistent with the health care team's structure and lines of authority.

- Manage conflict within the workplace by considering the points of view of other persons.

- Respect and value the expertise and contributions of all team members.

- Accept compromise as necessary to ensure the best outcomes.

Resource Management

Central Service Technicians must understand and practice principles and techniques of resource management. They ensure the careful use of available resources as they make timely decisions. Central Service Technicians manage resources effectively when they:

- Control costs and reduce waste.

- Provide quality service.

- Practice time management skills.

- Identify and solve potential problems and anticipate customers' needs.

- Know and use inventory appropriately.

- Practice recycling and waste management tactics.

Other Skills

Other skills are also required by Central Service Technicians. For example, they must:

- Assist in the selection of the materials, supplies, and equipment necessary to provide services.

- Follow manufacturers' warnings and instructions, and ask for clarifications, if needed.

- Continuously evaluate results and procedures.

- Practice prescribed techniques to prevent **nosocomial** infections.

- Maintain departmental work areas in good repair.

- Keep their work environment clean and organized.

New health care roles demand higher levels of skill than ever before for those working in Central Service. The complexities involved in Central Service technology continue to grow, and a new breed of health care professional is emerging.

BASIC JOB RESPONSIBILITIES

Learning Objective 4. Define job responsibilities of Central Service Technicians.

Central Service Technicians are accountable for many tasks. **Job descriptions** are used to define and communicate job duties and requirements to employees within an organization. They are intended to be overviews that capture the general purpose and major accountabilities of a job, and they are used for the following reasons:

Figure 1.16 Sample Job Description. Note: This example defines the work of a certified Central Service Technician for one organization. Other organizations' job descriptions may vary.

Central Processing
Competency Based Position Description

Date: _____

Department Name: Central Processing	Job Title: Technician II, Central Processing
Employee Name:	Employee Signature:
Supervisor Name:	Supervisor Signature:

Performance Rating Systems Definitions

Performance meets criteria less than 60% of the time. The employee may be having difficulty understanding the essential job responsibilities and is unable to perform the function without substantial assistance, monitoring, or training. Generally, the employee has received significant corrective counseling or discipline in this job area.

Performance meets criteria 61-79% of the time. The employee may have a basic understanding of the essential job responsibilities, but is unable to perform the standard without additional assistance, monitoring or training.

Performance meets criteria 80-100% of the time. The employee at this level has a complete understanding of the position and performs all aspects of the essential job responsibilities. The employee requires minimal supervision and is continually working on personal development.

Performance meets criteria 101-110% of the time. Performance at this level exceeds standard job accountabilities. The employee acts as a resource for both the management and staff in originating new ways of doing things and uses this influence to guide the work group / department to levels that otherwise would not be reached.

Position Description

Position Purpose: This position is responsible for ensuring that all surgical supplies, instruments and equipment are properly inventoried, decontaminated, assembled, inspected, packaged, sterilized, stored, distributed and tracked in a quality / timely manner throughout the hospital. Works independently with little supervision. Qualified to train others. Serves as a resource to Central Processing customers.

ESSENTIAL JOB RESPONSIBILITIES	EVALUATION METHOD	PERCENTAGE
Decontamination: Performs duties as a CP Technician independently, works proficiently without supervision and helps train new employees: Identifies and uses appropriate methods and solutions to sort, disassemble, decontaminate, rinse and disinfect instruments and clinical equipment. Operates and troubleshoots cleaning equipment. Appropriately handles garbage, linen and biohazardous materials. Maintains safety standards.	1. Direct Observation 2. Event Occurred 3. Peer Review	
Preparing Instruments: Performs duties as a CP Technician independently, works proficiently without supervision and helps train new employees: Consistently uses recipes to correctly assemble, protect, wrap containerize and/or peel package and label instruments. Identifies and inspects instruments for cleanliness and functionality.	1. Direct Observation 2. Event Occurred 3. Peer Review	
Storage: Performs duties as a CP Technician independently, works proficiently without supervision and helps train new employees: Properly handles and stores sterile supplies, equipment and instruments.	1. Direct Observation 2. Event Occurred 3. Peer Review	
Sterilization Process: Performs duties as a CP Technician independently, works proficiently without supervision and helps train new employees: Selects appropriate sterilization methods. Knows and follows correct principles of sterilization. Properly documents and verifies sterilization loads and biological tests to determine the efficacy of the sterilization process.	1. Direct Observation 2. Event Occurred 3. Peer Review	

Distribution: Performs duties as a CP Technician independently, works proficiently without supervision and helps train new employees: Accesses Doctor Preference Cards. Retrieves, disburses and tracks medical and surgical supplies and equipment to the customer in a quality/timely manner.	1. Direct Observation 2. Event Occurred 3. Peer Review	
Equipment: Performs duties as a CP Technician independently, works proficiently without supervision and helps train new employees: Knows, uses, maintains and operates the equipment specific to CP, i.e. steam, ETO, Sterrad and Steris System I sterilizers; cart washers; washer/disinfectors, ultrasonic cleaners and heat sealers as well as a variety of testing devices.	1. Direct Observation 2. Event Occurred 3. Peer Review	
Inventory Control: Performs duties as a CP Technician independently, works proficiently without supervision and helps train new employees: Knows and uses the processes involved in ordering, receiving, stocking, rotating delivering and monitoring usage of surgical supplies. Communicates supply issues to appropriate personnel in a timely manner.	1. Direct Observation 2. Event Occurred 3. Peer Review	
Environmental Standards: Maintains a clean orderly work area. Completes assigned housekeeping duties.	1. Direct Observation 2. Event Occurred 3. Peer Review	
Resource: Serves as a resource to customers on all Central Processing functions.	1. Direct Observation 2. Event Occurred 3. Peer Review	
Other: Performs other related job duties as required. Tracks his/her progress and compliance in regards to training, staff meeting and inservice education, etc.	1. Direct Observation 2. Event Occurred 3. Peer Review	

Minimum Qualifications:
- ✓ At least 18 years of age.
- ✓ High School Education / GED or possible work experience.
- ✓ Must have 6 months of applicable work experience in Central Processing.
- ✓ Basic computer knowledge.
- ✓ Good interpersonal skills. Ability to establish and maintain effective working relationships and the ability to receive and give constructive feedback.
- ✓ Good verbal and written communication skills (in English), being concise by phone, intercom and in person.
- ✓ Self-motivated, able to work independently with little or no supervision.
- ✓ Has learned concepts and applies them to his/her work.
- ✓ Able to work standing. Must be able to bend, twist, push, pull and lift up to 50 pounds without special equipment or assistance of others.
- ✓ Has successfully passed IAHCSMM certification test.
- ✓ Responsible to maintain professional competence and certification.
- ✓ Required to receive the Heptavax vaccination series upon hiring.

• To evaluate positions and determine compensation. They can be used in conjunction with other resources to establish a pay range for a given position.

• To clarify expectations. Job descriptions outline key job expectations which can be reviewed at the time of hire to clarify performance standards and expectations. They should be reviewed regularly (usually annually) by both the supervisor and those who occupy the position.

• To review performance. Job descriptions can be used during annual performance reviews to recognize exceptional performance, restate performance expectations, and to determine growth opportunities and establish goals.

Health care facilities use different formats for job descriptions, but they typically include the type of information noted in **Figure 1.16**, which is an example of a job description for a Central Service Technician.

BASIC CENTRAL SERVICE CONCERNS

Learning Objective 5. Discuss basic concerns of Central Service personnel:
- Career growth and professional development.
- Department organization.
- Compensation.

In this section, we will review three special concerns shared by Central Service professionals: Career growth and professional development, how their department is organized/structured, and the matter of compensation.

Career Growth and Professional Development

Many Central Service departments still use on-the-job training to fulfill job demands. However, as Central Service develops more fully into a profession, formal education and certification of Central Service Technicians will more frequently become a requirement for working in the department. Formal Central Service technology training courses are becoming more readily available through many post-secondary education systems. Many health care systems are developing their own training courses for teaching Central Service technology. Long distance learning courses are also available for those who do not have an organized training course readily available in their areas.

Career growth and professional development opportunities for Central Service professionals typically depend on their individual motivation to achieve departmental and personal goals. Many facilities offer career progression with more work responsibilities and higher compensation levels within the role of Central Service Technician. As knowledge and responsibilities increase, a qualified

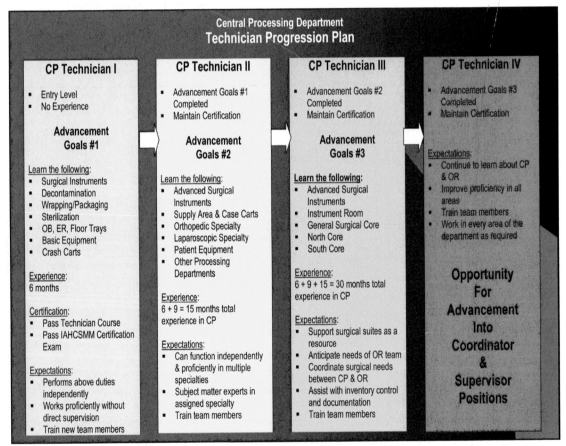

Figure 1.17 Many progressive Central Service departments implement a progression program for their technicians. As knowledge, experience and performance increase, technicians can advance. Wages increase with each advance-

and high performing technician can advance. (See **Figure 1.17**)

Now (and increasingly in the future) qualified, high-performing Central Service Technicians who have achieved **certification** status will be able to choose where they want to work. Selecting a department/health care system that provides for upward progression will be key to this decision. (**Figures 1.18, 1.19** and **1.20** provide examples

Education and Experience are Critical

To survive in today's dynamic and complex environment, it is necessary to be prepared, and education and experience become absolutely critical to do so. Qualified and educated professionals are in demand to meet the new challenges in Central Service departments. Upward mobility requires exploration of the experience, education, and skills required to qualify for supervisory and management positions within the field of Central Service.

of charts that can be developed to encourage and monitor technician progression.)

Department supervisors should have previous Central Service work experience that may include work as a surgical nurse or technologist, or other applicable clinical background. A more experienced Central Service Technician or Surgical Technologist may be prepared to master the more complex duties and responsibilities required of supervisory positions. Supervisory training will most likely be required. Completion of a formal Central Service technology course and certification are essential.

A growing number of health care facilities require managers to have a Bachelor's degree. Some larger

> *Certification – Association and industry recognition given to individuals with educational and/or work experience requirements who successfully complete an examination process that demonstrates their knowledge of subject-matter to be mastered for success in the position.*

Technician Progress Chart #1

Name:		CP Hire Date:		Employee #:

Central Processing Technician I		
Grade: SN 7	Job Code: 2056	Requirements: Entry Level; No Experience

TO

Central Processing Technician II		
Grade: SN 8	Job Code: 253	Requirements: Advancement Goals #1 Completed; Maintain Certification

Advancement Goals #1

Experience = 6 months:

Training Start Date:				Training End Date:	
☐ I month	☐ 2 months	☐ 3 months	☐ 4 months	☐ 5 months	☐ 6 months
Comment (More or less time required?):					

Training Module Completion:

☐ Surgical Instruments	☐ Decontamination	☐ Wrapping/Packaging	☐ Sterilization
☐ OB, ER, Floor Trays	☐ Basic Equipment	☐ Crash Carts	

Certification:

☐ Successfully complete Central Processing Technician Training Course	Date:
☐ Successfully complete IAHCSMM certification requirements	Date:

Successfully Completed Advancement Goals #1:

Expectations: Performs above duties independently; works proficiently without direct supervision; and can train new team members.			
Tech:	Date:	Super:	Date:

Figure1.18

Technician Progress Chart #2

Name:	CP Hire Date:	Employee #:

Central Processing Technician II		
Grade: SN 8	Job Code: 253	Requirements: Advancement Goals #1 Completed; Maintain Certification

TO

Central Processing Technician III		
Grade: SN 9	Job Code: 247	Requirements: Advancement Goals #2 Completed; Maintain Certification

Advancement Goals #2

Experience = Additional 9 months:

Training Start Date:				Training End Date:	
☐ 1 month	☐ 2 months	☐ 3 months	☐ 4 months	☐ 5 months	☐ 6 months
☐ 7 months	☐ 8 months	☐ 9 months	Comment (More or less time required?):		

Training Module Completion (Resource for one area or trained to cover absences in three areas.):

☐ Instrument Room	☐ Supply Area & Case Carts	☐ Patient Equipment
☐ Orthopedic Specialty	☐ Laparoscopic Specialty	☐ Other Processing Departments

Certification:

☐ Maintains certification

Successfully Completed Advancement Goals #2:

Subject matter experts in assigned specialty; can function independently & proficiently in multiple specialties; and trains team members.			
Tech:	Date	Super:	Date:

Figure1.19

Technician Progress Chart #3

Name:	CP Hire Date:	Employee #:

Central Processing Technician III		
Grade: SN 9	Job Code: 247	Requirements: Advancement Goals #2 Completed; Maintain Certification

TO

Central Processing Technician IV		
Grade: SN 10	Job Code: 2243	Requirements: Advancement Goals #3 Completed; Maintain Certification

Advancement Goals #3

Experience = Additional 15 months:

Training Start Date:				Training End Date:	
☐ 1 month	☐ 2 months	☐ 3 months	☐ 4 months	☐ 5 months	☐ 6 months
☐ 7 months	☐ 8 months	☐ 9 months	☐ 10 months	☐ 11 months	☐ 12 months
☐ 13 months	☐ 13 months	☐ 14 months	☐ 15 months	Comments:	

Training Module Completion (Resource for one area or trained to cover absences in three areas.):

☐ Instrument Room	☐ North Core	☐ South Core

Certification:

☐ Maintains certification

Successfully Completed Advancement Goals #2:

Support surgical suites as a resource; anticipate needs of OR team; coordinate surgical needs between SP & OR; assist with inventory control and documentation; and train team members.			
Tech:	Date	Super:	Date:

Figure1.20

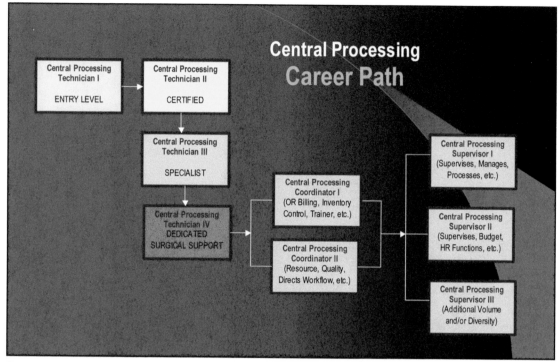

Figure 1.21 There are opportunities for career development within the modern Central Service department. Positions beyond the technician level may require special training and./or degrees.

teaching institutions prefer department heads to have a Master's degree. The emphasis on education in the management discipline is becoming more important as health care organizations become more business-oriented to survive in today's competitive economic environment. (See **Figure 1.21**)

Department Organization

The organizational structure of the modern Central Service department is much broader than it used to be. The title "Director" is most popular for the Central Service department head. Other popular terms are "Manager" and "Supervisor". Larger departments most frequently operate "24/7" (around the clock; seven days a week). In these facilities, each shift usually has a supervisor or coordinator. **Figures 1.22** and **1.23** provide

Career ladder – A plan projecting progressively more responsible professional positions that serves as a foundation for designing a professional development program.

examples of Central Service Department organizational charts.

The reporting relationship for department heads varies between facilities. Commonly, the Director of Central Service reports to persons with titles such as "Vice-President of Clinical (or Support) Services," "Vice-President (or Director) of Materiel Management," or "Vice-President (or Director) of Nursing (or Surgical) Services."

Technicians usually report directly to a shift or other supervisor and, increasingly, facilities have **career ladders** for technical staff members based on factors such as education, certification, and work experience.

Compensation

Compensation, including benefits, is influenced by many factors such as job descriptions (tasks performed), scope and span of responsibility, size of institution, organizational structure, job market, and geographic location. At the department head level, the Central Service Director should be fairly

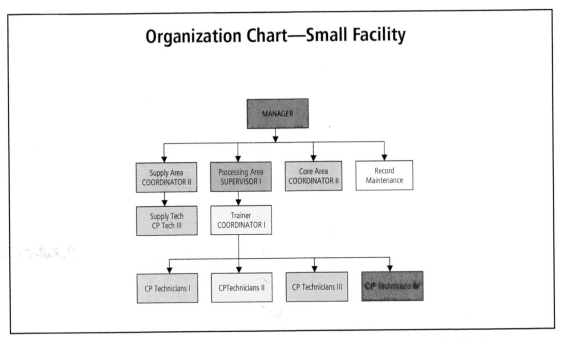

Figure 1.22 Smaller facilities have fewer opportunities for advancement beyond technician level.

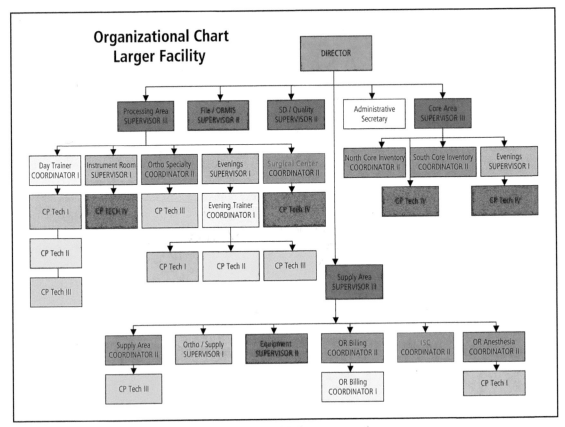

Figure 1.23 Larger facilities have more positions available for career options.

compensated relative to organizational peers. As previously mentioned, there are a growing number of health care facilities that compensate Central Service staff members with pay increments based on experience, high performance, additional education and training, and upon certification.

IN CONCLUSION

The Central Service environment is dynamic and fast-paced. The work is challenging, highly technical, and complex. The performance of this vital department has a major impact on the smooth operation of the many departments to which it provides products and services.

Inefficiencies in productivity, errors that create the need for re-work, and poor quality performance, are costly to hospitals. With the ever-increasing costs of health care, Central Service professionals must strive to conserve resources and minimize expenses. More importantly, however, is the safety and welfare of the patients who have entrusted us with their care. Negligence and carelessness in Central Service could cost a patient's life!

Conscientious Central Service professionals will find great satisfaction in knowing that their efforts, service, special skills, and caring are a part of every surgical procedure, each patient recovery, every birth, each patient discharge, and each happy family reunion.

Central Service is an evolving occupational discipline. Over the years, there have been dramatic changes ranging from the increased use of technology and support services provided to the job skills, training, and educational requirements needed to fulfill these job responsibilities. Changes continue at a fast pace!

REFERENCES

Colbert, Bruce J. *Workplace Readiness for Health Occupations.* Second Edition. Thomson Delmar Learning. 2006.

Booth, Kathryn A. *Health Care Science Technology: Career Foundations.* McGraw-Hill Companies, Inc., 2004.

For National Health Care Skill Standards; visit the National Consortium on Health Science & Technology Education (NCHSTE) website: *www.nchste.org.*

CENTRAL SERVICE TERMS

Integrated delivery network (IDN) *Cert. Exam*

Service 8 *pg. 8*

Decontamination 8

Case cart system 13

Doctor preference card 13

Case cart pull sheet 13

Materiel Management department 13

Negative air pressure 13

Positive air pressure *pg. 13*

Standard precautions 14

Nosocomial 14

Job description 14

Certification *pg. 21*

Career ladder *pg. 23*

Chapter Outline

WORD ELEMENTS IN MEDICAL TECHNOLOGY

ANALYSIS OF MEDICAL TERMS

MORE ABOUT SUFFIXES, ROOTS, AND PREFIXES

COMMON ABBREVIATIONS IN SURGERY SCHEDULES

ENDNOTES

CENTRAL SERVICE TERMS

Chapter 2
Medical Terminology

Chapter Learning Objectives:

As a result of successfully completing this chapter, readers will be able to:

1. Define the word elements "prefix," "root," and "suffix."

2. Analyze medical terms by their word elements.

3. Recognize suffixes, roots, and prefixes that relate to medical and surgical terms.

4. Identify common abbreviations used in surgery schedules.

Central Service Technicians require knowledge of medical terms to help them in their day-to-day work, because these words are part of the professional language utilized by health care personnel. The special terminology used to describe parts of the body, diseases, instruments, and surgical procedures is the topic of this chapter.

WORD ELEMENTS IN MEDICAL TECHNOLOGY

Learning Objective 1. Define the word elements "prefix," "root," and "suffix."

Central Service Technicians frequently encounter specialized medical terms in their daily work activities. Use of appropriate medical terminology can improve communication, for example, between central service and operating room personnel. As well, many medical and surgical supplies, instruments, and equipment have names driven by medical terminology principles. As Technicians learn the meanings of these names, they will have a greater understanding of what their work involves, and their job satisfaction will increase.

The majority of medical terms are of either Greek or Latin origin. Many terms combine both Greek and Latin **word elements** to form a single medical term; for example, the term, "claustrophobia," (meaning fear of enclosed spaces) joins the Latin word element, claustrum (enclosed space), to a Greek word element, phobia (fear).

Word elements – Parts of a word.

Root word element – Tells the primary meaning of a word; also called base word element.

Prefix word element – The word element that comes before the root word element.

Suffix word element – The word element that comes after the root word element.

Combining vowel – A letter, usually an "o," that is sometimes used to ease the pronunciation of a medical term.

At first, medical terminology may seem strange and overwhelming. However, after a working knowledge of these word elements is gained, it becomes easier to analyze words, and usage difficulties will be reduced.

Medical terminology changes with the dynamics of evolving technology in healthcare. New terms, abbreviations, and words are constantly being created to meet the needs of this new technology. However, through word association and memorization of basic medical terms and word elements, Central Service Technicians can establish a solid foundation upon which to build an extensive vocabulary.

After basic word elements are learned, more complex medical terms can be analyzed. You'll discover that they have an anatomy just like humans. As with the example of "claustrophobia" above, many words consist of word elements joined together to expand the meaning of a single term.

The anatomy of a medical word may consist of three types of word elements:

- *Root word element* – Tells the primary meaning. Many roots signify a procedure, disease, or body part. Example: the medical term for heart is" cardio."

- *Prefix word element* – Comes before the root, and may be one or two syllables. When added to a root, the prefix can alter or modify its meaning. Example: the medical term for the prefix, "around," is "peri." Therefore, the term, "pericardio," means "around the heart."

- *Suffix word element* – Comes after the root, and may be one or two syllables. When added to the root, the suffix can also alter or modify its meaning. Example: the medical term for the suffix that means, "inflammation," is "itis." Therefore, the term, "pericarditis," refers to "inflammation around the heart." Note: Sometimes a **combining vowel** (usually an "o") is used to ease pronunciation. However, not all medical terms have combining vowels.

Figure 2.1 shows additional examples of how word elements are combined to form medical terms.

ANALYSIS OF MEDICAL TERMS

Learning Objective 2. Analyze medical terms by their word elements.

The best way to learn the meaning of a medical term is to break it apart. Begin with the suffix since it most often gives a clue and meaning about the root, and how it is being used. Then consider the root and prefix. In other words, consider the overall relationship between each word element in the term.

When analyzing medical terms, you may encounter suffixes meaning "pertaining to." **Figure 2.2** provides several examples of suffixes, words in which they are used, and the meaning of the words.

Just as with the English language, certain rules of grammar apply to medical terminology. Making medical terms conform to the basic rules of spelling and pronunciation may result in letters in the word element being changed, dropped, or added. **Figure 2.3** shows some examples.

Figure 2.1 Word Elements are Combined to Form Medical Terms

Word Elements   **Word**

Prefix	Root	Suffix	
hemi- (half)	gastro (stomach)	-ectomy (surgical removal)	hemigastrectomy (removal of half of the stomach)
hemi- (half)	colo (colon)	-ectomy (surgical removal)	hemicolectomy (removal of half of the colon)
hemi- (half)	cardio (heart)		hemicardia (only two of the four chambers of the heart are formed)

An easy way to remember the difference between prefix (which comes before the root) and suffix (which comes after the root) is to put the words in alphabetical order: prefix, root, and suffix. This tells you that "prefix" is the first word element, and "suffix" is the last word element.

Note: Not all medical terms consist of all three word elements. A medical term may be formed by a root alone, by combining two roots, a root and suffix, or a prefix and root.

Figure 2.2 Suffixes that Mean "Pertaining To"

Suffix	Example		Meaning
-ac	cardi-ac	=	pertaining to the heart
-al	derm-al	=	pertaining to the skin
-ic	hem-ic	=	pertaining to blood
-eal	esophag-eal	=	pertaining to the esophagus
-ary	pulmon-ary	=	pertaining to lungs
-ous	cancer-ous	=	pertaining to cancer

Figure 2.3   Letters in Word Elements May Be Dropped or Added

Word Elements and Meaning			Word	Letter(s) Changed
Prefix	**Root**	**Suffix**		
	procto(rectum)	-itis(inflammation)	proctitis	O is dropped
endo(within)	artery(artey)	-ectomy(removal)	endarterectomy	O and Y are dropped
	chir(hand)	-plasty(surgical revision)	chiroplasty	O is added

Figure 2.4 Common Suffixes

Suffixes are word elements that come after the root word, and may be one or two syllables.

Common Medical Suffixes

Suffix	Meaning	Example	Meaning
-algia	pain	neuralgia	nerve pain
-cide	kill	germicide	destruction of germs
-emia	blood	hyperglycemia	high blood sugar
-genic	origin	osteogenic	originating in the bones
-itis	inflammation	tonsillitis	inflammation of the tonsils
-megaly	large or enlargement	cardiomegaly	enlargement of heart
-necrosis	death of tissue	arterionecrosis	tissue death of artery
-ology	study of	bacteriology	the study of bacteria
-oma	tumor	carcinoma	malignant tumor
-rrhage	flow	hemorrhage	uncontrolled flow of blood

Common Surgical Suffixes — Cards

Suffix	Meaning	Example	Meaning
-cise	cut	excise	to cut out
-ectomy	surgical removal	cystectomy	removal of a cyst
-oscopy	visual examination of an organ or joint	laparoscopy	visual examination of organs in the abdomen
-ostomy	creation of a new	colostomy	creation of new opening to colon on the body
-otomy	incision into an organ	gastrotomy	incision of the stomach
-pexy	surgical fixation	orchiopexy	surgically fixation of an undescended testicle to the correct location
-plasty	surgical restoration, plastic repair	rhinoplasty	surgical repair of the nose
-rrhaphy	to suture	myorrhaphy	to suture muscle wound
-tome	a cutting instrument	dermatome	an instrument used for cutting skin

Figure 2.5 Common Roots

Roots are base word elements that refer to the main body of a medical word.

Common Medical Roots

Root	Meaning	Example	Meaning
adeno	gland	adenoma	glandular tumor
aero	air	anaerobe	an organism that lives only in absence of air
arthro	joint	arthritis	inflammation of a joint
broncho	bronchus	bronchitis	inflammation of the bronchus
cardio	heart	electrocardiogram	electrographic record of the heartbeat
cerebro	brain	cerebrospinal	referring to the brain and spinal cord
chole	bile	cholecyst	gall bladder
chondro/io	cartilage	chondroma	cartilaginous tumor
costo	rib	intercosto	between the ribs
cysto	bladder	cyst	any fluid-filled sac
derma	skin	dermopathy	skin disease
gastro	stomach	gastrointestinal	pertaining to the stomach and intestines
gyne	woman	gynecology	the study of diseases affecting the female
hema or hemat	blood	hemophilia	inability of the blood to clot
hepat	liver	hepatitis	inflammation of the liver

Common Surgical Roots — cardo

Root	Meaning	Example	Meaning
arthro	joint	arthroscopy	visual examination of a joint
colo	colon	colectomy	removal of part of the colon
cranio	skull	craniotomy	surgical opening into the skull
herni	rupture	herniorrhaphy	surgical repair of a rupture
hyster	uterus	hysteropexy	abdominal fixation of the uterus
lipo	fat	liposuction	aspiration of fatty tissue
litho	stone	lithotripsy	crushing of a stone
oopher	ovary	oophorectomy	surgical removal of the ovary
rhino	nose	rhinoplasty	repair nose defect
tracheo	trachea	tracheostomy	surgical opening into trachea

Figure 2.6 Common Prefixes

Prefixes are word elements that are placed before the root to alter or modify its meaning.

Prefix	Meaning	Example	Meaning
a, an-	without	asepsis	without infection; sterile
ad-	toward (in the direction of)	addiction	toward dependence on a drug
anti-	against	antiseptic	preventing sepsis (infection)
dis-	apart, away	hip dislocation	displacement of femur from pelvic joint
dys-	painful	dysentery	painful inflammation of the intestine
hyper-	above, excessive	hyperacidity	excessive acid in the stomach
hypo-	below, deficient	hypoglycemia	low sugar content in the blood
neo-	new	neonatal	newborn
pre-	before	preoperative	before surgery
sub-	under, beneath	subcutaneous	beneath the skin
supra-	above	suprapubic	above the pubis

Common Surgical Prefixes   — Cards

Prefix	Meaning	Example	Meaning
bi-	two/ both sides	bilateral total hip reconstruction (THR)	two (both) total hip reconstructions
hemi-	half	hemigastrectomy	surgical removal of half of stomach
para-	beside, near	parathyroidectomy	surgical removal of tissue near thyroid
peri-	around, about	periosteal elevator	instrument used to remove tissue around the bone
post-	after	post partum	after delivery of a baby

Figure 2.7 Common Abbreviations for Surgical Procedures

Abbreviation	Surgical Procedure	Meaning
ACL	Anterior Cruciate Ligament	Reconstruction or repairing of the anterior cruciate ligament. In an ACL Reconstruction a graft is used to replace the ligament and in an ACL Repair the torn ligament is put back together.
BSO	Bilateral Salpingoooophorectomy	Surgical removal of both fallopian tubes and ovaries
BKA	Below the knee amputation	Surgical removal of the leg below the knee
CABG	Coronary Artery Bypass Graft	Creation of a new blood supply to an area of the heart with a clotted/blocked artery.
CR	Closed Reduction	Treatment of a fractured bone without a surgical incision.
D & C	Dilatation and Curettage	Dilate the uterine cervix and remove the inner lining of the uterus by scraping with a curette.
ORIF	Open Reduction Internal Fixation	Treatment of a fractured bone with an incision, and the use of plates and screws or pins to hold the fragments together.
TAH	Total Abdominal Hysterectomy	Surgical removal of the uterus through an incision in the abdomen
THA	Total Hip Arthroplasty	Hip joint reconstruction by removing the bone and placing a plastic/metal component in the femur.
TURP	Transurethral Resection of the Prostate	Surgical removal of part of the prostate gland by inserting instruments across the urethra to reach the prostate internally.

The ability to analyze medical terminology requires practice. This is accomplished by further reading, study, and experience in the health care work environment.

MORE ABOUT SUFFIXES, ROOTS, AND PREFIXES

Learning Objective 3. Recognize suffixes, roots, and prefixes that relate to medical and surgical terms.

Suffixes, roots, and prefixes relate to medical terms (for diagnosis and symptoms), to surgical terms (for operative procedures), and in conjunction with instrument names. **Figures 2.4 – 2.6** identify some commonly used word elements.

COMMON ABBREVIATIONS IN SURGERY SCHEDULES

Learning Objective 4. Identify common abbreviations used in surgery schedules.

Medical terminology involves numerous commonly-used abbreviations for surgical procedures with which Central Service Technicians must be familiar. Some frequently used surgical abbreviations are noted in **Figure 2.7.**

CENTRAL SERVICE TERMS

Word element

Root word element

Prefix work element

Suffix word element

Combining vowel

Chapter Outline

CELLS, TISSUES, AND ORGANS

- Cells
- Tissues
- Organs

BODY SYSTEMS

- Skeletal system
- Muscular system
- Nervous system including sensory organs
- Endocrine system
- Reproductive system
- Urinary and excretory systems
- Respiratory system
- Digestive system
- Circulatory system

IN CONCLUSION

REFERENCES

CENTRAL SERVICE TERMS

Chapter 3
Anatomy and Physiology

Chapter Learning Objectives:

As a result of successfully completing this chapter, readers will be able to:

1. Review the structure, function, activities, and role of cells, tissues, and organs in the body.

2. Identify and describe the structure and roles of each major body system, and indicate common surgical procedures that involve each system.
   - Skeletal
   - Muscular
   - Nervous
   - Endocrine
   - Reproductive
   - Urinary and excretory
   - Respiratory
   - Digestive
   - Circulatory

The human body is very complex and amazing. The study of its incredible structure began with the Greeks and Romans many years ago. The body consists of many parts, systems, and networks that work in harmony like a great orchestra to carry out the body's sustaining functions. While each movement seems effortless and somewhat unplanned, you'll discover that there are marvelous relationships between the body's parts, its systems, and their functions.

CELLS, TISSUES, AND ORGANS

Learning Objective 1. Review the structure, function, activities, and role of cells, tissues, and organs in the body.

The study of the human body requires an understanding of anatomy and physiology. Our study begins by considering cells, tissues, and organs.

Cells

Here are some facts about **cells**:

• They are the basic living unit of life. The human body is made up of more than one hundred trillion of these tiny structures.

• They vary in size, shape, and function depending upon the location in the body where they are found.

• They are so small that they can only be seen with the use of a microscope.

• Within each cell are still smaller structures called organelles: microscopic organs within a cell that perform specific functions.

• Functions of the cell include respiration, nutrition, energy production, waste elimination, reproduction, and much more.

• Living cells come only from other living cells.

• Cells reproduce by duplication and division into two new cells; each new cell is called a daughter cell, and is identical to the parent cell (see **Figure 3.1**).

Regardless of their size and shape, each human cell consists of three main parts:

• The **cell membrane** is porous and flexible, and surrounds the cell to keep it separated from the outside environment. The cell membrane allows and controls the passage of materials in and out of the cell. Examples include the absorption of oxygen and food, and the elimination of harmful waste products produced by the cell.

• The **cytoplasm** surrounds the nucleus, and contains within-cell fluid and organelles.

• The **nucleus** is surrounded and protected by the cytoplasm. This oval structure acts as the brain center of the cell to direct and control all activities including duplication into two new cells.

More About the Cell Nucleus

The nucleus contains three important components:

• DNA (deoxyribonucleic acid) – DNA stores the information needed to build proteins essential to restore cells, and it also transfers messages about organisms from parent to offspring.

• RNA (ribonucleic acid) – RNA translates the DNA messages, and guides the protein-making process.

• Chromosomes – These cell components are comprised of DNA, and pass on the traits of parent cells to new cells.

Cell – The basic unit of life; the smallest structural unit of living organisms capable of performing all basic functions of life.

Cell membrane – The outer covering of a cell that regulates what enters and leaves it.

Cytoplasm – The lining matter of a cell between the cell membrane and nucleus.

Nucleus – The functional center of a cell that governs activity and heredity.

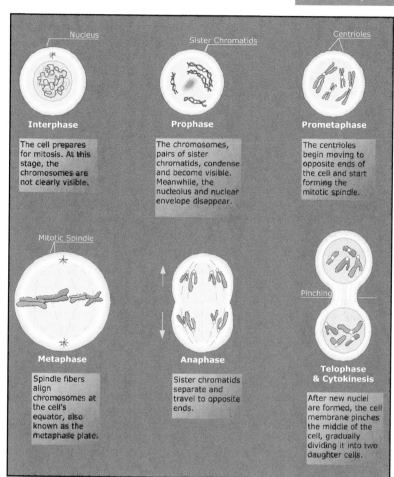

all waste products. A final example of connective tissue is cartilage, which provides framework and support to the human body.

- Muscular tissue – This tissue shortens as it contracts. When attached to bone, these contractions make body movement possible. Muscle tissues also line the inner walls of organs that contract to help food pass through the digestive system. As the cardiac muscles contract, blood is pumped through the body.

- Nervous tissue – This tissue of communication is located throughout the body. When stimulated, nervous tissue carries messages back and forth between the brain and every part of the body.

Figure 3.1 Cell Reproduction – The Development of Daughter Cells

Tissue

Two or more cells that are similar in structure and function are joined together to form **tissue**.

The four major primary tissues of the human body are:

- Epithelial tissue – This tissue covers the body's external surface (skin), and the linings of body cavities (the mouth, ears, nose, throat, stomach, chest, abdomen, pelvis and other body parts).

- Connective tissue – This tissue provides support, stores energy, and connects other tissues and parts. Bones provide protection, support, and shape to the body, and storage for calcium. Fat keeps the body warm, cushions organs, and stores nutrients. Blood transports food and oxygen to all body parts, and removes

Organs

Organs are formed when two or more different types of tissues are grouped together to perform a specific function.

Examples of organs include the:

- Brain – An organ in the central nervous system that is the primary receiver, organizer, and distributor of information in the body.

Tissue – A group of similar cells that perform a specialized function.

Organ - A part of the body containing two or more tissues that function together for a specific purpose.

- Heart – The organ that pumps blood throughout the body.

- Stomach – An organ that is part of the digestive system. It helps digest food by mixing it with digestive juices, and converting it into a liquid.

- Skin – The largest organ of the body that serves as the body's outer covering.

BODY SYSTEMS

Learning Objective 2. Identify and describe the structure and roles of each major body system, and indicate common surgical procedures that involve each system.
- Skeletal
- Muscular
- Nervous
- Endocrine
- Reproductive
- Urinary and excretory
- Respiratory
- Digestive
- Circulatory

A **system** is a group of organs working together in the body to carry out a particular activity.

While each body system provides a specific bodily function, none are independent of any other. Each system must work together to help the body function as a total organism. With the exception of the reproductive system, each body system and its organs work together to help maintain life. The remainder of this chapter will provide details about the body's major systems.

Skeletal System

Without the skeletal system (see **Figure 3.2**), the body would just be a mass of immovable tissue. There are approximately 206 bones that, collectively, comprise the body's skeletal system. They are arranged in an orderly manner, and are fastened together by tough connective tissue known as **tendons** and **ligaments**.

The five main functions of the skeletal system are to:

- Give the body shape and support.

- Allow movement.

- Protect vital organs.

- Produce blood cells.

- Store calcium.

Most bone is made from **cartilage** but, through a process known as **ossification**, cartilage is sometimes replaced by bone.

Cartilage is a flexible connective tissue that provides framework to the body. Its purposes include:

- To support body structures such as the ears and nose.

- To connect the ribs to the sternum.

- To serve as a cushion between bones to prevent them from rubbing together at junctures and joints.

A **joint** is any place where two bones meet. Some are immovable such as those found in the skull, and others are movable and allow the bones that they connect to move. (Examples are the knee and elbow joints.)

System – *A group of organs that work together to carry out a specific activity.*

Tendons – *A cord of fibrous tissue that attaches a muscle to a bone.*

Ligaments – *A band of connective tissue that connects a bone to another bone.*

Cartilage – *A type of flexible connective tissue.*

Ossification – *The process by which cartilage is replaced by bone.*

Joint – *Any place where two bones meet.*

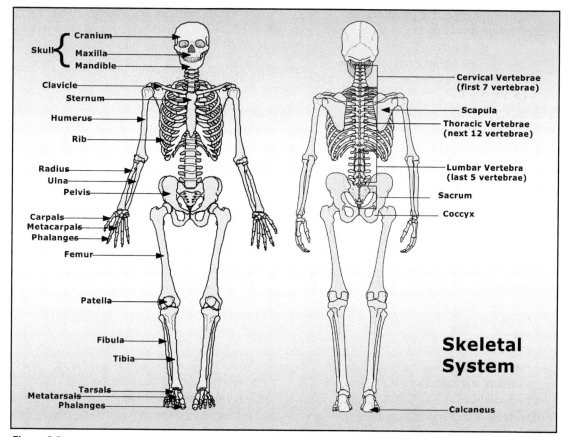

Figure 3.2

There are several types of joints:

- Gliding joints – allow us to lower our head as the vertebrae (bones in the spinal column) of the neck slide over one another.

- Ball and socket joints – such as in the shoulder and hip consist of a bone with a rounded head that fits into a rounded cup socket of another bone. These joints make possible movements like swinging one's arm around in a circle.

- Pivot joints – allow a turning motion such as the palm of the hand rotating from up to down when a bone rotates on another ring-shaped bone.

- Hinge joints – (found in one's knees, knuckles, and elbows) allow backward and forward bending motions like a door hinge.

The overall covering or lining of a joint is called a synovial membrane. It secretes or produces a fluid called synovial fluid to lubricate joint surfaces.

Bones are comprised of living tissue, and their strength and hardness come from chemical substances called minerals. A cross section of bone shows that it consists of two principal materials:

- A hard outer material called cortical or compact bone is dense and strong, and consists of calcium and phosphorous. This hard outer surface is surrounded by the periosteum: a tough membrane that contains bone-forming cells and blood vessels.

- The inner section of bone is porous, and is called spongy or cancellous bone. It is filled with material called marrow. A pipeline of blood vessels and nerves runs through the middle of thick bones.

Surgical procedures that involve the skeletal system include:

- Craniotomy – Making an opening into the skull bone to access the brain.

(FROnt)

- Anterior Cervical Fusion – Removing disc tissue pressing on a nerve in the neck area, inserting a piece of bone between the vertebrae, and fusing this area with plates and screws.

(Back)

- Posterior Lumbar Interbody Fusion (PLIF) – Removing disc tissue pressing on the lower spine area, inserting a piece of bone between the vertebra, and fusing this area with plates and screws.

- Open Reduction Internal Fixation (ORIF) – Making an incision in the skin, realigning a fractured bone, and inserting screws and plates to assure the bone ends do not move so healing can be promoted. (see Figure 3.3)

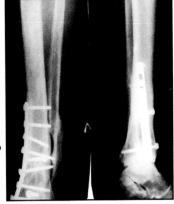

Figures 3.3 Open Reduction Internal Fixation

- Total Knee Arthroplasty (TKA) – Removing the bone at the end of the femur, and the bone at the proximal (nearest) end of the tibia, and replacing them with metal/plastic components. (see Figure 3.4)

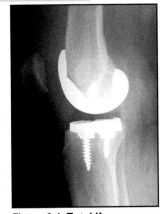

Figure 3.4 Total Knee Arthroplasty

- Total Hip Arthroplasty (THA) – Removing the head of the femur and the socket where it fits in the hip bone, and replacing these structures with metal, ceramic, and plastic components that mimic that original ones.

Muscular System

Even as one sleeps many of the more than 600 muscles in the body (of which 400 are skeletal) are actively at work to keep us alive (see **Figure 3.5**). For example:

- Heart muscles contract to pump blood throughout the body.

- Chest muscles contract to move air in and out of the lungs.

- Muscles in the digestive tract move food and fluid through the body.

- Muscles throughout the body contract to produce heat, and maintain the body's core temperature.

Muscles are made of up long, thin cells or fibers that run parallel to one another, and they are bundled together by connective tissue called **fascia.** Muscle fibers have the ability to contract (shorten), and this contraction causes body movements.

There are three types of muscle tissue: skeletal, smooth, and cardiac.

Voluntary

- Skeletal muscles – are attached to bones by tendons. As skeletal muscles contract, the arms, legs, head, or other body parts to which they are attached move. We consciously control skeletal muscles; they only move only when we want them to move.

- Smooth muscle – is organized into thin, flat sheets of tissue. Smooth muscles are called involuntary or visceral muscles, because they contract and function without our conscious control. They control breathing, movement of food and fluid in the digestive system, movement of

**Fascia** – A band or sheet of fibrous connective tissue.

blood throughout the circulatory system, and the movement of urine through the urinary system.

• Cardiac muscle – is similar to woven mesh fibers that branch out through the heart to give it more strength to pump blood. These involuntary muscle fibers contract and make the heart beat, and they are durable, and do not normally tire.

To function, these muscle fibers require energy and oxygen that are derived from the food consumed, and oxygen from the environment when we breathe. Their functions involve movement, support, the maintenance of posture and body position, and the production of body heat.

Surgical procedures involving the muscular system include:

• Fasciotomy – Making an incision into the fibrous membrane covering a muscle, usually to relieve pressure from an injured or swollen muscle.

• Herniorrhaphy – Repairing a cavity wall/muscle layer that is allowing all or part of an organ to project through the opening.

• Rotator cuff repair – Repairs to the muscles and ligaments of shoulder joints depend on the size and shape of the tear.

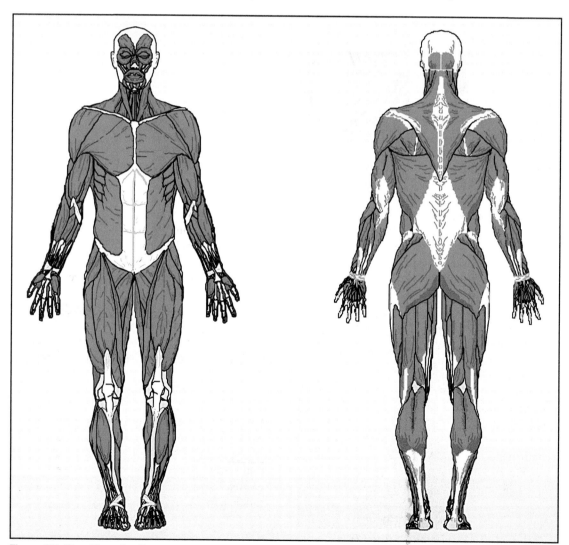

Figure 3.5 The Muscular System

Frequently used methods are the Bankart, Putti-Platt, and Bristow Procedures.

Nervous System Including Sense Organs

The nervous system (see **Figure 3.6**) is a vast communication network. It coordinates and carries messages between all parts of the body, and enables us to be aware of the changes in the environment and to react accordingly. A complex series of nervous tissues somewhat like electrical wiring runs from the brain and spinal cord throughout the entire body.

Functions of the nervous system include:

- It controls all body activities, and allows us to respond to stimuli. Many reactions are automatic such as blinking when a foreign object approaches the eye.

- Nerve tissue carries electrical messages from the brain and spinal cord that signal muscles to contract.

- Other actions are more conscious and involve emotion, reason, and memory. Like a computer, the brain stores learned information based on past experiences that can later be communicated to the body by the nervous system.

The nervous system is composed of two types of cells: neurons (also called nerve cells) are the functional unit that carry and transmit information throughout the body, and neuroglia that support and protect neurons as they work.

Anatomically, the nervous system is divided into two parts: **Central Nervous System (CNS)**, and the **Peripheral Nervous System**.

The CNS consists of the brain and spinal cord which are covered by protective membranes called meninges. The CNS is the body's control center, and it is the storehouse for information about what is happening or has happened within or outside the body.

The **brain** is the main control unit of the CNS. It is comprised of more than 100 billion nerve cells, and is a spongy, convoluted, and complex organ.

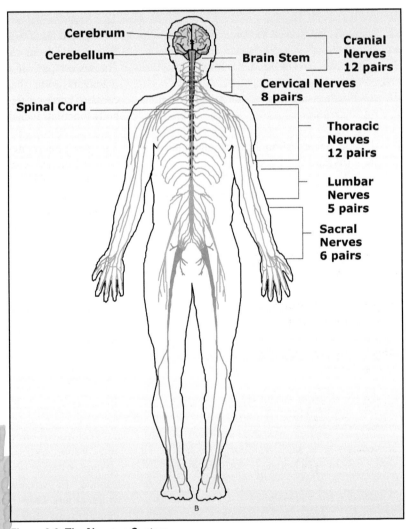

Figure 3.6 The Nervous System

Three membranes surround the brain, and provide nourishment and protection to it:

- The pia mater is the inner membrane that clings to the contour and many folds of the brain.

- The arachnoid mater is the middle membrane. It resembles a spider web. Between the inner membrane and middle membrane is a water-like fluid called the cerebral spinal fluid (CSF) in which the brain floats as a cushion against shock.

- The dura mater is the outer membrane. It is very thick and tough and it touches the inner skull.

The brain is divided into three parts, each of which carries out a specific function: **Cerebrum, Cerebellum**, and **Brain Stem**.

The cerebrum is the largest part of the human brain. It functions to:

- Manage the nerve impulses that allow us to think, speak, and remember.

- Control most voluntary muscle contraction.

Central Nervous System (CNS) – The part of the nervous system that includes the brain and spinal cord.

Peripheral Nervous System – All nerve tissue outside the central nervous system.

Brain – The main control unit of the Central Nervous System.

Cerebrum – The largest part of the brain. It controls mental activities and movement.

Cerebellum – The second largest part of the brain. It controls muscle coordination, body balance, and posture.

Brain Stem – This controls many automatic body functions such as heartbeat and breathing.

- Interpret information gathered by the senses.

- Influence the foundation of personality, emotions, and attitudes.

The cerebrum is divided into two halves (hemispheres). Each half controls different mental activities and movement on the opposite side of the body. A series of nerve pathways run between each half to facilitate communication.

The cerebellum is located inferior (below) and posterior (behind) the cerebrum. It is the second largest part of the brain, and its role is to adjust the motor impulses that control muscular coordination, body balance, and posture.

The brain stem is located at the base of the brain, and is formed by bundles of nerves that extend from the cerebrum and cerebellum. The lowest part of the brain stem (the medulla oblongata) joins the brain to the spinal cord. It contains nerve centers that control many automatic body functions including heartbeat and breathing.

The peripheral nervous system involves the network of nerves and sense organs that branch out of the CNS, and connect the CNS to other parts of the body. One part (the autonomic nervous system) controls all involuntary body processes like heartbeat and peristalsis (the rippling motion of muscles in the digestive tract that mixes food with gastric juices to form a thin liquid). Other nerves are under direct control of the conscious mind. When we tell our hand to wave, for example, a message is sent from the brain down the spinal cord through a peripheral nerve to our hand.

The Sense Organs

The sense organs (eyes, ears, nose, tongue, and skin) are accessory structures of the nervous system that provide a notion of all that surrounds us. They house special sensory receptors that are message-carrying structures. Most sense organs respond to stimuli from outside the body, while others keep track of the body's internal environment. They respond to light, sound, taste, chemicals, heat, and pressure.

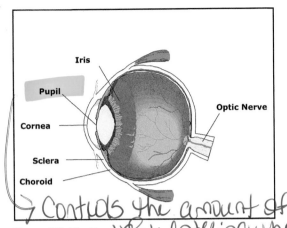

Figure 3.7 The Eye *Contols the amount of light entering the eye.*

Eyes (see **Figure 3.7**) are the organs of vision. They produce images by focusing light rays that are interpreted by the brain. The eyes consist of three layers of tissue:

- The sclera. This is the white portion of the eye that is an outer coat to provide protection. At the center front of the sclera is a transparent protective shield called the cornea.

- The choroid is the middle layer of the eye that furnishes nourishment to the eye via blood vessels. The choroid layer includes the iris: a muscle that is the colored portion of

the eye. A circular opening called the pupil is found at the center of the iris. It controls the amount of light entering the eye as it narrows or widens. Between the cornea and eye lens is the aqueous humor: a watery-like fluid that fills the compartment of the eye.

- The retina is the eye's third layer. It is located on the back surface of the eyeball. The eye lens focuses light onto the retina which contains light-sensitive cells (receptors) that receive and transmit impressions to the brain through the optic nerve. The vitreous humor is a fluid-filled compartment of the eye that gives the eyeball a round shape.

Ears are the organs of hearing. They are made of up three parts: the external, middle, and inner ear (see **Figure 3.8**). Sound waves travel through the ear to the auditory nerve that transmits nerve impulses to the brain. Here's how the ear allows us to hear:

- The external ear serves as a funnel that gathers sound waves, and passes them through the ear canal to the ear drum.

- The ear drum consists of a tightly stretched membrane that separates the outer ear canal from the middle ear. Vibrations of the ear drum enter the middle ear which contains three tiny bones: the malleus, incus, and stapes.

- The sound vibrations are then passed through these bones into the fluid-filled inner ear. There, vibrations are channeled through the fluid into a spiral-shaped tube called the cochlea which contains the receptors or nerve endings that transmit nerve impulses to the brain.

The inner ear also contains semi-circular canals consisting of three curved tubes filled with fluid. Body balance is regulated by this fluid as it shifts with body movement. As the fluid shifts, it presses against tiny hairs

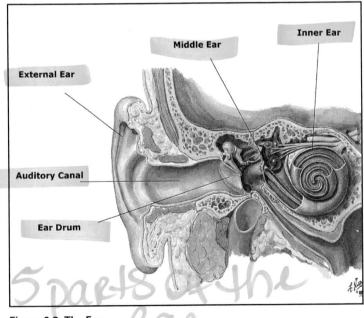

Figure 3.8 The Ear *5 parts of the ear*

stimulating nerve impulses that travel to the brain. The brain responds to these impulses by coordinating muscle movement.

The nose is the organ of smell, and consists of many sensory receptors or cells. These receptors are located in the mucous membranes of the nasal cavity, and are sensitive to chemicals carried through the air. The olfactory nerve endings extend to the receptors, and are stimulated by different odors. Olfactory bulbs are the enlarged portion at the ends of the olfactory nerves. (See **Figure 3.9**)

The tongue is the organ of taste, and is covered with taste buds (sensory receptors). (see **Figure 3.10**) The sense of taste, like smell, is a chemical sense. Chemicals are carried by the saliva throughout the mouth. Taste buds located in different areas of the tongue can distinguish four kinds of taste: sweet, sour, bitter, and salty. There are 80 different types of chemical odors, and the combination of taste and odors produces flavors.

The skin is the largest body organ. It contains many nerve endings at and below its surface. The skin, therefore, acts as an important sensory organ. Touch receptors near the skin's surface allow us to distinguish textures, and to respond to heat, cold, and rain. Further below the skin surface are receptors that respond to touch and pressure. The sense of pain stimulates nerves, and sends messages of potential danger to the brain.

There are numerous surgical procedures involving the nervous system:

- Craniotomy – Creating an opening in the skull to expose the brain to facilitate procedures such as the removal of tumors and clots.

- Carpal Tunnel Repair – Removing tissue or displaced bone in the wrist area to release pressure on the median nerve.

- Ulnar Nerve Transposition – Making an incision at the elbow area to allow the ulnar nerve to be moved to an area that provides protection and comfort.

- Cataract Extraction – Removing a clouded eye lens with a clear, artificial lens replacement.

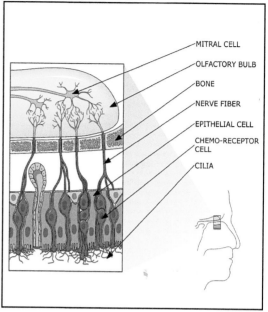

Figure 3.9 The Nose

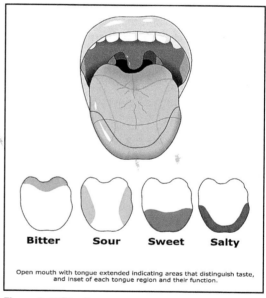

Figure 3.10 The Tongue

- Corneal Transplant – Grafting corneal tissue from one eye to another to improve vision when the cornea is damaged or scarred.

- Bilateral Myringotomy with Tubes (BMT) – Making an incision into the tympanic membrane (ear drum) to permit fluid to drain. Small tubes placed in the membrane allow continuous drainage. The tubes fall out as the membrane heals.

• Stapedectomy – Removing the stapes (an ear bone) when it has thickened and no longer transmits sound waves. It is replaced with an artificial implant to improve hearing.

• Tympanoplasty – Reconstructing the ear drum so sound waves can be sent to the middle and inner ear.

• Split-thickness Skin Graft (STSG) – Cutting the skin from a donor site, and using a graft mesher to expand the graft. The graft is then transplanted onto the surgical area.

Endocrine System

Think about a time when you were really excited, threatened, or in a suddenly stressful situation. How did your body react? Chances are your muscles tensed up, your heartbeat quickened, and your breathing rhythm changed. These rapid changes in body activities are set in motion by the **hormones** or secretions produced by the glands of the endocrine system (see **Figure 3.11**). These glands and the substances they produce have a profound influence on functions, **metabolism,** growth, and personality.

Following is some important information about the endocrine system:

• Since hormones are distributed through the body, the endocrine glands that produce them are not necessarily next to the organs they control. Regardless of where hormones enter the bloodstream, they continue their journey through the circulatory system until they reach their targeted organ. Tissue cells and organs recognize and accept hormones made for them, and reject others that are not for them.

• The nervous system and endocrine system work together. When the brain interprets information as a threat, it rapidly sends out nerve impulses that trigger certain endocrine glands to release their hormones into the blood stream. In a fearful situation, the hormones will cause the heartbeat to accelerate and

prepare muscles for action. In this state, one is ready for fight or flight (to defend or run).

• Endocrine glands are located throughout the body.

• Some glands of the endocrine system secrete more than one hormone.

The major glands of the endocrine system include:

• The pituitary gland – A small pea-shaped gland located at the base of the brain, it is considered the master gland because it helps control the activities of all other endocrine glands. Its secretions also stimulate skeletal and body growth, development of sex organs, regulation of blood pressure, the reproductive process, and muscle development.

• The thyroid gland – Located at the base of the neck just below the larynx (voice box), its hormones help to regulate the rate of metabolism, and maintain the body's levels of calcium and phosphorous.

• The parathyroid gland – Four pea-shaped glands located on or sometimes in the thyroid that control the blood's calcium level.

• The adrenal glands – During sudden stress, these glands located on top of each kidney release adrenalin that increases our heart rate and physical strength. Adrenalin also enhances our ability to think, and to respond more quickly than usual in emergency situations.

Hormones – Chemical messengers that travel through the blood and act on target organs.

Metabolism – The total chemical changes by which the nutritional and functional activities of an organism are maintained

Insulin – A hormone that reduces the level of sugar in the blood.

Glucagon – A hormone that can increase the blood sugar level.

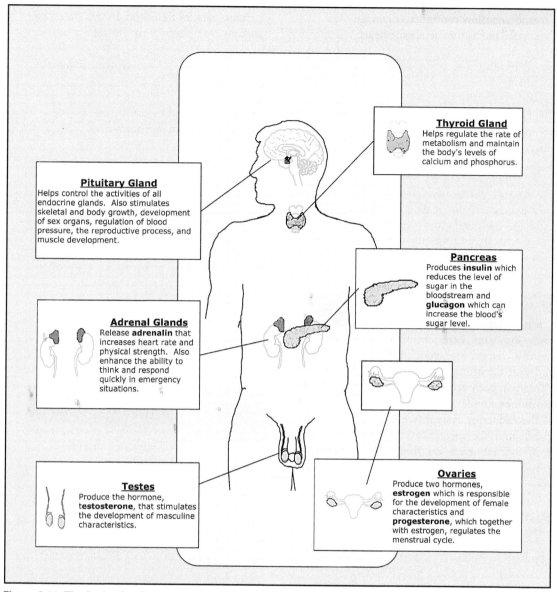

Thyroid Gland
Helps regulate the rate of metabolism and maintain the body's levels of calcium and phosphorus.

Pituitary Gland
Helps control the activities of all endocrine glands. Also stimulates skeletal and body growth, development of sex organs, regulation of blood pressure, the reproductive process, and muscle development.

Pancreas
Produces **insulin** which reduces the level of sugar in the bloodstream and **glucagon** which can increase the blood's sugar level.

Adrenal Glands
Release **adrenalin** that increases heart rate and physical strength. Also enhance the ability to think and respond quickly in emergency situations.

Testes
Produce the hormone, **testosterone**, that stimulates the development of masculine characteristics.

Ovaries
Produce two hormones, **estrogen** which is responsible for the development of female characteristics and **progesterone**, which together with estrogen, regulates the menstrual cycle.

Figure 3.11 The Endocrine System

- The pancreas – Located just below the stomach, this gland contains cells organized into groups known as the Islets of Langerhans. Two primary hormones are produced by the pancreatic islets: **insulin**, which reduces the level of sugar in the blood stream, and **glucagon** which can increase the blood's sugar level.

- The ovaries (female sex glands) – Produce two hormones: estrogen and progesterone. Estrogen is responsible for the development of female characteristics, and progesterone together with estrogen regulates the menstrual cycle.

- The testes (male sex glands) – Produce the hormone, testosterone, that stimulates the development of masculine characteristics.

Surgical procedures involving the endocrine system include:

- Thyroidectomy – Removing nodules and/or goiters (enlargement) on the thyroid.

- Oophorectomy – Removing an ovary.

- Orchiectomy – Removing a testicle.

Reproductive System

Everyone begins life as a tiny single cell formed when two other cells join together in a process called fertilization. The male sex cell is produced by the male reproductive system, and is called **sperm.** The female sex cell (egg) is called ovum (plural: ova), and is produced by the female reproductive system. Both sperm and **ovum** contain rod-shaped structures called chromosomes that are responsible for inherited characteristics passed on from parent to child. Each sex cell contains 23 **chromosomes;** therefore, a fertilized egg consists of 46 chromosomes, receiving 23 from the sperm and 23 from the ovum.

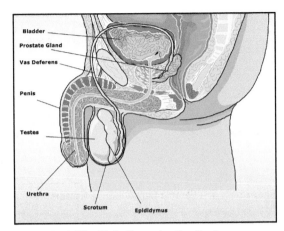

Figure 3.12 The Male Reproductive System

The male reproductive system (see **Figure 3.12**) consists of:

- Two **testes** – These oval-shaped glands are located in a skin-covered, pouch-like structure called the **scrotum.** Two tube structures are also in the scrotum. The **epididymus** is a tube that carries sperm cells from the testes to the **vas deferens** (a thick-walled tube structure approximately 18 inches long) where they mature. The vas deferens then carries sperm to a hollow chamber located behind the bladder called the **seminal vesicle.**

- The seminal vesicle joins with the vas deferens to form the **ejaculatory duct.** The secretions of the seminal vesicle are called **semen** which bathes and nourishes the sperm cells. In the ejaculatory duct, the semen-containing sperm, upon ejaculation, enter the **urethra,** a membranous canal running through the **penis** which transfers the sperm to the female's body.

- **Prostate gland** – A partly glandular and partly muscular gland surrounding the neck of the bladder. It secretes a fluid which is part of the semen, and stimulates the sperms' motility (movement).

Sperm – The male sex cell.

Ovum – The female sex cell.

Chromosomes – Rod-shaped structures responsible for inherited characteristics passed on from parent to child.

Testes – Male reproductive gland that forms and secretes sperm and several fluid elements in semen.

Scrotum – Sac in which testes are suspended.

Epididymus – A tube that carries sperm cells from the testes to the vas deferens.

Vas deferens – A duct that transfers sperm from the epididymus to the seminal vesicle.

Seminal vesicle – A gland that produces semen.

Ejaculatory duct – A duct formed by the joining of the seminal vesicles with the vas deferens, through which semen moves during ejaculation.

Semen – Mixture of sperm cells and secretions from several male reproductive glands.

Urethra – A tube that discharges urine and semen.

Penis – Male organ of urination and intercourse.

Prostate gland – Produces a fluid element in semen that stimulates the motility of sperm.

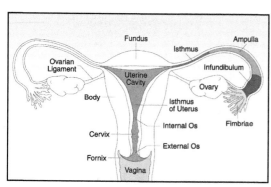

Figure 3.13 The Female Reproductive System

The female reproductive system (see **Figure 3.13**), unlike that of the male, is completely internal.

- The **vagina** is a muscular canal approximately 4-1/2 inches long through which a baby passes during birth. It extends from an external opening to the cervix (neck of the uterus).

- The **uterus** is located between the rectum and urinary bladder and is a hollow, pear-shaped organ. It is lined with a fluffy vascular layer of tissue called **endometrium**. The fertilized ovum embeds itself into the endometrium → *lining of uterus* which sloughs off (separates) during menstruation if an ovum is not fertilized.

- The **fallopian tubes** (oviducts) extend from two openings on each side of the anterior portion of the uterus. The distal (furthest) ends of the fallopian tubes are funnel shaped, and finger-like projections called **fimbriae** extend from them. They are located near, but not attached to, the **ovaries** (organs located at about hip level on each side of the female body that produce ova). The fimbriae draw the ovum into the fallopian tube, where it travels to the uterus.

Surgical Procedures involving the reproductive system include:

- Orchiectomy – Removing a testicle.

- Orchiopexy – Relocating a non-descended testicle to the correct location in the scrotum.

- Transurethral Resection of the Prostate (TURP) – Removing part of the prostate gland by inserting instruments across the urethra to reach the prostate internally.

- Radical Prostatectomy – Removing the prostate gland using an incision in the abdomen and also the urinary bladder. Frequently, additional tissue is biopsied for invasion of cancer cells.

- Hysterectomy – Removing the uterus.

- Bilateral Salpingoophorectomy – Removing both fallopian tubes and ovaries.

- Endometrial Ablation – Scarring or removing the inner lining of the uterus to treat abnormal bleeding.

- Dilatation & Curettage (D&C) – Widening of the cervix (opening of the uterus) to permit evacuation of the contents or scraping of the lining.

- Ectopic Pregnancy – Removing a fertilized ovum growing in the fallopian tube to prevent complications such as hemorrhage, shock, and scarring of the fallopian tube.

- Pelviscopy – Visualizing the pelvic cavity (lower abdomen) using an endoscope for diagnosis or treatment of female reproductive organs.

- Tubal Ligation – Cutting, burning, tying, or applying a clip on the fallopian tubes to prevent future pregnancies.

Vagina – The muscular canal in a female that extends from an external opening to the neck of the uterus.

Uterus – A female organ within which the fetus develops during pregnancy.

Endometrium – Lining of the uterus.

Fallopian tubes – Slender tubes that convey the ova (eggs) from the ovaries to the uterus.

Fimbriae – Finger-like projections extending from the fallopian tubes that draw ova (eggs) into the fallopian tube.

Ovaries – Female reproductive glands.

Urinary and Excretory Systems

The urinary system (see **Figure 3.14**) provides "pollution control" by eliminating body waste. This process takes place as blood is filtered by the urinary system. Urine is a water solution consisting of various waste substances that are products of metabolism. It obtains its color from excreted bile pigments, and may be a shade of amber, yellow, or clear. Depending on the amount of liquid intake or loss through respiration, an average adult may excrete between 1000cc-1800cc of urine during a 24-hour period. In males, the urinary and reproductive systems are closely related, and comprise the genitourinary system. In the female, however, the two systems are not interrelated.

Organs of the urinary system in both sexes include:

- The **kidneys** – Two bean-shaped organs containing a vast network of vessels and tubules called *nephron* that act as a filter to remove excess water and waste substances including salts and minerals from the blood. This process creates or produces urine.

- The **ureters** – Two tube-like structures that extend from each kidney and connect them to the urinary bladder. The *peristaltic* (automatic constriction and relaxation) action of the ureters moves urine from the kidneys to the urinary bladder.

- The **urinary bladder** – Serves as a reservoir for urine. It is a muscular, membranous sack located in the pelvis just anterior (front) of the *sigmoid colon* and posterior to (behind) the pubis. The bladder is flexible, and its size depends upon the amount of urine present. The average capacity ranges from between 300cc to 500cc in adults. As the amount of urine in the urinary bladder increases, it applies pressure on the bladder walls sending an impulse to the central nervous system. As the bladder wall contracts, the *sphincter muscle* at the junction of the urethra relaxes, and urine is released.

- The **urethra** – A membranous canal or tube that connects the urinary bladder to outside the body to eliminate urine. In the male, the urethra is approximately 20cm long, and passes through

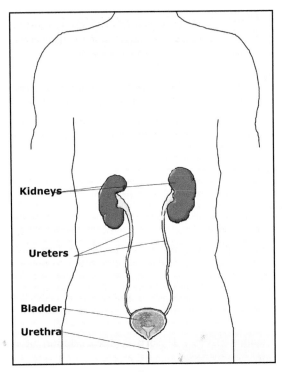

Figure 3.14 The Urinary System

Kidneys

Ureters

Bladder

Urethra

the prostate gland and pelvic wall and extends through the penis. The female urethra is about 4cm long, and it runs from the bladder through the sphincter muscles to the external meatus (opening) located at the anterior (front) of the vagina.

Now that we've discussed the urinary system, let's consider the excreting system that removes toxic

Kidneys – *Organs that remove excess water and waste substances from the blood in a process that yields urine.*

Ureters – *Tube-like structures extending from the kidneys to the urinary bladder that move urine between these organs.*

Urinary bladder – *The reservoir for urine.*

Liver – *An organ that filters the blood to remove amino acids and neutralize some harmful toxins.*

Skin – *This organ contains sweat glands that, through the process of perspiration, produces and eliminates sweat.*

(poisonous) waste substances. The kidneys (urinary system) and lungs (respiratory system) also perform excretory functions as do the liver and skin.

The **liver** is another filter for the blood; it removes amino acids, and can neutralize some harmful toxins. It can also convert *hemoglobin* from worn-out blood cells into substances the body requires.

The **skin** is the largest organ of the human body. It contains sweat glands, oils, hair, and nails. Dead skin cells form hair and nails. Sweat glands remove excess water, salt, and other bodily wastes. These are located in the dermis (inner layer of skin), and consist of coiled tubes connected to pores in the skin's surface. The sweat glands, through the process of perspiration, produce and eliminate sweat. Perspiration rids the body of waste, and it also helps to regulate the body's temperature by cooling its outside surface. The excretion of oil by the sebaceous glands keeps the skin soft, and prevents hair from becoming too dry or brittle.

Surgical procedures involving the urinary system include:

- Nephrectomy – Removing the kidney.

- Lithotripsy – Crushing stones that form in the kidney and become stuck in an ureter. The procedure involves decreasing the size of the stones with a laser or shock waves or removing them using a long, flexible instrument called a stone basket.

- Cystoscopy – Viewing the urinary bladder using an endoscope.

The Respiratory System

The respiratory system (see **Figure 3.15**) supplies the body with oxygen, and removes carbon dioxide that forms as a result of the body using oxygen in the blood.

This exchange of gases is accomplished automatically as one breathes in a two step process: *inspiration* (inhaling air into the lungs) and *expiration* (exhaling air from the lungs). Air contains other impurities

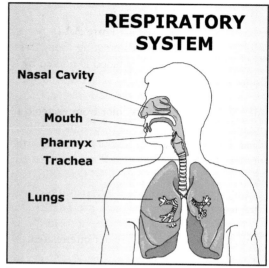

RESPIRATORY SYSTEM

Nasal Cavity
Mouth
Pharnyx
Trachea
Lungs

Figure 3.15 The Respiratory System

such as dirt, dust, and microorganisms, and these are filtered out by the respiratory system.

The primary organs of the respiratory system are:

- **Nose** (nasal cavity) and **mouth** – During inspiration air enters the nostrils (nasal openings) and mouth. Air in the nose is filtered, moistened, and warmed.

- **Pharynx** – Air passes to the pharynx (throat) which is the crossroads of the nose, mouth, voice box, and **esophagus**. Food continues down the esophagus, while air passes through the **larynx** (voice box) to the trachea.

- **Trachea** (windpipe) – The trachea divides into two tube-like structures, the right and left **bronchi**, that extend into the **lungs**.

- **Lungs** – The air continues through the bronchi to the *bronchioles:* a series of many smaller tubes extending from each bronchus somewhat like the branches of a tree. At the end of each bronchiole are small clusters of air sacs called *alveoli* that comprise the lungs' tissue. Alveoli and each alveolus are covered by a thin wall surrounded by a vast network of *capillaries* (tiny blood vessels). There the blood picks up oxygen from the inspired air, and releases the waste gas, carbon dioxide, during expiration.

More About the Lungs

The right lung consists of three lobes, while the left lung consists of two lobes to allow space for the heart.

The lungs are located in the thoracic cavity (chest), where they are covered by a thin membrane called the pleura, and protected by the skeletal rib cage and sternum. The pleura secrete a lubricating fluid that permits smooth movement of the lungs during the respiratory cycle.

The diaphragm is a muscle located below the lungs. It contracts, and causes the chest cavity to expand to allow more space for air. During expiration, the diaphragm relaxes, and air is forced out of the lungs.

Surgical procedures involving the respiratory system include:

- Thoracotomy – Making an opening into the thoracic cavity (chest) to give surgeons access to the lungs and heart.

- Thoracoscopy – Viewing the thoracic (chest) cavity with an endoscope for diagnosis or treatment.

- Pneumonectomy – Removing a lung.

- Tracheotomy – Making an opening into the trachea.

- Laryngectomy – Removing the larynx (voice box).

- Bronchoscopy – Visualizing the bronchus with an endoscope.

- Septoplasty – Straightening or removing cartilage and/or bone in the nose when the nasal septum is deformed, injured, or fractured.

- Endoscopic Sinus Procedures – Removing bone defects or inflamed tissue of the paranasal sinuses areas to allow the sinuses to drain.

The Digestive System

The human body, like any other complex piece of machinery, requires a source of energy or fuel to keep it functioning. Its fuel is from the chemicals (nutrients) in food.

The function of the digestive system (see **Figure 3.16**) is to convert food into energy for the body. The human body requires six basic categories of nutrients: proteins, carbohydrates, fats, water, minerals, and vitamins. A well-balanced diet is important to keep the body healthy and strong.

The process of digestion breaks food down mechanically and chemically so that it can be absorbed by body cells or discharged as waste. The pathway that food takes through the digestive system is called the **alimentary canal** (digestive tract). Here is some important information about it:

The alimentary canal is approximately 30 feet long, and consists of the **mouth, esophagus, stomach, small intestine, large intestine, rectum,** and **anus.**

Nose – Nasal cavity.

Mouth – The opening through which air, food, and beverages enter the body.

Pharynx – Throat.

Esophagus – Tube that carries food from the throat to the stomach.

Larynx – Voice box.

Trachea – Windpipe.

Bronchi – Tube that extends from the trachea into both sides of the lungs.

Lungs – The two organs of respiration.

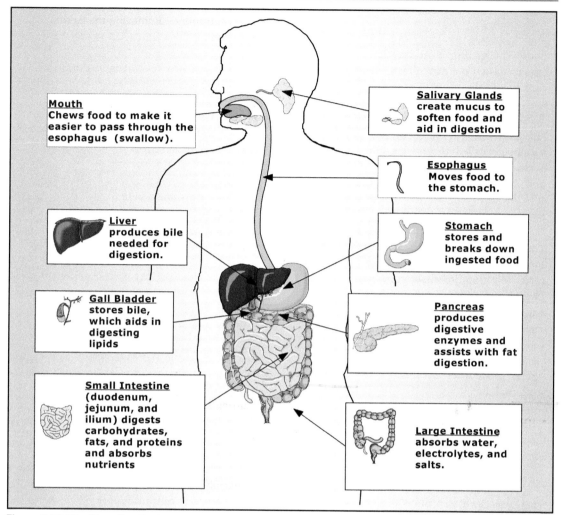

Mouth
Chews food to make it easier to pass through the esophagus (swallow).

Salivary Glands
create mucus to soften food and aid in digestion

Esophagus
Moves food to the stomach.

Liver
produces bile needed for digestion.

Stomach
stores and breaks down ingested food

Gall Bladder
stores bile, which aids in digesting lipids

Pancreas
produces digestive enzymes and assists with fat digestion.

Small Intestine
(duodenum, jejunum, and ilium) digests carbohydrates, fats, and proteins and absorbs nutrients

Large Intestine
absorbs water, electrolytes, and salts.

Figure 3.16 The Digestive System

The liver, gallbladder, and pancreas are accessory organs of the digestive system.

The salivary, gastric, and intestinal glands are accessory structures to the digestive system that contribute to the process of digestion.

A review of the components of the alimentary canal allows us to study the digestive process.

• **Mouth** – The digestive process begins in the mouth. There food is softened by saliva that is secreted by various salivary glands located throughout the mouth. The teeth tear and grind the softened food into smaller particles that allow it to be easily swallowed. The food then passes through the esophagus.

• The **esophagus** – This is a somewhat flexible muscular tube that produces peristaltic contractions that move food into the stomach.

• The **stomach** – An elongated and muscular J-shaped pouch that serves as a reservoir for food as gastric gland secretions (mucin, hydrochloric acid, and enzymes) convert the food into a semi-liquid material called chyme.

• **Small intestines** – From the stomach, the liquified food enters the small intestines which are approximately 20 to 23 feet long, and where the greatest amount of digestion and absorption of nutrients into the body cells occurs. The small intestines are divided into three portions: duodenum, jejunum, and ileum. Bile (produced by the liver and stored in the gallbladder) along with pancreatic and intestinal juices, facilitates digestion in the small intestines.

- **Large Intestine (colon)** – Material that is not absorbed by the small intestines enters the large intestine (colon), which is approximately 5 to 6 feet long. The first few inches of the large intestine are called the cecum from which the appendix vermiform extends. The large intestine consists of six portions: ascending colon, transverse colon, descending colon, sigmoid colon, rectum, and anus. Peristaltic action moves food through the large intestine where the absorption of water and electrolytes or salt occurs.

- **Rectum** and **anus** – The rectum is the last several inches of the large intestine where the remaining waste (feces) becomes dehydrated and is eliminated through the anus.

Surgical procedures involving the digestive system include:

- Appendectomy – Removing the appendix.

- Parotidectomy – Removing a salivary gland (parotid) because of tumor formation.

Alimentary canal – *The pathway that food takes through the digestive system; also called digestive tract.*

Mouth – *The beginning of the alimentary canal.*

Stomach – *A pouch that serves as a reservoir for food that has been consumed.*

Small intestines – *The organ in the digestive system where the greatest amount of digestion and absorption of nutrients into the body cells occurs.*

Large Intestine (colon) – *The digestive organ that dehydrates digestive residues (feces).*

Rectum – *The last several inches of the large intestine.*

Anus – *The lower opening of the alimentary canal.*

- Gastrectomy – Removing the stomach. This procedure includes hemi (half) or total (all) the stomach.

- Gastric Bypass – Isolating a small portion of the stomach, and suturing part of the small intestines to it to treat morbid obesity. (Food intake is then limited to the small part of the stomach.)

- Cholecystectomy – Removing the gallbladder with a surgical incision or by laparoscopy.

- Colectomy – Removing all or part of the large intestine.

- Laparoscopic Cholecystectomy – Removing the gallbladder with endoscopic instrumentation.

Close Look at Three Important Digestive Organs

- ***Organ 1:*** The pancreas – The pancreas is located next to the duodenum, where its duct is united with the common bile duct. They jointly enter the small intestine (duodenum), and assist with fat digestion. Pancreatic acinar cells produce pancreatic juice which is essential in carbohydrate, fat, and protein metabolism.

- ***Organ 2:*** The liver – The liver is the largest internal organ in the human body, and serves many important functions. It produces bile needed in the digestive process, regulates the volume of glycogen and glucose, manufactures heparin and antibodies, regulates blood volumes, stores iron and vitamins, and filters harmful substances.

- ***Organ 3:*** The gallbladder – The gallbladder is located under the liver, and serves as a reservoir for bile produced by the liver. The hepatic duct from the liver, and the cystic duct from the gallbladder join to form the common bile duct that connects to the duodenum.

pathrogenic –

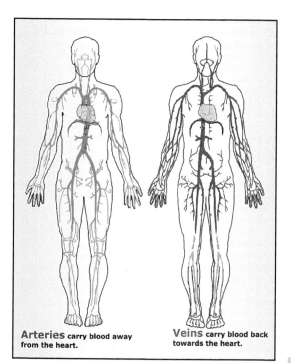

Arteries carry blood away from the heart.

Veins carry blood back towards the heart.

Figure 3.17   The Circulatory System

The Circulatory System

The circulatory system (see **Figure 3.17**) is the body's primary transportation network. It delivers nutrients and oxygen to body cells, and carries away carbon dioxide and other harmful waste products from them. This is accomplished as blood is pumped through 64,000 miles of blood vessels in the body.

The lymphatic system (see **Figure 3.18**) is a subsidiary of the circulatory system, and it serves a vital role in the body's defense against disease.

More About the Circulatory System

When the body is invaded by microscopic organisms, (bacteria or viruses), the circulatory system transports disease-fighting blood cells and chemicals to combat the invaders, and defend the body. It also transports chemical messages throughout the body. For example, the pancreas may send a chemical message through hormones in the blood to the liver to stimulate action that lowers the blood sugar level.

It consists of a series of tiny vessels located throughout the body that carry clear liquid fluid (lymph) that originates from blood plasma.

Large numbers of lymph nodes (tissue masses containing special cells [lymphocytes]) that filter bacteria and other harmful materials out of the lymph are located in the lymph and blood vessels. Lymph flows from the lymph vessels into two veins located in the neck region to return lost fluid back into the bloodstream.

Tonsils are one type of a lymph node, and they are located on both sides of the base of the tongue in the throat.

Sentinal lymph nodes are frequently identified during cancer surgery. The surgeon tries to find the first (sentinal) lymph node where the cancer cells have started to spread.

Blood is a type of connective tissue fluid that moves throughout the circulatory system and transports many important substances. The body contains an average of five to seven liters of blood. Blood is a mixture of plasma, red blood cells (erythrocytes), white blood cells (leukocytes) and platelets:

- Plasma – More than 55% of the blood is made up of plasma, a yellowish liquid that is composed of water (92%) and proteins. Plasma serves as the vehicle of transportation for dissolved nutrients, enzymes, waste, and other substances through the body.

- Red blood cells – These structures have thin centers that allow them to be pliable when moving through narrow capillaries. Red blood cells are rich in hemoglobin (an iron protein) that picks up oxygen in the lungs, transports it to all the body cells, and then transports carbon dioxide back to the lungs. These cells are produced in the bone marrow, and have a life span of approximately 120 days. Worn out or damaged red blood cells are broken down in the liver and destroyed by the spleen.

- White blood cells – Some white blood cells are twice as large as red blood cells, and their life span can range from hours to years. White

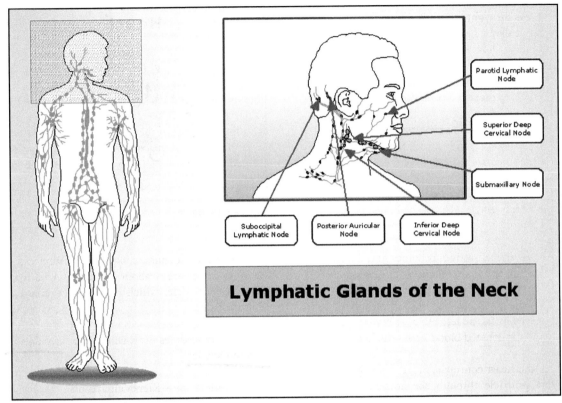

Figure 3.18 Lymphatic System

blood cells are also produced by bone marrow, and their purpose is to attack, destroy, and digest disease-producing organisms that enter the body.

• Platelets – These tiny cell fragments detach from bone marrow and enter the bloodstream. They have no color or nucleus, and last for a maximum of ten days. Enzymes released by the platelets act on other blood components to create fibrin. This chemical weaves across cells in blood vessels, and traps blood cells and plasma that will harden and clot.

Circulation in the body is a continuous process traveling the same route throughout the body all the time. Blood moves from the heart to the lungs, and back to the heart where it is pumped to all the cells of the body through a system of vessels. Blood then returns back to the heart to be re-circulated.

The vessels that carry blood away from the heart are called **arteries,** and **veins** are the vessels that carry blood back towards the heart. **Capillaries** are the tiny vessels abundant throughout the body that serve as connections between veins and arteries.

The **heart** (see **Figure 3.19**) is the muscular organ about the size of a fist that pumps five liters of blood through the body every minute while resting only between beats. Located in its upper right side is a "pacemaker" that signals the heart muscle to contract which controls the heartbeat. Here's how the heart works:

• The heart consists of four hollow chambers: two on each side.

• A thick tissue wall called the septum separates the right and left sides of the heart.

• The upper chambers of the heart are called **atria,** and the lower chambers are called **ventricles**.

• Deoxygenated blood (blood that has had oxygen removed by the cells) returns to the heart, and enters the right atrium.

- As the right atrium becomes full, a tissue flap called a heart valve opens. It allows the blood to flow into the right ventricle.

- When the right ventricle is full, the valve closes to prevent a back flow of blood.

- As the right ventricle contracts, the blood is forced out of the heart through the pulmonary artery into the lungs where it is oxygenated.

- The oxygenated blood (blood that now contains oxygen) leaves the lungs through the pulmonary veins and enters the left atrium.

- As the left atrium becomes full, the left atrium heart valve opens, and the blood flows into the left ventricle. As the left ventricle becomes full, the left atrium valve closes, the left ventricle contracts, and oxygenated blood leaves the heart.

As the heart contracts, blood is forced out of the left ventricle through the aortic valve into the **aorta**: the largest blood vessel in the body. The aorta is an artery that carries blood away from the heart, and it branches out into a vast network of smaller arteries throughout the body. Since

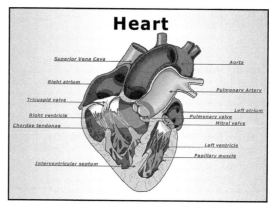

Figure 3.19 Heart

the left ventricle pumps blood throughout the entire body, it works about six times as hard as the right ventricle, which only pumps blood a short distance.

Surgical procedures involving the circulatory system include:

- Tonsillectomy – Removing lymph tissue in the pharynx (throat).

- Adenoidectomy – Removing tonsil tissue at the end of the soft palate (roof of the mouth).

- Arteriovenous (AV) Fistula – Suturing the radial artery and cephalic vein together in the lower arm to allow the dilated (enlarged) vein to be used for large bore needle insertion for renal dialysis.

- Abdominal Aortic Aneurysmectomy (AAA) – Obliterating a weakened, balloon-like area in the aorta and replacing it with a synthetic product.

- Hemorrhoidectomy – Removing anal arteries.

- CABG – Removing a vein from the lower limb to bypass the blocked coronary artery of the heart.

- Carotid Endarterectomy – Removing plaques from the carotid artery that cause lack of brain oxygenation.

Blood – A type of connective tissue fluid that transports many substances throughout the circulatory system.

Arteries – Vessels that carry blood away from the heart.

Veins – Vessels that carry blood back to the heart.

Capillaries – Vessels that serve as connections between veins and arteries.

Heart – The muscular organ that pumps blood throughout the body.

Atria – The two upper chambers of the heart.

Ventricles – The two lower chambers of the heart.

Aorta – The largest blood vessel in the body.

IN CONCLUSION

Having a basic understanding of the structure and function of the human body helps Central Service Technicians develop a better understanding of the terms they see and hear daily. Understanding basic information about common surgical procedures also helps them better understand the procedures that they prepare for and improves the communication process between Central Service and its customers.

REFERENCES

Brooks, M. *Exploring Medical Language: A Student-Directed Approach. Fifth Edition. Mosby, Inc. 2002.*

Davies, J. *Essentials of Medical Terminology. Second Edition. Delmar Publishers, Inc. 2002.*

Fremgen, B. *Medical Terminology: An Anatomy and Physiology Systems Approach. Prentice-Hall, Inc. 1997.*

Gylys, B. *Medical Terminology Simplified: A Programmed Learning Approach by Body Systems. F. A. Davis Company. 1995.*

Gylys, B; and Wedding, M. *Medical Terminology: A Systems Approach. Third Edition. F. A. Davis Company. 1995.*

Isler, Charlotte. *The Patient's Guide to Medical Terminology. Third Edition. Health Information Press. 1997.*

Lillis, C. *A Concise Introduction to Medical Terminology. Fourth Edition. Appleton & Lange. 1997.*

McCann, J; and Schilling. *Medical Terminology Made Incredibly Easy. Springhouse Corporation. 2001.*

CENTRAL SERVICE TERMS

Cell

Cell membrane

Cytoplasm

Nucleus

Tissue

Organ

System

Tendons

Ligaments

Cartilage

Ossification

Joint

Fascia

Central Nervous System (CNS)

Peripheral Nervous System

Brain

Cerebrum

Cerebellum

Brain Stem

Hormones

Metabolism

Insulin

Glucagon

Sperm

Ovum

Chromosomes

Testes

Scrotum

Epidilymus

Vas deferens

Seminal vesicle

Ejaculatory duct

Semen

Urethra

Penis

Prostate gland

Vagina

Uterus

Endometrium

Fallopian tubes

Fimbriae

Ovaries

Kidneys

Ureters

Urinary bladder

Liver

Skin

Nose

Mouth

Pharynx

Esophagus

Larynx

Trachea

Bronchi

Lungs

Alimentary canal (digestive tract)

Mouth

Stomach

Small intestines

Large Intestine (colon)

Rectum

Anus

Blood

Arteries

Veins

Capillaries

Heart

Atria

Ventricles

Aorta

Chapter Outline

Chapter 4

Microbiology for Central Service

Chapter Learning Objectives:

As a result of successfully completing this chapter, readers will be able to:

1. Define the term, "microbiology," and tell why Central Service Technicians must know about it.

2. Restate basic facts about microorganisms.

3. Identify common ways to identify and classify microorganisms:
   - By shape
   - By color change
   - By need for oxygen

4. Explain environmental conditions necessary for bacterial growth and survival.

5. Provide basic information about non-bacterial organisms:
   - Viruses
   - Protozoa
   - Fungi

6. Describe how microorganisms are transmitted between persons and places.

7. Review basic procedures to control and kill microorganisms.

Some Central Service Technicians are sometimes daunted by microbiology because much of its terminology is unfamiliar, and because it deals with a world that cannot be seen without a microscope. However, we can see the effects that microorganisms have on us. For example, we have all become sick with infections, colds, or the flu and, even though we didn't see the microorganisms that infected us, we felt their effects.

Periodically, outbreaks of Norovirus or E-Coli contamination make the news, as hundreds (or more) of persons become ill with a foodborne illness. Microscopic invaders can enter our bodies and cause serious illness and even death. How can something so small have such massive power over the human body? Why can anyone, even the strongest and healthiest person, become infected by microorganisms? Why does the risk of infection increase in people whose immune systems or natural body defenses are compromised? Central Service Technicians must have a clear understanding of basic information about microorganisms to answer these and related questions, and this chapter will help them to do so.

OVERVIEW OF MICROBIOLGY

Learning Objective 1. Define the term, "microbiology," and tell why Central Service Technicians must know about it.

Most people have a basic understanding of **microbiology.** They know that it's not wise to eat food that falls on the floor, or to touch a sick person's soiled facial tissues and share eating utensils. They know they should wash their hands before eating and after using the restroom, and they try to protect babies and small children who may put everything they can into their mouths. They understand that taking these precautions helps to protect against "germs." Still their understanding of the world of microbes is typically limited.

Central Service Technicians must have a basic understanding about microbiology for two reasons:

- They have the responsibility to protect patients from microorganisms in the healthcare environment.

- The nature of their job duties places them and their co-workers in harm's way for exposure to harmful microorganisms.

"Seeing" Microorganisms with the "Mind's Eye"

One reason that microbiology is daunting to some Central Service Technicians is that they must control an "enemy" they cannot see. A "mental picture" can help them to do so.

Let's compare microorganisms to seeds to draw some comparisons for our study of microorganisms. There are many varieties of seeds, and each produces a different plant. Seeds must have the right conditions to grow and continue living. Those in a paper

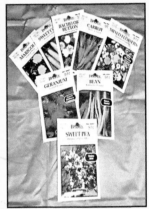

Figure 4.1

envelope at the store will not germinate and grow (see **Figure 4.1**). However, when they are placed in the right conditions with proper soil, water, fertilizer, warmth and sunlight, they grow and develop (see **Figure 4.2**).

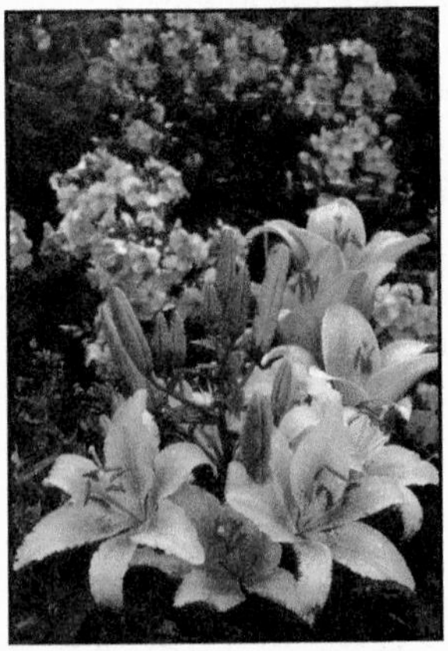

In the same manner, there are many varieties of microorganisms, and each can produce a specific effect (an infection or disease) when

Figure 4.2

they have the right conditions for growth and reproduction.

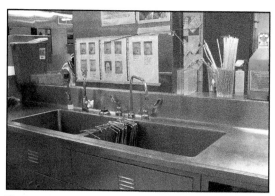

Figure 4.3

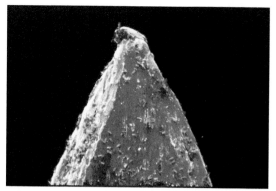

Figure 4.5

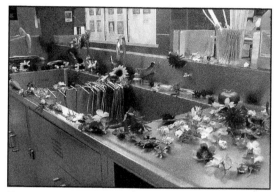

Figure 4.4

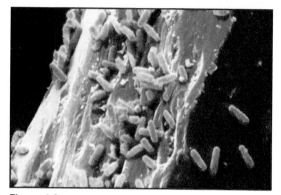

Figure 4.6

Central Service Technicians should be able to recognize the conditions that favor the growth of microorganisms, and learn to "see" microorganisms in the workplace. For example, the decontamination work station in **Figure 4.3** looks safe to the untrained eye. However, if microorganisms were as easy to see as plants that same work station might look like the photo in **Figure 4.4**.

The visual comparison of the two photos helps to illustrate **contamination**. Microorganisms present on objects cannot be seen with the naked eye. **Figures 4.5** and **4.6** are magnified photos of a contaminated needle. They illustrate that, even though we cannot see microorganisms,

Microbiology – The study of microorganisms. The science which treats the nature, life, and action of microorganisms.

Contamination – The state of being soiled or infected by contact with infectious organisms or other material.

they are present in our environment. The surgical instruments, equipment, and utensils processed by Central Service personnel everyday are loaded with microorganisms that pose a threat to patients, Central Service Technicians, and other facility personnel.

All Central Service Technicians should have a broad overview of microbiology including knowledge about:

• Basic facts about microorganisms.

• How those microorganisms are identified and classified.

• How they grow.

• What conditions they need to grow and reproduce.

• How they are transmitted from person-to-person and place-to-place.

• How they can be controlled and killed.

While the science of microbiology is vast, the remainder of this chapter provides Central Service Technicians with the above information that directly relates to their jobs.

BASIC FACTS ABOUT MICROORGANISMS

Learning Objective 2. Restate basic facts about microorganisms.

Microorganisms are nearly everywhere in nature and in our environment. This includes in untreated water, air and dust, on uncooked foods, in decaying matter, on the skin and hair of people and animals, in their intestinal tracts and feces, and in the body's fluid discharges. Even healthy humans harbor millions of bacteria and continually shed them into the environment by a careless cough or sneeze or from a draining sore.

Not All Microorganisms Are Harmful

Microbes are necessary for the existence of all plants and animals, and life could not continue very long in an environment without them. One function of microorganisms in nature involves the decay process. Without microbial activity, there would be no decay or disposal of animal carcasses and vegetation in forests. The accumulation of three or four seasons of non-decayed leaves would cover streets, and roads, and would stop business and farming.

Sewage treatment also depends on bacteria. Microorganisms convert waste materials and feces into soluble, odorless compounds for disposal. A great need of space travel is for microorganisms to effectively and rapidly treat waste within a confined area.

Microorganisms are also useful in food products (examples: in the production of some cheeses and vinegar), and they even help to contain oil spills in the oceans. In this chapter we will focus on one type of microorganism—bacteria—because they are responsible for more infections in humans than any other type of microbe. Also more is known about the laboratory techniques for the study and control of bacteria than for other microorganisms.

Size and Structure of Bacteria

Bacterial cells are very small, and the **micron** (1/25,000 of an inch; 1/1,000 of a millimeter) is used to measure them. Most bacteria are approximately 1 or 2 microns in size. It is estimated that one cubic inch (a volume that measures 1 inch x 1 inch x 1 inch) contains nine trillion (9,000,000,000,000) cells of the average rod-shaped bacterium. Further, four hundred million (400,000,000) of these cells would occupy the same space as one granule of granulated sugar. When bacteria are magnified 1,000 times, they may look no bigger than a dot on this page. To observe bacteria, one needs a microscope that can magnify at least 900 times. Magnifications of 80,000 to 150,000 times are possible with the electron microscope. Note: While this is a common instrument in many universities and research centers, it is seldom used in hospitals. An electron microscope is required to see viruses, which are much smaller than bacteria.

The term "**protoplasm**" describes all living materials in the cell. **Cytoplasm** (the fluid and all structures inside the cell except the **nucleus**) is a clear, thick, and jelly-like substance. Cytoplasm produces and

---

Micron – *A unit of measurement; 1/1000 of a millimeter or 1/25,000 of an inch; usually designated by the Greek letter u.*

Protoplasm – *A thick mucous-like substance that is colorless and translucent that forms the biochemical basis of life found within the cell nucleus.*

Cytoplasm – *The living matter of a cell between the cell's membrane and nucleus.*

Nucleus – *The functional center of a cell that governs activity and heredity.*

Phagotization – *The process by which some cells can ingest bacteria or other foreign particles.*

DNA – *Deoxyribonucleic Acid. The protein found in the chromosomes of a cell nucleus which is the basis of heredity.*

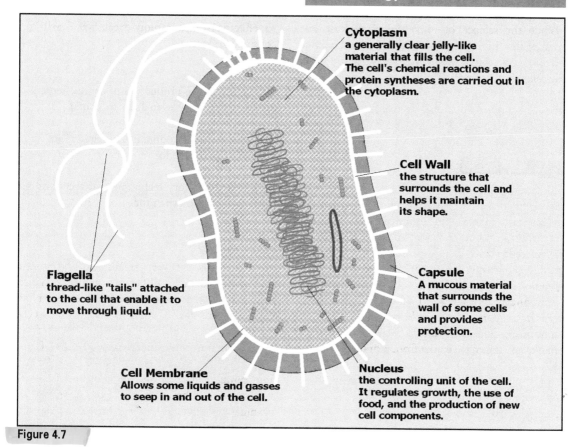

Cytoplasm
a generally clear jelly-like material that fills the cell. The cell's chemical reactions and protein syntheses are carried out in the cytoplasm.

Cell Wall
the structure that surrounds the cell and helps it maintain its shape.

Flagella
thread-like "tails" attached to the cell that enable it to move through liquid.

Capsule
A mucous material that surrounds the wall of some cells and provides protection.

Cell Membrane
Allows some liquids and gasses to seep in and out of the cell.

Nucleus
the controlling unit of the cell. It regulates growth, the use of food, and the production of new cell components.

Figure 4.7

transports proteins, nutrients, and energy so the cell can perform all necessary functions for life.

Figure 4.7 shows the components of a typical cell. Note: some cells may not contain all these components.

• Cell wall – The cell wall is a tough, rigid structure that helps maintain the cell's shape. It protects the cell from bursting in a solution that is less salty than the cell, or from becoming dehydrated in a solution that is saltier than the cell.

• Cell membrane – This layer is located just beneath the cell wall which is semi-permeable. It has small pores or openings that allow some liquids and gasses to seep in and out of the cell.

• Cytoplasm – This is the jelly-like protein located between the cell membrane and nucleus, and it is much like the white of an egg. All of the cell's chemical reactions and protein syntheses are carried out in the cytoplasm.

• Capsule – Some (but not all) bacteria have a slime layer around the cell wall. This capsule is a mucus material that protects the bacteria from the host cells that try to destroy it. Example: white blood cells in humans destroy bacteria by engulfing them in a process called **phagotization**. The capsule makes it harder for the white blood cells to engulf the bacteria.

• Flagella – These are thread-like "tails" attached to the cell that enable the bacteria to move through liquids.

• Nucleus – The nucleus is the controlling unit of the cell. It regulates growth, the use of food, and the production of new cell components. The nucleus is composed of one strand of **DNA**, a chromosome or chain of genes. The bacterial nucleus has no nuclear membrane (sack) enclosing the DNA. Instead, the bacterial chromosomes (DNA strand) float freely in the cytoplasm. Plants and animals have many chromosomes, and they are enclosed in a nuclear membrane.

Some cells protect themselves in a hostile environment by developing a thick coat around their nucleus called a **spore**. The rest of the cell will eventually disintegrate, but the spore can rejuvenate itself when the environment improves. Spores are of special concern to Central Service Technicians because they are very difficult to kill.

More About Cells

Cells are the basic units of all living organisms (plants, animals, and bacteria), and they are the smallest unit that can live, grow, and reproduce. They differ in size and shape, but they all have a nucleus, cytoplasm, and cell membrane. Plants and animals are comprised of many cells that form different tissues to perform specific tasks. Bacteria perform all life tasks within a single cell.

Bacterial cells differ from both plant and animal cells because they have no membrane to separate the nucleus (one strand of DNA) from the cytoplasm. Plants and animals have a nuclear membrane surrounding many strands of DNA.

Animal and most bacterial cells do not contain **chlorophyll**, a chemical in plant cells which enables them to change energy from sunlight into energy that makes food for the cell.

IDENTIFICATION AND CLASSIFICATION OF MICROORGANISMS

Learning Objective 3. Identify common ways to identify and classify microorganisms:
- By shape
- By color change
- By need for oxygen

Some people have trouble pronouncing and spelling the names of microorganisms. Although the names may be unfamiliar, there is a prescribed method for naming them. The first word in a microorganism's name (always capitalized) is the genus (tribe) of the microorganism and the second word is the specific name of the organism (called the species). There are also specific methods used to classify them into categories to help reduce the confusion that can arise when one reads or talks about them.

Bacteria Are Classified By Shape.

Bacteria are divided into three main groups according to their shape:

- Cocci are round or spherical shaped, and can occur in pairs, clusters, or chains.

- Rods may be large and brick-shaped, or small and stick-like.

- Spirals vary from comma-shaped to longer bacteria with many twists.

Figures 4.8, 4.9, and **4.10** illustrate the three main shapes of bacteria.

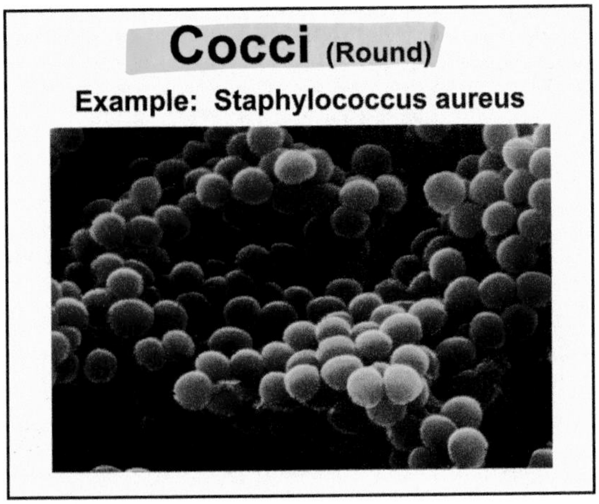

Cocci (Round)
Example: Staphylococcus aureus

Figure 4.8

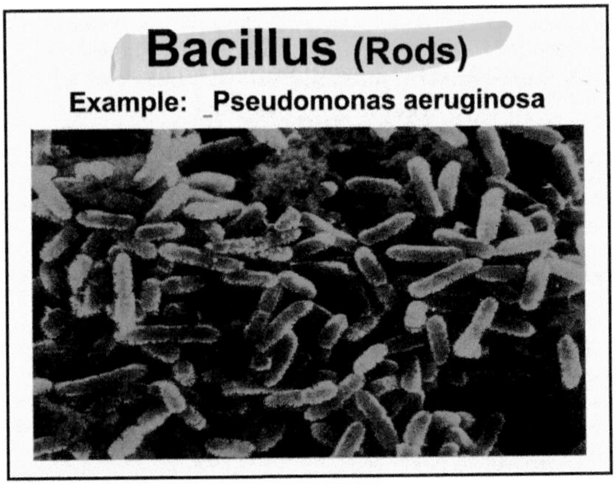

Bacillus (Rods)
Example: _Pseudomonas aeruginosa

Figure 4.9

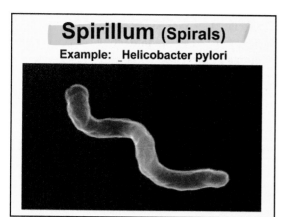

Spirillum (Spirals)

Example: _Helicobacter pylori_

Figure 4.10

Bacteria Are Classified By Color Change

Bacteria can be classified by the visual (color) change that occurs when they are subjected to specific tests (stains).

Bacteria are normally clear and colorless organisms, and they cannot be seen even when viewed under the microscope unless they are dyed with a stain so the shape of each individual organism can be seen. Two common stains that help identify bacteria are the Gram stain and the Ziehl-Neilson stain. Both stain processes help identify bacterial traits to assist physicians with diagnostic processes. _will not change color_

Christian Gram developed the Gram stain process in 1884, and it divides bacteria into two groups. Bacteria that stain purple with a special dye are called gram-positive, and they will retain this color even when a decolorizer is used. A small amount of the material to be stained is placed on a glass slide. It is passed through a flame to kill the microbes, and to make the bacteria adhere to the slide so they do not wash away during the staining process. When gram positive bacteria are stained with crystal violet (the primary stain), and are then treated with an iodine solution (mordant). the cells form a bond with the

Spore – _Microorganisms capable of forming a thick wall around themselves enabling them to survive in adverse conditions; a resistant form of bacterium._

Chlorophyll – _A molecule in plants that absorbs sunlight, and converts it to energy in process called photosynthesis._

stain. This cell and purple stain combination cannot be removed by the decolorizer.

By contrast, other bacteria have the purple color removed when the decolorizer is used, and they will be stained red when another dye is added. This second group of bacteria is called Gram-negative because they do not retain the original dye. The second dye cannot stain the Gram-positive bacteria because they are completely colored purple.

changes color

The Ziehl-Neilson stain is also known as an acid-fast stain. When most bacteria are stained with a certain chemical (carbolfuchsin) and the slide is heated, they stain easily. Then when the smear is treated with an acid-alcohol, some bacteria cells are completely decolorized. It is difficult to stain some bacteria with carbolfuchsin but, once stained, they retain the dye even when they are decolorized with an acid. Microbes that retain the red stain are called acid-fast. The acid-fast characteristic is probably caused by the presence of waxy substances within the cell wall. The bacteria that are decolorized by the acid wash are then stained by use of a second stain (methylene blue). Nonacid-fast organisms turn a deep blue when all their stain is removed by the acid.

There are two important acid-fast bacteria that most commonly cause disease: Mycobacterium tuberculosis causes tuberculosis, and Mycobacterium leprae causes leprosy.

Figure 4.11 reviews common microorganisms relative to the two characteristics just discussed: shape and gram stain results.

Bacteria Are Classified By the Need for Oxygen

Atmospheric oxygen is a requirement for the growth of the **aerobic bacteria** which require air with oxygen just as humans do. They may grow in liquids, but the liquid must have oxygen dissolved in it, because oxygen is needed for respiration and metabolism. By contrast, **anaerobic bacteria** (examples: tetanus and botulism) obtain their oxygen from another source, and their enzymes are inactivated by free oxygen. Oxygen must be

Name	Classification	Gram-Stain Results
Staphylococcus	Cocci (Round)	Gram-Positive
Streptococcus	Cocci (Round)	Gram-Positive
Enterococcus	Cocci (Round)	Gram-Positive
Mycobacterium tuberculosis	Bacillus (Rods)	Gram-Positive
Mycobacterium leprae	Bacillus (Rods)	Gram-Positive
Clostridium tetani	Bacillus (Rods)	Gram-Positive
Clostridium botulinum	Bacillus (Rods)	Gram-Positive
Clostridium perfringes	Bacillus (Rods)	Gram-Positive
Bacillus anthracis	Bacillus (Rods)	Gram-Positive
Geobacillus species	Bacillus (Rods)	Gram-Positive
Neisseria meningitis	Cocci (Round)	Gram-Negative
Neisseria gonorrheae	Cocci (Round)	Gram-Negative
Escheria coli (E. coli)	Bacillus (Rods)	Gram-Negative
Proteus	Bacillus (Rods)	Gram-Negative
Klebsiella	Bacillus (Rods)	Gram-Negative
Pseudomonis	Bacillus (Rods)	Gram-Negative
Salmonella typhi	Bacillus (Rods)	Gram-Negative
Shigilla dysenteriae	Bacillus (Rods)	Gram-Negative

Figure 4.11

eliminated from the environment for them to grow. An example of this is a deep-puncture wound preceding tetanus or lockjaw. The bacteria are introduced deep into the flesh by a nail or similar object. Then, when it is removed, the tissue and tissue juices close the wound, oxygen is removed from the environment, and the anaerobic bacteria can grow.

HOW BACTERIA LIVE AND GROW

Learning Objective 4. Explain environmental conditions necessary for bacterial growth and survival.

Suitable environments for specific bacteria may be as different as the bacteria themselves. Pathogenic (disease-causing) bacteria show variation in their nutritional requirements, and they are most likely to thrive where their specific nutritional requirements can be met. Some, like Staphylococci, can grow on and in many areas of the body, skin, blood, and hair follicles. Other bacteria such as Neisseria gonorrhea, (which cause a sexually-transmitted disease) are more delicate. They require a special environment such as that on the mucous membranes of the reproductive system where they can live and invade deeper tissue.

Temperature requirements vary widely among different kinds of bacteria. The **psychrophiles** grow best at 59°F – 68°F (15°C – 20°C) while the **thermophiles** can grow at 122°F – 158°F (50° – 70°C). Most of the bacteria pathogenic to humans are **mesophiles** and require body temperature 68°F – 113°F (20°C – 45°C) for optimum growth. Others such as soil bacteria and certain strains of water bacteria grow only at room temperature or below. (See **Figure 4.12**)

Moisture and relative humidity play a major role in the growth and survival of microorganisms. Those which inhabit our skin, other bacteria that produce spores, and the TB bacillus can survive for years in a dry state. Other species such as gonorrhea bacteria cannot survive for more than thirty seconds when subjected to complete drying.

Temperature Requirements for Bacteria

Name	Description	Optimum Growth Temperatures	
Psychrophiles	Likes Cold Temperatures	59° F to 68° F	(15° C to 20° C)
Mesophiles*	Likes Moderate Temperatures	68° F to 113° F	(20° C to 45° C)
Thermophiles	Likes Warm Temperatures	122° F to 158° F	(50° C to 70° C)

*Mesophiles are often pathogenic to humans and grow well at body temperature.

Figure 4.12

With the exception of the bacteria used in the fermentation process (vinegar and sauerkraut, for example), most species will not grow in an acid pH of 4.4 or lower. Microorganisms that are pathogenic to humans have an optimum pH range of 7 to 7.8: the same pH as blood.

Sunlight is lethal to the **vegetative stage** of pathogens. (A vegetative organism is in the actively growing rather than resting stage.) The spore of gram-positive Bacilli is in a resting stage, and is one of the most resistant to sunlight. Ultraviolet light in the range of 2537 **Angstrom** is the most lethal, and it has been used to disinfect air and purify the environment. Some facilities employ ultraviolet light in their operating rooms. Ultraviolet light and sunlight kill bacteria by causing breaks in the nuclear DNA.

Bacteria that grow on human skin and mucosa and in our gastrointestinal tract are typically not harmful, and they are called normal flora. However, normal flora can produce disease when these organisms are introduced into a normally sterile tissue. Example: when an appendix ruptures an abscess is formed by previously enclosed bacteria such as E. Coli and anaerobic bacteria living in the area.

Under optimal conditions, most bacteria and other microorganisms reproduce (multiply by dividing into two cells) approximately every twenty minutes. They do so in a process called **binary fission** in which the original "mother" cell divides into two "daughter" cells. **Figure 4.13** illustrates how E. coli multiplies (grows) by dividing. As bacteria divide they often adhere to each other in typical arrangements.

Aerobic bacteria – Capable of growing in the presence of free oxygen. Requiring oxygen.

Anaerobic bacteria – Capable of growing in the absence of free oxygen. Not requiring oxygen.

Psychrophiles (bacteria) – Cold–loving bacteria whose optimum temperature for growth is 59°F – 68°F (15°C – 20°C) or below.

Mesophiles (Bacteria) – Bacteria that grow best at moderate temperatures: 68°F – 113°F (20°C – 45°C).

Thermophiles (bacteria) – Bacteria which grow best at a temperature of 122°F – 158°F (50° – 70°C).

Vegetative stage – State of active growth of microorganisms (as opposed to the resting or spore stages.)

Angstrom – A unit that measures visible light.

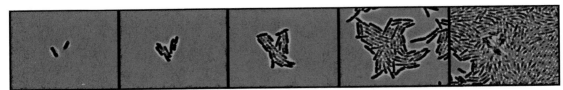

Figure 4.13 E. coli multiply by dividing.

Groups of microbes have specific requirements for growth and survival which tend to limit the location where they may be found, or the host in which they may invade. For example, a microbe that lives and thrives in the soil may not grow well in the vital organs of humans; the reverse is also true.

In some cases, microorganisms adapt and change as a means of survival. For example, **Methicillin-Resistant Staphylococcus Aureus (MRSA)** and **Vancomycin-Resistant Enterococcus (VRE)** have become an increasing problem in hospitals. Healthcare personnel must consistently use proper procedures for decontamination and sterilization to help prevent the spread of these antibiotic-resistant bacteria. Infection prevention and control policies must be strictly followed to protect patients from these resistant strains of bacteria.

NON-BACTERIAL ORGANISMS

Learning Objective 5. Provide basic information about non-bacterial organisms:

- Viruses
- Protozoa
- Fungi

Viruses   1,000 times smaller

The term, **virus,** is derived from the Latin word for poison. Viruses are about 1,000 times smaller than bacteria, and can only be seen with an electron microscope. To compare the size of viruses to bacteria, the American Society for Microbiology shares this analogy; If you were to enlarge an average virus to the size of a baseball, the average bacterium would be the size of a pitcher's mound and one single cell from the millions in the human body would be the size of the entire ballpark. (Source: www.MayoClinic.com) Viruses can only

be grown in cell cultures and not on artificial media such as agar plates.

A virus enters a living plant or animal cell, and then reproduces itself within the cell. It usually destroys the cell, and then enters another cell to survive. It has no means of movement, and depends on air, water, insects, humans, or other animals to carry it from one **host** to another. Some viruses survive away from the host for many hours or days when in organic material such as scabs, blood, and body wastes.

Viral diseases include smallpox, rabies, yellow fever, influenza, measles, mumps, polio, common colds, shingles, cold sores, warts, acquired immune deficiency syndrome (AIDS), and hepatitis. It is estimated that 60,000 new cases of HBV (hepatitis B) are reported annually in the United States, and there are an estimated 1.25 million chronically infected Americans.[1]

At least five distinct viruses are responsible for hepatitis: viruses (A), (B), (C), (D), and (E). Hepatitis A is often implicated in foodborne illness, and Hepatitis B, C, D, and E can be transmitted in body fluids. There are vaccines available for both Hepatitis A and B, and the vaccine for Hepatitis B is strongly recommended for most hospital workers.

Herpes simplex (HSV) is a viral disease which causes fever blisters and cold sores. These recurrent skin or mucous membrane infections are characterized by single or multiple clusters of small vesicles which are filled with clear fluid on slightly raised, inflammatory bases. There are two herpes virus strains. HSV Type 1 causes mouth and lip blisters. HSV Type 2 is associated with genital infections. The Herpes virus survives one-and-one-half to four hours on toilet seats, up to seventy-two hours on cotton gauze, and eighteen hours on plastic. Since many microorganisms survive in the dry state for days, healthcare workers should use standard precautions at all times for all patients.

Another virus that has caused infections in the United States is the West Nile encephalitis virus. This virus is a bird pathogen that can cause flu-like symptoms and encephalitis in humans, horses, and other animals. It is carried by mosquitoes from bird to man, and has also been transmitted from organ donors to organ recipients.

AIDS disease is caused by the human immunodeficiency virus (HIV). The only way an individual can acquire this disease is if the AIDS virus invades the individual's bloodstream. AIDS is considered a fatal, contagious, and incurable disease. Over one million cases have been reported in the U.S. with 83,000 deaths. Worldwide, eight to ten million cases have been reported.

Protozoa

A **protozoan** (plural: protozoa) is a one-celled animal organism. Protozoa have a well-defined nucleus, cytoplasm, and cell wall and, often, granules, and vacuoles.

Entamoeba histolytica is the most frequently encountered pathogenic protozoa. It is found in feces, intestinal ulcers, and liver abscesses of infected persons. It constantly changes its shape, is about 18-25 microns in size, and exhibits **amoeboid movement** by means of blunt pseudopodia (false feet). It engulfs particles and food by flowing around a particle and taking it into itself.

Cryptosporidium is another protozoan that can cause diarrhea and abdominal pain. This organism causes a severe, life-threatening diarrhea in AIDS or cancer patients, and organ transplant recipients.

Fungi

Fungi are a large group of plant-like organisms including molds, mushrooms, and yeasts without chlorophyll. They live by feeding on living or dead organisms. Some fungi such as yeasts occur as single cells that require a microscope to see. Others such as mushrooms are quite large.

Fungi and bacteria are often found together in nature. Many fungi are useful and, for example, are necessary to produce bread, cheese, wine, and beer. Some such as mushrooms are used as food. Other types are troublesome because they cause decay and mildew. Fungi grow on a wide variety of natural and industrial products. In addition, they are involved in the production of most kinds of antibiotics. For example, the mold Penicillium notatum produces the antibiotic penicillin.

Molds are composed of many-celled organisms that usually grow in compact masses of intertwining, branching, and hair-like filaments. They reproduce in a variety of ways including the formation of spores, fruiting bodies, and binary fission.

Several species of fungus cause respiratory diseases in humans who acquire these infections by inhaling spores from dust, bird droppings,

[handwritten: Bacteria needs 3 things to grow; mosture, food, temperature.]

Binary fission – *The typical method of bacterial reproduction in which a cell divides into two equal parts.*

Methicillin-Resistant Staphylococcus Aureus (MRSA) – *Staphylococcus aureus bacteria that have developed a resistance to Methicillin, the drug of choice. MRSA usually occurs with patients who have been on antibiotic therapy for a long time.*

Vancomycin-Resistant Enterococcus (VRE) – *Enterococcus bacteria that are no longer sensitive to Vancomycin. Transmission can occur either via direct contact or indirectly via hands of personnel.*

Virus – *One of a group of minute infectious agents that grow only in living tissues or cells.*

Host – *The animal, plant, or human that supports the growth of microorganisms.*

Protozoan – *Any one-celled animal-like microorganism of the sub-kingdom protozoa.*

Amoeboid movement – *The crawling movement of cells brought about by the cell successively becoming longer and then retracting.*

---

soil, and other sources. Certain fungi including Coccidioides immitis are not widely distributed in nature, but appear to be found only in particular geographic regions. The fungus disease coccidioidomycosis is also called desert fever, San Joaquin fever, and valley fever.

The fungus disease, histoplasmosis, is caused by Histoplasma capsulatum, and it occurs throughout the world with a relatively high incidence in certain countries. While the disease is widespread, it is generally mild, and may affect one or several organs. It may be difficult to diagnose this disease since it presents a broad spectrum of effects ranging from an asymptomatic (mild) infection to an acute, severe disease. It can also cause chronic pulmonary diseases.

Some fungi mainly attack the epidermis, hair, nails, and mucosal surfaces, and are called superficial fungi. They are further classified by the location of the effects produced. For example, ringworm of the scalp is Tinea capitis; that of the feet (Tinea pedis) is more commonly known as athlete's foot. Diseases caused by these agents also include various forms of ringworm (from the Latin word meaning "worm" or "larval"), and candida infections of mucosal surfaces such as thrush and vulvovaginitis.

Cryptococcus neoformans is yeast that causes cryptococcosis. Primary infections of the lungs may resemble tuberculosis or neoplasm, and systemic infections originating in the lungs may spread throughout the body. There they invade the skin, bones, viscera and, ultimately, the meninges and brain. Infection of the brain and meninges may resemble tuberculous meningitis, brain abscess, or brain tumor.

TRANSMISSION OF MICROORGANISMS

Learning Objective 6. Describe how microorganisms are transmitted between persons and places.

Microorganisms cannot move by themselves. However, they are called the "world's great hitchhikers." Their very small size enables them to be moved by air currents, on particles of dust, in liquids, and on solid objects such as patient care equipment and surgical instruments.

People are another very common method for transmitting microorganisms. Not only do they transmit microorganisms that naturally are found on their bodies, but they also transmit microorganisms from other sources (i.e. a contaminated piece of patient care equipment) that contaminate their bodies and clothes.

Humans and lower animals come in contact with thousands of different types of microorganisms, but only 1% (those that grow at human body temperature) are harmful to humans. The remaining 99% of organisms are sometimes pathogenic for plants and lower animals. However, microbes that survive in the environment can shift from pathogenic to nonpathogenic (and back again). One cannot rely on any microbes in the hospital environment to be nonpathogenic since they can change under favorable conditions. Also, any microbe can be harmful to patients whose defenses are compromised due to illness, injury, or invasive procedure. Therefore, infection prevention is the goal of every Central Service Technician as he/she works diligently to prevent the transmission of microorganisms to patients.

A Brief History of Infection Control

Since ancient times, scientists have proposed theories about transmissible and invisible infectious agents. In the mid-1800's, Louis Pasteur, a French scientist, helped establish the foundation of a "germ theory of disease" that suggested microorganisms caused infectious diseases. Robert Koch, a German bacteriologist, supported Pasteur's work with his own theory that proposed the need for a source, a method of transmission, and a susceptible host to acquire an infection.

Both of these great scientists influenced the understanding of disease transmission. Then, in the late 1800's, Ignaz Semmelweis, Joseph Lister, Florence Nightingale, and other medical pioneers contributed to the modern understanding of infectious disease transmission. Their efforts led to procedures designed to reduce infection risks in healthcare facilities. Although major progress has been made in understanding the principles of disease transmission, some healthcare workers still do not apply them. Over the past forty years, formalized infection control programs have evolved to ensure the safety and well-being of patients, visitors, and staff in healthcare facilities throughout the United States and the rest of the world.

The Chain of Infection

The infectious disease process is a complex interrelationship between source (agent), host, and environment. This process must be understood to develop strategies for prevention and control, and to recognize the key role of Central Service Technicians in the delivery of safe healthcare.

Infection control experts often illustrate the infectious disease process with the "Chain of Infection"[2] (see **Figure 4.14**). Consider a chain with six links, each of which is necessary and must be intact (unbroken) for an infectious disease to be spread. If only one link in the chain of infection is removed or broken, the spread of an infectious

disease cannot occur. The six links in the chain of infection are:

- Causative agent.
- Reservoir of the agent.
- Portal of exit of the agent from the reservoir.
- Mode of transmission of the agent.
- Portal of entry into the host.
- Susceptible host.

Let's examine each of these links, and identify methods used to break or interrupt the chain of infection.

The **causative agent** or pathogenic microorganism is the first link in the chain of infection. Infections are caused by a variety of microorganisms including bacteria, fungi, viruses, protozoa, and parasites. Characteristics that make these organisms capable of causing disease include:

- Invasiveness – The ability of an organism to invade the host and cause damage.

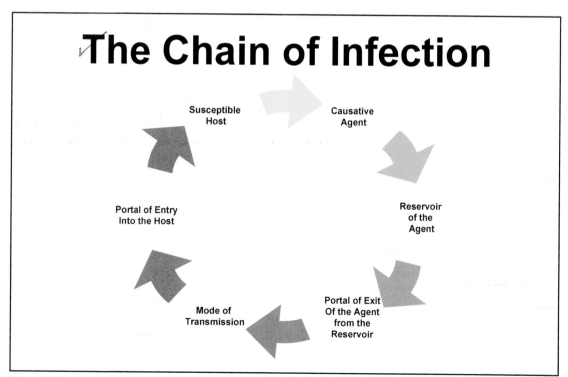

The Chain of Infection

Susceptible Host

Causative Agent

Portal of Entry Into the Host

Reservoir of the Agent

Mode of Transmission

Portal of Exit Of the Agent from the Reservoir

Figure 4.14

- Pathogenicity – The ability of an organism to gain entry into the host and cause disease.

- Virulence – The degree of pathogenicity.

- Infectious dose – The quantity of organisms required to cause disease.

- Viability in a free state – The ability of the organism to survive outside the host.

- Ability to develop resistance to antimicrobial agents – The ability of the microorganism to change itself to resist destruction by antibiotics. This occurs by mutation and through exchange of genetic material with other microorganisms.

Eliminating the infectious agent will interrupt the transmission of an infectious disease. Ways to do so include rapid identification by culture and prompt treatment of the infection, use of techniques to avoid cross contamination, the physical removal of contaminated substances (cleaning), and the use of effective disinfection and sterilization procedures.

The **reservoir of the agent** is a place in which an infectious agent can survive (although it may or may not be able to multiply or "divide"). The most common reservoirs are humans, animals, and the environment including fomites (inanimate objects such as patient care equipment, endoscopes, and hospital linen). The reservoirs most often associated with healthcare-associated infections are patients, healthcare workers, healthcare equipment, and the environment. Human reservoirs can be patients or staff with active infections, and others who are **carriers** of infectious agents. (Carriers are individuals who harbor infectious agents, but who are not affected by them.) Persons with active infections but without obvious symptoms, and those who are carriers represent the greatest risk to other patients and healthcare workers because the presence of disease-producing organisms may go undetected.

Good personal hygiene and health habits, the use of appropriate housekeeping measures and the proper cleaning, decontamination, disinfection, and sterilization of hospital equipment can eliminate reservoirs.

The **portal of exit** is the path by which an infectious agent leaves the reservoir. Portals of exit associated with human and animal reservoirs include:

- Respiratory tract – Through coughing and sneezing.

- Genitourinary tract – Though urine, vaginal secretions or semen.

- Gastrointestinal tract – Through vomit or stools.

- Skin/mucous membrane – Through mucous or wound drainage.

- Blood – Blood transfusions and contact with blood.

- Transplacental – Through the placenta from mother to baby.

The use of facial tissues, hand hygiene, wound dressings, control of secretions and excretions, trash and waste disposal, and the proper use of personal protective equipment can be effective ways to block the path of infections agents.

Mode of transmission describes the method of transfer of an infectious agent from the reservoir to a susceptible host. There are four major modes of transmission:

- Contact – Contact spread can be direct with immediate transmission of an agent from person-to-person. Example: the transfer of MRSA from one patient's wound drainage to another patient's mouth while performing mouth care with contact made by the hands of a care giver. It can also be indirect contact. Example: cross contamination from using contaminated patient care equipment when equipment used for one patient is not properly processed prior to its use with another patient. Droplet contact is also possible when a care giver's eyes, nose, or mouth comes in contact with large droplets that rapidly settle within three feet of a coughing or sneezing patient. An example occurs as a respiratory therapist develops the flu after an infected patient coughs in his/her face.

- Common vehicle – Active or direct transmission occurs when infectious agents are present in a vehicle such as food (salmonella), blood (HIV) or water (pseudomonas).

- Airborne – Infectious agents found in tiny droplets called droplet nuclei or dust that may remain suspended in the air for a long time, and travel great distances through a building's ventilation system.

- Vector-borne – (rarely occurs in hospitals in the United States. Agents can be carried on insects (for example, on the feet or wings of flies) or by the bites of insect or arthropods (mosquitoes, ticks and fleas).

Breaking this link in the chain of infection involves hand hygiene, cleaning and decontamination, disinfection and sterilization, proper food handling, water treatment, proper maintenance of heating and air conditioning systems with airflow control, isolation, and the use of Standard Precautions.

Portal of entry is the path used by an infectious agent to enter a susceptible host. Portals of entry associated with a human host include:

- Respiratory tract – Bypassing the normal airway defense mechanisms (for example, saliva in the mouth, the cough and gag reflex, and the cilia lining the respiratory tract) with an endotracheal tube.

- Genitourinary tract – Bypassing the flow of urine and normal secretions by the insertion of a foley catheter.

- Gastrointestinal tract – Eating and drinking contaminated food and water.

- Skin/mucous membrane – Through intentional (surgery) and accidental or traumatic breaks in the skin or mucous membranes. While intact skin is a barrier to bacteria, intact mucous membranes are not a barrier to many viruses.

- Transplacental – (from the mother to a fetus) Some infectious agents can pass from the mother through the placenta to the fetus, and cause infection in the fetus before birth.

- Parenteral – (percutaneous [via blood]) Bloodborne pathogens can pass through needle punctures in the skin.

Maintaining clean or sterile techniques when performing patient care procedures, and proper hand hygiene can alter the access of an infectious agent to a susceptible host. Other practices involve using only properly disinfected/sterilized equipment for invasive procedures, keeping devices off the floor, and safe handling and disposing of sharps.

The final link in the chain of infection, the **susceptible host**, is a person or animal that lacks the ability to resist infection by an infectious agent.

Causative agent (chain of infection) – *The microorganism that causes an infectious disease.*

Reservoir of agent (chain of infection) – *The place where an infectious agent (microorganism) can survive.*

Carrier – *An individual who harbors and disseminates specific pathogenic microorganisms without manifesting any clinical symptoms, and who serves as an intermediary in the transfer of diseases to a susceptible person.*

Portal of exit (chain of infection) – *The path by which an infectious agent leaves the reservoir.*

Mode of transmission – *(chain of infection) The method of transfer of an infectious agent from the reservoir to a susceptible host.*

Portal of entry (chain of infection) – *The path used by an infectious agent to enter a susceptible host.*

Susceptible host (chain of infection) – *A person or animal that lacks the ability to resist infection by an infectious agent.*

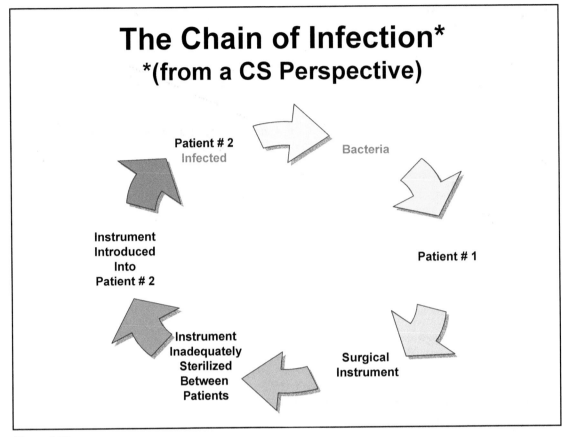

The Chain of Infection*
*(from a CS Perspective)

Bacteria

Patient # 2
Infected

Patient # 1

**Instrument
Introduced
Into
Patient # 2**

**Instrument
Inadequately
Sterilized
Between
Patients**

**Surgical
Instrument**

Figure 4.15

Several characteristics affect the susceptibility of a host to and the severity of a disease including:

- Age – The very young or elderly are more susceptible.

- Disease history/underlying disease – For example, cancer, diabetes and heart disease.

- Nutritional status – Inadequate nutrition.

- Compromised immune status – This includes patients undergoing chemotherapy or radiation therapy, those taking steroids, and patients with other infectious diseases such as HIV.

- Trauma – The injury itself and the measures used to treat the injury increase the risk of infection.

Measures used to alter host susceptibility include treatment of the primary disease (for example, keeping blood sugars under control in diabetics), administering vaccines (such as pneumonia and influenza vaccines), and recognizing that patients are at high risk for infection (and, therefore, providing antibiotics during surgery).

There are many opportunities for Central Service Technicians to interrupt the chain of infection, and to play an active and important role in preventing and controlling infectious diseases. **Figure 4.15** provides an example of how the Chain of Infection can be impacted by the Central Service Department.

CONTROL AND DESTRUCTION OF MICROORGANISMS

Learning Objective 7. Review basic procedures to control and kill microorganisms.

The primary purpose of the Central Service department is to control the spread of microorganisms. Infection prevention is a key component of patient safety. Many patients in healthcare facilities have compromised immune systems due to their age (newborn, extremely young, or elderly persons), or because of other disease factors or medical treatments. Patients that are otherwise healthy and strong can have their immune systems compromised by invasive or minimally invasive procedures that introduce supplies, implants, and instruments into their bodies.

Instruments and supplies enter a patient's body during invasive or minimally invasive procedures. The risk of infection is increased because many equipment, utensil, and instrument items used in patient care and treatment are reprocessable: they are used on one patient, reprocessed, and then used on another patient.

Central Service personnel must ensure that microorganisms from one patient are not transferred to the next patient. In Chapter 6, Infection Control and Prevention, we will address specific techniques that can be used to prevent the transmission of microorganisms.

Just as microorganisms differ in their needs for growth and reproduction, they also die at different rates. Some are more difficult to kill than others, and that is one reason why disinfection and sterilization processes are so complex. The vast array of items that must be processed is another reason why no single disinfection or sterilization process can kill all microorganisms. The cleaning, disinfection and high- and low-temperature sterilization chapters in this book will describe the tools and tactics needed to effectively control and kill bacteria.

The management of microorganisms and the prevention of infection is the primary purpose for the Central Service Department. Patients depend on the protection that Central Service provides. Whether Central Service Technicians are transporting items, processing items in the Decontamination area, assembling and packaging items for sterilization, performing sterile processing duties, or maintaining the sterility of items after sterilization, the knowledge and skills that they use to control the spread of microorganisms is critical to patient safety.

ENDNOTES

1. *Centers for Disease Control. National Center for Infectious Diseases. Hepatitis Home Page: www.<cdc.gov/hepatitis/*

2. *APIC Text of Infection Control and Epidemiology. Association for Professionals in Infection Control and Epidemiology. Washington, D.C. 2000.*

REFERENCES

Heritage, J; Evans, E; and Killington, R. Microbiology in Action. Cambridge University Press.

Ricciuti, E. Microorganisms: The Unseen World. Blackbirch Press, Inc. 1994.

Bender, L. Atoms and Cells. Gloucester Press. 1990.

Needham, C; Hoagland, M; McPherson, K; and Dodson, B. Intimate Strangers: Unseen Life on Earth. ASM Press (American Society for Microbiology). 2000.

Huys, J. Sterilization of Medical Supplies by Steam. Vier–Turme GmbH Benedict Press, Munsterschwartzach, Germany, 2004.

Tierno, P. The Secret Life of Germs. Pocket Books, New York, NY, 2001.

WEBSITES

Association of Practitioners in Infection Control: www.apic.org
U.S. Centers for Disease Control Center: www.cdc.gov
www.cellsalive.com

CENTRAL SERVICE TERMS

Microbiology

Contamination

Micron

Protoplasm

Cytoplasm

Nucleus

Phagotization

DNA

Spore

Chlorophyll

Aerobic bacteria

Anaerobic

Psychrophiles (bacteria)

Mesophilics (bacteria)

Thermophiles (bacteria)

Vegetative

Angstrom

Binary fission

Methicillin-Resistant Staphylococcus Aureus (MRSA)

Vancomycin-Resistant Enterococcus (VRE)

Viruses

Host

Protozoan

Granules (protozoa)

Vacuoles (protozoa)

Amoeboid movement

Causative agent (chain of infection)

Reservoir of agent (chain of infection)

Carriers

Portal of exit (chain of infection)

Mode of transmission

Portal of entry (chain of infection)

Susceptible host (chain of infection)

Chapter 5

Regulations and Standards

Chapter Learning Objectives

As a result of successfully completing this chapter, readers will be able to:

1. Tell the difference between regulations and voluntary and regulatory standards.

2. Provide basic information about the U.S. Food and Drug Administration (FDA), and review its regulations applicable to:
   - Medical device classification
   - Pre- and post-market requirements
   - Medical device reporting requirements
   - Medical device recalls
   - FDA labeling document
   - Re-use of single-use medical devices

3. Explain the roles and responsibilities of other federal governmental agencies that impact Central Service, and discuss important aspects of the regulations and standards they administer:
   - Centers for Disease Control (CDC)
   - Department of Transportation (DOT)
   - Environmental Protection Agency (EPA)
   - Occupational Safety and Health Administration (OSHA)

4. Discuss the assistance provided by professional associations that develop regulations and standards affecting Central Service:
   - Association for the Advancement of Medical Instrumentation (AAMI)
   - American National Standards Institute (ANSI)
   - Association of Operating Room Nurses (AORN)

- Association for Professionals in Infection Control and Epidemiology (APIC)
- International Standards Organization (ISO)
- The Joint Commission
- National Fire Protection Association (NFPA)
- United States Pharmacopoeia – National Formulary (USP-NF)
- World Health Organization (WHO)
- Society of Gastroenterology Nurses and Associates (SGNA)

REGULATIONS AND STANDARDS

Learning Objective 1. Tell the difference between regulations and voluntary and regulatory standards.

Regulations and **standards** impact all of us in our daily lives. They establish minimum levels of quality, safety, reliability, efficiency, and interchangeability for the products and services we want and need. As well, these safeguards make it possible for us to have access to those products at the most economical cost. Typically, we take standards and regulations for granted. It is only when they are not followed, and the resulting products and services are of poor quality, unreliable, dangerous, or non-economical, that we realize their necessity.

Regulation – A mandatory law or rule that is issued by a governing body.

Standard – A uniform method of defining basic parameters for processes, products, services, and measurements.

Standards (regulatory) – A comparison benchmark that is mandated by a governing agency and, if not complied with, may cause a facility to be in violation and liable for legal penalty.

Standards (voluntary) – A comparison benchmark that is strongly recommended by a governing agency or professional organization that provides recommendations and guidelines to provide better patient care.

Statute – A written and enforceable law enacted by a governing body.

Health care regulations and standards provide guidelines to assist health care professionals, including those in Central Service, in providing optimal patient care while protecting themselves, others, and the environment. They provide information to help assure consistency in departmental activities by outlining minimal performance expectancies and requirements for quality monitoring.

Standards may be **regulatory** or **voluntary.** Regulatory standards are those that provide requirements imposed by governmental agencies that can yield legal penalties if they are not followed. Voluntary standards are strongly suggested for better patient care, but not mandated with legal consequences for non-compliance. Voluntary standards may be incorporated into federal, state or local **statutes,** and they may be considered by courts of law. Central Service personnel are affected, directly or indirectly, by the regulations and standards developed by many federal, state, and local governmental agencies and by professional organizations. They must be familiar with applicable regulations and standards for several reasons:

- Compliance with regulations is mandatory, and failure to comply may lead to serious legal consequences for the health care facility.

- Many regulations and voluntary guidelines focus on ensuring workplace safety. Knowledge about required and recommended practices will help Central Service Technicians to protect themselves and others from exposure to infectious agents, toxic substances, and accidents.

- Awareness of regulations and standards applicable to disinfection and sterilization agents and to medical devices and equipment is helpful in the pre-purchase evaluation of products and in the effective on-going use of these products.

- The professional growth and advancement of Central Service personnel is enhanced as they gain knowledge about regulatory requirements and the "state of the art" in professional practices.

- The goal of patient welfare is best-served by careful compliance with regulations, and by adherence to widely accepted consensus guidelines (standards) for infection control and sterility assurance.

Regulations and regulatory and voluntary standards are issued by federal, state, and local governing agencies. However, voluntary standards are also issued by professional organizations. They provide significant assistance to health care personnel because they are developed by many experts whose combined knowledge and experience across numerous disciplines yield better judgments than that of a single person in one health care facility.

Professional Central Service Technicians and their managers have no interest in "doing the least they can" to avoid legal issues. Instead, they are concerned about "doing the most they can" to help protect their patients, themselves, and others. To do so, they willingly comply with regulations and standards developed by governmental agencies and private organizations.

The remainder of this chapter will provide basic information about important regulations and standards that should be understood and followed by all Central Service Technicians.

U.S. FOOD AND DRUG ADMINISTRATION

Learning Objective 2. Provide basic information about the U.S. Food and Drug Administration (FDA) and review its regulations applicable to:
- Medical device classification
- Pre- and post-market requirements
- Medical device reporting requirements
- Medical device recalls
- FDA labeling document
- Re-use of single-use medical devices

The FDA is the federal agency responsible for ensuring that foods, cosmetics, human and veterinary drugs, biological products, medical devices, and electronic products that emit radiation are safe and effective for the public's use. Its staff members also ensure that these products are honestly represented to the public. The FDA functions within the Public Health Service of the U.S. Department of Health and Human Services. The FDA regulates the manufacture of all medical devices, and requires the pre-market clearance of new medical devices. It also regulates the sterilants and high level disinfectants used to process critical and semi-critical devices. Rigorous testing with a broad range of microorganisms is required prior to marketing these chemicals.

Medical Device Classification

The level of regulation placed on any device depends upon how the FDA has classified that device:

- **Class I Devices** – These include low risk devices such as most hand-held surgical instruments and ultrasonic cleaners. These items are subject to "general controls" which include registration and device listing, medical device reporting, and quality system regulation and labeling. Most Class I devices are exempt from a pre-market notification approval (510k). Note: 510(k) submission requirements are discussed in the next section of this chapter.

- **Class II Devices** – These are devices considered to pose potential risks great enough to warrant a higher level of regulation. Class II devices include most types of sterilization equipment, and biological and chemical indicators. Manufacturers are required to submit a pre-market notification application (510k) before they can sell these products. Class II devices are usually subject to performance standards, post-market surveillance studies, and specific guidelines or special labeling.

- **Class III Devices** – These are the most stringently regulated devices, and include heart valves, pacemakers, and other life-sustaining devices. Manufacturers of new Class III devices must obtain a pre-market approval (PMA) from the FDA to demonstrate the safety and effectiveness of these products.

Pre- and Post-Market Requirements

Unless a device is listed as exempt from regulation, a 510(k) submission is required for Class I and II devices. Class III devices may require either a 510(k) or a PMA. A 510(k) application is a comprehensive package of information designed to demonstrate that the new product is "substantially equivalent" to one or more medical devices already being marketed. By contrast, a PMA is required for most Class III devices which are new to the health care market. A PMA is more complicated to complete because it must prove the device has a reasonable assurance of safety and effectiveness for its intended use based on valid scientific evidence. Sometimes submission of clinical data is also necessary to prove safety and effectiveness. The FDA requires a satisfactory inspection of a health care facility before the PMA application can be approved.

Post-market device requirements that apply to third party and hospital reprocessors include FDA mandates applicable to:

- Registration and listing.

- Medical device reporting, tracking, corrections, and removals.

- Quality system regulation.

- Labeling.

Personnel from the hospital's Risk Management Department should be involved in the completion of these packets of information if the CS Department is submitting a PMA applicable to reprocessing single-use devices.[1]

Medical Device Reporting Requirements

The Safe Medical Devices Act of 1990 requires health care facilities to become subject to user reporting requirements. Before the passage of this Act, medical device manufacturers were required to notify the FDA whenever they learned of a patient death or serious injury that may have been caused by or was attributed to their devices, and whenever they learned of a device malfunction that, if it recurred, could cause a death or serious injury.

Beginning in 2000, Medical Device Reporting regulations require user facilities (hospitals, ambulatory surgical facilities, nursing homes, and outpatient treatment facilities) to report suspect medical device-related deaths to the FDA and the manufacturers within 10 work days. User facilities must report medical device-related serious injuries only to the manufacturer within 10 work days. If the manufacturer is unknown, the injury should be reported to the FDA.

A serious injury is defined as an injury or illness that is life-threatening; resulting in permanent impairment of a body function or permanent damage to body structure; or necessitates medical or surgical intervention to preclude permanent impairment of a body structure. An annual report of deaths and serious injuries must also be submitted to the FDA on January 1st of each year.

Since direct patient care givers are more likely to be directly affected by this law, it is conceivable that certain sterilization failures may have to be reported if they can be linked to patient illness. As this occurs, the Central Service department will be affected.

FDA's *MedWatch Program* is designed for the voluntary reporting of device related problems. It provides a vehicle by which health care professionals can notify the FDA about medical device malfunctions, labeling inadequacies, and other problems including those involving other products regulated by the FDA including drugs and biologicals.[2]

In recent years, the FDA has used both voluntary and mandatory reporting programs to collect information about specific potential problems. **Figures 5.1** and **5.2** show the FDA forms that are used for, respectively, voluntary and mandatory reports.

MedWatch Program – *A safety information and adverse event reporting system that serves healthcare professionals and the public by reporting serious problems suspected to be associated with the drugs and medical devices they prescribe, dispense, or use.*

Figure 5.1 FDA MedWatch Voluntary Reporting Form

U.S. Department of Health and Human Services

MEDWATCH

The FDA Safety Information and
Adverse Event Reporting Program

For VOLUNTARY reporting of
adverse events, product problems and
product use errors

Page ____ of ____

Form Approved: OMB No. 0910-0291, Expires: 10/31/08
See OMB statement on reverse.

FDA USE ONLY

Triage unit
sequence #

PLEASE TYPE OR USE BLACK INK

A. PATIENT INFORMATION

1. Patient Identifier	2. Age at Time of Event, or Date of Birth:	3. Sex	4. Weight
In confidence		☐ Female ☐ Male	_____ lb or _____ kg

B. ADVERSE EVENT, PRODUCT PROBLEM OR ERROR

Check all that apply:

1. ☐ Adverse Event ☐ Product Problem *(e.g., defects/malfunctions)*
☐ Product Use Error ☐ Problem with Different Manufacturer of Same Medicine

2. Outcomes Attributed to Adverse Event
(Check all that apply)

☐ Death: _____ *(mm/dd/yyyy)*
☐ Life-threatening
☐ Hospitalization - initial or prolonged
☐ Required Intervention to Prevent Permanent Impairment/Damage (Devices)

☐ Disability or Permanent Damage
☐ Congenital Anomaly/Birth Defect
☐ Other Serious (Important Medical Events)

3. Date of Event *(mm/dd/yyyy)*	4. Date of this Report *(mm/dd/yyyy)*

5. Describe Event, Problem or Product Use Error

6. Relevant Tests/Laboratory Data, Including Dates

7. Other Relevant History, Including Preexisting Medical Conditions *(e.g., allergies, race, pregnancy, smoking and alcohol use, liver/kidney problems, etc.)*

C. PRODUCT AVAILABILITY

Product Available for Evaluation? *(Do not send product to FDA)*

☐ Yes ☐ No ☐ Returned to Manufacturer on: _____ *(mm/dd/yyyy)*

D. SUSPECT PRODUCT(S)

1. Name, Strength, Manufacturer *(from product label)*
#1
#2

2. Dose or Amount	Frequency	Route
#1		
#2		

3. Dates of Use *(if unknown, give duration) from/to (or best estimate)*	5. Event Abated After Use Stopped or Dose Reduced?
#1	#1 ☐ Yes ☐ No ☐ Doesn't Apply
#2	#2 ☐ Yes ☐ No ☐ Doesn't Apply

4. Diagnosis or Reason for Use *(Indication)*
#1
#2

8. Event Reappeared After Reintroduction?
#1 ☐ Yes ☐ No ☐ Doesn't Apply
#2 ☐ Yes ☐ No ☐ Doesn't Apply

6. Lot #	7. Expiration Date
#1	#1
#2	#2

9. NDC # or Unique ID

E. SUSPECT MEDICAL DEVICE

1. Brand Name

2. Common Device Name

3. Manufacturer Name, City and State

4. Model #	Lot #	5. Operator of Device
Catalog #	Expiration Date *(mm/dd/yyyy)*	☐ Health Professional ☐ Lay User/Patient
Serial #	Other #	☐ Other:

6. If Implanted, Give Date *(mm/dd/yyyy)*	7. If Explanted, Give Date *(mm/dd/yyyy)*

8. Is this a Single-use Device that was Reprocessed and Reused on a Patient?
☐ Yes ☐ No

9. If Yes to Item No. 8, Enter Name and Address of Reprocessor

F. OTHER (CONCOMITANT) MEDICAL PRODUCTS

Product names and therapy dates *(exclude treatment of event)*

G. REPORTER *(See confidentiality section on back)*

1. Name and Address

Phone #	E-mail

2. Health Professional?	3. Occupation	4. Also Reported to:
☐ Yes ☐ No		☐ Manufacturer

5. If you do NOT want your identity disclosed to the manufacturer, place an "X" in this box: ☐

☐ User Facility
☐ Distributor/Importer

FORM FDA 3500 (10/05) Submission of a report does not constitute an admission that medical personnel or the product caused or contributed to the event.

Figure 5.1 FDA MedWatch Voluntary Reporting Form (continued)

ADVICE ABOUT VOLUNTARY REPORTING

Detailed instructions available at: http://www.fda.gov/medwatch/report/consumer/instruct.htm

Report adverse events, product problems or product use errors with:

- Medications *(drugs or biologics)*
- Medical devices *(including in-vitro diagnostics)*
- Combination products *(medication & medical devices)*
- Human cells, tissues, and cellular and tissue-based products
- Special nutritional products *(dietary supplements, medical foods, infant formulas)*
- Cosmetics

Report product problems - quality, performance or safety concerns such as:

- Suspected counterfeit product
- Suspected contamination
- Questionable stability
- Defective components
- Poor packaging or labeling
- Therapeutic failures (product didn't work)

-Fold Here-

Report SERIOUS adverse events. An event is serious when the patient outcome is:

- Death
- Life-threatening
- Hospitalization - initial or prolonged
- Disability or permanent damage
- Congenital anomaly/birth defect
- Required intervention to prevent permanent impairment or damage
- Other serious (important medical events)

Report even if:

- You're not certain the product caused the event
- You don't have all the details

How to report:

- Just fill in the sections that apply to your report
- Use section D for all products except medical devices
- Attach additional pages if needed
- Use a separate form for each patient
- Report either to FDA or the manufacturer *(or both)*

Other methods of reporting:

- 1-800-FDA-0178 -- To FAX report
- 1-800-FDA-1088 -- To report by phone
- www.fda.gov/medwatch/report.htm -- To report online

If your report involves a serious adverse event with a device and it occurred in a facility outside a doctor's office, that facility may be legally required to report to FDA and/or the manufacturer. Please notify the person in that facility who would handle such reporting.

-Fold Here-

If your report involves a serious adverse event with a vaccine call 1-800-822-7967 to report.

Confidentiality: The patient's identity is held in strict confidence by FDA and protected to the fullest extent of the law. FDA will not disclose the reporter's identity in response to a request from the public, pursuant to the Freedom of Information Act. The reporter's identity, including the identity of a self-reporter, may be shared with the manufacturer unless requested otherwise.

The public reporting burden for this collection of information has been estimated to average 36 minutes per response, including the time for reviewing instructions, searching existing data sources, gathering and maintaining the data needed, and completing and reviewing the collection of information. Send comments regarding this burden estimate or any other aspect of this collection of information, including suggestions for reducing this burden to:

Department of Health and Human Services *Food and Drug Administration - MedWatch* *10903 New Hampshire Avenue* *Building 22, Mail Stop 4447* *Silver Spring, MD 20993-0002*	*Please DO NOT* *RETURN this form* *to this address.*	*OMB statement:* *"An agency may not conduct or sponsor, and a person is not required to respond to, a collection of information unless it displays a currently valid OMB control number."*

U.S. DEPARTMENT OF HEALTH AND HUMAN SERVICES
Food and Drug Administration

FORM FDA 3500 (10/05) (Back) Please Use Address Provided Below -- Fold in Thirds, Tape and Mail

---

DEPARTMENT OF HEALTH & HUMAN SERVICES

Public Health Service
Food and Drug Administration
Rockville, MD 20857

Official Business
Penalty for Private Use $300

NO POSTAGE
NECESSARY
IF MAILED
IN THE
UNITED STATES
OR APO/FPO

BUSINESS REPLY MAIL

FIRST CLASS MAIL   PERMIT NO. 946   ROCKVILLE MD

MEDWATCH
The FDA Safety Information and Adverse Event Reporting Program
Food and Drug Administration
5600 Fishers Lane
Rockville, MD 20852-9787

Figure 5.2 FDA MedWatch Mandatory Reporting Form

Form Approved: OMB No. 0910-0291, Expires: 10/31/08
See OMB statement on reverse

U.S. Department of Health and Human Services
Food and Drug Administration

For use by user-facilities,
importers, distributors and manufacturers
for MANDATORY reporting

MEDWATCH

FORM FDA 3500A (10/05)

Mtr Report #

UF/Importer Report #

Page ____ of ____

FDA Use Only

A. PATIENT INFORMATION

1. Patient Identifier	2. Age at Time of Event:	3. Sex	4. Weight
	or ————	☐ Female	___ lbs
In confidence	Date of Birth:	☐ Male	or ___ kgs

B. ADVERSE EVENT OR PRODUCT PROBLEM

1. ☐ Adverse Event   and/or   ☐ Product Problem (e.g., defects/malfunctions)

2. Outcomes Attributed to Adverse Event
(Check all that apply)
- ☐ Death: _____ (mm/dd/yyyy)
- ☐ Life-threatening
- ☐ Hospitalization - initial or prolonged
- ☐ Required Intervention to Prevent Permanent Impairment/Damage (Devices)
- ☐ Disability or Permanent Damage
- ☐ Congenital Anomaly/Birth Defect
- ☐ Other Serious (Important Medical Events)

3. Date of Event (mm/dd/yyyy)

4. Date of This Report (mm/dd/yyyy)

5. Describe Event or Problem

6. Relevant Tests/Laboratory Data, Including Dates

7. Other Relevant History, Including Preexisting Medical Conditions (e.g., allergies, race, pregnancy, smoking and alcohol use, hepatic/renal dysfunction, etc.)

PLEASE TYPE OR USE BLACK INK

C. SUSPECT PRODUCT(S)

1. Name (Give labeled strength & mfr/labeler)
#1
#2

2. Dose, Frequency & Route Used	3. Therapy Dates (If unknown, give duration) from/to (or best estimate)
#1	#1
#2	#2

4. Diagnosis for Use (Indication)
#1
#2

5. Event Abated After Use Stopped or Dose Reduced?
#1 ☐ Yes ☐ No ☐ Doesn't Apply
#2 ☐ Yes ☐ No ☐ Doesn't Apply

6. Lot #	7. Exp. Date
#1	#1
#2	#2

8. Event Reappeared After Reintroduction?
#1 ☐ Yes ☐ No ☐ Doesn't Apply
#2 ☐ Yes ☐ No ☐ Doesn't Apply

9. NDC# or Unique ID

10. Concomitant Medical Products and Therapy Dates (Exclude treatment of event)

D. SUSPECT MEDICAL DEVICE

1. Brand Name

2. Common Device Name

3. Manufacturer Name, City and State

4. Model #	Lot #	5. Operator of Device
Catalog #	Expiration Date (mm/dd/yyyy)	☐ Health Professional ☐ Lay User/Patient
Serial #	Other #	☐ Other:

6. If Implanted, Give Date (mm/dd/yyyy)	7. If Explanted, Give Date (mm/dd/yyyy)

8. Is this a Single-use Device that was Reprocessed and Reused on a Patient?
☐ Yes   ☐ No

9. If Yes to Item No. 8, Enter Name and Address of Reprocessor

10. Device Available for Evaluation? (Do not send to FDA)
☐ Yes   ☐ No   ☐ Returned to Manufacturer on: _____ (mm/dd/yyyy)

11. Concomitant Medical Products and Therapy Dates (Exclude treatment of event)

E. INITIAL REPORTER

1. Name and Address	Phone #

2. Health Professional?	3. Occupation	4. Initial Reporter Also Sent Report to FDA
☐ Yes ☐ No		☐ Yes ☐ No ☐ Unk

Submission of a report does not constitute an admission that medical personnel, user facility, importer, distributor, manufacturer or product caused or contributed to the event.

Figure 5.2 FDA MedWatch Mandatory Reporting Form (continued)

Medical Device Recalls

A recall is an action taken to address a problem with a medical device that violates FDA regulations. This action can be enforced when a device is defective, and/or poses a risk to health. Recalls can be instituted voluntarily by the manufacturer, distributor, or another interested party, or they can be mandated by the FDA. A recall does not always mean the affected product can no longer be used. Instead, it could mean that the product must only need to be checked or repaired. For example, if an implant such as a pacemaker is recalled, it may not have to be removed; however, the risks of the removal decision should be discussed with the patient. The FDA monitors all mandated recalls to ensure the actions taken by manufacturer are adequate to protect the public health.

There are three categories of FDA recalls.

- **Class I: High Risk** – There is a reasonable chance the product will cause serious health problems or death. The manufacturer must notify customers, and direct them to notify the product recipients. The notification must include the name of the device being recalled, the lot or serial numbers, the reason for recall, and instructions to correct, avoid, or minimize the problem. The company must also issue a press release to notify the public. In addition, the FDA may also issue its own press release or public health notice, and FDA posts applicable information on its Medical Device Recalls web site.

- **Class II: Less Serious Risk** – There is a possibility that the product will cause a temporary or reversible heath problem, or there is a remote chance that the device will cause serious health problems. The manufacturer must notify customers and, sometimes, asks them to inform the product's recipients. Generally neither the FDA nor the manufacturer issues a press release .

- **Class III: Low Risk** – There is little chance that using or being exposed to the product will cause health problems. However, because the product violates FDA law, there is a need to take an action to address the

problem. The manufacturer must notify customers, and neither the FDA nor the manufacturer will issue a press release.

Medical Device Recalls

Product recalls in 2006 included the following items:

- Automated external defibrillators
- Teething Rings
- Volumetric infusion pumps
- Vascular grafts
- Coronary Stents

To learn about recently-recalled items including the manufacturer and the product status, check out the FDA website: www.fda.gov. When you reach the site, type "medical device recalls data base" into the site's search box. When you reach the data base, click on "search" to review all products.

FDA Labeling Document

The FDA has expressed concern about the potential for the transmission of infectious diseases caused by improper reprocessing of medical devices. In April, 1996, it released a document, "Re-labeling Reusable Medical Devices for Reprocessing in Health Care Facilities," to provide guidance for FDA reviewers who evaluate pre-market approval applications for medical devices.[3]

This document requires manufacturers to comply with seven new criteria, mostly involving reprocessing instructions, when they submit medical device applications to the FDA for evaluation. It clearly places the responsibility for safe and effective reprocessing of medical devices with both the manufacturer and the users.

The manufacturer is responsible for:

- Supporting the claim of reuse with adequate labeling; the labeling must provide sufficient instructions about how to prepare the device for the next patient.

- The documentation of tests which show that the instructions are adequate, and can be reasonably executed by the users.

The users are responsible for:

- Confirming that they have the facilities and equipment to execute the instructions.

- Ensuring that the instructions are followed.

This is a major step toward providing health care professionals with manufacturers' reprocessing recommendations, which are necessary resources that have often been difficult to obtain. These recommendations are also useful for users as they select equipment needed to successfully reprocess the devices used in their facility. Due to industry demand, the FDA is considering re-addressing the Labeling Document to improve the quality of information given from the manufacturer to the user.

Re-Use of Single-Use Medical Devices

Reprocessing a medical device labeled for single use dates back to the 1970s when it was common practice to reuse **hemodialyzers**. (The major difference in that practice and what is being done today is that the reprocessed hemodialyzers were re-used on the same patient.) Even in those early days, the FDA was involved in the re-use issue. For example, in 1979, it responded to the increased reprocessing of devices labeled for single use by issuing a Compliance Policy Guide that was re-issued in 1980 and 1981, and then revised in 1987. The principles of this Compliance Policy Guide are reflected in FDA's current enforcement document. It concluded that any institution or practitioner who re-uses a single-use device (SUD) should be able to demonstrate that (a) the item can be adequately cleaned and sterilized, (b) the quality of the device will not be adversely affected, and (c) the device will remain safe and effective for its intended use.

In the 1980s, health care facilities began to feel the full impact of managed care, decreased insurance reimbursements, and non-reimbursed patient care. The practice of re-using disposable medical devices increased, as did the FDA's concern for public health and safety. There were estimates that almost 50% of hospitals were reprocessing SUDs, but specific data was not readily available. It was difficult to trace an infection to a reprocessed SUD, and adverse events were thought to be under-reported.

In 1999, the FDA and the Association for the Advancement of Medical Instrumentation (AAMI) co-sponsored a conference of health care professionals, device manufacturers, third-party reprocessors, physicians, scientists, medical ethicists, government representatives, and interested parties to solicit viewpoints and gain assistance in developing a strategy to address the re-use issue. In the months that followed, other meetings were held to obtain further feedback, and draft documents were released for public review and comment.

FDA Enforcement Requirements for Hospitals Reprocessing Single-Use Devices

In August, 2000, the FDA released its final guidance document, Enforcement Priorities for Single-Use Devices Reprocessed by Third Parties and Hospitals, which included a timetable for compliance.[4] Barring future exceptions, as of August, 2002, the phase-in period had ended, and all hospitals and third-party reprocessors who reprocessed SUDs were required to be in compliance with the pre-market and post-market requirements outlined in the enforcement document. The enforcement document does not currently apply to permanent pacemakers, hemodialyzers, health care facilities that are not hospitals, and unopened but unused SUDs.

Hospital Re-use Options

Ideally, a multi-disciplinary hospital committee should make the decision about reprocessing

Hemodialyzers – Equipment used to remove impurities and waste products from blood before returning it to the patient's body.

devices labeled for single-use. Input from legal/administrative, infection control, central service/sterile processing, surgical services, risk management, finance, and materiel management personnel is necessary to evaluate the legal, ethical, and economic issues involved. Each member of the committee must be educated in the new FDA regulatory requirements for hospitals reprocessing SUDs. **Figure 5.3** gives an overview of the steps needed to consider single-use items for re-use. It should be understood that receiving an FDA 510(k) to reprocess SUDs subjects the health care facility to stringent FDA regulations and on-site surveys.

Faced with the new FDA regulatory requirements, hospital administrators may consider outsourcing their SUD reprocessing to a third party-reprocessor. While outsourcing does relieve the hospital of the burden of the actual work, it does not relieve the facility of legal and ethical responsibilities applicable to the reprocessing of SUDs. It is obviously necessary to provide safe and effective medical devices regardless of who does the processing or where the processing takes place.

Third-Party Reprocessors

The hospital's reuse committee should decide what SUDs will be reprocessed, and how many times the device will be reprocessed before disposal. Committee members should also evaluate the level of liability insurance needed to be carried, and they should select the third-party reprocessing company after, among numerous other tasks, a selection sub-committee visits the company's facilities.

The FDA suggests that potential third-party reprocessors answer the following questions:

- When did FDA last inspect your facility? What were the results of that inspection? (Ask to see a copy.)

- Do you have documentation that demonstrates your company has been cleared/approved by the FDA to reprocess

SUDs? (Ask to see the documentation and copies of filed PMAs and 510[k]s.)

- How do you monitor manufacturing processes, and what records do you maintain to comply with FDA's Quality System Regulations? (Ask to see the records, and learn what you will be receiving with the returned SUD that confirms its sterility.)

- What aspects of your overall process (for example, cleaning, packaging, and sterilization) have been validated? (Ask to see proof of the validation.)

- Has your company set limits on the number of times a SUD can be reprocessed? If yes, how did you determine that number? What procedures do you have in place to ensure that a SUD is not reprocessed beyond the specified number of times? (Ask to see where this is taking place. Talk with the technician.) Note: this relates to the decision noted above about the number of times the device will be reprocessed.

FDA's web site for frequently-asked questions including those which address third-party reprocessors of single-use devices is: http://www.fda.gov/reuse/reuse-faq.shtml#1

The Association of Medical Device Reprocessors recommends asking if the sterilization system is commissioned and certified according to AAMI recommendations, and if the sterilization system is re-qualified annually and routinely calibrated. Also, determine if the residual sterilant level is routinely tested, and request the documentation.

Other suggested questions to ask potential third-party reprocessors include:

- Does the company have a tracking system and, if so, how does it work? (Some reprocessors track the device through the system; some can track a device to the actual patient's use. Ask to see policies and procedures related to the tracking process.)

Figure 5.3 Steps in Consideration of Single-Use Items for Reuse

Step 1: Preliminary Evaluation

- Is the single use item now being purchased at the lowest possible cost?
- Is there a belief that reuse of this item will save money?

Step 2: Evaluation of Reuse Alternatives

- Is a reusable device available?
- Are there scientific studies to support reuse of the single use device?

Step 3: Initial Cost Analysis

- Does an initial cost analysis suggest an acceptable savings over the continued use of the single use device?

Step 4: Risk Assessment

- Assess patient and employee safety if device is reused.
- Assess that risk is manageable.

Step 5: Consideration of Reprocessing Protocols

- Study feasibility of reuse including cleaning, reconditioning, inspection/testing, packaging and sterilization.

Step 6: Examine Facility Requirements

- Staff expertise.
- Equipment availability.
- Time necessary for reproducing single use items.

Step 7: Develop Procedures

- How will single use devices be reprocessed?
- Validate by testing each proposed reprocessing step in compliance with FDA requirements.

Step 8: Undertake Potential Cost Assessment

- Estimate current costs.
- Estimate costs of reprocessing single use items with procedures developed and validated in step seven.

Step 9: Obtain any Necessary Approval

- Comply with current FDA pre-market submission requirements.

Step 10: Conduct Clinical Study

- Assess results: What is the likelihood of adverse effects compared to single use of the item?

Step 11: Undertake Actual Cost Assessment

- Consider costs based upon clinical study.

Step 12: Implement Reprocessing of Single Use Items

- This step requires approval of the pre-market submissions (PMA or 510[k]) and compliance with post-market requirements.

- What is the estimated turnaround time for a device? Will this time be addressed in the contract?

- How many technicians are certified? (Ask to see the certificates.)

- Are the company's policy and procedure manuals and the quality manual available for review?

The more information acquired during on-site visits to potential third party reprocessors, the better equipped will the re-use committee be to make an effective third-party reprocessor selection decision.[5]

For more information about the FDA, go to: www.fda.gov

OTHER FEDERAL REGULATORY AGENCIES

Learning Objective 3. Explain the rules and responsibilities of other federal government agencies that impact Central Service, and discuss important aspects of the regulations and standards they administer:
- Centers for Disease Control (CDC)
- Department of Transportation (DOT)
- Environmental Protection Agency (EPA)
- Occupational Safety and Health Administration (OSHA)

Centers for Disease Control (CDC)

The CDC is an agency of the federal government agency that is organized within the Department

Prions –*Virus-like infectious agents that cause a variety of neurodegenerative diseases of humans and animals, including scrapie in sheep and goats, bovine spongiform encephalopathy (BSE) in cattle, and Creutzfeldt-Jakob disease (CJD) in humans. Prions are thought to differ from viruses by containing neither DNA nor RNA, only protein. They are extremely resistant to inactivation by heat and disinfecting agents.*

of Health and Human Services. It works to promote the health and quality of life by preventing and controlling disease, injury, and disability, and by responding to health emergencies. CDC personnel developed the first practical recommendations for isolation techniques, and guidelines for infection control are established based on this research data. Although CDC guidelines are not considered regulatory, other agencies rely heavily on them, and review health care facilities for compliance with them. Many CDC guidelines are incorporated into the policies and procedures of health care facilities including their protocols for instrument processing following exposure to **Prions** (http://www.cc.gov/ncidod/diseases/cjd/cjd.htm), and their Bioterrorist Readiness Plan (http://www.cdc.gov/mcodpd/hip/bio/13aprAPIC-CDC) developed in conjunction with the Association for Professionals in Infection Control and Epidemiology (APIC).

Note: this voluntary international professional association is discussed later in this chapter.

For more information about the CDC, go to; www.cdc.gov

Department of Transportation (DOT)

The DOT is a federal government agency dedicated to ensuring a fast, safe, and efficient transportation system. Laws relating to health care include those concerning the transportation of minimally-processed instrumentation for repair/labeling, and the transportation of hazardous and radioactive wastes. The DOT inspects and cites organizations for statute violations. Central Service Technicians who are responsible for transporting and/or storing hazardous wastes or shipping minimally-cleaned instrumentation should be aware of the DOT's requirements.

Note: state or local regulations may be more restrictive than federal regulations and, in all cases, regulations with the most stringent provisions apply.

For more information about the DOT, go to: www.dot.gov

Environmental Protection Agency (EPA)

Congress created the EPA as a regulatory agency in 1970 to create and enforce laws relating to cleaner water, air, and land. This federal agency is responsible for minimizing **greenhouse gases** and toxic emissions, for regulating the re-use of solid wastes, for controlling indoor air pollution, and for developing and enforcing pesticide regulations. The EPA administers two acts that are very important to the Central Service Technicians: The Federal Insecticide, Fungicide, and Rodenticide Act (FIFRA), and the 1990 Clean Air Act Amendments.

The Federal Insecticide, Fungicide, and Rodenticide Act regulates pesticide safety and effectiveness, and it impacts all anti-microbial products including disinfectants and sanitizers. Every disinfectant and sanitizer manufacturer must obtain an EPA registration number for every covered product. The manufacturer must submit data relating to labeling claims, effectiveness, and safety data to a division of EPA's Office of Pesticide Program. If the data is approved and accepted, a registration number is issued. All EPA- approved products must contain the following label information:

- Product ingredients.

- Directions for use.

- Product precautions and warnings.

- Directions for storage and disposal.

- The EPA registration number.

Central Service Technicians must always read and consistently follow the information provided on all chemical labels.

EPA also administers the 1990 Clean Air Act Amendments which created a regulatory program to protect the earth's ozone layer. In 1996, the

Greenhouse gases – *Any gas such as carbon dioxide (CO2,) methane (CH4), halogenated fluorocarbons (HCFCs), and ozone (O3) which contributes to potential climate change.*

production of chlorofluorocarbons (CFCs), an ozone-depleting chemical used in the 12/88 mixture of Ethylene Oxide sterilant, was phased out. The EPA approved an alternate mixture using hydrochloroflurocarbons (HCFCs).

The Clean Air Act Amendments also established National Emission Standards for Hazardous Air Pollutants (NESHAP). These regulations established emissions standards for industrial ethylene oxide (ETO) sterilization facilities. To date, there are no national emission standards for ETO sterilization within the health care industry; however several states have developed standards.

The Clean Air Act Amendments also include a regulation passed in 1997 that affects the use of medical waste incinerators. Since the cost of retrofitting existing incinerators is usually financially prohibitive, some hospitals are returning to reusable items such as basin sets and floor procedure trays to reduce waste. This in turn, creates an increased workload in these Central Service Departments.

For more information about the EPA, go to: www.epa.gov

Occupational Safety and Health Administration (OSHA)

Created in 1971, OSHA is organized within the U.S. Department of Labor. Its primary role and responsibility is to protect workers from occupationally-caused illnesses and injuries. Many of OSHA's regulations and standards are represented in laws passed by the U.S. Congress. The OSHA regulations of most direct relevance to Central Service personnel are those that pertain to the Occupational Exposure to Bloodborne Pathogens Standard, and guidelines for the use of Ethylene Oxide Sterilization.

The Occupational Exposure to Bloodborne Pathogens Standard is a comprehensive guideline which outlines employee safety in all areas of the facility as they relate to potential exposure from bloodborne pathogens. This guideline is addressed in the Infection Control Chapter.

The Guidelines for the use of Ethylene Oxide Sterilization addresses the safe use of ETO, and this guideline is addressed in the Low Temperature Sterilization Chapter.

The General Duty Clause of the Occupational Safety and Health Act requires that, "each employer furnish to each of his employees employment and a place of employment which are free from recognized hazards that are causing, or are likely to cause, death or serious physical harm to his employees."[6] This means that OSHA may intervene in a matter of worker protection even if there is no specific regulation that covers the situation.

OSHA personnel conduct announced and unannounced inspections of facilities. The need for inspections is based on complaints through the OSHA Whistle Blower Program, the rate of workplace accidents, high hazard targets, referrals, and follow-ups of previous visits. OSHA violations are rated as:

• Willful – A violation that the employer intentionally and knowingly commits. These carry fines and penalties of $5,000 to $70,000 per incident.

• Serious – A violation in which there is substantial probability that death or serious physical harm could result, and that the employer knew or should have known of the hazard. These carry penalties of up to $7,000.

• Repeat – A violation of any standard, regulation, or rule where, upon reinspection, a substantially similar violation is found. These penalties range up to $70,000.

• Failure to abate – Failure to correct a prior violation may result in penalties of up to $7,000 per day.

OSHA representatives may enter a facility for a specific reason; however, once inside the facility, they have the right and obligation to investigate any violation in any department they may find. Recent penalties and citations can be viewed by assessing the OSHA web site.

State Agencies May Regulate Healthcare Facilities

State agencies may also be involved in the regulation of healthcare facilities and the Central Service departments within them.

• Department of Health Services (DHS). Many states look to their DHS to establish local health safety standards that may mirror federal standards or be more stringent. A few states include DHS surveyors in the The Joint Commission survey process. DHS surveys do not need to be scheduled and, in fact, are often random and unannounced.

• Department of Transportation (DOT). Several states have their own regulations for transporting healthcare wastes from the facility to landfills or other final disposal sites. This state agency may affect Central Service Technicians working in the decontamination area.

• Environmental Protection Agency (EPA). Some States have EPA offices to more closely regulate issues which concern their jurisdiction. State regulations regarding biohazardous waste and drain discharge are important to Central Service Technicians. State EPA offices monitor chemicals poured into the main sewer lines, and there may be regulations against pouring blood and disinfectants into sink drains in Central Service decontamination areas.

• Occupational Safety and Health Administration (OSHA). Approximately twenty-six states have State OSHA offices. These offices typically follow the same penalty criteria as those at the federal level.

Standards and regulations of state agencies may be more restrictive than, but cannot be less restrictive than, those of their Federal counterparts. In other words, the requirements of the most restrictive agency always apply. Central Service Technicians must be aware of and consistently comply with applicable state and other localized standards and regulations.

For more information about OSHA, go to: www.osha.gov

PROFESSIONAL ASSOCIATIONS

Learning Objective 4. Discuss the assistance provided by professional associations that develop regulations and standards affecting Central Service:

- Association for the Advancement of Medical Instrumentation (AAMI)
- American National Standards Institute (ANSI)
- Association of Operating Room Nurses (AORN)
- Association for Professionals in Infection Control and Epidemiology (APIC)
- International Standards Organization (ISO)
- The Joint Commission
- National Fire Protection Association (NFPA)
- United States Pharmacopoeia – National Formulary (USP-UF)
- World Health Organization (WHO)
- Society of Gastroenterology Nurses and Associates (SGNA)

The above sections of this chapter have discussed the impact of regulations and voluntary standards developed by government agencies on the important work of Central Service Technicians. We now turn our attention to professional associations that develop and promote voluntary standards that provide a foundation for how "things are done" in Central Service operations.

Recommended Practices and Standards (AAMI) – *Voluntary guidelines representing a consensus of AAMI members that are intended for use by healthcare facilities to help ensure that medical instrumentation is safe for patient use.*

Standards (AAMI) – *Recommendations representing a consensus of AAMI members that provide guidance to device manufacturers that address design, performance, labeling, and other factors applicable to the instruments they manufacture.*

Association for the Advancement of Medical Instrumentation (AAMI)

Founded in 1967, AAMI is a voluntary consensus organization whose membership is comprised of over 6,000 individuals and 375 organizations. Committees of manufacturers, health care professionals, regulators, scientists, academics, and other interested parties research and develop new or revise existing **Recommended Practices and Standards** that address the use, care and processing of devices and systems. Committees also develop **Standards** for manufacturers which recommend the labeling, safety, and performance requirements to be met by the products they produce.

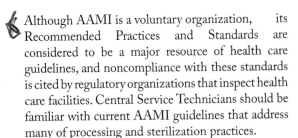
Although AAMI is a voluntary organization, its Recommended Practices and Standards are considered to be a major resource of health care guidelines, and noncompliance with these standards is cited by regulatory organizations that inspect health care facilities. Central Service Technicians should be familiar with current AAMI guidelines that address many of processing and sterilization practices.

For more information about AAMI, go to: www.aami.org

American National Standards Institute (ANSI)

Founded in 1918, ANSI's primary mission is to "enhance the global competitiveness of U.S. business and the American quality of life by promoting and facilitating voluntary consensus standards and ensuring their integrity." ANSI represents the interests of more than 125,000 companies and 3,500,000 individuals. ANSI does not develop American standards; however, it provides a neutral arena for interested parties to work toward agreement. ANSI's committee membership is similar to that of AAMI (discussed above).

Standards are submitted to ANSI for approval from other organizations such as AAMI. Examples of ANSI-approved standards include the Recommended Practices and Standards developed by AAMI. ANSI is the sole U.S. representative to the International Standards Organization (ISO).

Note: ISO is discussed later in this section.

For more information about ANSI, go to: www.ansi.org

Association of Operating Room Nurses (AORN)

AORN is a professional organization consisting of Perioperative nurses and others who are dedicated to providing optimal care to the surgical patient. AORN committees comprised of allied association members including the International Association of Healthcare Materiel Management (IAHCSMM) develop nationally-recognized Standards, Recommended Practices, and Guidelines. AORN, like all the professional associations being discussed, is not a regulatory agency. However, regulatory officials look for compliance with AORN standards as they interact with health care facilities. Central Service Technicians should be aware of AORN Standards, Recommended Practices, and Guidelines that relate to instrument processing.

For more information about AORN, go to: www.aorn.org

The Association for Professionals in Infection Control and Epidemiology (APIC)

APIC is a voluntary international organization whose members are dedicated to the prevention and control of infections and related outcomes. APIC members work in conjunction with other agencies such as the Centers for Disease Control to adopt standards for infection/disease prevention. Examples include the Bioterrorist Readiness Plan and Guidelines for Infection Prevention and Control in Flexible Endoscopy.[4] Central Service

Medicare – *A federal medical insurance program that primarily serves those over 65 years of age (regardless of income), and younger disabled persons and dialysis patients; medical bills are paid from trust funds into which covered persons have paid.*

Medicaid – *A federal and state assistance program that pays covered medical expenses for low-income persons. It is run by state and local governments within federal guidelines.*

Technicians may interact with their facility's Infection Control professionals who conduct departmental surveys to ensure compliance with APIC Standards, Practices, and Guidelines.

For more information about APIC, go to: www.apic.org

International Standards Organization (ISO)

ISO is a non-governmental organization with a network of National Standards Institutes representing 156 countries. The standards it issues are voluntary, and the organization has no legal enforcement authority. However, many ISO standards have been adopted by some countries, or are referred to in legislation which makes them regulatory in these jurisdictions. Proposed standards are submitted from members such as AAMI to the general membership, and are granted ISO status based on consensus of the entire membership. Central Service Departments may, in the future, increasingly follow regulatory ISO standards.

For more information about ISO, go to: www.iso.org

The Joint Commission

The Joint Commission is a private, independent not-for-profit organization that develops standards for health care facilities. The Joint Commission personnel evaluate 15,000 health care organizations and programs in the U.S. by conducting on-site surveys at least every three years. The Joint Commission teams may arrive unannounced at a facility, and spend two–five days studying virtually every aspect of care within it. Joint Commission standards are voluntary; however, they carry significant weight. Failure to comply with these standards as evaluated through the The Joint Commission survey process can result in the loss of accreditation by the federal and state governments. This, in turn, can result in the forfeiture of millions of dollars in **Medicare** and **Medicaid** program payments.

Central Service Technicians must understand and cooperate with their facility's procedures to comply with The Joint Commision requirements. They must know and promote the hospital's mission, and consistently comply with all safety standards including those specific to their department. They must attend all mandatory hospital in-service sessions, assist with quality improvement tactics for their specific functions, and follow all directives of Infection Control personnel. The Joint Commision emphasizes continuous improvement in the quality of patient care, and Central Service personnel play a key role in improved patient outcomes. Standards issued by The Joint Commision may be incorporated by reference into federal, state and/or local statutes, and then become binding on health care facilities.

For more information about The Joint Commision, go to: www.jointcommission.org

National Fire Protection Association (NFPA)

NFPA is an international organization that works to reduce the burden of fire and other hazards around the world. NFPA members represent nearly 100 nations and organizations, and use a consensus process to develop codes and standards that influence building safety in the U.S. and in other countries.

NFPA is important to Central Service Technicians because of the fire safety standards used for the buildings in which they work. As well, NFPA standards address the fire burden of all disposable packaged items stored and used within the facility, the fire standards for patient drapes utilized in the Operating Room, and wrappers utilized in the Central Service processing area.

For more information about NFPA, go to: www.nfpa.org

United States Pharmacopoeia – National Formulary (USP-NF)

The USP creates and revises standards for medicines, dosages, forms, drug substances, and dietary supplements. These standards are published in the USP National Formulary (NF). Standards are set for packaging, labeling, bacteriological purity, pH, and mineral content. The USP is important to Central Service Technicians who work with purified water or sterilizing water for irrigation.

For more information about USP-NF, go to: www.usp.org/uspnf

World Health Organization (WHO)

WHO is an agency of the United Nations, and was established in 1948 to further international cooperation in improving health conditions. Its major task is to combat disease, especially key infectious diseases, and to promote the general health of the peoples of the world. Its staff members coordinate international efforts to monitor outbreaks of infectious diseases such as Severe Acute Respiratory Syndrome (SARS), Malaria, and Acquired Immune Deficiency Syndrome (AIDS). This agency provides a central clearing house for research services and international standards. Agencies such as the CDC base many standards on the research and direction provided by the WHO.

For more information about WHO, go to: www.who.org

European Commission for Standardization (ECHN)

This organization sets the health care standards for Europe in much the same way that AAMI sets standards for the U.S. Recent attention has focused on the comparison of ECHN standards to their U.S. counterparts.

Society of Gastroenterology Nurses and Associates (SGNA)

SGNA is a non-profit organization with a membership of over 7,500. It collects information and establishes standards and guidelines relating to the processing of flexible endoscopes.

For more information about SGNA, go to: www.sgna.org

ENDNOTES

1. *Pre-market requirements are found in the Food, Drug and Cosmetic Act (the Act), Sections 510, 513, and 515, and in 21 CFR Parts 807 and 814. Note: "The Act" provides the regulation; the CFR indicates the classification and tells what is needed to comply with the regulation.*

Information concerning the substantial equivalence decision-making process can be found on-line at http://www.fda.gov/cdrh/k863. html. Information for successfully completing a 510(k) notification is available on the web site: http://www.fda.gov/cdrh/devadvice/314. html.

PMA information is contained in Sections 513 and 515 of the Act, and 21 CFR Part 814. Guidance for preparation of a PMA may be obtained from www.fda.gov/cdrh/ode/448.pdf.

Additional information about each post-market requirement is available through the CDRH home page: http://www.fda.gov/ cdrh/; select "Post-market requirements". Guidance documents are also available on these post-market requirements by accessing the CDRH home page and selecting "Device Advice"; http://www.fda. gov/cdrh/devadvice/.

2. *Health care personnel who wish to voluntarily report device problems or potential hazards can call Medwatch (1-800-FDA-1088) or use the web site, http://www.fda.gov/medwatch/report/ hcp.htm, to report on-line or to obtain additional information and/ or forms.*

3. *Labeling Reusable Medical Devices for Reprocessing Health Care Facilities: FDA Reviewer Guidance, Office of Device Evaluation, April, 1996. (page 2)*

4. *Current FDA reuse information is found on its website: www.fda.gov/cdrh/reuse/index.shtml.*

5. *Current FDA re-use information is found on its web site: www. fda.gov/chrh/reuse/index.shtml*

6. *OSHA Employer responsibilities, http://www.osha.gov/as/opa/ worker/employer-responsibility.html*

REFERENCES

Code of Federal Regulations, Title 21, Part 813 — Medical Device Reporting, Subparts A, B, C. U.S. Government Printing Office. Washington, DC. 2000.

EPA. "Data Requirements for Registration." Federal Register 49 No. 207 (October 24, 1984): 42881-42905.

"Clarification of HIV (AIDS Virus) Labeling Policy for Antimicrobial Pesticide Products." Federal Register 54, No. 26 (February 9, 1989): 6288-6290.

National Emission Standards for Hazardous Air Pollutants for Source Categories, Code of Federal Regulations, Title 40, Part 63, Subpart 0 (Updated 1996). Washington, D.C.: EPA, 1994.

Centers for Disease Control. "Section 2: Cleaning, Disinfecting, and Sterilizing Patient Care Equipment." Guidelines for Hand-washing and Hospital Environmental Control. Atlanta: CDC, 1985.

Occupational Safety and Health Administration. "Occupational Exposure to Formaldehyde." Federal Register 52, No. 233: 46168-46312. Code of Federal Regulations, Title 29, Part 1910. Washington, D.C.: OSHA, 1987.

"Occupational Exposure to Ethylene Oxide." Federal Register 49, No. 122 (June 22, 1984): 25734-25809. Code of Federal Regulations, Title 29, Part 1910.1047. Washington, D.C.: OSHA, 1984.

"Occupational Exposure to Ethylene Oxide." Federal Register 53, No. 66 (April 6, 1988): 53:11414-11438. Code of Federal Regulations, Title 29, Part 1910.1047. Washington, D.C.: OSHA, 1988.

"Hazard Communication Standard." Code of Federal Regulations, Title 29, Part 1910.1200.

"Occupational Exposure to Blood-borne Pathogens: Final Rule." Federal Register 56 No. 235 (December 6, 1991): 56:64004. Code of Federal Regulations, Title 29, Part 1910.1030.

29CFR Part 1910.1030 Occupational Exposure to Bloodborne Pathogens; Final Rule; effective March 6, 1992; 29 CFR Part 1910.1030 Occupational Exposure to Bloodborne Pathogens; Needlestick and Other Sharp Injuries; Final Rule. Amended and effective April 18, 2001; and 29CFR 1910.1035 Occupational Exposure to Tuberculosis, Proposed Rule, October 17, 1997.

CENTRAL SERVICE TERMS

Regulation

Standard

Regulatory (standards)

Voluntary (standards)

Statute

MedWatch Program

Hemodialyzers

Prions

Greenhouse gases

Recommended Practices and Standards (AAMI)

Standards (AAMI)

Medicare

Medicaid

Chapter Outline

Chapter 6

Infection Prevention and Control

Chapter Learning Objectives:

As a result of successfully completing this chapter, readers will be able to:

1. Explain the role of Central Service Technicians in a healthcare facility's infection prevention and control efforts.

2. Discuss personal hygiene and personal protective equipment precautions that enable Central Service Technicians to protect patients and themselves.

3. Define the term, Standard Precautions, and review its role in preventing the transmission of infectious organisms.

4. List key elements in the Bloodborne Pathogens Standard published by Occupational Safety and Health Administration (OSHA).

5. Describe basic environmental concerns as Central Service work areas are designed.

6. Review environmental aspects of Central Service work procedures that impact infection control:
   - Traffic control
   - Work area cleanliness
   - Workflow

7. Define the terms, "asepsis," and "aseptic technique," and review the five basic principles of asepsis.

Infection Prevention is a critical mission of everyone in the Central Service department as they prepare, process, store, and distribute medical and surgical supplies and equipment.

CENTRAL SERVICE AND INFECTION PREVENTION AND CONTROL

Learning Objective 1. Explain the role of Central Service Technicians in a healthcare facility's infection prevention and control efforts.

Central Service personnel must assume several important responsibilities in their facility's **infection** prevention and control efforts. The infection prevention and control goals of the Central Service department are to:

- Eliminate and/or destroy all potentially infectious contaminants present on reusable instruments and equipment.

- Safely distribute reusable and single-use items required for the delivery of patient care.

- Establish and enforce standards for decontamination, disinfection, and sterilization in various healthcare settings.

The importance of these responsibilities is clear. The use of medical devices that have not been properly handled, disinfected or sterilized, can cause infections in patients and staff.

Each year, approximately two million patients (about 10% of those hospitalized) in U.S. hospitals develop healthcare facility-associated infection. These result in an estimated 90,000 deaths, immeasurable suffering and disability, and are associated with billions of dollars in increased healthcare costs. Most of these infections can be attributed to the increasing use of invasive medical devices and/or surgery.[1] In response, regulatory agencies and professional organizations representing various healthcare disciplines and perspectives have imposed regulations and developed guidelines for practice.

Approximately 27,000,000 surgical procedures and more than 10,000,000 gastrointestinal endoscopic procedures are performed in the U.S. annually.[2] Each involves the use of a medical device or instrument that has contact with a patient's sterile tissues or mucous membranes, and infection is a major risk of all these procedures. Additionally, bloodstream infections caused by intravenous and other vascular catheters, pneumonia caused by ventilators and respiratory therapy equipment, and urinary tract infections secondary to the use of foley catheters are reported in significant numbers in U.S. hospitals. It is ironic that this life-saving technology can result in the spread of healthcare-associated organisms, and can greatly increase a patient's risk of infection.

Despite the introduction of vaccines and antibiotics, infectious diseases remain a major health problem for most people around the globe. Although many have been eliminated or controlled, there are new and re-emerging threats. Additionally, there are a growing number of organisms that have developed resistance to commonly-used antibiotics that create treatment challenges that were previously never considered.

Infection prevention principles and practices are based on knowledge about the nature and characteristics of disease-producing microorganisms, and on an understanding about how they are transmitted in the healthcare environment.

The primary purpose of the Central Service Department is to stop the spread of disease-producing microorganisms in the healthcare facility. Central Service Technicians must assure that items used in patient care including instruments, utensils, supplies, and equipment are free from microorganisms that can harm patients and hospital staff. In chapter 4, you learned about microorganisms: how they live, grow, and are transmitted from person-to-person and place-to-place. In this chapter, you'll discover how Central Service personnel control the spread of

Infection – *Invasion of human body tissue by microorganisms which multiply and produce a reaction.*

microorganisms and prevent infection. Then, in subsequent chapters, you will examine various methods that Central Service Technicians use to remove, reduce, and destroy microorganisms on patient care items.

GETTING READY FOR INFECTION PREVENTION AND CONTROL

Learning Objective 2. Discuss personal hygiene and personal protective equipment precautions that enable Central Service Technicians to protect patients and themselves.

For Central Service Technicians, the process of infection prevention and control begins before they enter their work area, and continues throughout the time they are performing their duties in the workplace.

Before Work Practices

Infection prevention and control begins in the staff locker room where employees change from the clothing worn from home (commonly referred to as street clothes) into hospital issued surgical scrub uniforms. Because they will be entering a controlled environment, they need to help maintain that environment by wearing appropriate attire. **Figure 6.1** shows a Central Service Technician dressed appropriately for the Central Service department.

The basic attire worn by Central Service Technicians includes:

- A facility-issued scrub uniform.

- Hair covering that covers all head and facial hair except eyebrows and eyelashes.

- Shoes with non-skid soles.

Changing into clean attire before beginning work reduces the amount of microorganisms introduced into the Central Service Department and other restricted areas of the healthcare facility. It also insures that staff members do not carry potentially pathogenic microorganisms home on their own clothes when they leave the facility.

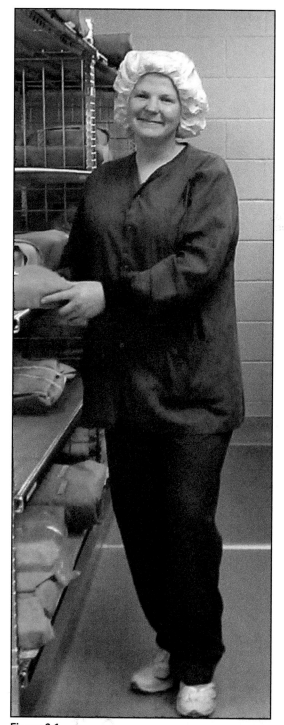

Figure 6.1

Before beginning work, Central Service Technicians must also remove watches and other jewelry because they can harbor microorganisms which can then be transmitted into and out of the Central

Handwashing Procedure:

1. Remove all jewelry.

2. Turn on faucet using a paper towel.

3. Wet your hands and apply liquid soap.

4. Work soap into a lather and scrub hands for at least 15 seconds.

5. Keep your hands at a lower angle than your elbows to prevent the dirty water from running back onto your arms.

6. Interlace your fingers to clean between them.

7. Dry your hands with clean paper towels.

8. Turn off the faucet using a clean paper towel.

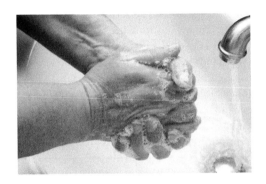

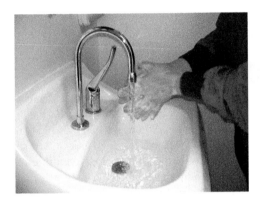

Figure 6.2 Handwashing

Service Department. Also, rings worn under gloves may compromise their barrier effectiveness by puncturing or weakening the glove where it comes in contact with the ring.

Central Service Technicians must make one final preparation before entering the work area: they wash their hands.

important procedure to prevent and control the transmission of microorganisms from one person to another or from one site to another.

Central Service Technicians should wash their hands upon entering and leaving their work area, and whenever their hands become soiled or contaminated. Infection control experts recommend

Hand Hygiene Practices

Hand hygiene (washing hands with soap and water or using an alcohol-based hand rub) is the most

Hand hygiene – The act of washing one's hands with soap and water or using an alcohol-based hand rub.

that hands be washed immediately and thoroughly if they become soiled with blood, body fluids, secretion, or excretions. In the absence of visible soil (such as following contact with contaminated items without visible soil or after gloves are removed), an alcohol-based hand rub should be used following the manufacturer's recommendations.

Effective hand washing consists of wetting, soaping, lathering, and vigorously rubbing one's hands together (make certain to lather between fingers and around nails) for at least 15 seconds. Washing should be followed by rinsing with running water and thorough drying with a disposable towel. (See **Figure 6.2**) Recent evidence also supports the use of lotions after hand washing to keep the skin healthy, and to minimize skin irritation and excessive drying.[3]

Fingernails of personnel working in high-risk areas should be maintained at a length of ¼ inch or less because they may harbor microorganisms. Also, long nails increase the risk of tearing gloves. Note: fingernail polish and artificial nails should not be worn in the Central Service Department.

Personnel with open or weeping wounds or excessive skin irritations should refrain from handling any patient care equipment until medically evaluated, and/or the condition is resolved.

Every Central Service Technician must consistently follow dress codes and hand washing protocols to help maintain the integrity of the environment for infection control.

Use of Personal Protective Attire

In addition to the dress code for all Central Service Technicians noted above, more stringent requirements apply for anyone working in the decontamination area. Those who are assigned to (or enter) the decontamination area must also wear:

- General purpose utility gloves. These provide the hands with a protective barrier, and prevent contamination when handling applicable items. Gloves do not replace the need for hand hygiene, because they may have slight imperfections, and one's hands may become contaminated when

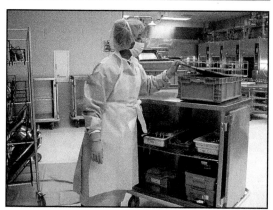

Figure 6.3

gloves are removed. The thickness and durability of gloves should be sufficient to prevent them from being easily torn when performing normal duties.

- A fluid-resistant covering with sleeves. A covering such as a jumpsuit, backless gown, or apron made of a fluid-resistant material should be worn to prevent the contamination of clothing, and to protect the Central Service Technician's skin from exposure to blood and body fluids. Arms should be completely covered.

- Full face protection. A full-length face shield or a combination of mask and eye goggles should be worn as a protective barrier during cleaning procedures to prevent mucous membrane exposure from splashes, sprays, and/or aerosolized contaminated fluids.

- Shoe covers. These may be necessary to protect shoes from becoming wet and contaminated during cleaning procedures.

The above specialized attire, commonly referred to as **Personal Protective Equipment (PPE)**, is designed to protect the worker from exposure to harmful microorganisms that may be present in the Decontamination area. (See **Figure 6.3**)

> ***Personal Protective Equipment (PPE)*** – *Specialized clothing or equipment worn by an employee for protection against a hazard.*

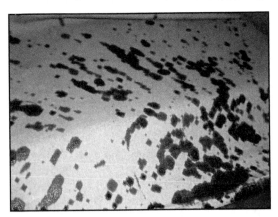

Figure 6.4

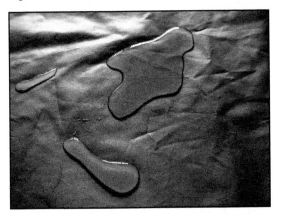

Figure 6.5

All persons working in the decontamination area must comply with dress code requirements for personal protective equipment. This requirement is mandated by the Occupational Safety and Health Administration (OSHA), and was established to insure that workers are protected from potential pathogens from all patients.

The risk of exposure to pathogenic microorganisms can be reduced by following dress codes in decontamination areas. For example, fluid-resistant gowns provide protection from splashes that may soak into and contaminate regular scrub attire. **Figure 6.4** shows liquid splashed on a standard surgical scrub top. Note: the liquid quickly soaked into the fabric upon contact. **Figure 6.5** shows the same amount of liquid splashed onto a fluid-resistant gown. You can see how the water beads up, and does not soak into the gown. These photos illustrate how wearing a fluid-resistant gown can protect your skin from contaminated splashes and spills.

Use of PPE is a Must!

Standard Precautions drive the infection prevention and control procedures that Central Service Technicians must use because they are exposed to contaminated instrumentation and equipment. Failure to wear the appropriate personal protective equipment (PPE) increases the individual's risk of acquiring an infection.

The revised guideline uses a variety of infection control measures designed to reduce the transmission risk of bloodborne and other pathogens from both recognized and unrecognized infection sources in a hospital.[4]

OVERVIEW OF STANDARD PRECAUTIONS

Learning Objective 3. Define the term, "Standard Precautions" and review its role in preventing the transmission of infectious organisms.

In the early 1970's, the Centers for Disease Control (CDC) established the first practical recommendations for isolation technique. The origins of isolation precautions date back to the days of quarantine, a control measure used in infectious disease epidemics of earlier times. With the new recommendations, infections and communicable diseases were categorized based upon the likely mode of transmission. This method required a diagnosis or suspected diagnosis, and often resulted in the "over isolation" of most patients.

One limitation of isolation was that it was diagnosis-driven, and did not provide for patients who, while infected and posing a risk to others, did not have visible signs or symptoms of the infection or disease. Further, the handling and processing of contaminated equipment and supplies was not addressed by these earlier recommendations.

The CDC revised its isolation manual in 1983 and included the recommendation to centralize an area for the decontamination and reprocessing of patient care equipment by appropriately-trained personnel.

In 1987, as a result of the HIV epidemic, a new strategy for isolation precautions was introduced.

It addressed the issue of patients with bloodborne diseases who did not demonstrate signs or symptoms of infection. This new strategy, known as Universal Precautions, provided guidance for healthcare workers involved in the care of all patients, including those with bloodborne infections (the majority of which are not readily recognized).

OSHA adopted the use of Universal Precautions as a major component of its Bloodborne Pathogens Standard that was finalized and published in 1991.

From an infection control standpoint, there was major limitation of Universal Precautions: it only applied to body fluids associated with the transmission of bloodborne diseases such as hepatitis B and C and HIV rather than to all body fluids encountered when providing patient care. It was also recognized that the use of Universal Precautions could prevent the transmission of other infections and communicable diseases and epidemiologically-significant microorganisms (those that are most often involved in the incidence and spread of disease). To eliminate confusion, the name was changed to Standard Precautions and, in 1996, the CDC incorporated the concept of Standard Precautions into its recommendations.

Standard precautions place emphasis on the use of blood and body fluid precautions for all patients. The most important principle in following these guidelines is to treat all items used with all patients as contaminated. Exposure prevention by the careful handling of needles and other sharps and by the use of gowns and gloves is emphasized as well. Masks with eye protection to prevent mucous membrane exposures of the eyes, nose, and mouth during certain procedures are also included.

Standard precautions – Method of using appropriate barriers to prevent transmission of infectious organisms from contact with blood and all other body fluids, non-intact skin, and mucous membranes. It applies to all patients, regardless of diagnosis or presumed infectious status.

OSHA BLOODBORNE PATHOGENS STANDARD

Learning Objective 4. List key elements in the Bloodborne Pathogens Standard published by Occupational Safety and Health Administration (OSHA).

OSHA published the Bloodborne Pathogens Standard in 1991 in response to concerns and recognizing the potential for occupational exposure to bloodborne diseases (hepatitis B and C and HIV). The Standard places the responsibility for providing a safe work environment on the employer, and contains several key elements:

- A written Exposure Control Plan (the plan) that summarizes the employer's program for the protection of workers from occupational exposure to bloodborne diseases. The plan must be reviewed annually and updated whenever new tasks or procedures affecting occupational exposures are instituted.

- Training upon initial hire and annually thereafter. If significant changes are made to the plan, additional training is required to address the changes.

- The provision of hepatitis B vaccine at no cost. Employees who choose not to take the vaccine must sign a declination (refusal) form, and they may reconsider at any time during their employment.

- Observance of Standard Precautions. All patients should be considered to be infected with bloodborne diseases.

- The use of engineering (to physically remove the hazard) and development of work practice controls (policies and procedures) to prevent occupational exposure and transmission of bloodborne pathogens.

- Provision of PPE including gloves, fluid resistant gowns, masks or face shields, eye protection, and laboratory coats to prevent occupational exposure to infectious materials. PPE must be available in appropriate sizes, and at no cost to employees. This equipment must be used whenever an employee may come in contact with blood or other potentially infectious materials, and is not optional or at the discretion of the employee.

• Provision of a clean and sanitary working environment including scheduled cleaning using hospital germicides (disinfectants) approved by the EPA.

• The use of fluorescent orange or orange red "BIOHAZARD" labels to identify contaminated items or regulated waste that may be stored or transported in refrigerators, freezers, or other containers. Labels are not required when using red bags or containers.

• Disposal of all sharp items in rigid, puncture-proof containers that can be sealed.

• Any contaminated item must be transported in covered, rigid, puncture-proof containers that are properly labeled or color-coded.

• Provision for medical evaluation and treatment when an employee experiences an exposure incident.

• The need to maintain medical as well as training records.

ENVIRONMENTAL CONCERNS IN CENTRAL SERVICE AREAS

Learning Objective 5. Describe basic environmental concerns as Central Service work areas are designed.

In addition to specific guidelines for dress codes and Standard Precautions, there are environmental mechanisms designed to help Central Service Technicians promote infection control. Some are evident and others, while not as evident, still play an important role in maintaining an environment that is safe for patients and employees.

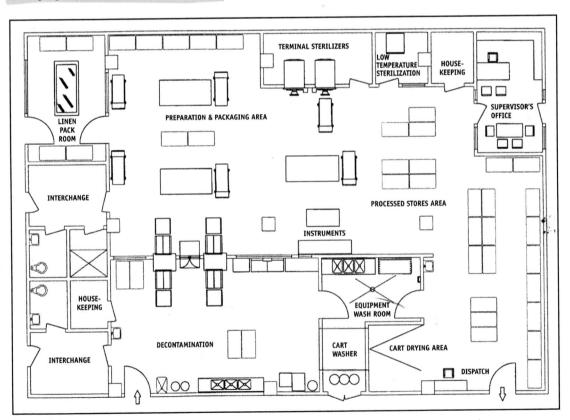

Figure 6.6

The Use of Air Pressure to Control Airborne Bacteria

Clean Area	Decontamination Area
Positive Air Pressure	Negative Air Pressure

Airflow ▶

Figure 6.7

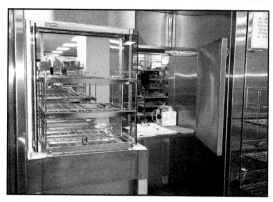

Figure 6.8

Physical Design

Central Service departments are physically designed to separate clean items from their dirty counterparts. This is especially important because there must be a physical barrier between decontamination (the work area where contaminated equipment, instruments, and utensils are returned for processing) and the sterile storage area (where items that are safe and ready for patient use are stored). **Figure 6.6** illustrates a typical floor plan in a small Central Service department. Note the physical separation of the decontamination area from all other work areas.

In addition to walls separating the decontamination from the rest of the department, the area is designed to reduce the likelihood that airborne bacteria can be transmitted from the decontamination area to the clean area. This is accomplished with use of positive and negative air pressures. The decontamination area has a negative (lesser) air pressure than the clean area. This means that, when a door or window is opened

between the separate work areas, air tends to flow from the clean (positive pressure) area to the dirty (negative pressure) area. This minimizes the risk of airborne bacteria, if present in the decontamination area, being carried to the clean area. **Figure 6.7** illustrates the airflow created by the use of positive and negative air pressures. To maintain the balance necessary for air pressure systems to function correctly, access windows and doors between the decontamination and clean areas must remain closed when not in use. Note: **Figure 6.8** shows an access window between the decontamination area and the clean area.

Environmental Controls

Central Service areas must also meet specific temperature, humidity and air exchange requirements. These vary by work area, and Central Service Technicians must be familiar with the requirements for each specific area. **Figure 6.9** outlines the requirements for each basic work area.

Work Area	Temperature	Humidity	Air Exchanges
Decontamination	60°F to 65°F (16°C to 18°C)	30% to 60%	10 per hour
Preparation and Packaging	68° F to 73° F (20° C to 23° C)	30% to 60%	10 per hour
Clean/Sterile Storage	75° F or lower (24° C or lower)	Less than 70%	4 per hour

Figure 6.9 Central Service Temperature, Humidity, and Air Exchange Requirements*

These standards are based on ANSI/AAMI ST79:2006; Comprehensive Guide to Steam Sterilization and Sterility in Healthcare Facilities.

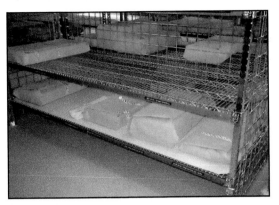

Figure 6.10

Other Requirements

Central Service departments are equipped with hand washing sinks conveniently located for easy access. Central Service Technicians should wash their hands only in dedicated hand washing sinks (not in those used for decontamination purposes).

The fixtures and furniture in Central Service departments must be constructed of materials that can be washed, and they must be cleaned on a regularly scheduled basis.

The area designated for sterile storage may consist of either open (rack) or closed (cabinet) storage units. The decision about the type of storage used is based on the types of items to be stored, and the amount of traffic in the area. For example, closed cabinets may be used in high traffic areas, and open shelving (racks) may be used in more controlled, low traffic areas.

 Open rack systems should have a solid bottom so that items stored on the lower shelves are protected from contamination during housekeeping tasks. (See **Figure 6.10**)

Note: more detailed standards for design requirements for Central Service work areas can be found in ANSI/AAMI ST79:2006.

MAINTAINING CENTRAL SERVICE ENVIRONMENTS

Learning Objective 6. Review environmental aspects of Central Service work procedures that impact infection control:
- Traffic control
- Work area cleanliness
- Workflow

Engineering and design activities cannot prevent and control infection by themselves. The effective management of microorganisms relies on those who work within the Central Service department. Central Service Technicians must understand the infection control protocols within their facility, and they must adhere to them at all times. Failure to do so puts patients and employees at risk. Each infection control protocol is designed to protect patients and employees, and to maintain the integrity of the Central Service environment.

Traffic Control

The first step in maintaining environmental integrity is to control the traffic that enters and passes through the Central Service department. The dress codes discussed earlier in this chapter apply to all persons entering the Central Service department. Department dress standards for visitors (examples: sales representatives, maintenance personnel and clinical engineering staff) vary between facilities. In some facilities, they must change into surgical scrubs; in others coveralls (worn over their street clothes) are required. Central Service Technicians must protect the integrity of the environment by enforcing traffic control guidelines. This may sometimes mean educating visitors about dress code and traffic control protocols.

Dress code requirements may change as Central Service Technicians move from one area to another. For example, surgical scrubs and hair coverings may be appropriate for the clean assembly area, but OSHA-required PPE is necessary for the decontamination area. Dress codes are an important part of traffic control. Therefore, Central Service Technicians must understand what attire is appropriate in different areas. (See **Figure 6.11**)

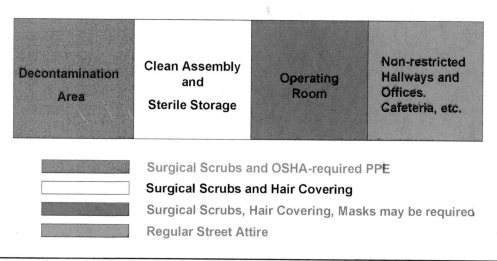

What to Wear
CS Dress Requirement Review

Decontamination Area	Clean Assembly and Sterile Storage	Operating Room	Non-restricted Hallways and Offices. Cafeteria, etc.

Surgical Scrubs and OSHA-required PPE

Surgical Scrubs and Hair Covering

Surgical Scrubs, Hair Covering, Masks may be required

Regular Street Attire

Figure 6.11

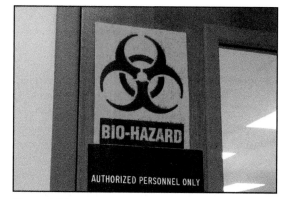

Figure 6.12

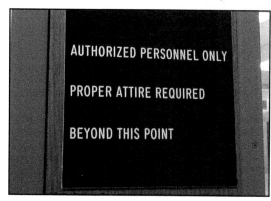

Figure 6.13

Areas that Central Service Technicians routinely travel through may have four separate traffic control/dress code requirements:

• Biohazard – These areas may be contaminated from used equipment, utensils, and instruments. OSHA-required PPE is required in these areas.

• Unrestricted – These areas include normal traffic areas such as hospital corridors, most offices, locker rooms, and general public areas such as the cafeteria and waiting rooms. Street clothes may be worn in unrestricted areas.

• Semi-restricted – These areas include peripheral support areas to the OR, such as Central Service clean assembly and sterile storage areas, and access corridors to operating rooms. Surgical scrub attire and hair coverings are required in these areas.

• Restricted – These areas are those where sterile procedures are performed. Surgical scrub attire, hair coverings, and masks are required in these areas. Persons working within the sterile field (examples: surgeons, surgical technologists, and nurses) have additional requirements of a sterile surgical gown and gloves.

Central Service departments use signage to assist in traffic control. All biohazard areas are designated with biohazard signs (symbols) that indicate the need for Standard Precautions and protective attire (See **Figure 6.12**). All restricted and semi-restricted areas also have signage that informs people entering the area about the need for specific dress codes (See **Figure 6.13**).

Work Area Cleanliness

Central Service Technicians must minimize the amount of contaminants such as dust, lint, and bacteria in their work areas. They know that, the cleaner the work area, the more likely that the products they prepare will be safe. For example, dust and lint particles not only carry bacteria but, in some cases, lint remaining in a sterile set may enter the patient's body during surgery.

Central Service Technicians also know that bacteria can be transmitted by contact with contaminated items. This is easy to envision in the decontamination areas. However, items in clean assembly areas can also be contaminated, and that contamination can be transmitted to other objects. Inanimate objects that can transmit bacteria are called **fomites**. Common fomites that become contaminated in Central Service areas include door handles, computer pads and keyboards, telephones, and other items routinely handled by several people. **Figure 6.14** uses the example of flowers that was introduced in Chapter 4 to help us visualize some common fomites that may harbor bacteria in work areas. Central Service Technicians know that by routinely cleaning these items and their general work areas (work stations), they can control the unwanted spread of bacteria within their workplace.

Fomite – An inanimate object that can transmit bacteria.

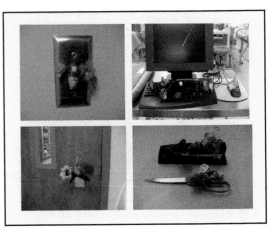

Figure 6.14

Environmental cleaning (housekeeping) is a vital component in the department's overall infection prevention and control process. Central Service departments are routinely cleaned to insure that the microbial population is minimized. Basic housekeeping procedures used in Central Service should be the same as those used in operating and delivery rooms and cleaning guidelines include:

• Floors should be cleaned (wet mopped) at least daily. They should never be swept or dust-mopped because dust can rise and be redistributed on items in the area. When sterile packages are opened, the dust that has accumulated on them may fall onto the package contents. Separate and dedicated cleaning equipment that is not used in other areas such as mops and buckets should be used in the decontamination area.

• Horizontal work surfaces such as counters and worktables should be cleaned at least daily.

• Light fixtures or their covers should be cleaned at least every 6 months.

• Other surfaces (including walls, cabinets, and racks) should be cleaned on a regularly scheduled basis.

Many Central Service housekeeping functions are performed by environmental services personnel. However, routine cleaning of sterile storage cabinets, carts, and racks is usually the responsibility of Central Service Technicians who have been

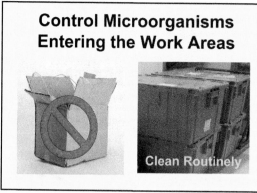

Control Microorganisms Entering the Work Areas

Clean Routinely

Figure 6.15

trained to properly handle sterile items, and who know specific product names and locations.

When cleaning sterile storage areas, it is important to keep in mind the types of "events" that can contaminate a sterile package. Although sterile packaging is referred to as "barrier" packaging, it is not indestructible. It can be torn, punctured, contaminated by moisture or rough handling, and contaminated by soil. Several guidelines can help to insure that sterile items are not compromised during routine housekeeping:

• Remove all sterile items from the storage unit (cart, rack, or cabinet) to be cleaned, and place them on a clean, dry surface. Avoid rough handling.

• Thoroughly clean the storage unit using the cleaning solution recommended by the facility. Be sure to wear gloves and the appropriate PPE, and to clean storage bins as well as shelves and drawers.

• Allow the storage unit to dry thoroughly.

• With clean, dry hands, return the sterile items to the exact place on the rack where they were before being removed.

• Record the cleaning date in the department's designated cleaning log.

Corrugated boxes and external shipping containers may harbor microorganisms. Corrugated boxes should not be allowed in work areas, and shipping containers like plastic tote boxes must be cleaned routinely. (See **Figure 6.15**)

Avoid Food and Drink in Work Areas

Food and beverages should not be allowed in Central Service work areas. This standard is well-understood for decontamination areas. However, why is this also necessary in clean areas of the department?

Beverages should not be allowed because they may spill and contaminate sterile items, or they may spill onto items that need to be sterilized and impact sterilization outcomes. Foods should not be allowed because they may also contaminate items. Central Service Technicians should not handle (eat) food in their work areas because their hands may be soiled, and they could transmit bacteria. Also, if their fingers become coated with oils (examples: residues from snack chips or chocolate), they could transmit that oil on to instruments to be sterilized. This oil may impede the contact of the sterilant with the entire surface of the instrument. Finally, food and beverages attract insects, and may increase the chance of insects invading the work area.

Workflow

The workflow in a Central Service department is designed to avoid cross-contamination and insure that items efficiently flow through the process from decontamination to storage. If one considers the journey that a surgical instrument makes from the end of use on one patient to the start of use on the next patient, it is easy to visualize the changes that take place. **Figure 6.16** illustrates the journey an instrument makes from its use, or contaminated state to its ready for use, or sterile state. The red shading illustrates the reduction of bacteria as the instrument moves through the process, from contaminated, to safe to handle, to sterile.

That journey also illustrates the workflow process within the Central Service department, where contaminated items enter into the decontamination area, are made safe to handle, passed through to the preparation area and prepared for sterilization, are sterilized and placed into sterile storage where their sterility is maintained until their next use.

Progression from Contaminated to Sterile

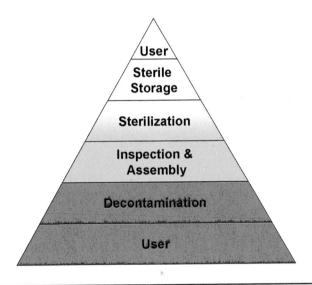

Figure 6.16

The department's physical design should facilitate this process, and work patterns should be designed that create a one-way flow of goods.

Central Service Technicians work with items at all stages of the decontamination, sterilization, storage, and distribution processes, so they must be well-versed in basic infection control theory. To insure that the workflow is maintained, and

that items are handled appropriately at each stage in the processing cycle, they must understand the principles of asepsis.

PRINCIPLES OF ASEPSIS

Learning Objective 7. Define the term, "asepsis," and "aseptic technique," and review the five basic principles of asepsis.

Definitions

Asepsis can be defined as the absence of microorganisms that cause disease, and an **aseptic technique** includes any activity or procedure that prevents infection or breaks the chain of infection.

There are two types of aseptic techniques:

- **Medical asepsis** (clean technique) – Procedures performed to reduce the number of microorganisms to minimize their spread.

Asepsis – *The absence of microorganisms that cause disease.*

Aseptic technique – *Any activity or procedure that prevents infection or breaks the chain of infection.*

Asepsis (medical) – *Procedures performed to reduce the number of microorganisms to minimize their spread.*

Asepsis (surgical) – *Procedures performed to eliminate the presence of all microorganisms, and/or to prevent the introduction of microorganisms to an area.*

Examples: hand washing and decontamination of equipment.

- **Surgical asepsis** (sterile technique) – Procedures to eliminate the presence of all microorganisms, and/or to prevent the introduction of microorganisms to an area. Examples: sterilization of instrumentation, and operating room techniques which prevent contamination of sterile instruments and supplies.

Principles of Asepsis

There are five basic principles of asepsis:

- **Principle One: Know What is Dirty** – Any items that have been used for patient care or that are visibly soiled are considered contaminated. In general, there is no difference between a "little contaminated" and a "lot contaminated." An item is considered to be either "contaminated" or "not contaminated." For the Central Service Technician, the terms "dirty" and "contaminated" mean the same thing.

Microbial contamination cannot be seen with the naked eye; it can be present even when it is not seen. If persons have been in contact with used patient care items and have not washed their hands, their hands must be considered contaminated. Examples of contaminated items include operating room instrument trays, used linens, and suction machines.

- **Principle Two: Know What is Clean** – Cleanliness is the basis of aseptic technique. Mechanical cleaning removes soil and most microorganisms. Any item that has been mechanically cleaned (thoroughly washed) is considered clean. If that item has been cleaned with a detergent disinfectant, it is considered clean and "decontaminated." The task of washing physically removes soil and most microorganisms. The detergent disinfectant will kill or prevent the growth of any microorganisms that have not been removed by the washing.

- **Principle Three: Know What is Sterile** – Sterility is defined as the absence of all microbes. Sterility is impossible to see with the naked eye; one cannot look at a specific item and determine its sterility. Absence of microbes can only be achieved by use of steam, dry heat, ethylene oxide, or other sterilization methods including peracetic acid, irradiation, ozone, and vapor phase hydrogen peroxide.

- **Principle Four: Keep the Three Conditions Separate** – There must be separation between dirty, clean, and sterile areas to allow a margin of safety. Clean or decontaminated items must not come in contact with dirty items. If they do, they must again be considered dirty. Sterile items must not contact non-sterile items, or they must also again be considered non-sterile. Sterile items should not be stored near the sink, or in any location where there is a risk that they will become wet or soiled. The presence of moisture allows the passage of microorganisms through wrappers resulting in contamination of sterile supplies.

- **Principle Five: Remedy Contamination Immediately** – When dirty, clean, and sterile areas or items have not been separated, the situation must be corrected immediately. Central Service Technicians must accept this principle as a special concern. One who observes a procedure has as much responsibility for maintaining proper aseptic technique as does the person who performs the procedure. There are times when only a Central Service Technician will know or suspect that something may be contaminated. Even though taking action may result in more work, this must be done to protect the patient.

Asepsis has its basis in a conscious-careful attitude ("sterile conscience"). A careless attitude may lead to an increased risk of infection, so always be aware of actions taken. By adhering to the principles of asepsis, the risk of infection will be reduced for patients and the facility's employees. The responsibility of Central Service Technicians to provide safe items for use can never be compromised.

Important! Important!

Central Service Technicians face the on-going challenge of insuring that the sophisticated instruments and equipment they process are safe for patient use. Advances in technology and the emergence of new microbiological challenges have increased the difficulty in meeting this challenge. Every Central Service Technician must appreciate the importance of infection control and prevention, and must thoroughly understand their role in the process.

REFERENCES

1. Mayhall, C. ed. Hospital Epidemiology and Infection Control. Third Edition. Baltimore, Maryland: Williams and Wilkins. 2004.

2. Rutala, W; et. al. Draft Guideline for Disinfection and Sterilization in Healthcare Facilities." CDC. 2002.

3. Boyce, J., et. al. "Guideline for Hand Hygiene in Health Care Settings." 2002.

4. Centers for Disease Control and Prevention. Hospital Infection Control Practices Advisory Committee. "Draft Guidelines for Isolation Precautions in Hospitals." Infection Control Hospital Epidemiology. CDC, 2006.

ANSI/AAMI ST79:2006: "Comprehensive Guide to Steam Sterilization and Sterility Assurance in Healthcare Facilities" , 2006.

The Joint Commission. Accreditation Manual for Hospitals. Oakbrook Terrace, Illinois: Joint Commission for the Accreditation of Health Care Organizations. 2006.

Pommerville, ed. Alcamo's Fundamentals of Microbiology. Seventh Edition. Redwood City, CA: Jones and Bartlett Publishing. 2004.

APIC Text of Infection Control and Epidemiology. Association for Professionals in Infection Control and Epidemiology. Washington, D.C. 2006.

Smith, S, et. al. Clinical Nursing Skills: Basic to Advanced. Sixth Edition. Upper Saddle River, New Jersey: Prentice-Hall, Inc. 2000.

U.S. Department of Labor. Occupational Safety and Health Administration. Occupational Exposure to Bloodborne Pathogens, Final Rule. Federal Register 1991; 56 (235): 64175-64182.

ADDITIONAL RESOURCES

Abrutyn, E, et. al. The Expert's Guide to the Guidelines. Second Edition. Philadelphia, Pennsylvania: W.B. Saunders Company. 2001.

Block, S. Disinfection, Sterilization and Preservation. Fifth Edition. Philadelphia, Pennsylvania: Lippincott, Williams & Wilkins. 2001.

Centers for Disease Control and Prevention. "Guideline for Environmental Infection Control in Healthcare Facilities." 2001.

CENTRAL SERVICE TERMS

Infection

Hand hygiene

Personal Protective Equipment (PPE)

Standard precautions

Fomite

Asepsis

Aseptic technique

Asepsis (medical)

Asepsis (surgical)

Chapter 7

Tools For Cleaning

Chapter Learning Objectives

As a result of successfully completing this chapter, readers will be able to:

1. Explain the importance of using purified water in the cleaning process, and review procedures to test for water purity.

2. Discuss factors that impact water purity.

3. Provide an overview of components and products that are important in water purification systems.

4. Explain the basics of distillation, deionization, and reverse osmosis water purification systems.

5. Identify common cleaning chemicals, and review basic protocols for their use.

6. Note the importance of bushes, cloths, and sponges in an effective cleaning process.

Significant pre-work is needed before the cleaning process can begin. Water must be purified, and systems must be in place to assure that the water used for this purpose is consistently of the correct quality. Numerous chemicals are also needed in the proper concentrations, and they must be safely used. Finally, cleaning utensils must be appropriate and ready to use when the cleaning process begins. The above and related pre-cleaning activities are the subject of this chapter.

TESTING FOR WATER QUALITY

Learning Objective 1. Explain the importance of using purified water in the cleaning process, and review procedures to test for water purity.

Regardless of whether the water used by a health care facility comes from a municipal water source, a natural aquifer, or is surface water, it must be purified to provide the proper quality of final rinse water for the instrument cleaning process. There are many impurities in water, even if it is tap water that had been treated at a municipal water treatment plant. Water from any source typically contains minerals, dissolved solids, particles, gases, and organic and non-organic chemicals. Some water sources also contain bacteria, algae, and parasites. These contaminants may impede cleaning and biocidal processes and in some cases, certain contaminants may shorten the life of instruments by harming the finish of instruments. Therefore, water used as a final rinse in any cleaning process should be purified to reduce or eliminate these elements.

It is important that tests of water samples be made at each site where it is used as a final rinse in manual and mechanical (ultrasonic, washer sterilizer, cart washer, and washer decontaminator/disinfector) processes. Tests can be performed by facility personnel or, alternatively, manufacturers and distributors of cleaning products, cleaning machines, and water treatment products often provide these tests free of charge.

Procedures to conduct a water sample test include:

• Obtain a sterile plastic container to collect the sample. Note: sterile urine specimen containers can be used for this purpose.

• Locate the source where the final rinse enters the sink (manual system) or cleaning equipment. Note: maintenance, biomedical, or service contractor personnel may need to disconnect water lines to obtain the test samples.

• Let the water flow for several seconds, and then fill the collection container.

• Close the lid tightly, and send the container to the testing facility as quickly as possible to minimize changes that can occur over time with levels of gases in the water.

• A report about water quality including conductivity, total dissolved solids, pH, chlorides, silicates, and particle count will be returned by the testing facility.

FACTORS THAT IMPACT WATER QUALITY

Learning Objective 2. Discuss factors that impact water purity.

Factors that impact water quality include its conductivity, total dissolved solids, acidity or alkalinity, chlorides, and other particles.

Conductivity

The **conductivity** of the water is an important measurement that indicates its ionic (electrical) charge. The greater the ionic charge, the more elements there are in the water. When these elements are removed, the water loses its electrical charge, and more aggressive attempts to regain these charges occur. This is the principal reason that water should not be purified to the highest possible degree because, as it becomes aggressive, it will strip weaker metals from their source (such as instruments being processed) to bind with the water. Today's technology provides water that is resistant to a minimum of 300,000 **ohms** (the preferred standard), and **deionization** and **reverse osmosis** are the systems most commonly used to treat the final rinse water used for cleaning.

Total Dissolved Solids

Total dissolved solids include elements such as iron, silicates, calcium, and magnesium. While there are many others, these are the ones about which Central Service Technicians are most concerned because they affect the appearance of processed items after they are cleaned. Hard water stains (water spots), and bluish or rainbow-color and powdery stains result from these dissolved solids. Hard water stains that arise after the items are dry appear as water spots or gray areas on the inside chamber of cleaning machines and on instruments. Bluish or rainbow-type stains are caused by iron and silicates in the water. Powdery stains or chalky build-ups on surfaces of cleaning machines result from the calcium and magnesium in the water. These elements act like plaque in our body's arteries, and can have the same effect on pipes and valves in a plumbing system.

Silicates are natural minerals found in soil and, therefore, in water. The silicate-level of tap water

---

Conductivity (of water) – A measurement of the ability of water to carry an electrical current.

Ohm – A unit of measurement that expresses the amount of resistance to the flow of an electric current.

Deionization – The process by which ions with an electrical charge are removed from water.

Reverse osmosis – The diffusion (flowing) of water through a semi-permeable membrane to eliminate impurities that it contains.

Silicate – A mineral commonly found in water that is derived from silca found in quartz and other components.

Chloride – A compound commonly found in water that is created when chlorine is combined with another element or radical. (Examples: a salt or hydrochloric acid.)

---

is usually 400 parts per million (ppm) or more. The ideal level in water used for cleaning is 100 ppm or less. Silicates can leave a bluish or rainbow stain on stainless steel that can be removed by reducing the concentration of silicates in the water before continued processing. It is important to conduct daily tests for a few weeks to assure the silicate level is consistently at 100 ppm or less.

It is important to remove dissolved solids from the water before they become visible on the instruments and cleaning machines used for processing. Why? It doesn't make sense to use dirty water in the cleaning process to rinse instruments that have just been cleaned.

Acidity or Alkalinity

The acidity or alkalinity (pH) of the water plays an important role in cleaning because the water interacts with products that also have a specific pH level. If the pH of water and the product being cleaned are the same, the pH will not change. However, if they are different, they will change. Purified water should have a pH of 6.5 – 7.5.

Chlorides — *Cause Rusting on instruments.*

Chlorides are always found in treated water. There are many types of chlorides including sodium chloride, potassium chloride, and ammonium chloride. Most tap water has a chloride concentration of 400 ppm or more. The goal: 100 ppm or less. In high concentrations, chloride will attack the instruments being cleaned, eventually find a weak spot in the finish, and expose the core metal and allow corrosion to accelerate. Chloride test kits are available that use a measured number of drops of a testing agent in a bottle containing a specified amount of the water being tested. The water will turn to a specific color that can then be compared to a color chart to determine the concentration (ppm) of chloride in the water.

Other Particles

Particles are usually small solid objects such as pieces of rusted piping, and minuscule pieces of rubber, plastic, filter elements, and other materials.

Water can also contain sediment: small solid objects usually from the bottom of the water source such as sand, clay, and dirt. These and other elements in the water can cause it to look cloudy or dirty. Water professionals use their eyes to determine the **turbidity** of the water, and to note any materials at the bottom of a collection device. Gases in the water can also make the water look turbid; however, after a period of time, the water will degas, and become more clear. Particles and sediment in water make it dirty, and the cleaning ability of the detergents used with dirty water is greatly reduced.

OVERVIEW OF WATER PURIFICATION SYSTEMS

Learning Objective 3. Provide an overview of components and products that are important in water purification systems.

Many different system components play a role in an effective water purification process, and each must be in good working order. Filters, granular activated carbon (GAC), softeners, and deionization products are required to purify the water, and cost effectiveness is important as this is done. For example, the main component of a reverse osmosis system is an expensive membrane material. If tap water flows over this membrane without being pre-treated, the membrane will require more frequent maintenance and replacement. Water in a reverse osmosis system is usually run through a pre-filter, softener, another pre-filter, the reverse osmosis membrane, and then still another filter.

When a deionization system is used, if tap water entering the deionization tanks has not been pre-treated, the tanks will not be able to effectively remove the positive and negative charged elements in the water. Also, more frequent service to and replacement of the tanks will be necessary. In a typical deionization system, the water usually flows through a pre-filter, GAC, another filter, the deionization tanks, and then a post (after) filter.

Filters

Filters are made of numerous materials for the different applications for which they are used. They are used on sterilizers for air and steam, to treat water in the cleaning process, and for peracitic acid in the peracitic acid processes. Steam filters are usually made of a solid ceramic or steel mesh, while filters for treating water and air are usually made of different types of plastics or textile fibers. Both are usually inside a cartridge housing that is snapped or bolted into the plumbing or air line.

Filter manufacturers must be consulted about length of use before replacement, but most filters are replaced according to the results of pressure gauge tests on the water or before it enters and after it leaves the filter. When filters are new, the pressures on both gauges are almost the same. When the gauge measuring the steam or water after it leaves the filter indicates a drop in pressure, this indicates that the filter is getting clogged, and must be replaced. Some manufacturers require steam filter replacement as frequently as every six weeks, so it is important to read and follow the manufacturer's replacement recommendations.

The size of filters to be used is also important. The filter size is measured in **microns**. For steam, filtering is not done to eliminate bacteria but, rather, to eliminate particles that might otherwise break free in the steam lines. Some filters eliminate chemicals that might be transferred in the steam. The size of steam filters vary from 1, 5, or 25 microns in size.

Turbidity – *Occurs when water contains sediments or solids that, when stirred, make the water appear cloudy.*

Tap water – *Water that has been treated, and is acceptable for drinking.*

Microns – *Unit of measurement; 1/1000 of a millimeter or 1/25,000 of an inch, or one millionth of a meter. (Note: a meter equals 39.37 inches.)*

Cation resin tank – *A tank into which untreated hard water flows, and in which sodium ions are exchanged for calcium and magnesium ions to produce soft water.*

Water purification usually involves a pre-and post-filter. The pre-filter is larger than the post-filter. The size of filters for deionization or reverse osmosis systems range from a 1–.5 micron pre-filter to a .5–.2 micron post-filter. Steam sterilizers use only one air filter, and it is usually a sub-micron filter (below 1 micron).

Granular Activated Charcoal (GAC)

Granular Activated Charcoal (GAC) is used to remove chlorides in water. A common example of its usage occurs in a fresh water fish aquarium. GAC filters (most people call this charcoal) must be placed in a holder through which the aquarium water runs. Without the GAC, the fish would die from excessive chlorides. GAC is also used to treat water in a deionization or reverse osmosis system. The GAC cartridge or tank is placed before the system to reduce the chlorides that would otherwise inhibit the effectiveness of a deionization system or dissolve the membrane in a reverse osmosis system. Testing the water with a chloride test kit can determine when the tank needs to be changed, or when the cartridge needs to be replaced. An acceptable amount of chlorides in the final water is 100 ppm or less.

Softeners

Softeners are used to remove the calcium and magnesium in the water, and the word, "softened," describes the result of the process. Calcium and magnesium are the main elements that contribute to the "hardness" of water. When they are removed, the water is softened. The process involves use of a **cation resin tank**. The resin contains positively-charged (cation) ions that attract the negatively charged (anion) ions of calcium and magnesium. When the resin has attracted all the negatively charged minerals it can hold, the tank needs to be recharged or back-washed. This process strips and washes away the minerals that have been attracted, and allows the resin to be recharged (renewed) with a positive charge.

DISTILLATION, DEIONIZATION, AND REVERSE OSMOSIS SYSTEMS

Learning Objective 4. Explain the basics of distillation, deionization, and reverse osmosis water purification systems.

In the past, distillation was the only process used in purifying water, and produced the quality of water that was used to prepare and sterilize solutions. While the United States Pharmacopeia (USP) dictates the water quality used to prepare solutions, it does not address the quality of water needed for decontamination purposes. Distillation removes dissolved solids, gasses and organics, along with particles, bacteria, pyrogens (pus-producing organisms,) and endotoxins. Because the sterilization of water is more commercialized these days, the use of the still is often limited to making fill water for filling heating/cooling therapy units. Stills used to make distilled water can become the source of contamination because of limited use and maintenance.

Distillation

When distilled water became less expensive to buy than to produce, most Central Service Departments discontinued the use of stills. Reverse osmosis systems became more affordable for many

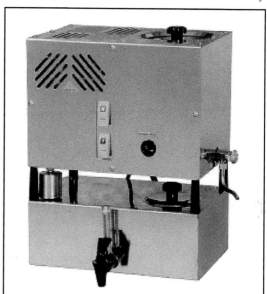

Figure 7.1

decontamination purposes, and type 1 or type 2 deionized water systems were recommended for washer decontaminators. Small and reasonably inexpensive stills can still be purchased for use with heating/cooling therapy units. (See **Figure 7.1**) However, most water treatment systems contain a valve that can be turned to obtain water for these units so the purchase of a still for this purpose is not necessary.

Deionization

Deionization systems are used for heating/cooling therapy units, and for the final rinse water in manual and automated cleaning processes. They use a combination of a pre-filter, GAC, another filter, cation resin tank (or tanks), and a post-filter to remove the ionic-charged elements in the water. A single bed tank includes a single cation and single anion tank, or one mixed tank which includes both the cation-and anion-charged resins. A dual bed tank contains two cation-and two anion-charged tanks or two mixed tanks. One advantage of a dual bed system: when tanks must be changed, the water can flow through another set of tanks, so water quality is not interrupted. By contrast, when the tank in a single bed system must be charged, one must either call the replacement source, and/ or send the tanks out to be recharged. With either option, the quality of water is interrupted, but the decision is usually based on available storage space.

A resistivity light is included at the end of the last tank to detect the water's ionic charge. If an ionic charge is detected, the electricity to the light is interrupted, and the light will not stay on. Note:

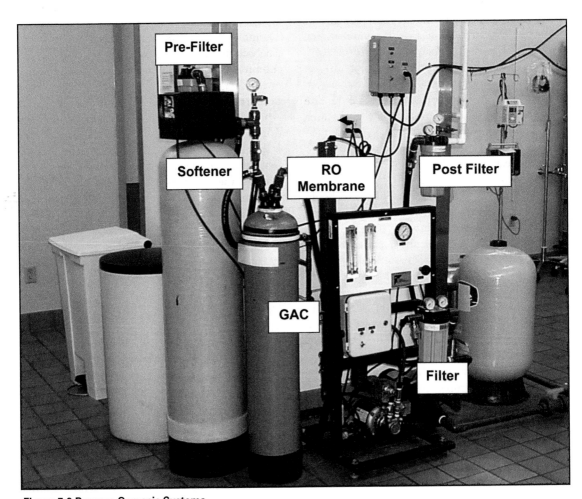

Figure 7.2 Reverse Osmosis Systems

If water has not flowed through the tanks for a period of time, the light might also go out. This can occur, for example, on the morning after a day when the water was not used and the water settled. Then it is necessary to allow water to flow through the tanks for a few minutes to assess whether the sensor re-lights.

Running water through the tank system helps prevent the need for premature changing of the tanks. Plumbing for the system must be specially manufactured for deionization systems because the use of other materials allow plumbing materials to leech into (cling to) the water. No metal of any kind should be used in the plumbing system unless it has no contact with the water. While the deionization process does remove dissolved solids and gases, it provides for little or no removal of organics, particles, bacteria, pyrogens, and endotoxins. This is why filters must be part of the system.

Reverse Osmosis

Reverse Osmosis systems (see **Figure 7.2**) require the water to be treated by (in sequence) a pre-filter, softener, GAC, and another filter. The water then flows across a vertical membrane filter. When the osmotic pressure on the side of the membrane increases, water passes through the membrane before going through a post-filter. The water should be circulating continuously. Plumbing and system components through which water passes, must be manufactured for reverse osmosis systems because other products can leech into the water.

Testing the quality of water for total dissolved solids, pH, conductivity, chlorides, silicates, and particles will determine if the system is working correctly. Maintenance on the system should be performed by someone qualified in reverse osmosis systems, because the expensive membrane can be damaged if it is not handled correctly. Reverse osmosis can remove a large percentage of dissolved solids and organics, and it is capable of removing all particles, bacteria, pyrogens, and endotoxins. However, it removes little, if any, dissolved gases.

CLEANING CHEMICALS

Learning Objective 5. Identify common cleaning chemicals, and review basic protocols for their use.

Different types of chemicals are used in the cleaning process including enzymatic products, detergents, descalers, and pre-soaks. Each has a specific purpose in efficiently processing reusable supplies and equipment, and each must be used according to the manufacturer's instructions. It is also against Federal Law to use these products for unintended purposes.

Close Look at Cleaning Chemicals

Enzymatic products – There are different types of enzymatic products. Some can be used at the point of use to decontaminate and loosen the soil on instruments, and others are used in manual or automatic washing processes. Enzymes are catalysts that can accelerate the speed of chemical reactions without being consumed by the reaction or becoming part of the product formed. Enzyme products contain protease enzymes that are especially useful in removing proteins such as dried-on blood and tissue. The role of temperature is very important when dealing with enzyme-based products. Temperatures should not exceed 140° F because the enzymes become inactive. Multi-enzymatic products contain protease (for protein soils), lipase (for fats), and amylase (for starches).

Detergents take longer to clean if they are not used in conjunction with protease enzymes or multi-enzymes. When mixed with water, detergents enhance the water's ability to remove soil. Detergents do not kill microorganisms; however, germicidal detergents do have this capability.

Detergents contain emulsifiers and chelating agents. Chelating agents have an ionic charge that allows soils with the opposite charge to break away and attach to the chelating agent. An emulsifier surrounds these particles to prevent them from re-attaching, and they also help to break bonds that oils can create to trap soil. Alkaline detergents (pH 10–11.5) are effective at removing organic soils; however, they can leave an alkaline residual film. When they are used, an acidic detergent (pH 3–4.5) wash should follow.

Acidic detergents work well on inorganic soils, neutralize alkaline residues, and make stainless steel shine. However, concentrations must be monitored because the use of improper amounts hinders effective cleaning, and instruments can be damaged. Products such as colored anodized aluminum should not be cleaned with high acid detergents because the coloring will be removed. Use of neutral-to-moderately alkaline pH detergents (ph 7–8.5) can help to prevent this problem. Neutral pH detergents, however, require more mechanical action than their higher alkaline pH counterparts to remove soils.

Descalers – Descalers are not typically required if the water quality and soap/detergent mixtures are correct, and if equipment is operating properly. However, this is not always the case, and problems can go unnoticed until a chalky-powdery, hard-to-remove substance appears on the walls of equipment and sinks. Then an acidic detergent or a descaler is needed to remove the scale. Note: acidic detergents can also be used, but they must be reapplied to improve the surface of the metal. Descalers are specifically made to remove this scale. A smaller quantity of this product will be needed than if an acidic detergent is used; however, both are the products of choice to remove scale.

Pre-soaking chemicals – Pre-cleaning or pre-soaking products are used in the first step in the decontamination process. Some commonly used pre-cleaning agents are plain water, detergent solutions, enzymatic detergents, and combination enzyme-germicide detergents.

The process of pre-cleaning should begin immediately after the completion of any invasive procedure. Blood and other visible debris, if left on an instrument, serve as a reservoir for microbial growth, and may damage an instrument's finish. If not removed, the corrosive agents in blood and body tissue can penetrate the protective outer layer of an instrument, and cause rusting or pitting of the stainless steel. The manufacturers' directions must be followed when using these pre-cleaning products, because exceeding the time allowed for the instruments to be immersed in the solution can damage and corrode them. These products are extremely helpful in reducing the time to remove soil in the cleaning process.

Manual cleaners – These products, when mixed properly, make the water "wetter," and help it to penetrate under the soil and break the bond that attaches the soil to the instruments. Their main function, then, is to remove soil, not kill microorganisms. Manual cleaners should be low-foaming and free-rinsing. The manufacturer's directions should be followed for proper dilution in the quality of water being supplied. This source should also be consulted to determine the proper water temperature when using the product for manual cleaning. However, hot water is a common temperature for manual cleaning.

Mechanical cleaning processes for ultrasonic washers, washer sterilizers, washer decontaminators/disinfectors, cart washers, and automatic endoscopic reprocessors, require the use of products such as enzymatics, multi-enzymes, detergents, and soaps. The equipment manufacturer's written instructions (not those of the solution's manufacturer), must be referenced for recommended cleaning solutions for the equipment. If the wrong product is selected, possible premature replacement or damage to the equipment's components may occur, and it may be impossible to properly clean the instrumentation. Chemicals that are used should be low-foaming, and easily removed with rinsing. Water temperatures are usually controlled by the machine, but some equipment allows Central Service Technicians to make adjustments that enable them to more closely follow temperature usage instructions for specific cleaning products. As with any chemical, no matter what it is used for, the manufacturer's directions must be understood and followed. Failure to do so can cause injury and/or damage to the equipment/instruments.

Safety Precautions

Central Service Technicians working with chemical solutions and around blood and body fluids must be protected, and even those who are not working with these materials but who are in the area must still wear personal protective equipment (PPE).

Forearm-length gloves made specifically for decontamination, a fluid-impervious gown, face shield, and rubber shoes or decontamination shoe covers should be worn when performing cleaning duties including pre-cleaning, cleaning, and loading automated machines.

Never mix chemicals unless the product is an activator or catalyst for another product that requires mixing. Doing so can cause injury or even death. Some chemicals when mixed together can create a gas that might not be noticeable until one has become overcome by fumes and passes out. Always follow the manufacturer's dilution instructions when mixing chemicals with water. Problems associated with improper dilution range from an irritated nose, throat or eyes, to nose bleed, dizziness, chemical burn, and even asphyxiation. Always read the precautions and warnings of any product you use. Material Safety Data Sheets (MSDS) are required for these products, and must be available for Central Service Technicians to read and study. The temperature of the water and products used with it are important for effective cleaning. For example, cold (not hot) water should be used to remove blood. When cleaning blood from instruments, first run cold water over them to help remove the visible blood. Then the selected cleaning process should be used while following the manufacturer's water temperature instructions for the products.

Some products are more effective in hot water because molecules move more quickly. Temperatures for hot water range from 120°F–165°F. Water heaters must be used to increase the temperature of water to these levels. While the temperature of the tap water coming into the sink cannot be increased, automated machines have steam-or electrically-heated coils to raise the temperature to a pre-determined setting. Steam will heat the water more quickly than an electric coil if time is an important concern.

Product Disposal Concerns

Manufacturer's labels and MSDS materials always indicate that city, county, and state laws concerning disposal should be followed. Note: Federal laws require that cleaning products be used in the ways for which they are intended. Begin by learning about city laws as they can be more stringent than county or state requirements. Conversely, county and state regulations must also be reviewed because they may be more stringent. City, county, and state environmental or hazardous waste departments are excellent sources for applicable regulations in these jurisdictions.

Never pour chemicals down a sink, because they usually enter the sewer system, and this can be very dangerous. As well, city, county, state, or Environmental Protection Agency (EPA) inspectors may take water samples down from the flow direction of the facility. Concentrations of chemicals that are too high can lead to significant fines, and it is important to never mislead officials about chemical problems.

CLEANING TOOLS

Learning Objective 6. Note the importance of brushes, cloths, and sponges in an effective cleaning process.

Brushes, cloths, sponges, and other items including stylets and high pressure nozzles for water and air are also required for the cleaning process. Brushes are available in many different diameters and lengths to accommodate special needs. Some must be rigid, and others must be flexible to properly clean the many different lumens and channels in modern instruments.

Brushes used for cleaning are usually made of nylon bristles; however, cloth and cotton varieties are also available. Some are impregnated with enzymes, and help with the decontamination process while they are used to clean scopes. Brushes should be disposable. However, if reused, they should be cleaned of visible soil, and be subjected to a cold or hot sterilization process at least daily to assure they are not a source of contamination.

Abrasive brushes should never be used because they can scratch the surface of the instrument and accelerate corrosion. If metal or wire brushes are used for instrument cleaning, they should be approved for use on surgical instruments. Note: numerous types of buffing wheels can be used on a bench grinder to help remove stains, and are just as effective as a wire brush without causing instrument damage. Repair vendors often use these types of grinders to remove stains from instruments.

Brushing should be done under water by following the grain, if any, on the instrument to prevent the formation of aerosols. Instrument manufacturers should be consulted, and their recommendations should be followed to maintain any potential warranty.

Wash cloths are made of textiles. Some have lint and others are low-or-lint free. If cloths similar to rest room washcloths are used, they must be inspected for lint fibers that might become entrapped on the instrument. Use of a lint-free or low-lint cloth such as a surgical towel reduces this risk. Cloths should be changed regularly, or when visibly soiled or stained. When using a cloth towel, verify that the cleaning chemicals used will not be deactivated by the cloth product.

Sponges can be used to clean basins, containers, and trays. They should be replaced daily to assure they will not become a source of contamination. Unfortunately, their structure makes them virtually impossible to completely clean and sterilize for reuse, and their low cost makes this recommendation very feasible.

CENTRAL SERVICE TERMS

Ohm

Conductivity (of water)

Deionization

Reverse osmosis

Silicate

Chloride

Turbidity

Tap water

Microns

Cation resin tank

Chapter Outline

Chapter Learning Objectives

Chapter 8

Decontamination; Point of Use Preparation and Transport

As a result of successfully completing this chapter, readers will be able to:

1. Review the three priority goals of soiled item transport.

2. Identify the sources of contaminated items.

3. Explain point-of-use preparation procedures.

4. Review basic procedures to transport soiled items from user areas to the Central Service decontamination area.

5. Discuss safety guidelines for transporting soiled items to the Central Service decontamination area.

6. Provide basic sources for education and training information applicable to the transport of contaminated items.

Reusable instruments, equipment, and utensils processed in the Central Service Department are transported to patient care and treatment areas where they are then used in a wide variety of procedures and care applications. After use, they must be transported back to the Central Service decontamination area to be reprocessed for subsequent reuse. Sometimes the transport distance is only a few feet between the user department and Central Service. In other cases, however, items may need to be transported a few miles (or more) between facilities. This chapter reviews recommended protocols and requirements for these transportation activities.

GOALS OF SOILED ITEM TRANSPORT

Learning Objective 1. Review the three priority goals of soiled item transport.

Regardless of transport distance, there are always three priority goals of soiled item transport:

- To prepare contaminated items so that they will not be damaged after use, and before return to the Central Service department in the decontamination area.

- To transport the soiled items without cross-contaminating the environment between the point-of-use and the decontamination area.

- To assure that all individuals who may come in contact with contaminated items remain safe during the transportation process.

The remainder of the chapter explains basic methods to achieve these goals.

SOURCES OF CONTAMINATED ITEMS

Learning Objective 2. Identify the sources of contaminated items.

There are two common points-of-use for devices that will require preparation and transport (return) to Central Service. High volumes of contaminated items will be used in surgery, and lesser numbers of items will be used in other departments including Labor and Delivery, Emergency Services, Endoscopy, and the Cardiac Catherization Lab.

In many facilities, the Central Service decontamination area is located close to the Surgery department. That is the logistical choice because Surgery is the source of the majority of soiled items transported to Central Service. Sometimes the decontamination area is adjacent to Surgery. Enclosed carts filled with contaminated instruments, equipment, and utensils, can be easy, quickly, and safely transported to the decontamination area through a connecting hallway. If the Central Service department is located on another level of the facility, items can be transported between floors using a dedicated elevator or dumbwaiter system that is designed and used exclusively to transport contaminated items. Soiled (contaminated) items from other departments may be retrieved and returned to the Central Service decontamination area after a telephone or computer request is made by user department personnel. Sometimes soiled items may be delivered to the decontamination area by employees of the user department. For example, Surgery staff return case carts to the decontamination area after surgical procedures. Generally, however, contaminated items are placed in a designated holding area to be picked-up by Central Service Technicians at designated times.

Holding Items Until Return to Central Service

All departments that use and store reusable items for later transport to the Central Service Department need a designated holding area for contaminated items until they can be retrieved. These areas should be clearly designated with **biohazard signage**, and should not be accessible to visitors or other unauthorized personnel. The contaminated holding area should have contaminated trash and linen receptacles, and a dedicated hand washing sink. Areas where liquid waste (blood, suction canister contents, etc.) may be an issue, will also need a shielded flush-type commode for liquid waste disposal.

POINT-OF-USE PREPARATION

Learning Objective 3. Explain point-of-use preparation procedures.

Instrument decontamination begins at point-of-use, and is then continued in the Central Service decontamination area. Central Service personnel must enlist the help of user departments to insure that instruments and equipment are prepared for the decontamination process immediately after use.

Reasons for Point-of-Use Preparation

There are two important reasons that the preparation process should begin in the user department at point-of-use:

• Point-of-use preparation helps prolong the life of instruments. Common substances such as blood and saline to which instruments are exposed during procedures can break down the devices' protective finish, and hasten their decomposition.

• Soil and debris that dry on instruments are much more difficult to remove than moist soil and debris, especially in instruments with lumens and hard-to-reach crevices. Those substances also break down the instruments' protective finishes.

Sometimes more aggressive cleaning methods must be used, and instruments with dried soil also take longer to clean. This can increase processing time, and that delay may impact their availability for subsequent use.

The proper care and handling of instruments and equipment is the responsibility of everyone who comes in contact with them, and these concerns begin with personnel at the point-of-use.

✳ *Biohazard signage –Notices posted in easily-seen locations that alert persons in the area about the presence of harmful bacteria, viruses, or other dangerous biohazardous agents or organisms.*

✳ *Gross soil –Tissue, body fat, blood, and other body substances.*

Point-of-Use Preparation Guidelines

Point-of-use preparation does not replace the cleaning process. Instead, its purpose is to begin the cleaning process. The following guidelines should be followed when users prepare items for transport to the Central Service decontamination area:

• Remove gross soil. **Gross soil** should be removed immediately after use.

• Follow manufacturer's instructions for point-of-use cleaning. Some manufacturers provide instructions for point-of-use cleaning. For example, flexible fiberoptic endoscope manufacturers typically suggest that water be suctioned through the scope's suction channel at the end of a procedure to preclean the suction channel and to remove loose debris. Information for proper point-of-use cleaning and preparation of instruments should be provided by the manufacturer of the instruments.

• Keep soiled instruments moist. Keep instruments moist to prevent soil from drying on their surface. This can be accomplished by spraying them with an enzyme product, soaking them in an enzyme solution or water, or placing a moist towel over them. Instruments should be arranged in an orderly fashion with their box locks (hinges) in the open position. Note: if instruments are placed in a soak basin or solution, they should not be exposed to the solution for an extended period of time, because this may damage the instruments' surface. Also, the soak solution must be removed before transport to reduce the risk of spills.

• Remove disposable components; use proper disposal methods. Remove disposable components such as blades, disposable tubing, and canisters. Sharp items should be placed in a hard-sided container labeled biohazard. Separating disposable from reusable components reduces the amount of contaminated items that must be transported, and it also reduces the risk of injury from "**sharps**" such as knife blades and needles. When separating disposable items, watch closely to insure that reusable items are not removed and discarded with disposable components (Example: metal drape clamps are sometimes left attached to disposable drapes.)

- **Separate reusable linen.** Reusable linen should be removed, and placed into an appropriate bag or container. Users should use extra caution to insure that small instruments are not mistakenly included with the linen.

- **Empty fluids from containers.** If a contaminated device has a reusable fluid container, bottle, or receptacle, fluid should be removed and disposed of according to the facility's protocols. Disposable fluid containers should also be handled according to required facility procedures.

- **Separate reusable sharps from other instruments.** Place instruments with sharp points or edges such as reusable needles, cutting edges, and skin hooks in a separate container so they can be easily identified, and to reduce the risk of injuries from sharps.

- **Keep items together.** Instrument sets or multi-part items should be kept together for their transport to the Central Service decontamination area. If items are separated or left behind, re-assembly will be delayed. Failure to keep items together also increases the risk that components will be misplaced or lost.

- **Notify the Central Service Department about items needing repair.** If instruments or equipment are in need of repair, tag them so they can be removed from the system for repair or refurbishing. (See **Figure 8.1**)

Central Service departments must work together with end users to insure that point of use preparation is carried out according to specific requirements. In many cases, departments will need to develop joint procedures for the handling of used items to insure that everyone involved understands their role in the process.

TRANSPORT OF SOILED ITEMS

Learning Objective 4. Review basic procedures to transport soiled items from user areas to the Central Service decontamination area.

Contaminated items should be contained before transport through the facility to minimize airborne or contact spread of microorganisms, and to reduce the risk of cross-contamination and infection. Instruments from surgical procedures can be transported in enclosed carts (see **Figure 8.2**). If a transport cart that is not enclosed is used, the cart must have a solid bottom shelf to prevent drips and spills, and the cart should be covered during transport. Smaller numbers of instruments from other departments can be transported in dedicated transport containers (see **Figure 8.3**), or in plastic bags that are clearly labeled, "Biohazard". Large items such as suction units and other types of patient care equipment can be transported in special carts designed for soiled item transport. (See **Figure 8.4**)

The goal of all enclosed transport is to transfer the contaminated items to the Central Service decontamination area while minimizing the risk of cross-contamination. All transport devices must be free from external gross contamination (such as blood) before transport to reduce the risk of environmental contamination and personnel exposure.

Sometimes contaminated items may need to be transported between buildings or campuses of multi-campus health care systems to a centralized decontamination area. When it is necessary to

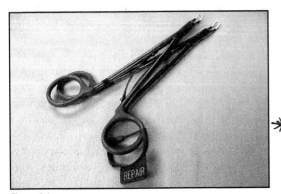

Figure 8.1

Sharps—*Cutting instruments including knives, scalpels, blades, needles, and scissors of all types. Other examples includes chisels and osteotomes, some curettes, dissectors and elevators, rongeurs and cutting forceps, punches, saws, and trocars.*

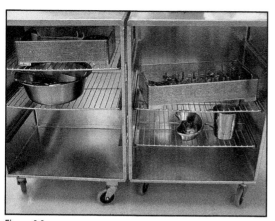

Figure 8.2

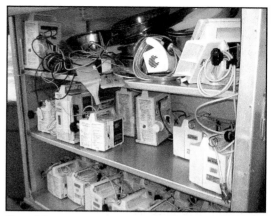

Figure 8.4

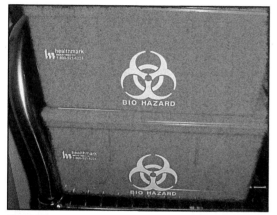

Figure 8.3

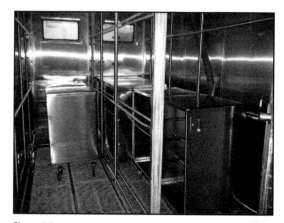

Figure 8.5

transport contaminated items using a truck or van, facility personnel must consult U.S. Department of Transportation (DOT) guidelines, and follow applicable state and local requirements for the safe transport of biohazard materials.

Personnel transporting contaminated items should be trained in and must consistently follow safe handling procedures. These include methods to safely load transport devices to avoid spillage, and to assure that items are securely contained.

The transport of contaminated items should be kept physically separate from the transport of their clean and sterile counterparts. Containers and carts used for transporting contaminated items should not be used to transport and deliver clean items unless they are thoroughly decontaminated between uses. For example, surgical case carts are used to transport soiled instruments from surgery to the decontamination area and then decontaminated so

they can be used to transport sterile packages back to surgery. **Figure 8.5** is a photo of a mechanical cartwasher used to decontaminate carts after they have transported soiled items..

Ideally, items from surgery should be transported to the Central Service decontamination area immediately after use. As you've learned, this reduces the opportunity for soil to dry on the instruments, and this practice also allows the items to be returned to service in a timely manner.

Contaminated items from other departments are often placed in a holding area for pick-up on a scheduled basis by Central Service Technicians who then return them to the decontamination area for processing. These rounds should be conducted as scheduled, because failure to perform soiled item pick-ups can lead to equipment and instrument shortages. All health care facilities have limited numbers of instrument sets and patient care equipment. The instrument and equipment replenishment system relies on items moving through the system (from storage to use to processing and back to storage) on a timely basis to maintain an adequate supply of available instruments and equipment.

SAFETY GUIDELINES FOR SOILED ITEM TRANSPORT

Learning Objective 5. Discuss safety guidelines for transporting soiled items to the Central Service decontamination area.

All instruments, utensils, and equipment used in patient care and treatment processes should be considered contaminated, and they should be handled as such. Central Service Technicians who transport contaminated items should wear a protective gown or coat over their scrubs. They should also wear gloves to handle the items as they are picked- up and placed into the transport cart. The gloves should then be removed and hands should be washed.

Whenever there is a danger of splashes, spills, or aerosol exposure, Central Service Technicians should wear the appropriate Personal Protective Equipment (PPE) required by Occupational Safety and Health Administration (OSHA) regulations. Central Service Technicians who are assigned to clean and decontaminate the soiled items must also follow OSHA regulations for PPE.

Transporting equipment and carts through corridors can also pose significant safety concerns. Central Service Technicians must maintain control of transport carts at all times and should refrain from moving them at excessive speeds. Patients, visitors, other health care providers, and movable equipment share the same hallways as transport carts and excessive speed or inattention could lead to accidents. Central Service Technicians should maintain control of their carts and pay particular attention to hallway intersections and doors that may open into the path of the cart. Many facilities install safety mirrors at hallway junctions to help prevent accidents. (See **Figure 8.6**)

In addition to maintaining safe control of their transport carts, Central Service Technicians should always yield to patients and visitors in hallways and at elevators. In any health care facility, the routine transport of soiled items never takes precedence over the transport of patients.

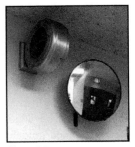

Figure 8.6

EDUCATION AND TRAINING

Learning Objective 6. Provide basic sources for education and training information applicable to the transport of contaminated items.

When performed improperly, the transport of contaminated items can pose a threat to the safety of patients, visitors, and employees. Carefully thought out procedures must be developed to help assure that all contaminated items are appropriately handled. The development of these procedures should be done with the input and/or support of the facility's Infection Control and Hazardous Materials committees.

Recommended practices for contaminated item transport are provided by the Association for the Advancement of Medical Instrumentation (AAMI).[1] Procedures should also reflect Occupational Safety and Health Administration (OSHA) regulations.[2] Additional information regarding soiled instrument preparation and transport can be obtained from the Association for periOperative Nurses (AORN).[3]

Everyone who may have contact with contaminated items must be educated about the dangers associated with biohazardous items. In addition to education and training for Central Service Technicians, this includes Environmental Service employees, courier and transport technicians, and drivers. Their education should include proper handling of biohazardous items, and the correct application and use of PPE.

IN CONCLUSION

Point-of-use instrument preparation requires a partnership between the Central Service and user departments. Good communication and training can help personnel in both departments to protect their facility's instruments, and to better serve the patients. By understanding and following the recommended guidelines for the preparation and transport of contaminated items, Central Service Technicians help to protect patients, visitors, and their health care worker peers.

ENDNOTES

1. AAMI. Comprehensive Guide to Steam Sterilization and Sterility Assurance in Health Care Facilities. ANSI/AAMI ST79: 2006. (pp. 38-41 and Appendix G). (Information is available at: www.aami.org)

2. U.S Department of Labor, Occupational Safety and Health Administration, Regulations Standards CFR 1910.1030, Bloodborne Pathogens. (Information is available at: www.osha.gov)

3. Recommended Practices for Cleaning And Caring For Surgical Instruments And Powered Equipment. In Standards, Recommended Practices and Guidelines (Denver: AORN, Inc, 2006) p. 555-557. (Information is available at: www.aorn.org)

CENTRAL SERVICE TERMS

Biohazard signage

Gross soil

Sharps

Chapter Outline

Chapter 9
Cleaning and Decontamination

Chapter Learning Objectives

As a result of successfully completing this chapter, readers will be able to:

1. Discuss basic factors that impact cleaning and decontamination:
    - Design and location of decontamination area
    - Environmental design and controls
    - Housekeeping concerns
    - Staff safety and personal attire
    - Staff education and training

2. Describe important selection and usage concerns for cleaning agents (water, detergents, enzymes, and enzymatic detergents) and for lubricants.

3. Explain details about cleaning and decontamination, and review manual procedures and mechanical methods to complete both processes.

4. Discuss procedures to clean basic types of instruments:
    - General cleaning protocols
    - Delicate and hard-to-clean instruments
    - Instrument containers and basins
    - Power equipment
    - Mobile patient care equipment
    - Verification and quality control tactics

5. Review procedures to manage infectious waste.

Cleaning refers to the removal of all visible and non-visible soil, and any other foreign material from the medical device being reprocessed. It is the most important step in the disinfection/sterilization process. Instruments must be thoroughly cleaned and rinsed for subsequent reprocessing steps to be effective. *Decontamination* relates to removing or reducing contamination by infectious organisms or other harmful substances. Together, cleaning and decontamination are important early steps in reprocessing. The use of established principles and procedures is required to assure that these steps in the sterilization process will be effective. The cleaning task is the topic of this chapter.

BASIC FACTORS THAT IMPACT CLEANING AND DECONTAMINATION

Learning Objective 1. Discuss basic factors that impact cleaning and decontamination:
- Design and location of decontamination area.
- Environmental design and controls.
- Housekeeping concerns.
- Staff safety and personal attire.
- Staff education and training.

Design and Location of Decontamination Area

Several design-related factors must be considered as the decontamination area is planned. First, since effective decontamination is an expensive process, it is more cost-effective to centralize processing to one area. (If this is not done, principles discussed throughout this book should be duplicated in other areas where decontamination/reprocessing occurs.)

The location of the decontamination area should consider the needs to transport contaminated devices to/from the points of use, and for efficient and effective cleaning and decontamination after items to be processed reach the area. Contaminated devices should be contained from the point of use to the decontamination area. This requires direct accessibility to the area through corridors or dedicated dumbwaiters or elevators.

The square footage of required floor space for decontamination is at least as much as the floor space dedicated to the clean/sterile preparation area. When it is not, slowed decontamination can disrupt the flow of instrument processing. This space must allow several Central Service Technicians to perform required work tasks.

The Association for the Advancement of Medical Instrumentation (AAMI) has specific and detailed guidelines relating to the design, structure, and general considerations for the decontamination workspace, and for the safe handling of medical devices. Working with the American National Standards Institute (ANSI), it has developed ANSI/AAMI Standard ST79: 2006: "Comprehensive guide to steam sterilization and sterility assurance in health care facilities". This document addresses requirements for decontamination areas and should be used as a template when decontamination areas are designed. There are many health care design firms that specialize in designing sterile reprocessing centers that can assist with new or rehabilitated workspace projects. The American Institute of Architects (AIA) consults with the United States Department of Health and Human Services, and other federal regulatory agencies to develop recommendations for basic design elements of reprocessing workspaces.

Cleaning – The removal of all visible and non-visible soil, and any other foreign material from the medical device being reprocessed.

Decontamination – Removing or reducing contamination by infectious organisms or other harmful substances.

Relative humidity – The amount of water vapor in the atmosphere expressed as a percentage of the total amount of vapor the atmosphere could hold without condensation.

Biohazardous – A term relating to infectious agents that present a risk or potential risk to human health either directly through infections or indirectly through the environment.

Cleaning is Fundamental

Manufacturers of reusable medical devices provide instructions about how to reprocess their devices between patient uses. Disease transmission between patients or from environmental sources to a patient is a problem that can be caused by improperly processed medical devices. Other problems resulting from improper processing include inadequate and unacceptable device performance, or even failure (breakage), since instruments cannot perform if they have debris such as soil or rust on them.

Cleaning is the first step in reprocessing a device after use. Failure to properly clean an instrument may permit foreign material (for example, soil, organic materials including microorganisms, and inorganic matter and lubricants) located outside and inside of the device to hinder the disinfection and/or sterilization processes. Cleaning is normally accomplished by manual wiping, brushing, or flushing, or by using mechanical aids such as water and detergents to remove foreign material.

Environmental Design and Controls

Floors and walls in the decontamination area should be constructed with materials that can tolerate harsh chemicals. Walls should not be constructed of particulate or fiber-shedding materials. Spills and splashes are a common occurrence in the decontamination area, and this can create a need for frequent cleaning/disinfecting. Floor drains should be positioned and designed to provide adequate drainage.

The ventilation system should allow for no less than 10 air exchanges per hour, and the area should be under negative pressure from other areas within the Central Service department. Temperature should be regulated between 16°C and 18°C (60°F and 65°F). This low temperature is needed because Central Service Technicians working in the decontamination room require fluid-resistant attire that, when worn for extended periods of time, becomes hot. A low temperature also helps inhibit the growth of microorganisms. **Relative humidity** is also important, and should range from 30% to 60%.

Lighting is essential to a safe work environment, and is a key element in the cleaning process. Lighting in the decontamination area should be adequate for detailed cleaning and inspection. The Illuminating Engineering Society of North America (IES) recommends that lighting be based on three main factors; the age of the workers, the importance of speed or accuracy, and the amount of light reflection in the work area. Adequate lighting can improve cleaning processes and reduce worker eye strain.

Traffic should be restricted to personnel working in the area, and access to the area should be controlled. Emergency eyewash/shower equipment (See **Figure 9.1**) should be placed so these safety stations are accessible within 10 seconds or 30 meters of potential chemical exposure. Note: An eye wash station may be installed on a sink faucet (See **Figure 9.2**). Hand washing stations should also be provided, and they should be designed so hand contact with the faucet during operation is not necessary. Hand wash stations should not be used to clean medical devices.

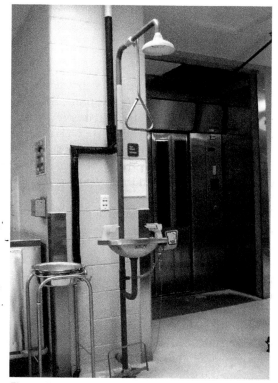

Figure 9.1

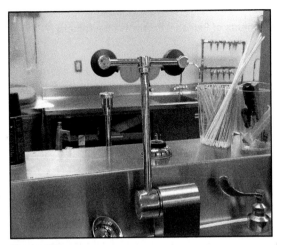

Figure 9.2

Housekeeping Concerns

The decontamination area is the central point for handling contaminated devices, and there will be a high microbial count in the environment. The first line of defense for reducing contaminates is cleaning, and special attention should be given to the cleaning procedures used in this area. For example:

- Horizontal work surfaces should be cleaned and disinfected at the beginning and end of each shift.

- Spills should be spot-cleaned immediately.

- Floors should be cleaned and disinfected daily.

- **Biohazardous** waste should be removed at frequent intervals.

Adequate storage for equipment used to clean the decontamination area should be available, and tools such as mops used in this area should not be used in other areas of the department.

Staff Safety and Personal Attire

Employee safety is a very important concern at all times including during cleaning and decontamination. Since Central Service Technicians do not know the origin of the contamination, they must assume that every item received in the decontamination area can pose a potential

risk to them. To protect personnel who perform cleaning and decontamination tasks, Occupational Safety and Health Administration (OSHA) requirements for Occupational Exposure to Bloodborne Pathogens must be followed. Applicable procedures impact environmental controls, personal attire, equipment/supplies, effective work practices, and the training of personnel working in the decontamination area.

Personal Protective Equipment (PPE) (See **Figure 9.3**) is required in the decontamination area because this attire is designed to protect employees from splashes and other means of contamination. Employers should provide a variety of PPE to meet cleaning process needs. PPE should be latex-free, be generally easy to use, and be easily available. **Figure 9.4** lists components of proper PPE.

PPE that becomes soaked with blood or other potentially infectious material, and gloves that are nicked or torn should be discarded immediately. Jewelry should not be worn because it harbors bacteria. Also, since acrylic fingernails can support the growth of microorganisms, they should not be permitted, and no food or drink should enter the decontamination area.

Personal Protective Equipment (PPE) – According to OSHA, "specialized clothing or equipment worn by an employee for protection against a hazard.

Standard Precautions – Method of using appropriate barriers to prevent transmission of infectious organisms from contact with blood and all other body fluids, nonintact skin, and mucous membranes. It applies to all patients, regardless of diagnosis or presumed infectious status. The precautions consist of appropriate handwashing, gloves when touching the above materials, facial protection when there is a chance of splashing body substances into one's face, and gowns when there is a chance of splashing of body substances onto one's clothing. Precautions also include appropriate disinfection of patient-care equipment, appropriate handling of soiled linen, prevention of needlesticks and other injuries from sharps, and appropriate handling and disposal of sharps, all without regard to the patient's diagnosis. (ANSI/AAMI ST79 2006)

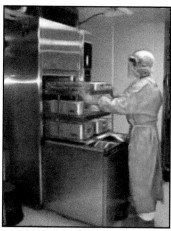

Figure 9.3

Figure 9.4 Components of Personal Protective Equipment (PPE)

- Hair covering.

- Eye protection such as goggles or eyeglasses with solid side shields or a chin-length face shield.

- Fluid-resistant facemask

- A gown with reinforced sleeves, and a front that acts as a barrier to fluids.

- Strong general-purpose utility gloves that cover the sleeves of the reinforced gown, and that can resist cuts and tears.

- Decontamination shoe covers that are skid-resistant.

- Employer-provided cloth scrub attire that is discarded at the end of each shift.

Hand washing and the frequent use of appropriate hand germicidal agents should be mandated. Whenever Central Service Technicians complete tasks, remove PPE, or move from one area to another, they should properly wash their hands, because this is the most important element in the prevention of nosocomial (hospital-acquired) infections. A "hand wash only" sink should be provided within the decontamination area, and it should be separate from sinks used to sort and pre-prepare instruments for processing.

The U.S. Centers for Disease Control (CDC) has developed guidelines for handling contaminated items. They are known as "**Standard Precautions**," and address the concern that all body fluids and items that have contacted body fluids are potentially infectious. These guidelines should be used as a basis for the safe handling and cleaning of all medical devices entering the decontamination area, and this philosophy should be an integral part of staff education and training. Central Service Technicians should consider all items entering the decontamination area contaminated.

Staff Education and Training

Effective and on-going education and training is critical to the safe processing of medical devices to protect patients, and safety training is the on-going responsibility of both the employer and the Technicians.

ANSI/AAMI ST79: 2006, 4.2.2 states: "Advances in surgical and information technology, the emergence of new diseases and microorganisms, and the increased responsibility for all aspects of sterile processing have brought into focus how important it is for sterile processing personnel to be knowledgeable and competent. The protection of patients, employees, and other individuals in the hospital environment depends on the implementation of procedures designed to reduce the risk of exposure to potentially pathogenic microorganisms." Before any new staff member is assigned to the decontamination area, he/she must receive a thorough and comprehensive orientation. Topics including the use of PPE, general staff safety, hand washing, and the proper use and

Policies for Hepatitis B Immunization and Employee Injuries

Personnel should be required to be immunized against Hepatitis B. If they decline, OSHA requires that a Hepatitis B vaccine declination statement be signed. Written policies relating to the need for and process to report employee injuries are also needed to address reporting, treatment, and follow-up procedures. Detailed information about both of these policies should be part of new-employee orientation programs, and should also be provided during on-going in-service education.

handling of contaminated patient care equipment must be addressed and documented as part of on-going staff competency evaluation. Experienced Central Service Technicians require regular safety updates to stay focused on patient safety. Tactics including the use of in-services, handouts, checklists, policy reviews, and demonstrations can address critical safety points, and help to assess employee competence.

On certification test

SELECTION AND USAGE CONCERNS FOR CLEANING AGENTS AND LUBRICANTS

Learning Objective 2. Describe important selection and usage concerns for cleaning agents (water, detergents, enzymes, and enzymatic detergents) and lubricants.

Overview

There are several important considerations in the selection and use of cleaning agents and lubricants. First, written cleaning recommendations of the original equipment manufacturer (OEM) should be consulted. Improper usage and/or use of the wrong cleaning agent can damage and/or compromise the operation of a medical device. Sometimes the use of the wrong cleaning agent or process can even harm the patient on which the device is used. Technicians must receive training in the proper processing of all new medical devices or instruments. This should include the provision of detailed, written directions that are archived and immediately accessible to all Central Service staff.

Mobile patient care equipment has different processing needs than surgical instrumentation, and all equipment and instruments should be handled in a safe, effective, and consistent manner. Every cleaning agent and cleaning process must help to render the medical device safe for handling during subsequent processing steps.

Effective cleaning agents:

- Are non-abrasive.

- Are low-foaming.

- Are free-rinsing (the cleaning agent is completely removed with proper rinsing).

- Are biodegradable.

- Allow for rapid soil dispersion.

- Are non-toxic.

- Are effective on all types of soil.

- Have long shelf-life.

- Are cost-effective.

- Can be monitored for effective concentration and useful life.

Central Service Technicians commonly use several cleaning agents, each of which is formulated for a specific action: water, detergents, enzymes, and enzymatic detergents.

Water

Water quality is a broad concept covering several characteristics. Water is a **wetting agent** that is the primary vehicle used in the cleaning process. Without water, the best detergent would be ineffective. The relevant measurable characteristics of water are **pH level**, hardness, temperature and purity. To be pure, water must be free of particulates, total dissolved solids, microbes, and pyrogens (fever-producing substances.) Note: we'll discuss water pH level and hardness here. Water temperature and purity were considered in Chapter Seven.

Wetting agent – A substance that reduces the surface tension of a liquid, and allows the liquid to penetrate or spread more easily across the surface of a solid.

pH level – A measure of alkalinity or acidity.

Chelating agents – Chemicals that hold hard water minerals in solution, and prevent soaps or detergents from reacting with the minerals.

Sequestering agents – Chemicals that remove or inactivate hard water minerals.

The pH level of water is important because it influences the effectiveness of enzyme and detergent cleaners. Cleaning agents have optimal pH levels of performance and, at extreme pH levels, these cleaners are completely inactivated.

Hard water minerals such as calcium and magnesium can cause deposits or scale formation during the cleaning process because of their inverse solubility (lower solubility at higher temperatures). The presence of **chelating** or **sequestering agents** helps minimize formulation of insoluble deposits, and prevents both instrument spotting and equipment scaling. Tactics to minimize the formation of insoluble scale include the use of softened water for wash water, and the installation of steam line filters on washer equipment. Softened water does not contain hard water minerals, so its use reduces the formation of mineral scale. The use of steam filters prevents steam contaminants from being carried into the washer and deposited on instruments and equipment. A final rinse with distilled or de-ionized water will prevent mineral deposits.

Detergents

Water is not an effective cleaning agent by itself, so a detergent must be used with it. Traditionally soaps were made from animal fats combined with minerals such as sodium or potassium hydroxide. However, these soap compounds should never be used for cleaning instruments because they leave behind a residue and can damage stainless steel.

Detergents are substances that can dislodge, remove, and disperse solid and liquid soils from a surface being cleaned. They work by:

- Lowering surface tension so the cleaning liquid can penetrate the soil and the object being cleaned.

- Deflocculating (breaking up and dispersing) soil, separating clumps of dirt and dissolving or suspending small particles in the cleaning fluid (usually water containing the detergent.)

- Keeping soils and dirt clumps in suspension or solution so they can be washed and rinsed away rather than be re-deposited on the material or object being washed.

Many detergents are formulated for specialized applications (for example, in ultrasonic cleaners or for hard water). Some detergents may form precipitates (other chemicals made from minerals) in hard water, and special hard water cleaning formulations are then necessary. Detergents must be compatible with the cleaning equipment with which they are used. For example, a foaming detergent will hinder the operation of a washer-disinfector that uses high-pressure jets. They should also be compatible with the materials used to construct the medical device being cleaned, and the materials used in the cleaning equipment itself. Detergents used should not cause corrosion or promote electrolytic action between the equipment and the medical device being cleaned.

The pH level of a detergent measures its acidity or alkalinity. A detergent with a low pH (0-6) is acidic; one with a high pH (8-14) is alkaline. Examples of acidic substances include vinegar and lemon juice, and soap is an alkaline substance. For most cleaning applications, neutral or mildly alkaline pH detergents are preferred. Note: **Figure 9.5** reviews the pH scale.

Water quality and chemical use are critical factors in producing an effective cleaning cycle. Therefore, these factors should be checked when cleaning equipment is initially used and periodically thereafter. In addition, it is important to check water quality to ensure it has not changed over time

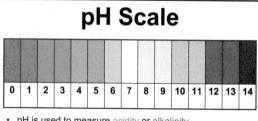

pH Scale

0 1 2 3 4 5 6 7 8 9 10 11 12 13 14

- pH is used to measure acidity or alkalinity.

- Acids turn litmus paper RED.

- Alkalies (sometimes called bases) turn litmus paper BLUE.

Figure 9.5

(for example, because of building construction and remodeling or environmental changes). Detergent companies should also test their products to determine which is best for a specific use. Detergents are available in many forms, from liquids (ranging in size from small bottles to large drums) to solid (block) detergents that are mixed with water as they are dispensed. Each facility makes detergent selections based on its specific cleaning needs and cleaning equipment requirements.

Enzymes

Enzyme products are commonly used to clean heavily soiled items. They are very helpful for processing difficult-to-clean devices such as instruments with lumens. Enzymes break down or "digest" large organic molecules to facilitate their removal. They do so by finding a specific site on the substance or material, interacting with it, and breaking it apart. The enzymes are not consumed as this occurs, so they can repeat the process on another molecule.

Enzymes are very specific in their action. For example, a protein enzyme will not recognize fat molecules. In fact, a protein enzyme will not even recognize a chemically altered protein (one that has already undergone a chemical reaction); it only recognizes proteins in their natural state.

Popular enzymes used in Central Service Departments include:

- Protease enzymes – Break down blood, mucous, feces, and albumin.

- Lipase – Break down fatty deposits such as bone marrow and adipose tissue.

- Amylase – Catalyzes (changes) starch.

Elements in soil can gradually degrade enzymes during use, and reduce their cleaning efficiency. Dried soil on a device must be re-hydrated before enzymes that facilitate its removal can be effective. Re-hydration to restore fluid is time-dependent, and will limit the enzyme's soil contact time. Pre-cleaning can reduce these problems. After pre-cleaning, the instrument should remain moist to maintain the hydration needed to optimize the enzyme's efficiency.

Enzymatic Detergents

Enzymatic detergents usually consist of a detergent base with a neutral pH to which one or more enzymes and a surfactant is added. After the detergent breaks down organic materials, it removes the dissolved particles from the instrument's surface. Enzymatic detergents are biodegradable, and can replace high alkaline or acidic products that may harm instruments. Always follow the manufacturer's recommendations about the proper amount and temperature of water. Temperatures above 40°C (140°F) can affect the chemical reaction, and cool temperatures may not activate the enzyme. Therefore, it is very important to monitor water temperature.

When selecting an enzymatic detergent, consider the following:

- Water temperature in the decontamination area.

- Room temperature in the decontamination area.

- Useful life and stability of the product being considered.

- Expiration date of product.

- The material used to construct the device to be cleaned.

- Whether the detergent is approved and registered with the Environmental Protection Agency (EPA).

Detergents for Ultrasonic Cleaners

Only detergents that have been specially formulated for use in ultrasonic cleaners should be used in them. They must be low-foaming to prevent interference with the cleaning process. These detergents are usually formulated with **surfactants** and chelating agents to prevent the re-deposit of soil. **Figure 9.6** illustrates an ultrasonic cleaner with low-foaming detergent.

Surfactant – A surface-acting agent that lowers the surface tension of a liquid so it can penetrate deeper, and prevents debris from being re-deposited on the item to which the soil was attached.

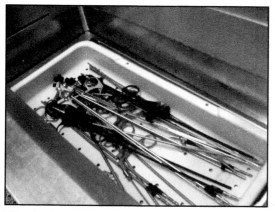

Figure 9.6

Lubricants

✳Water-soluble lubricants (often called "instrument milk") designed for surgical instruments were originally developed as rust inhibitors for carbon-steel dental drills, and were used to pre-coat them prior to sterilization. Today, lubricants are an important part of the instrument maintenance program, because they help to maintain the integrity of instruments, and keep them in good working order. Instrument lubrication also prolongs the life and action of stainless steel and tungsten carbide scissors, prevents abrasion on blades moving against each other, and increases their cutting action.

Lubrication is performed after cleaning. Lubrication may be performed mechanically as one of the final steps in the mechanical wash process, or it can be applied manually in the clean assembly area using a spray bottle. In the past, instrument baths (pans filled with instrument lubricating solution) were commonly used, but instrument baths run an increased risk of contamination. Instrument lubricant is often referred to as "instrument milk" because of its white, milky appearance. Always use the lubrication according to the manufacturer's recommendations to assure the proper soak time and dilution concentration. It is also important to insure that the lubricant is designed for use with the surgical instruments to be cleaned, and compatible with specific sterilization processes that will follow.

Always Follow Cleaning Guidelines

ANSI/AAMI ST79:2006 details the requirements for the entire cleaning process from point-of-use to the sterilization of the medical device prior to next use. This standard should always be followed by Central Service Technicians to provide consistency and to ensure the safety of workers and the public.

CLEANING AND DECONTAMINATION PROCESSES AND METHODS

Learning Objective 3. Explain details about cleaning and decontamination, and review manual procedures and mechanical methods to complete both processes.

Process Overview

The terms, "cleaning" and "decontamination," were briefly defined at the beginning of this chapter. More technical definitions will now help to explain the processes.

Cleaning involves the removal, usually with a detergent and water, of both visible and non-visible soil (for example, blood, protein substances, and other debris) from the surfaces, crevices, serrations, joints, and lumens of instruments, devices, and equipment. Gross soil should be removed as soon as possible to:

- Reduce the number of microorganisms on the item.

- Reduce the nutrient material that can support microbial growth.

- Reduce the potential for environmental contamination by aerosolization or spillage.

- Minimize damage to devices from blood and other substances.

Cleaning is the first and most important step in the sterilization process. **One can clean without sterilizing, but one cannot sterilize without cleaning. As well, one can clean without**

disinfecting, but one cannot disinfect without cleaning. The sterilization process cannot produce a sterile device that has not first been cleaned. Dead organisms in soil or organic debris left on medical devices can cause pyrogenic or foreign body reactions. They can also create a breeding site for an infection if the device is used for an invasive procedure. Also, residual debris can affect an instrument's ability to function properly (for example, hemostats, ronguers, and other instruments may not open or close properly).

Decontamination involves the use of physical or chemical procedures to remove, inactivate, or destroy bloodborne pathogens on an item's surface. This is necessary so these pathogens can no longer cause infection, and so the surface of the item will be safe for handling, use, or disposal. The purpose of decontamination is to make devices safe for people who are not wearing gloves, and to reduce the bioburden to make the next processing steps easier. Some instruments are safe for handling after they have been thoroughly cleaned; however, others require exposure to a microbiocidal process. The level of decontamination required depends on:

- How the item was last used.
- How the item will next be used.

How an item was, or will be used determines the level of decontamination required. For example, infusion pumps/heating pads are not exposed to broken skin, and they should be safe to handle after cleaning. By contrast, surgical instruments have been exposed to blood and body tissues. Manufacturers of reusable medical devices provide written reprocessing instructions, and these should be obtained before the device is first used. The instructions should be provided to the Central Service Technicians who will be responsible for reprocessing the device, and this information should be consistently and carefully followed. This will help reduce risks of exposure to personnel working in the preparation and packaging areas who are not usually wearing gloves.

Technology Creates Cleaning Challenges

Advancements in technology have created new and more sophisticated types of instruments that are very complex in design, and made from a variety of different materials. These devices create processing challenges because they often contain:

Long, narrow lumens and channels in instruments that were not designed for easy cleaning. (See **Figure 9.7**)

- Multiple internal channels.
- Channels that are not freely accessible.
- Valves.
- Crevices, joints, or surface pores. (See **Figure 9.8**)
- Clamps that cannot be opened for cleaning.
- Components that cannot be readily dismantled (A primary rule of cleaning is that anything that can be disassembled must be disassembled.)
- Rough, irregular surfaces that can entrap or retain bioburden and impurities (See **Figure 9.9**)
- Porous materials.
- Luer-locks (such as those on syringes and adaptors) (See **Figure 9.10**)
- Junctions between insulating sheaths and activating mechanisms.
- Heat-sensitive materials.
- Electrical components.

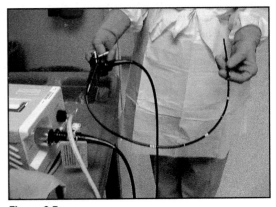

Figure 9.7

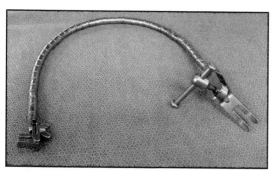

Figure 9.8

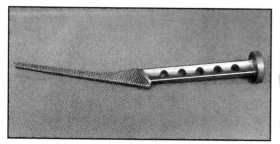

Figure 9.9

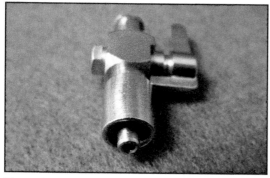

Figure 9.10

Manual Cleaning

The purpose of manual cleaning is to physically remove deposits that were not removed, or were only softened during the pre-soak. This is done by use of friction.

Manual cleaning may be done:

• Prior to mechanical cleaning.

• When the decontamination area does not have an ultrasonic cleaner or washer sterilizer-washer decontaminator.

• For delicate or complex instruments that cannot be processed in mechanical equipment.

• To clean powered equipment that cannot be immersed in water.

• For instruments with lumens.

To facilitate the cleaning process, the water temperature should be below 43°C (110°F). This will help prevent the **coagulation** (denaturing) of proteins.

Water hardness, temperature, and the type of soil to be removed can impact the effectiveness of the detergent. Excessive amounts of detergents can be difficult to rinse off, and will eventually begin to deteriorate the instrument. Therefore, it is important to use the correct amount as specified by the manufacturer.

When cleaning aluminum or stainless steel, a "to and fro" motion in the direction of the grain should be used rather than a circular motion. This will help to prevent scratching the surface of the item and causing damage. All instruments should be cleaned in a wide-open position to allow cleaning of the box-lock or hinged areas. (See **Figure 9.11**) Always brush instruments under the water's surface to prevent aerosol contamination. (See **Figure 9.12**)

A three-sink arrangement (See **Figure 9.13**) used for manual cleaning should consist of:

• A wash sink with water and a detergent solution.

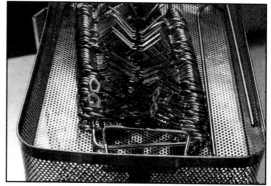

Figure 9.11

Coagulation - *to cause to become viscous or thickened into a coherent mass; to clot*

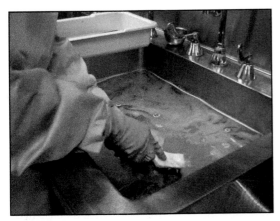

Figure 9.12

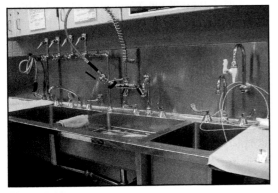

Figure 9.13

- A second sink (intermediate rinse) that contains plain or softened (de-ionized) water.

- A third sink (final rinse) with distilled/de-ionized water to help prevent instrument spotting, to rinse off pyrogens, and to prevent the re-deposit of minerals, microbes, and pyrogens.

Vertical soaking cylinders are used to soak instruments with lumens so all surfaces will be contacted by the cleaning solution. By contrast, when luminal instruments are soaked horizontally, air bubbles will likely become entrapped in the lumens.

Mechanical Cleaning

Ultrasonic (sonic) cleaners, automated **washers,** and automated cart washers are in common use in Central Service Departments, and will be discussed in this section.

What About Cleaning Brushes?

The correct brush must always be used. Consider the need to clean a lumen. If the brush is too large, it will not fit into the lumen. If the brush is too small, it will not have complete contact with the lumen walls, and will not thoroughly clean them. As well, the brush must be long enough to extend through the lumen. **Figure 9.14** illustrates the need for several different sized brushes to meet specific lumen cleaning needs.

Brushes must be cleaned and disinfected/ sterilized, and those showing wear should be discarded. Prompt cleaning of brushes and cleaning tools reduces the number of or eliminates microorganisms that create biofilms.

There is a risk of cross-contamination from one medical device to another when reusable cleaning brushes are used. A cleaning process requiring reusable components such as brushes must include the cleaning process for these components. Reusable brushes should be cleaned, and disinfected or sterilized at the end of the shift, or when heavily soiled. Disposable and reusable brushes that are worn should be discarded.

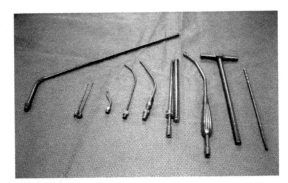

Figure 9.14

Washers – Automated equipment used to clean, decontaminate, or disinfect (low, intermediate, or low-level) and dry medical devices.

Cavitation – The process used by an ultrasonic cleaner in which low-pressure bubbles in a cleaning solution burst inward, and dislodge soil from instruments.

Ultrasonic (Sonic) Cleaners

The term, "ultrasonic," is an appropriate name for this type of mechanical cleaner. "Ultra" means beyond, and "sonic" means sound. When an ultrasonic wave passes through a liquid, it makes the liquid vibrate very fast. Hospital sonic cleaners produce from 20,000 to 38,000 vibrations per second. The vibrations are transmitted through the detergent bath and create **cavitation**: ultrasonic waves pass through a cleaning solution, the molecules of the solution are set in very rapid motion, and small gas bubbles develop. As the bubbles become larger, they become unstable until they implode (not explode). This creates a vacuum in the solution that draws minute bits of foreign matter (including microorganisms) from cracks and crevices such as hinges and serrations on instruments. This vacuum action results in a thorough cleaning of the instruments including hard-to-reach areas. Note: **Figure 9.15** illustrates the cavitation process.

Ultrasonic cleaning is superior to manual scrubbing because the cavitation action can reach small areas in the instrument that brushes cannot reach. After cavitation, rinsing is necessary to remove any scum or sediment (including detergent) that remains on the instruments. Since the ultrasonic cleaning process lifts grease, fat, and lipids from instruments, sediments in the ultrasonic cleaner similar to a ring in the bathtub may remain. It is important to always use the correct solution in the tank, and to routinely clean it according to the manufacturer's instructions.

Instruments to be processed must be pre-cleaned to remove gross soil such as blood and tissue debris, and to keep the ultrasonic solution clean. In addition, coagulated protein absorbs sound, and reduces the cleaning action in the sonic cleaner. Bath temperatures for cleaning instruments should be between 27°C (80°F) and 43°C (109°F). Be sure to use cleaners specifically designed for use in the ultrasonic equipment, and always follow the manufacturer's specific recommendations for dilution and water temperature. Temperatures above 60°C (140°F) will coagulate protein, and make it more difficult to remove. Water should be changed when it is visually soiled, or at regularly scheduled intervals to prevent the redeposit of soiled particles onto other instruments. Orthopedic instruments may have fatty deposits on them that can soil the water quickly. Therefore, water should be changed more often when these devices are cleaned. The unit's tank should be cleaned, and drain-checked for debris at each water change.

An ultrasonic unit may have one, two, or even three chambers. The first chamber is for the detergent bath; the second is for rinsing; the third is for drying. (**Figures 9.16** and **9.17** illustrate examples of single and dual chamber ultrasonic cleaners.)

Water must be degassed each time it is changed in the sonic cleaner. Excess bubbles in the water are present during filling, and these gas bubbles fill the cavitation bubbles and reduce the energy released during the implosion. To degas a unit, fill the sonic cleaner, close the lid, and run it for 5-10 minutes. Degassing should only be done after the tank is filled, and not while it is being filled to avoid damage to the equipment.

The lid of the sonic cleaner should be closed at all times when the unit is operating to prevent aerosols from being dispersed.

All lumens must be completely filled with fluid so the cavitation process can be effective inside the lumen. All instruments must be completely submerged in the solution so they are exposed to the cavitation process.

Instruments placed in the sonic cleaner should be opened. Even instruments that do not appear

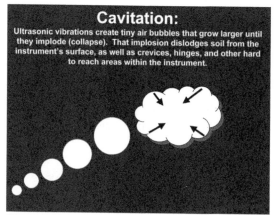

Cavitation:
Ultrasonic vibrations create tiny air bubbles that grow larger until they implode (collapse). That implosion dislodges soil from the instrument's surface, as well as crevices, hinges, and other hard to reach areas within the instrument.

Figure 9.15

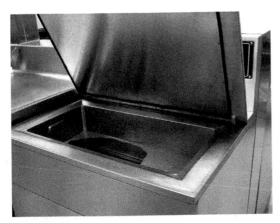

Figure 9.16

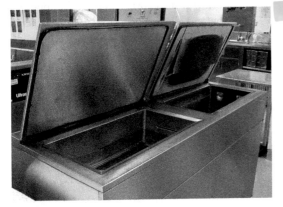

Figure 9.17

used should be processed as if they had been, and these should also be cleaned in the open position. Instruments should be placed in trays designed for use in the machine. They are typically of small wire construction with 8 openings per inch to allow transmission of sonic energy.

Items that should not be placed in a sonic cleaner include chrome-plated and ebonized instruments, and those made of plastic, cork, glass, wood, chrome, and rubber. Also, needles should not be cleaned with the sonic method. Be sure to consult the instrument manufacturer's recommendations for specific cleaning information before placing a device in an ultrasonic cleaner. Ultrasonic energy can loosen the tiny screws of delicate instruments, and destroy the glues or amalgam in other devices. Endoscopy instrumentation or instruments that contain fiber optic components will be damaged if placed in an ultrasonic cleaner.

Stainless steel instruments should not be mixed with their aluminum, brass, or copper counterparts. Sonic detergents can turn aluminum light handles a dull gray color. Do not overload or stack instruments over three inches high in the trays, and do not put more than one tray into the sonic cleaner at the same time. It is important to test ultrasonic washers for effectiveness, and commercially available test kits are available for this purpose.

As with all processing equipment, the manufacturer's operating and maintenance recommendations should always be carefully followed.

Automated Mechanical Washing

Washers have been utilized for many years in Central Service Departments, and they are effective to clean instrumentation, instrument containers, basins, bowls, and pitchers. Automated mechanical washers are not appropriate for washing electrical, battery, or pneumatic devices. The cleaning of these devices must be done manually following the written instructions of the Original Equipment Manufacturer (OEM). Note: Methods used to clean these devices will be covered later in this chapter. (**Figures 9.18** and **9.19** illustrate examples of single chamber and multi-chamber mechanical washers.)

Washers work on the principle of **impingement**. They are an effective means to disinfect instruments because of their thermal action (see the following chapter), and because enzymatic detergents can be used. As discussed earlier, detergents used in automated washers must be approved for use in the equipment, and must consider the instrumentation to be cleaned.

In some ways, impingement washers work like a dishwasher. They rely on a combination of water temperature, special detergent, and a spray force action to remove the soil from devices being processed. To clean effectively, items must be

Impingement – The spray-force action of pressurized water against instruments being processed to physically remove bioburden.

properly prepared, and placed in a manner that facilitates the mechanical cleaning process.

Mechanical impingement washers typically use several successive steps during the wash cycle. The first step is a pre-rinse to wet the instruments, and to prepare them for the detergent cycle. The second step is a detergent cycle with water at a higher temperature to maximize the effectiveness of the detergent action. The third step is typically a lubrication cycle followed by a rinse cycle to remove any remaining detergents. Many automated mechanical washers have a dry cycle.

Washers can only be effective when they are properly used, loaded, and serviced in compliance with the manufacturers' recommendations. Operator's manuals and detailed instructions about the basic operation and loading of instrument racks should be provided. Central Service Technicians should be familiar with these instructions, and staff must be in-serviced about compliance with them.

Washer racks should never be over-loaded, and spray arms should move freely during operation. Instruments that are sticking up and/or out of their perforated baskets must be relocated to rest below the spray arms' travel paths. Instruments should be disassembled, and their box-locks should be opened to permit direct contact of the water and detergent. Trays or sets with multiple levels should be opened, and each tray should be placed separately on the washer rack. Failure to separate multi-level trays can cause the wash process to fail, because tray layers impede contact between the spray action and the items within the tray Figure 9.20 illustrates how tray layers can impede cleaning. Also, trays with lids/covers should be opened so that contents may be exposed to the washer spray Figure 9.21 illustrates how the lid of an instrument tray can impede the cleaning process. Figures 9.22 and 9.23 also illustrate how improper loading of trays can protect soil by impeding contact with spray action. Delicate instruments may be dislodged from the racks due to the blunt force of the spray action. These instruments should be confined in small-perforated baskets with lids or hold-downs. Figure 9.24 shows a properly loaded instrument rack.

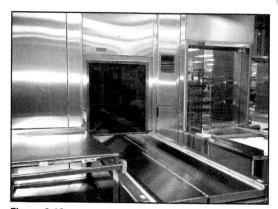

Figure 9.18

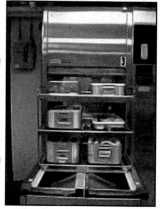

Figure 9.20

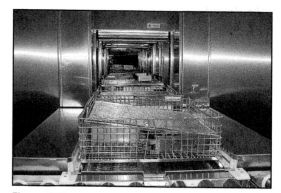

Figure 9.19

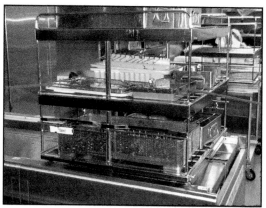

Figure 9.21

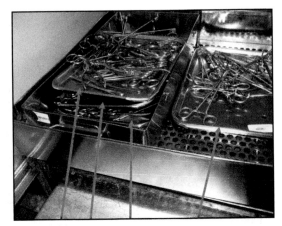
Figure 9.22

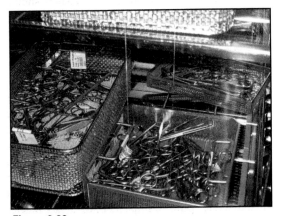
Figure 9.23

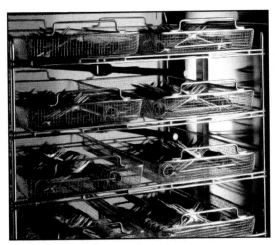
Figure 9.24

Instrument washer racks should be inspected daily. Routine cleaning of washers should include inspection and cleaning of spray arms and washer jets. Mineral build-up will hinder spray action, and

disrupt cleaning effectiveness. Washer traps need special attention, should be inspected daily for debris, and must be cleared of any obstructions.

Washer detergent levels should be frequently monitored. If detergent drums are allowed to run dry, a column of air may enter the detergent feed line. Priming the lines each day will help to prevent washer cycles with inadequate detergent levels.

Automated washers have pre-set factory installed cycles for use with different cleaning situations. Instrument cycles generally are the longest cycle because they have multiple rinse, wash, lubrication, and drying times to meet the instruments' cleaning needs. Basins and containers are generally run on a utensil cycle, and have a shortened cycle time because the cleaning challenge is not as great as that with complex instruments. Some washer manufacturers offer special cycles for delicate instruments. When running a mixed load of containers and instruments, the instrument cycle should normally be utilized for maximum effectiveness. Central Service Technicians should be familiar with different washer cycles, and should be able to select the appropriate cleaning cycle for the items to be processed. Some washers have optical scanning systems that scan washer basket bar codes, and then adjust the equipment for the proper cleaning cycle. These systems can help reduce employee errors.

Automated Cart Washers

The use of cart washers has automated the cleaning of surgical case carts, rigid containers, and other miscellaneous medical devices. (**See Figure 9.25**) Several manufacturers offer cart washers with design features and special washer racks to facilitate the reprocessing of basins, pans, bedside commodes, and surgical stainless steel tables. Processing rigid containers and surgical basins in a cart washer can yield operational speed and efficiency. **Figure 9.26** shows a cart washer with a rack designed for rigid container systems, bowls, and basins.

Cart washers operate in a manner similar to automated instrument washers, but on a larger scale. Spray arms travel in a vertical motion, and deliver high temperature water and detergent

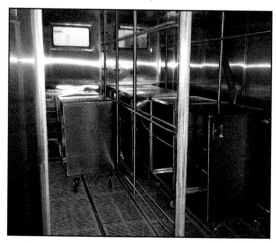

Figure 9.25

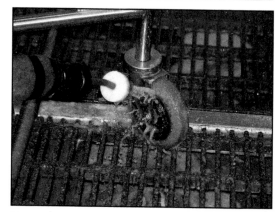

Figure 9.27

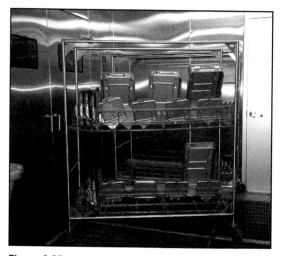

Figure 9.26

under higher pressure. Successive steps provide rinse water and hot air drying cycles. Cart washes resemble automated car washes in their cleaning process. However, cart washers include a high temperature process to reduce bacteria, and to facilitate drying.

Detergents selected for cart washing should be formulated for use in cart washers, and should have the ability to rinse off freely.

Since a cart washer may require Central Service Technicians to enter the chamber of the washer to load or unload it, extreme caution should be taken to avoid injury. High water temperatures make the chamber walls hot to the touch, and chamber doors could be inadvertently closed while someone

is in the chamber. Automatic cart washers should be equipped with an emergency shutoff that is regularly tested. Extensive in-service and education sessions should be conducted prior to operation, and should include an emphasis on safety.

Many manufacturers offer case carts designed for use in automated cart washers. Features of these carts include the ability to drain off residual water, and wheels that can tolerate high temperatures. Older-style carts may lack these features, and can be damaged if processed in an automated washer. Always check with the applicable surgical case cart manufacturer prior to implementing a cart washer program for cleaning case carts.

Carts that cannot be processed using a mechanical cart washer can be processed manually using a spray gun over a floor grate. **Figure 9.27** illustrates the cleaning of a cart wheel using a manual cart cleaning gun over a floor grate.

What Is Free-Rinsing?

Free rinsing refers to the removal of any residue of cleaning agents and chemicals remaining after the cleaning process, and is necessary regardless of whether a manual or automated cleaning process is used. Residual cleaning chemicals affect instrument performance, pose risk of infection, and/or have corrosive effects on the finish of instruments.

Ideally, de-ionized water should be utilized as the free rinsing agent to minimize the deposit of minerals that appear as water spots when dry.

BASIC INSTRUMENT CLEANING PROCEDURES

Learning Objective 4. Discuss procedures to clean basic types of instruments:
- General cleaning protocols.
- Delicate and hard-to-clean instruments
- Instrument containers and basins
- Power equipment.
- Mobile patient care equipment
- Verification and quality control tactics.

General Cleaning Protocols

Every instrument and medical device entering the decontamination area requires attention and respect, and it must be assumed that each is potentially hazardous. The use of PPEs and Standard Precautions must be mandatory and enforced. Central Service Technicians deserve the respect of the entire health care team, as they are at the front line in patient safety and infection control. How they clean the instruments they receive will affect others, and will potentially touch the lives of many who follow them after this process. Cleaning efforts must be focused, and they must be done consistently, efficiently, and effectively.

The best time to begin the instrument cleaning process is within 15 minutes to one hour after the procedure for which it was used. Prolonged delays in cleaning can have detrimental effects on the instrumentation. Sets can begin to stain, pit, rust, and become dull. Dried blood becomes more difficult to remove. Instruments to be cleaned should never be left to stand without being covered with a moistened towel. Alternatively, if they can be immersed, they can be placed in a soak basin with water containing presoak or time-monitored enzymatic detergents.

When instruments are received, Central Service Technicians must visually and cautiously inspect them for sharps and disposables. Technicians are at the heart of the quality control process during cleaning. Pre-cleaning errors must be identified, communicated, and addressed as part of the quality improvement process. Error reports should be viewed as opportunities for staff education and process improvement.

Instruments such as tissue retractor systems that must be taken apart for effective cleaning should be disassembled. Those with jaws and box hinges need to be opened and inspected for gross tissue and bioburden. Large amounts of bioburden can be removed manually before automated washing. Those with deep serrations and crevices can be cleaned manually with brushes, pipe cleaners, and/or forced water and air.

Instruments such as suction tubes with lumens require special attention. These devices should be placed under water to prevent aerosolizing of contaminated water droplets. Then they can be cleaned with brushes, and/or have water forced through them with a plastic syringe filled with water and enzymatic detergent. Consult the OEM for recommended brush sizes to effectively clean these channels.

Curettes and other orthopedic instruments can conceal bone and bioburden. Scraping out material with bristle brushes should be an initial step in the cleaning process.

Instruments tagged for repair must still be cleaned and decontaminated. Central Service Technicians must inform their peers assembling the sets prior to sterilization about any instrument issue. The use of repair tags and wrapped pipe cleaners are effective means to indicate that an instrument has repair issues. When instruments are returned from repair, they must be considered contaminated. They must be cleaned, decontaminated, and inspected before being returned to their respective sets.

Delicate and Hard-to-Clean Instruments

Delicate instruments are a cleaning challenge. They must be separated from regular or heavy instruments during cleaning. A dedicated sink arrangement can be used to do so. Devices used for delicate surgical procedures are generally lightweight with fine points and tips. Mixing them with heavy instruments, or placing heavy devices on top of them, invite damage and misalignment.

Delicate instruments such as skin hooks can slip through perforated baskets, and become entangled.

They should be placed in perforated baskets with fine holes to prevent damage to the tips.

Instruments used for ophthalmic surgeries can rust because of the extensive use of saline solutions during operative procedures and frequent flash sterilizations. It is important to rinse and lubricate these instruments often.

Devices with cabling systems pose a unique challenge because of their construction. They must be inspected for nicks and breaks in insulation during the cleaning process. Often, electrical cabling systems require that end caps be placed over gold-plated pins during cleaning and decontamination. Consult the OEM for special considerations, and to determine if these devices can withstand automated washers.

Orthopedic surgery has many instrument sets that require extended preparation and inspection prior to and during cleaning. Joint replacement cutting guides, rasps, reamers, and broaches hide (and usually are loaded with) gross amounts of blood, bone, and tissue. This can occur with the best point-of-use care in the operating room, and these instruments must be cleaned with brushes and extensive hand detailing. Pre-soaking with enzymatic detergents can help to remove much of the bioburden from the crevices. Some washer manufacturers have designed special washer racks to hold and to flush out these challenging devices. **Figures 9.28** to **9.30** show common cleaning challenges associated with orthopedic instrumentation.

Instrument Containers and Basins

Cleaning rigid instrument containers and basins requires procedures that differ from those used for instruments. A neutral pH detergent is recommended, because acidic or alkaline pH detergents will etch or damage aluminum and some composite materials. These items need not be placed in, and may not even fit on, conventional instrument racks. Instead, they will require special racks designed for this purpose.

Handles, locking mechanisms, and basin rims should be inspected for cracks, missing pieces, and "lost" components.

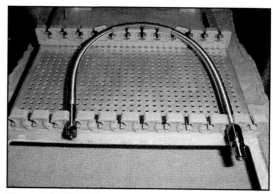

Figure 9.28 Flexible Reamer

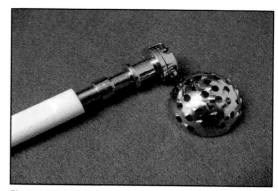

Figure 9.29 Acetabular Reamer

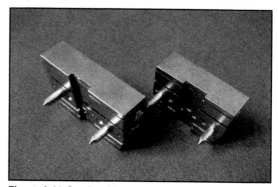

Figure 9.30 Cutting Blocks

Power Equipment

Power equipment presents challenges to Central Service Technicians. These devices are powered by batteries, pneumatic air, and/or electric power cords. They are not designed for cleaning in an automatic washer, and they must be manually cleaned and decontaminated. The OEM's written guidelines should be consulted for cleaning and sterilization instructions.

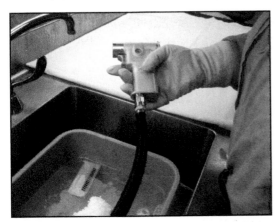

Figure 9.31

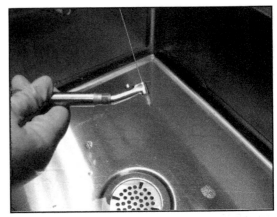

Figure 9.33

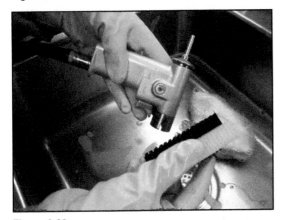

Figure 9.32

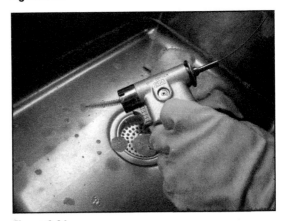

Figure 9.34

In general, these devices can be surface-wiped with a clean, soft cloth, water, and an approved neutral pH enzymatic detergent. Care should be taken to prevent exposure of the connection points and battery contacts to harsh chemicals. These connection areas can react with chemicals to cause damage and loss of electrical contact with the power source. Note: Chapter 12 provides a more detailed discussion of this type of damage.

Cannulated drills must have their lumens cleaned out with running tap water, and the chucks must be brushed out with pipe cleaners and a soft brush. A plastic syringe filled with water and enzymatic detergent can assist in delivering cleaning agents to these hard-to-reach areas. Then the channels must be flushed with distilled or deionized water to remove any residual detergent. **Figures 9.31** though **9.37** illustrate cleaning practices for orthopedic drills and saws and their accessories.

Orthopedic saws frequently have residual bone chips and impacted bioburden in their working parts. They must be flushed and brushed clean under running water. The use of forced air could be used, but extreme caution is necessary to prevent exposure due to aerosolization.

Mobile Patient Care Equipment

Mobile patient care equipment presents cleaning challenges that are substantially different from those posed by surgical instruments. Many of these devices are constructed from a mix of plastics, polymers, and stainless steel metals, and require cleaning agents that will not harm their surface. OEM instructions should be consulted for specific cleaning instructions.

In general, the use of mild cleaning agents and germicidal disinfectants can be utilized to clean

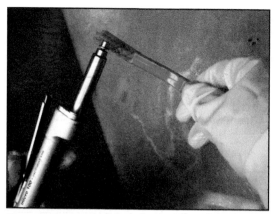

Figure 9.35

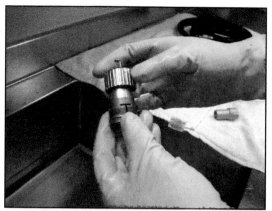

Figure 9.37

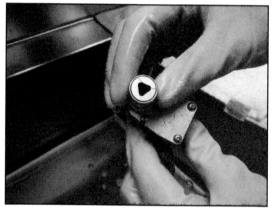

Figure 9.36

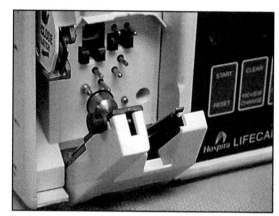

Figure 9.38

exterior components of this equipment. Use of the incorrect cleaning agent may affect product warranties and device functionality. Some chemicals may cause cosmetic changes in plastic and other materials. It is important to consult the OEM instructions before using any cleaning chemicals. Gross soil may be removed with warm water and enzymatic detergents. Bleach should be avoided, as it may affect the device's finish and surface material.

Some devices have access doors and hatches that must be opened to clean intricate parts. Extreme care is needed to avoid damage to these critical parts. Soft materials and applicators may be used to clean these crevices. **Figure 9.38** shows a piece of equipment with an access door. Care must also be taken to thoroughly clean around switches and cleaning cords. It is important that the cloth used for cleaning not be overly wet (dripping) as water may damage the equipment.

Central Service Technicians must clean many pieces of mobile equipment such as isolation, latex allergy, and special procedure carts. Carts must be cleaned after each use. Do not clean the inside drawers of these carts while they are in the decontamination area because, to do so, would expose the supplies in the carts to the area's bioburden. Instead, remove the clean contents of the cart, and place them in plastic bags. Transport the empty cart to the decontamination area, and clean all surfaces inside and out. Then transport the cart to a clean room, and complete the cleaning and re-stocking tasks. Note: Supplies that are exposed to contamination should be discarded.

All mobile equipment should be inspected and, if recommended by the manufacturer, tested prior to issuing to the next patient. Central Service Technicians must be familiar with the cleaning and testing requirements for the device. Mobile equipment that is damaged or broken, or identified as incomplete should be "tagged out" of service until the specific issue has been resolved.

Verification and Quality Control Tactics

The most common method of verifying the cleaning process is a meticulous visual inspection after completing the cleaning process. This task is the responsibility of all Central Service staff, and must be performed prior to sterilization. Sites where soil is located in complex devices may make this difficult; therefore, manufacturers of these devices have a responsibility to provide instructions for process inspection and verification.

A commercial monitoring product is available that mimics dried blood, and tests the effectiveness of automated washers. It is designed to parallel worse case scenarios of instruments processed in mechanical cleaning equipment, and to monitor the machine's ability to remove bioburden. After the cycle has completed, the monitor is inspected for residual bioburden. If any residue is present, there is a clear indication that some parameters needed for cleaning are not being achieved.

Failure of this quality assurance check can alert one about the need to investigate each variable, and it can also assist in identifying and resolving the problem. The product is similar in principle to a biological indicator used in sterilizers. In the same way that biological monitors monitor the process (but do not prove sterility), this product monitors the cleaning process, but will not prove that all instruments are cleaned. If the instruments are not disassembled and positioned correctly in the machine, debris can remain on them. With more emphasis being placed on the cleaning process, these types of monitors may become the standard of care in the future.

INFECTIOUS WASTE

Learning Objective 5. Review procedures to manage infectious waste.

Central Service Technicians should be especially concerned about handling regulated medical waste, and they should be familiar with their state and local requirements to do so. The Environmental Protection Agency (EPA) regulates infectious medical waste management.

Medical waste is any solid or liquid waste generated in the diagnosis, treatment, or immunization of human beings or animals, in applicable research, or in the production or testing of biologicals. Note: "biologicals" include soiled or blood-soaked bandages, culture dishes and other glassware, discarded surgical gloves and surgical instruments, needles, lancets, and cultures.

Definitions of "infectious waste" used by federal and state regulatory agencies that govern its handling are not the same. Some states require that all waste associated with a surgical procedure or which is recognized as medical disposable products (whether or not bloody) must be treated as infectious waste.

Waste is categorized as follows:

- General trash – garbage disposed of as municipal solid waste.

- Regulated medical waste or infectious waste – defined as waste capable of transmitting infectious diseases. This waste must be red-bagged.

- Hazardous waste – may cause mortality or serious illness if disposed of improperly, and must be red-bagged.

- Low-level radioactive waste – exhibits radiologic characteristics such as radioactive decay. If radioactive material is received in Central Service, call the facility's assigned nuclear or radiologic officer, or handle as per facility policy.

Regulated medical waste represents a risk to the public health and the environment. Examples include:

- Sharps (used and unused). These are discarded medical devices capable of puncturing or cutting the skin, and creating a portal of entry. Examples include needles, syringes with needles attached, trocars, pipettes, scalpel blades, and broken glassware. (See **Figure 9.39**)

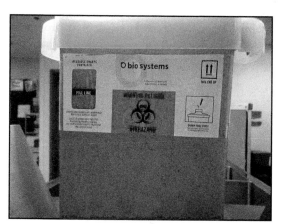

Figure 9.39

- Selected isolation waste. This is biological waste and discarded materials contaminated with blood, excretion, exudates, or secretions from humans who are isolated to protect others from certain highly virulent diseases.

- Pathological waste. Examples include human tissue, organs, and body parts removed during surgery, autopsy, or other medical procedures.

- Human blood, blood products, and body fluids. This category includes discarded free-flowing human blood and blood products.

Unfortunately, employees handling infectious waste are sometimes not protected with the appropriate Personnel Protective Equipment (PPE). It is the joint responsibility of the employee and the employer to provide and to appropriately use PPE. Staff cannot take shortcuts that violate appropriate waste management practices.

Technicians working in the decontamination area must be knowledgeable about waste management and disposal practices. Policies and procedures should detail how waste collected during cleaning and processing are safely handled. EPA and state guidelines should be consulted when these policies and procedures are written.

Central Service personnel should work with the facility's infection control officer in policy development, training, and process monitoring activities. Technicians require regular infection control updates as part of their vigilance for patient safety, and to continue compliance with The Joint Commission concerns. The infection control team should perform spot checks of the cleaning environment for cleanliness and staff safety. To insure that safe work practices are being followed, staff should be frequently monitored and observed during all phases of cleaning and decontamination to validate consistent and accurate compliance with required procedures.

Production and handling procedures for contaminated medical devices should insure consistency and cleaning effectiveness. Successful reprocessing facilities use this approach as they provide excellence to their customers.

Challenges! Challenges!

There will always be challenges as complex medical devices and instrumentation are cleaned and decontaminated. When failures occur, the best tactic is to undertake a thorough analysis of the process to determine why it occurred. When discovered, intervention in the form of action plans can yield changes that address the problems.

IN CONCLUSION

Cleaning is a complex multi-step process. If not performed properly, disinfection and sterilization standards discussed throughout this book will not be achieved. Regulatory agencies have standards and recommended practices that should always be followed. The manufacturer's recommendations about operation of cleaning equipment should be consulted prior to cleaning any medical devices. Technicians must perform the final inspection step to assure that medical devices are cleaned. This inspection includes complete removal of debris and detergent residues. Cleaning is the most important and most challenging step in medical device processing because, if a device is not clean, it cannot be sterile.

ENDNOTES

ANSI/AAMI ST79: 2006: Comprehensive Guide to Steam Sterilization and Sterility Assurance in Health Care Facilities", Association for the Advancement of Medical Instrumentation, www.aami.org October, 2006.

Talikwa, L. Facing Up to Wearing Facial Protective Equipment. Managing Infection Control. July, 2002.

Barnes, R. Enzymes. Communiqué. May/June, 2000.

Carlo, A. and Frieze, M. Challenges Impacting the Reprocessing of Reusable Medical Devices. Managing Infection Control. September, 2003.

Ryan, P; and Romey, S. Instrument Milk – The Controversy Continues: Survey on Instrument Lubrication. Journal of Healthcare Materials Management. August/September, 1989.

Cain, M. Washer/Disinfectors for Tomorrow's Healthcare Market. Infection Control Today. January, 1999.

Barnes, R. To Sonic or Not to Sonic. Communique. January/ February, 2000.

Vrancich, A. Proper Care and Handling of Surgical Instruments. Managing Infection Control. June, 2002.

Schultz, R. Surgical Instrument Cleaning Manual. Spectrum Surgical Instruments Corp. 1993.

OSHA Directives CPL 2-2.44D. Enforcement Procedures for the Occupational Exposure to Bloodborne Pathogens. Effective date: November 5,1999.

Pyrek, K. Infectious Medical Waste Management. Infection Control Today. January, 2002.

Dunn, J. Let's Talk Trash. Infection Control Sterilization Technology. February, 1999.

CENTRAL SERVICE TERMS

Cleaning

Decontamination

Relative humidity

Foot candle

Biohazardous

Personal protective equipment (PPE)

Standard precautions

Wetting agent

pH level

Chelating agents

Sequestering agents

Surfactant

Cavitation

Washers

Impingement

Chapter 10

Disinfection

Chapter Learning Objectives

As a result of successfully completing this chapter, readers will be able to:

1. Define the term, "disinfection," and explain how disinfection differs from sterilization.

2. Review factors that impact the effectiveness of a disinfectant.

3. Discuss the relationship between the risk level (intended use) of the device to be disinfected and the selection of a disinfectant.

4. Explain disinfectant activity levels as they relate to the resistance of microorganisms to germicidal agents:
   - high-level disinfection
   - intermediate-level disinfection
   - low-level disinfection

5. Review factors which affect the chemical action of and other important selection considerations for disinfections.

6. Provide basic information about the types of disinfectants commonly used in health care facilities: quaternary ammonium compounds, phenolics, alcohol, halogens, glutaraldehyde, ortho-phthalaldehyde, and formaldehyde.

7. Review safety requirements that should be followed when using chemical disinfectants.

8. Define the term, "thermal disinfection," and note key points to ensure that it is occurring.

Central Service departments use chemical disinfectants for many tasks including disinfecting instruments, cleaning equipment, and wiping surfaces. Knowledge about the protocols for their use is important for all Central Service Technicians, and basic information about disinfectants is provided in this chapter.

BASIC TERMINOLOGY

Learning Objective 1. Define the term, "disinfection," and explain how disinfection differs from sterilization.

A **disinfectant** is a chemical used on inanimate objects such as medical instruments to kill all organisms except spores. Unless a sterilant claim is made on the label, disinfectants cannot make something **sterile** (free from all living organisms). Disinfectants are not the same as **antiseptics** (chemicals used on living tissue such as skin to slow the growth of microorganisms). The process of **disinfection** can also be done by heat (**thermal disinfection**).

Sterilization is the use of physical or chemical procedures to completely destroy all microbial life. Steam-pressure autoclaving, dry heat, and low temperature methods (ethylene oxide gas, hydrogen peroxide [gas plasma], ozone, and liquid parasitic acid) are used to accomplish sterilization. Note: before items are disinfected or sterilized, they must be thoroughly cleaned. You learned in Chapter 9 that cleaning and decontamination renders contaminated items safe to handle with reasonable care. Cleaning is the first process used to protect

employees from risk of infection when items are returned to Central Service.

To select the most appropriate disinfectant for a given purpose, one must understand some basic characteristics of alternate chemical disinfectant groups (called "**families**"). As will be seen, some chemical families have members which appear to be dissimilar even though they share certain characteristics.

Disinfection is an often misunderstood and misused process. Knowledge about numerous factors that impact effective disinfection is important if the process is to be done correctly.

FACTORS IMPACTING EFFECTIVE-NESS OF DISINFECTANTS

Learning Objective 2. Review factors that impact the effectiveness of a disinfectant.

Thorough cleaning of items is the first and most important step in any sterilization or high-level disinfection process. Organic matter (soil) such as serum, blood, pus, and fecal material can dilute or inactivate the active ingredient in a liquid disinfectant. It can also hinder the contact of the disinfectant's ingredients with microorganisms on the surface of the device. Therefore, items should be cleaned until no visible tissue residue, fluid, or soil remains on them.

Excessive moisture must be removed from items before they are disinfected, because the disinfectant solution can be diluted by water that remains on

Disinfectant – A chemical which kills most pathogenic organisms, but does not kill spores, and is not a sterilant.

Sterile – Completely devoid of all living microorganisms.

Antiseptics – A solution which inhibits the growth of bacteria. Usually used topically and only used on animate objects.

Disinfection – The destruction of nearly all pathogenic microorganisms on an inanimate surface.

Thermal disinfection – The use of heat to kill all organisms except spores.

Sterilization – A process by which all forms of microbial life including bacteria, viruses, spores, and fungi are completely destroyed.

Families (chemicals) – A group of chemicals that have similar characteristics.

Bactericidal – Relating to the destruction of bacteria.

surfaces and in the lumens of items. Then the concentration of the active ingredient is lowered, and it is unable to kill certain microorganisms within the recommended exposure time.

Effectiveness of disinfectants also depends upon other factors besides excessive moisture including:

- Type and level (number) of microorganisms. Some microorganisms are more resistant to aqueous (liquid) disinfectants than are others. For example, the tubercle bacillus is much more resistant than some common vegetative organisms. The number of microorganisms is also important. This bioburden or microbial load can impede the ability of the disinfectant to do its job.

- Direct contact with the item. An item to be disinfected must come in direct contact with the disinfecting agent for a specified time. "Direct contact" means that there can be nothing including oils, protein soil, and detergent films between the disinfecting agent and the surface of the item being disinfected.

- Time. Direct contact by the disinfecting agent for a required amount of time is essential to achieving the desired **bactericidal** effect. This can, however, cause operating concerns. For example, if 70% isopropyl alcohol is used as a disinfectant, the alcohol may evaporate before the necessary contact time has elapsed.

- The temperature of the disinfectant. Some disinfectants are more effective when they are heated to an optimal temperature.

- pH. Disinfectants are formulated over a range of pH values at which they will be most effective. However, some disinfectants work better in an alkaline pH (greater than 7), while others work best under acetic or acid conditions (a pH of less than 7).

- Hardness of water. Minerals such as calcium and magnesium can affect the efficacy of the disinfectant by tying up its active ingredients. Most products are tested in hard water. Check the manufacturer's label for the disinfectant's claim of effectiveness and know the water quality of the water used for mixing disinfectant solutions.

- Material compatibility. Medical devices are designed from many different types of materials, and the disinfectant that is used must be appropriate for the material to be disinfected.

- Positioning of the devices. The position of some devices during disinfection is critical. (Example: lumens must be soaked vertically and items should be positioned so that no air pockets impede contact of the disinfectant solution during soaking).

DISINFECTANTS AND RISK LEVELS

Learning Objective 3. Discuss the relationship between the risk level (intended use) of the device to be disinfected and the selection of a disinfectant.

In the United States, chemical germicides utilized in health care are regulated by two federal agencies: the Environmental Protection Agency (EPA), and the Food and Drug Administration (FDA). Note: Risk levels are based upon the Spaulding Classification system which has been adopted for use by the Centers for Disease Control and Prevention (CDC).

The selection of a disinfection agent must be based, in part, upon the intended use of the device, and the degree of disinfection required for that device. Patient care items are divided into three categories based on the degree of risk of infection when the items were used on patients. The CDC and the Association for the Advancement of Medical Instrumentation (AAMI) use this system in their

hando chaet

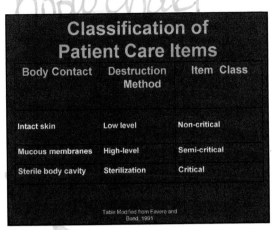

Figure 10.1

guidelines and recommendations. (See **Figure 10.1**) The three categories are:

* Critical items – Instruments or objects introduced directly into the blood stream or into other normally sterile areas of the body. Examples are surgical instruments, cardiac catheters, implants, pertinent components of a heart-lung oxygenator, and the blood compartment of a hemodialyzer. Sterility at the time of use is required for these items. One of several accepted sterilization procedures rather than disinfection is usually recommended.

* Semi-critical items – Examples include non-invasive flexible fiberoptic endoscopes, endotracheal tubes, anesthesia breathing circuits, and cystoscopes. Although these items come in contact with intact mucous membranes, they do not ordinarily penetrate body surfaces. Sterilization, although desirable, is not absolutely essential.

Nonlipid virus – A virus whose nucleic acid core is not surrounded by a lipid envelope. These viruses are generally more resistant to inactivation by disinfectants.

Lipid virus – A virus whose core is surrounded by a coat of lipoprotein. Viruses included in this structural category are generally easily inactivated by many types of disinfectants, including low level disinfectants.

* Semi-critical items should be subjected to a high-level disinfection procedure that can be expected to destroy vegetative (growing) microorganisms, most fungal spores, tubercle bacilli, small or **non-lipid viruses**, and medium-sized or **lipid viruses**. In most cases, meticulous physical cleaning followed by an appropriate high-level disinfection treatment will yield a reasonable assurance that the items are free of pathogenic microorganisms.

* Non-critical items – These items usually come into direct contact with the patient but, in most instances, only with unbroken skin. Examples include blood pressure cuffs, crutches, bed boards, most neurologic or cardiac diagnostic electrodes, and other medical accessories.

DISINFECTANT ACTIVITY LEVELS

Learning Objective 4. Explain disinfectant activity levels as they relate to the resistance of microorganisms to germicidal agents:
* high-level disinfection
* intermediate-level disinfection
* low-level disinfection

Disinfectants are classified into three levels of activity when microorganisms are grouped according to their resistance to physical or chemical germicidal agents. These three activity levels are:[1]

High-level disinfection – Process that utilizes a sterilant for a shorter contact time than that used for sterilization, and that kills all microbial organisms but not necessarily large numbers of bacterial spores. (AAMI TIR No. 7: 1999).

Intermediate-level disinfection – Process that utilizes an agent that kills viruses, mycobacteria, fungi, and vegetative bacteria, but not bacterial spores. (AAMI TIR No. 7: 1999).

Low-level disinfection – Process that utilizes an agent that kills vegetative forms of bacteria, some fungi, and lipid viruses. (AAMI TIR No. 7: 1999).

• High-level disinfection. Sterilization of devices is desirable; however, if this is not possible, **high-level disinfection** is the minimum treatment recommended by the CDC. High-level disinfection will destroy all vegetative microorganisms, tubercle bacilli, most fungi, non-lipid and small viruses, and lipid and medium-sized viruses with the exception of high numbers of bacterial spores.

• Intermediate-level disinfection. Disinfectants used for **intermediate-level disinfection** kill vegetative microorganisms, Mycobacterium tuberculosis, var. bovis (which is significantly more resistant to aqueous germicides than are vegetative bacteria), fungi, lipid and non-lipid and medium-sized and small viruses, but not necessarily bacterial spores.

• Low-level disinfection. Disinfectants used for **low-level disinfection** cannot be relied on to kill bacterial endospores, Mycobacterium, all fungi, and small or lipid viruses.

Figure 10.2 shows disease producing agents, and how they can be destroyed.

Hierarchy of Disease Producing Agents

Organism Producing Disease	Destruction Method
Prions	Extended Sterilization Times
Bacterial spores	Sterilization
Mycobacteria	High Level Disinfection
Nonlipid and small viruses (Poliovirus)	Intermediate-level Disinfection
Fungi	Intermediate-level Disinfection
Gram Positive & Negative Vegetative Bacteria	Low-level Disinfection
Lipid or medium sized viruses (Hantavirus, Herpes Simplex Virus)	Low-Level Disinfection

Table Modified from Favero and Bond, 1991

Figure 10.2

(handwritten notes:)
OPA — Solution
OPA — min. of 12 min.
14 days — open use life
75 days After opening
6 mo. on test strips

CHEMICAL ACTION AND SELECTION CONSIDERATIONS

Learning Objective 5. Review factors which affect the chemical action of and other important selection considerations for disinfectants.

The effectiveness of the disinfectant which is selected depends upon several factors that must be considered prior to use:

• The types of materials or devices on which the disinfectant is used.

• Whether items are partially or completely disassembled before exposure to the disinfectant.

• The manufacturer's recommended disinfection parameters to ensure effectiveness. For high-level disinfectants that require dilution, the quality and temperature of the water to be used is important, as is the number of times and/or length of time that the disinfectant is reused.

• The positioning of the device in the disinfectant.

• Test results which enable the effectiveness of the process to be measured or monitored including how the tests are used, and how frequently they are used.

• Whether the disinfectant has an expiration date for **shelf life** and **use life**.

• Whether mixing or other preparation method is required.

• Reuse factors including dilution, time, temperature, organic soil, and bio-burden.

Shelf life (disinfectants) – *The length of time a disinfectant can be properly stored after which it must be discarded.*

Use life (disinfectants) – *The length of time or number of times used after which the efficiency of a disinfectant is diminished.*

- Whether the manufacturer recommends additional inspections to assure device functionality. (If so, one must know if special instrumentation is needed to perform these inspections or tests.)

The first step in selecting a disinfectant is to consider the use of the item according to the Spaulding System to determine the required disinfection level. Other disinfectant selection factors are also important, and should be considered as the following and related questions are addressed:

- Is a dedicated container or other equipment needed for use?

- How can the efficacy of the product or process be measured? How often?

- What are the limitations of the product or process?

- Before exposing a device to the product or process, how should it be cleaned?

- How much time is required for the "complete" disinfection process?

- Is the disinfectant user friendly? For example, how many steps are involved in the process? Must high-level disinfection parameters (for example, time, temperature and concentration) be selected?

- Are there special preparations needed to ready the medical devices for the disinfection process?

- Is control of water quality critical to the process?

- Is the disinfectant potentially toxic to those that handle it?

- Are there specific instructions which explain how toxic conditions or reactions can be avoided during use?

- Should a local exhaust hood be used?

- Are special storage conditions necessary?

- Does the disinfectant leave residues on processed items that could be toxic to patients or staff members? If so, is there a method for reducing residues on processed items to nontoxic levels?

- Are there potential physical hazards such as fire or explosion?

- Can heat or other environmental conditions cause chemical changes in the disinfectant?

DISINFECTANTS USED IN HEALTH CARE FACILITIES

Learning Objective 6. Provide basic information about the types of disinfectants commonly used in health care facilities: quaternary ammonium compounds, phenolics, alcohol, halogens, glutaraldehyde, ortho-phthalaldehyde, and formaldehyde.

Critical, semi-critical, and non-critical items must be sterilized or disinfected using high-level, intermediate, or low-level disinfectants before reuse. The disinfectants which are used must be suitable for applicable risk categories, and must address the selection concerns just noted. The discussion in this section provides specific information about the proper selection and use of each of the disinfectants commonly used in health care facilities in the United States.

Quaternary Ammonium Compounds

Quaternary Ammonium Compounds (commonly called "quats") are a low-level disinfectant. Most hospital personnel are acquainted with one member of this family: benzalkonium chloride. Another member of this group is cetylpyridinium chloride.

Quats are cationic surface-active compounds also known as "wetting agents." They lower surface tension of the solution which allows greater penetration of the disinfectant into the soil. Since

Figure 10.3 Summery of Quats

- Mode of action: inactivates energy-producing enzymes, denatures essential cell protein, and disrupts cell membranes.

- Advantages:
  - Bactericidal, fungicidal, and virucidal against lipophilic viruses.
  - Cationic surface-active compounds or wetting agents with built-in detergent properties.

- Disadvantages:
  - Not sporicidal.
  - Generally not tuberculocidal or virucidal against hydrophilic viruses.
  - Inactivated (absorbed or neutralized) by cotton and charcoal.
  - Cationic, and not compatible with soap (which is anionic).
  - Not effective against some gram-negative organisms commonly found in hospitals.

- Uses:
  - Environmental sanitation of non-critical surfaces such as floors, walls, and furniture.

these compounds are **cationic**, they carry a positive ionic charge, and they are incompatible with soap which is **anionic** (that possesses a negative charge).

The germicidal action of quats is reduced in the presence of organic materials. These compounds also possess another unique property: they are absorbed by some materials including cotton, wool, filter paper, and charcoal. This absorption markedly depletes its concentration. Historically, this created significant risks because it was a customary practice to soak items in a pan which had a cotton towel or gauze covering its bottom.

The presence of calcium or magnesium ions hinders the action of quats, and serious problems can develop if quats are mixed with hard tap water.

Cationic – Compounds that contain a positive electrical charge on the large organic hydrophobic molecule. Cationic detergents exhibit germicidal properties.

Anionic – Compounds which have a negative electrical charge on the large organic portion of the molecule which is relatively hydrophobic and lipophilic. These form the large group of synthetic detergents.

Another serious limitation to the use of quats is their lack of activity against the pseudomonas, especially Pseudomonas pyocyanea. Also, in aqueous solution, quats cause rusting of instruments after prolonged soaking unless sodium nitrate or a related chemical is added to the solution as a rust inhibitor.

Quats compounds are not the disinfectants of choice for use in Central Service because of their lack of activity against tubercle bacilli, and some other gram-negative Pseudomonas bacilli. There is a high percentage of hospital-acquired infections caused by gram-negative organisms, so this is a serious limitation. Other concerns relate to their fungicidal activity, and to their corrosive effect on stainless steel.

Figure 10.3 summarizes basic information about quats.

Phenolics

Phenols are intermediate- to low-level disinfectants containing phenol (carbolic acid) which has a long history of distinction and use. For example, during the 1880's, Lister used phenol in efforts to develop aseptic surgical techniques.

Figure 10.4 Summary of Phenolics

- Mode of action: penetrates cell wall, and precipitates cell protein

- Advantages:
  - Broad spectrum of use: bactericidal for gram-negative and gram-positive bacteria, fungicidal and tuberculocidal; active against lipophilic viruses.
  - Residual activity. Note: this can also be a disadvantage

- Disadvantages:
  - Not sporicidal.
  - Inactivated by organic material (but less than some other disinfectants).
  - Corrosive to rubber and some plastics.

- Uses:
  - Housekeeping usage for walls, floors, countertops, and furnishings.
  - Phenolics are recommended for use in the decontamination area for disinfection of hard surfaces. Copious rinsing is required to eliminate the potential for skin burns.

Depending upon their concentration, all phenolic compounds can act either bactericidally (to destroy bacteria) or bacteriostatically (to inhibit or retard bacterial growth). Accurate preparation of mixtures is important since small changes in dilution can produce large differences in bactericidal activity. Phenolic compounds have long been the agent of choice for housekeeping services because a residual phenolic film is left after use which can be reactivated later by damp mopping. However, this same residual film can be a problem when left on Central Service equipment. Note: the film can be removed by copious rinsing, although this may not be consistently done in many facilities.

Skin irritation (minor burns of sensitive skin) and even skin depigmentation can occur after exposure to phenolic residues on equipment if it comes in close contact with a patient's skin or mucous membrane. This problem should be addressed when phenolic compounds are considered for use in Central Service. For example, their use should be discouraged for items such as K-pads, alternating pressure pads, hypothermia blankets, and other items that have intimate contact with skin for long periods of time.

Phenolic compounds can be inactivated by the presence of organic material. For example, there is a decrease of up to 90% in bactericidal activity of some compounds in the presence of milk, serum, or feces. For maximum disinfectant effectiveness, most phenolics require wet contact for twenty minutes. However, this step is often overlooked even though it is part of the usage directions for these items.

Stainless steel instruments should not be subjected to strong phenolics for any prolonged period of time because these compounds are markedly corrosive. While phenolic compounds have many anti-microbial applications, they should also not be used on rubber or certain plastic items.

Figure 10.4 reviews basic information about phenolics.

Alcohol

Both ethyl and isopropyl alcohol have good disinfecting properties. Many experts believe that 70% isopropyl alcohol possesses the most effective disinfecting properties, especially when it is applied to inanimate objects, and this concentration is widely used in U.S. hospitals. Note: While ethyl or isopropyl alcohol products are available in 60-90% concentrations, high percent solutions are not necessarily better, and they can even be less effective since water is needed to carry alcohol into the cells

Figure 10.5 Summary of Ethyl or Isopropyl Alcohol

• Mode of action: denatures (changes the structure of) proteins.

• Advantages:

  • Rapid bactericidal agent against vegetative microorganisms; tuberculocidal, fungicidal, and virucidal. (Ethyl isopropyl is not effective against hydrophilic viruses.)

  • Fast-acting; no residue.

  • Non-staining

• Disadvantages:

  • Requires wet contact of at least five minutes to achieve a reasonable level of disinfection.

  • No residual activity.

  • Volatile; flammable.

  • Inactivated by organic material.

  • Can dissolve lens mountings on certain optical instruments.

  • Tends to harden and swell plastic tubing, including polyethylene.

  • Non-sporicidal.

• Uses:

  • To disinfect countertops and fixed equipment after cleaning, and for patient-use items such as earpecula, stethescopes, and thermometers. The addition of iodine to alcohol is helpful when disinfecting thermometers.

which it destroys. However, these concentrations do not typically kill bacteria which are encased in blood or pus because residual proteins interact with and deactivate most disinfectants. Note: this confirms a concern noted in other chapters: "One can clean without disinfecting, but one cannot disinfect without cleaning."

To achieve a reasonable level of disinfection, the alcohol must remain in wet contact with the surface of the object being disinfected for a minimum of five minutes. On vertical surfaces, this step may be accomplished by wrapping the item with a towel saturated with isopropyl alcohol.

The Society of Gastroenterolgy Nurses and Associates (SGNA) suggests that, if tap water is used to rinse flexible fiberoptic endoscopes after disinfection, a 70% isopropyl alcohol rinse be used. The Society also recommends that the channels be flushed with 70-90% ethyl or isopropyl alcohol to facilitate drying, and to discourage growth of residual microorganisms.

Under optimum conditions, alcohols can disinfect relatively fast (2 - 10 minutes), especially against vegetative organisms. However, it may take much longer (up to several hours) to destroy viruses, because they are always suspended in proteins which precipitate in alcohol and, in turn, provide some protection to the virus.

Figure 10.5 summarizes basic information about ethyl or isopropyl alcohol.

Halogens

Halogens are intermediate-level disinfectants that have similar elements possessing some unique properties. The family is known for its reactivity, and two members (chlorine and iodophors) possess disinfecting and sterilizing properties.

Figure 10.6 Summary of Chlorine

- Mode of action: inhibits some key enzymatic reactions within the cell, denatures protein,and inactivates nucleic acids.

- Advantages:
  - Extremely active as free chlorine.
  - Effective against gram-positive and gram- negative (vegetative) microorganisms; tuberculocidal, fungicidal, and virucidal.
  - Rapid-acting.

- Disadvantages:
  - Inactivated by organic matter.
  - Corrosive to metals.
  - Non-sporicidal.
  - Stains fabrics, plastics, and other synthetic materials.
  - Relatively unstable.

- Uses:

  - Widely used for disinfection of dialysis machines, hydrotherapy baths, toilets, lavatories, and bathtubs; also used as a bleach for laundry, and as a sanitizer for dishwashing.

  - A 1:10 dilution of 5.25% sodium hypochloride has been recommended by the CDC for cleaning blood spills.

Chlorine

Inorganic chlorine is most valuable for the disinfection of water, sewage, swimming pools, and food and drinking utensils. Many authorities believe that it has limited application for disinfection in a hospital setting, particularly in Central Service. Chlorine is not considered a disinfectant of choice because quality control is a concern, and there can be variations in chlorine release caused by the hardness of water and other factors. A hypochlorite solution (for example, sodium hypochlorite) can be useful, however, for bleaching stains from some materials.

Figure 10.6 reviews basic information about chlorine.

Figure 10.7 Summary of Buffered Iodine

• Mode of action: poisons cells of nucleic acids; quickly penetrates the cell walls of microorganisms.

• Advantages:

• Bactericidal, virucidal, and tuberculocidal.

• Rapid action against vegetative bacteria.

• Disadvantages:

• Corrosive to metals unless combined with anti-corrosive agents when formulated.

• Detrimental to rubber and some plastics.

• May burn tissue.

• Stains fabrics and other materiel.

• May require long contact time to kill some fungi.

• Uses:

• Used in skin preparations, thermometers (especially elemental iodine units combined with alcohol), and for disinfection of some equipment. The corrosive nature of iodine on metals, rubber, and some plastics limits its use as a primary disinfectant in Central Service.

Iodophors

Iodophors are a reactive member of the halogen family, and an iodophor compound results from mixing iodine with a detergent and other ingredients. An iodophor, then, is a buffered iodine which is water soluble. Its disinfecting properties are very depressed (inactivated) in the presence of organic (especially protein) matter.

Figure 10.7 summarizes basic information about iodine.

Glutaraldehyde

Glutaraldehyde is a high level disinfectant used for semi-critical devices such as endoscopes and ultrasonic probes used in radiology. Conditions including times and temperatures for its use as a high-level disinfectant vary by manufacturer, and it is always best to consult the product's manufacturer for this information. The time for sterilization is extended to 10 hours or more depending upon the concentration and the manufacturer's recommendations. Activation of the solution is usually accomplished by mixing the solution with a pre-measured activator.

Heavy Metals as Disinfectants

Some metals possess disinfecting properties. An example is mercury in the form of bichloride of mercury. In the early 1900's, it was used extensively for disinfection, especially in nurseries. Its use came into question, however, when researchers learned that mercury can be absorbed by intact human skin, and can cause brain damage. Mercury is no longer used in Central Service as a disinfecting agent.

Silver, in the form of silver nitrate, is another metal with disinfecting properties. It is used as drops in the eyes of newborn infants to prevent blindness which might be caused by gonorrhea. Silver nitrate also has had application in the treatment of burns. Example: catheters are treated with silver nitrate to decrease infections.

There are a few other metals, notably copper and tin, which possess some microbiocidal activities. However, there is no practical use for any heavy metal as a disinfectant in Central Service.

Glutaraldehyde is compatible with a wide range of materials. It kills microorganisms by alkylation of protein. Glutaraldehyde is usually a clear liquid that turns green when activated, and it has a sharp, pungent odor which is typical of all aldehydes. It is a strong irritant to the skin, eyes, and respiratory system, and vapor inhalation has been implicated as a possible cause of occupational asthma.

Glutaraldehyde should be used in separate designated areas where control can be exercised over ventilation, traffic, and proper equipment installation, operation, and maintenance. Rooms in which glutaraldehyde is used should be well-ventilated (a minimum of 10 air changes per hour), and large enough to ensure adequate dilution of the vapor. Local exhaust ventilation should be installed to control the vapor. *at least 200 sq. feet*

Although automated glutaraldehyde processing equipment is designed to reduce exposures, adequate ventilation is still necessary. Vapor can escape into the work area when the solution is activated and loaded into the reservoir, and it may become necessary for the Central Service Technician to open the system during the cycle.

Unused glutaraldehyde solution should be stored in a cool, secure, and properly marked location in tightly closed, properly marked containers labeled with the activation date.

Glutaraldehyde-based products can be used in automated or manual high-level disinfection processes. Many automated reprocessors are equipped with temperature-control devices, and feature computerized reprocessing cycles, bacteria-retentive filters for rinse water, and filters for removing suspended materials from the reused disinfectant.

Glutaraldehyde is compatible with materials used in many modern medical devices, and can be used to process medical devices containing heat-sensitive materials. Most glutaraldehyde-based instrument sterilants are labeled for reuse for 14 to 28 days. During the recommended reuse period, the concentration of the glutaraldehyde in the solution should be tested with test strips recommended by the manufacturer. If the solution falls below its minimum recommended concentration, it should

be discarded regardless of how many days the solution has been in use.

Solution test strips provide a fast and easy way to ensure that the glutaraldehyde solutions are safe (effective) to use without excessive dilution or heavy contamination. They work quickly and are simple to use: a test strip with an indicating pad is dipped into the glutaraldehyde solution for a few seconds. Wait for a color change. Note: It is important to confirm that staff members who perform the test have adequate color perception. Then enter the result in the log book to establish a permanent record. Always follow the manufacturer's written recommendations.

Glutaraldehyde fumes should be monitored for employee safety. The recommended maximum ceiling exposure limit is 0.20 ppm as a **ceiling limit** which must not be exceeded. Suitable eyewash units must be available for immediate emergency use within 10 seconds' travel time, and/or 100 feet travel distance of all glutaraldehyde usage locations. Note: one easy and inexpensive way to comply with this requirement is to mount a small eyewash that fits directly onto a water faucet.

Glutaraldehyde vapors increase whenever the solution is agitated such as when it is poured into or dumped out of a soaking bin, when instruments are placed into and removed from the solution, and when instruments are rinsed. Employees should be trained to minimize agitation of the solution during these work procedures. If exposure monitoring indicates that these procedures result in excessive exposure levels, the work process should be enclosed in a glutaraldehyde fume hood system. Exposure levels for Central Service Technicians during disposal can be greatly reduced by adding a glutaraldehyde-neutralizing agent to the solution immediately prior to disposal.

Ceiling limit – *According to OSHA, "the employee's exposure (to an air contaminant) which shall not be exceeded during any part of the work day. If instantaneous monitoring is not feasible, then the ceiling shall be assessed as a 15-minute time-weighted average exposure which shall not be exceeded at any time over a working day."*

Figure 10.8 Summary of Glutaraldehyde / Cidex

- Mode of action: A 2% alkaline solution with a pH of 7.5 - 8.5 kills microorganisms by alkylation of protein.

- Advantages:
  - Kills vegetative bacteria (within 2 minutes).
  - Bactericidal (gram-positive and gram-negative), tuberculocidal, fungicidal, virucidal, and sporicidal. For sterilization (killing spores), the soak time is 6 - 10 hours, and the manufacturer's label for recommendations should be followed.

- Disadvantages:
  - Noxious odors; good ventilation is required to prevent nausea for some healthcare workers.
  - Unstable (14 or 28-day product life).
  - Dilution of product reduces the activity necessary for high-level disinfection.
  - Vaporizes.
  - No cleaning ability. (Items must be thoroughly cleaned before use.)
  - Required rinsing process is always necessary.

- Uses:
  - Semi-critical items such as laryngoscope blades, flexible scopes, etc.

All employees who work with or around glutaraldehyde should receive thorough safety training including a discussion of OSHA regulations, safe work practices, proper protective clothing, and safe spill clean-up procedures. They must also be informed about specific steps the employer has taken to minimize exposure levels, the methods they can use to identify a release of glutaraldehyde, and how to determine when an over-exposure situation has occurred.

Disposable latex surgical or exam gloves do not provide adequate glutaraldehyde protection. These gloves are usually only 5 - 6 millimeters thick, and can quickly deteriorate. Nitrile or butyl gloves should be used when working with glutaraldehyde.

Figure 10.8 presents basic information about glutaraldehyde.

Ortho-Phthalaldehyde

Ortho-phthalaldehyde (commonly called OPA) is a relatively new high-level disinfectant that provides a fast and effective way to disinfect a wide range of instruments and endoscopes. It is compatible with a variety of materials including metal, plastic, elastomers, and adhesives commonly used in the construction of reprocessable medical devices. An OPA solution (0.55%) is effective at room temperature, and has excellent tuberculocidal and high-level disinfection capabilities. However, it is not classified as a sterilant. Even though OPA does not have an odor, the area of its use should still be well-ventilated, and its containers should have lids. (In other words, what you cannot smell can still hurt you!)

Soak time is 12 minutes at room temperature (usually 68°F; 20°C) in a manual system, or 5 minutes at 77°F (25°C) in an automatic endoscope reprocessor (AER) to destroy all pathogenic microorganisms. Note: always check with the product manufacturer for exact temperature recommendations.

Following immersion in OPA solution, the device should be thoroughly rinsed by completely immersing it in a large volume (for example, 2 gallons) of water. Repeat this procedure twice with fresh rinse water. Each rinse should be for a minimum of 1 minute unless otherwise noted by the device or equipment manufacturer. Discard the water down the drain after each rinse. Do not reuse the water for rinsing, or for any other purpose, as

Figure 10.9 Summary of OPA

• Mode of action: kills by protein alkylation.

• Advantages:
  • High level disinfection in 12 minutes at room temperature (usually 68°F; 20°C) in manual system or 5 minutes at 77°F (25°C) in an automatic endoscope reprocessor.
  • Provides a user-friendly environment.
  • Solution is compatible with a wide range of endoscopes and other medical devices.
  • Requires no activation or mixing.
  • 14-day reuse life, and two-year shelf life.
  • Can be discarded down hospital and office drains in accordance with local regulations.

• Disadvantages:
  • Improper rinsing can result in staining of patient tissues.
  • Does not have a sterilant label claim.

  • Patients with a history of bladder cancer should not be exposed to items processed by OPA.[2]

• Uses:
  • Semi-critical items such as laryngoscope blades, flexible fiberoptic endoscopes, etc.

it will be contaminated with OPA. Note: several reports have alleged the presence of black stains and/or burns appearing on the patient's skin after a transesophageal imaging examination. These are consistent with the presence of residual OPA on the transducer as a result of insufficient rinsing during the disinfection process. This reinforces the need for required rinsing procedures to be strictly followed to avoid residual OPA, and any other resulting undesirable effects.

The concentration of OPA solution during its use-life must be verified by use of OPA Solution Test Strips to assure that the **minimum effective concentration (MEC)** of 0.3% is present. The OPA solution may be used and reused within the limitations indicated above for up to 14 days.

It must then be discarded even if the test strip indicates a concentration above the MEC.

The OPA solution should be tested with test strips prior to each reuse to ensure that it is of the appropriate concentration. Visually inspect the solution during the reuse life for the presence of precipitates which may result from the use of hard water. Discard the solution if precipitation occurs.

Figure 10.9 provides a summary of basic information about OPA.

Minimum effective concentration (MEC) – The percentage concentration of the active ingredient in a disinfectant (or chemical sterilant) that is the minimum concentration at which the chemical meets all its label claims for activity against specific microorganisms.

Basic information about formaldehyde is presented in **Figure 10.10**

Figure 10.10 Summary of Formaldehyde

- Mode of action: inactivates microorganisms by alkylation.
- Advantages:
  - Bactericidal, tuberculocidal, fungicidal, and virucidal.
  - Sporicidal (8% formaldehyde + 70% alcohol).
- Disadvantages:
  - Inactivated by organic material.
  - May stain fabrics, plastics, and other synthetic materials.
  - Not sporicidal.
  - Carcinogen (1ppm, 8 hour TWA).
  - Irritating fumes.
  - Corrosive.

Formaldehyde

Formaldehyde (formalin) is available in different concentrations for use as a high, intermediate, and low-level disinfectant:

- High-level (8% formaldehyde + 70% alcohol).
- Intermediate-level (4 to 8% formaldehyde in water).
- Low-level (less than 4% limited activity against TB).

Since formaldehyde is not corrosive to hemodialysis equipment, it is used in concentrations of 4% to disinfect dialysis systems. To minimize a potential health hazard to dialysis patients, equipment must be rinsed thoroughly, and tested for residual formaldehyde. A minimum contact time for disinfection of used dialyzers is 24 hours.[3]

Preparing and Using Activated High-Level Disinfectant Solutions

When preparing activated solutions, the user should follow the instructions of the liquid chemical sterilant/high-level disinfectant manufacturer. Some liquid chemical sterilants are labeled for use as both sterilants and high-level disinfectants with sterilization requiring a longer contact time. The appropriate conditions for use are provided by the manufacturer on the product's label and are based upon FDA-recommended testing protocols. It is essential that users carefully follow label usage instructions to avoid a process failure.

Recommendations about the type of container used to prepare the activated solution should be followed to ensure that there is no interaction between the container and the active or inert ingredients of the liquid chemicals. Containers for high-level disinfectants should be covered to prevent exposure to fumes, to avoid evaporation, and to prevent particles such as dust from falling into them.

Gloves should always be worn when using a disinfectant. Skin is living tissue, and effective disinfectants are made to harm living things. Severe skin reactions can occur when strong disinfectants are used inappropriately.

Only high-level disinfectants labeled for reuse should be reused; the specified use-life, number of reuses, and/or expiration dates must not be exceeded. All items processed with high-level disinfectants should be thoroughly rinsed to reduce chemical residues to safe levels. Users should follow the recommendations of the device and the disinfectant manufacturers relating to the microbial quality of the rinsing solution. Manufacturers of high-level disinfectants provide chemical indicators to monitor their product's effectiveness, and these should be used according to recommendations.

The tasks of verifying EPA registration and FDA cleared disinfection solutions is also critical. All products must have labels with a registration number, and information that identifies the organism against which it is effective. Check for the most recent information on the FDA web page (Cleared Sterilants and High Level Disinfectants with General Claims for Processing Reusable Medical and Dental Devices): http://www.fda.gov/cdrh/ode/germlab.html

Sample Glutaraldehyde Spill Containment Plan

A written plan to contain glutaraldehyde spills should be prepared by the hospital. Procedures should specify:

- Clean-up equipment needed.
- Placement of equipment for easy access.
- A plan for alerting personnel.
- Recommendations for avoiding exposure.
- Evacuation of non-essential personnel.

The plan should include:

- Procedures for evacuating personnel in the event of a spill.
- Procedures for medically treating persons who may have been over-exposed to the solution or vapor.
- Procedures for reporting an emergency to appropriate authorities.
- Procedures for material clean-up which specify necessary equipment including that required for personal protection.
- Description of the employee training program, and method(s) used to verify competency.
- The known rate of air exchanges in the spill area.
- The potential for the general ventilation system to carry the vapor to other areas, and a prescribed course of action to prevent it from doing so.

- Product manufacturer's recommendations for emergency procedures as specified in the MSDS.
- Appropriate disposal methods for materials used for spill clean-up that meet the state's EPA requirements.

Several chemicals including sodium bisulfite, dibasic ammonium phosphate, household ammonia, and ammonium carbonate powder can be used to decrease the glutaraldehyde concentration in solutions, and/or to reduce ambient vapor levels in spill situations. Remember that the chemicals are hazardous. Specific storage, training, and utilization techniques are required. There are also commercially available products designed for this purpose.

Drips and splashes should be immediately wiped-up with a sponge, towel, or mop which should then be thoroughly rinsed with large amounts of water. The water can then be discarded down a drain.

Large spills should be contained and neutralized, or contained and collected for disposal. After the glutaraldehyde solution is collected and disposed of, the area contaminated by the solution should be thoroughly rinsed. Clean-up tools should also be thoroughly rinsed with water which can then be carefully flushed down a drain or discarded.

Maintain a Log Book

A log book should be maintained when using high-level disinfectants (glutaraldehyde and OPA). Central Service Technicians using these products should record the date the solution was poured from the original container into a secondary container. Other information to be recorded includes that shown in the column headings in **Figure 10.9**. Solutions should not be used if their concentration of high-level disinfectant falls below the minimum effective concentration (MEC) as indicated by solution test strips. Disinfected reusable devices should be either immediately used or stored in a manner that minimizes recontamination. Refer to the reusable device manufacturer's labeling for additional storage and/or handling instructions.

Figure 10.11 is an example of a high-level disinfectant solution log sheet.

Figure 10.11 High-Level Disinfectant Solution Log Sheet							
Location/Department:		High-Level Disinfectant:					
Warning: DO NOT USE SOLUTION BEYOND ITS STATED REUSE LIFE.							
Date Solution Opened	Date Solution Expires	Date Test Strips Expire	Test Date	Location	Test Results (+) Pass (-) Fail	Tested By (Initials)	Comments

SAFETY CONCERNS

Learning Objective 7. Review safety requirements that should be followed when using chemical disinfectants.

Safety is always a special concern when using chemical disinfectants. Basic safety concerns to be followed when Central Service Technicians perform disinfection tasks include:

• Staff must wear the necessary personnel protective equipment (PPE).

• An exhaust hood (see the photo in **Figure 10.12**) is needed since some disinfectants produce fumes that irritate the respiratory tract.

• Develop a spill plan and routine disposal procedures for each solution.

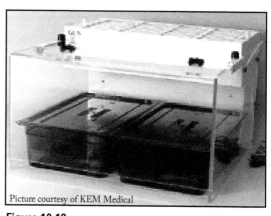

Picture courtesy of KEM Medical

Figure 10.12

- Provide an eye wash shower and other first aid supplies in close proximity to applicable work areas in case of an emergency.

- Provide easy access to a phone and phone numbers in case of emergency.

Additional safety procedures include the implementation of training programs.

- Provide yearly staff training that addresses chemical disinfectant usage.

- Provide yearly staff training (including for those in the housekeeping department) about safety issues.

- Monitor disinfectants (including air sampling if required), and share the results with staff.

It is also important to keep manufacturer's information on file, and staff should know where the resources are located. Material safety data sheets (MSDSs) should also be kept on file where staff members can easily locate them, and all applicable national, state, and local guidelines for each solution should be consistently followed.

Environmental Evaluation

Whenever possible, Central Service personnel should be aware of the impact that chemical disinfectants have on the environment. They can ask if a product's formulation contains materials that are confirmed as GRAS (Generally Recognized As Safe). The chemical disinfectant does not itself contain or produce adverse health effects, and is stable and fast-acting. Products can also receive what is known as the Green Seal when they meet certain criteria. Note: information about Green Seal-approved products can be found at: http://www.greenseal.org

THERMAL DISINFECTION

Learning Objective 8. Define the term, thermal disinfection, and note key points to ensure that it is occurring.

Disinfection can also be done by heat in a process called thermal disinfection. This is commonly accomplished with automated equipment such as automatic washer-sanitizers/disinfectors, pasteurization equipment, and automatic endoscope reprocessors. **Figures 10.13** and **10.14** provide examples of washers that use thermal disinfection processes.

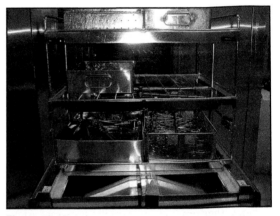

Figure 10.13

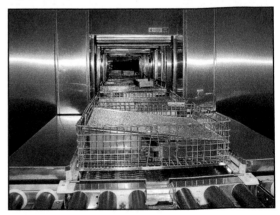

Figure 10.14

Water temperature is the key source of disinfection in any automatic washer equipment that claims thermal disinfection. The time and temperature required to achieve the specified disinfection level differs by brand. Since the target of thermal disinfection is the instrument's surface, it is critical to monitor the surface temperature of instruments to know if disinfection has occurred.

Water temperature needs be monitored and documented independent of the machine. Medical automatic washers usually monitor temperature in the washer's drain area, rather than at the instrument's surface level. Thermal couplers and heaters can also fail, and irreversible thermometers and remote sensing equipment are now available to monitor and document the temperature of the thermal disinfection rinse of medical automated washers.

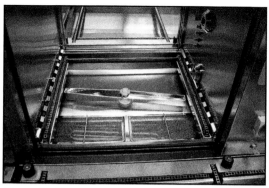

Figure 10.15

For thermal disinfection to be achieved, Central Service Technicians must visually inspect the instruments such as scopes and surgical tools that are being processed. This task must be performed prior to high level disinfection because bioburden left on the item can reduce the thermal disinfection process.

Commercially available products can enhance the visual inspection process. Some are soil tests to help assure that equipment is functioning properly. These tests involve attaching the test product to the equipment, and reading results after the cycle is run. Other products are specific tests for various types of bioburden that might not be noted by visual inspection of the instruments when they are processed.

Thermal disinfection equipment that uses spray arms should be checked at least daily to ensure that the arms are completely free-turning, and that the

spray nozzles are not clogged. (See **Figure 10.15**) If the equipment has strainers, they should be cleaned at least daily, or when there is visible debris. Regular preventive maintenance should be performed in compliance with the manufacturer's instructions by a factory-trained, qualified person on all thermal disinfection equipment. If nozzles are clogged, an ineffective thermal disinfection process is likely.

Central Service Technicians must be trained to properly operate all equipment, and must understand all necessary factors to help ensure that thermal disinfection has occurred. A quality improvement process that monitors thermal disinfection is important, and its use should be an integral part of the daily activities of all Central Service staff.

AAMI and The Joint Commission Support Verification Procedures

The Association for the Advancement of Medical Instrumentation (AAMI) emphasizes the need for Central Service staff to use appropriate methods to verify the decontamination process. For example, both the user and the manufacturer are alerted to the importance of following proper verification methods. (AAMI TIR 12). AAMI also advocates that departments should implement methods to verify that cleaning and thermal disinfection have taken place.[4]

The Joint Commission states the need for medical equipment to be maintained, tested, and inspected. (Standard E.C.6.20).

The Food and Drug Administration (FDA) and Disinfection Equipment

Medical washers or washer disinfectors are medical devices used to process medical devices. As such, they are regulated by the FDA when they are transported in interstate commerce. A medical washer-disinfector intended to clean and provide high level disinfection of medical devices must have an FDA cleared pre-market notification [510(k)] submission before it can be sold. By contrast, a medical washer intended to clean medical devices, or a medical washer-disinfector intended to clean and provide either low or intermediate level disinfection of medical devices, is exempt from 510(k) requirements.[6] The majority of medical automatic washers used in U.S. hospitals to clean surgical instruments provide low-to-intermediate level disinfection and are, therefore, exempt from the 510 (k) requirements. On the other hand, many automatic endoscopic reprocessors (AERs) are Class II medical devices. It is important to know how the FDA classifies equipment in a specific facility, and it must then be used according to the manufacturer's guidelines.

ENDNOTES

1. Block, S. Disinfection, Sterilization and Preservation. Fourth Edition. 1991.

2. The Q-Net"! Monthly ;Volume 12,Numbers 7,8 ; July August 2006.

3. Information about federal safety regulations applicable to formaldehyde is available in OSHA 29 CFE-1910.1048.

4. ANSI/AAMI ST79:2006: "Comprehensive Guide to Steam Sterilization and Sterility Assurance in Healthcare Facilities", Association for the Advancement of Medical Instrumentation, www.aami.org, October 2006 http://www.fda.gov/cdrh/ode/guidance/1252.html

ADDITIONAL RESOURCES

Chemical sterilants and high-level disinfectants: A guide to selection and use. AAMI Technical Information Report #7:1999 Approved October 18, 1999, 2000.

Glutaraldehyde Safety Action Plan. Purdue University/IAHCSMM Self Study Series. Lesson #32.

Association for the Advancement of Medical Instrumentation (AAMI). Safe Use and Handling of Glutaraldehyde-based Products in Health Care Facilities. March, 1997.

CENTRAL SERVICE TERMS

Disinfectant

Sterile

Antiseptics

Disinfection

Thermal disinfection

Sterilization

Families (chemicals)

Bactericidal

High-level disinfection

Intermediate-level disinfection

Low-level disinfection

Shelf life (disinfectants)

Use life (disinfectants)

Cationic

Anionic

Ceiling limit

Minimum effective concentration (MEC)

Chapter 11

Surgical Instrumentation

Chapter Learning Objectives:

As a result of successfully completing this chapter, readers will be able to:

1. Review the process by which surgical instruments are manufactured.

2. Define basic categories of surgical instruments based upon their functions, and identify the points of inspection, anatomy (features) of, and procedures to measure the following types of instruments:
   - Hemostatic Forceps
   - Needleholders
   - Tissue Forceps
   - Dressing Forceps
   - Retractors
   - Scissors
   - Suction Devices
   - Single and Double Action Rongeurs
   - Kerrison/Laminectomy Rongeurs
   - Nail Nippers
   - Graves and Pederson Vaginal Speculums

3. Identify solutions that can damage stainless steel instruments.

4. Explain procedures to test instruments for sharpness, and to identify (mark) them.

5. Emphasize the importance of instrument lubrication, and review tray assembly safeguards.

Instrument Manufacturing Process

Learning Objective 1. Review the process by which surgical instruments are manufactured.

Surgical instruments are manufactured differently than most Central Service Technicians might expect. In this era of high technology, they may imagine that instruments are stamped out on a high speed assembly line, packaged, and then shipped to the customer. However, this is far from the actual process, and their manufacture requires time-consuming and hands-on labor from highly skilled crafts persons.

Types of Stainless Steel

The study of the surgical instrument manufacturing process begins by considering the raw materials used to create them. Most are produced from stainless steel; however, other materials like titanium, copper, and silver are also widely used.

Several types of stainless are steel used to produce surgical instruments. One type (400 series stainless steel) is hard, and it is used when sharp cutting edges are needed. Instruments produced with 400 series steel include **scissors, osteotomes, chisels, rongeurs, forceps, hemostatic forceps,** and **needleholders.** This hardened steel is known as **Martensitic stainless steel.**

The second most popular steel used to manufacture surgical instruments is 300 series stainless steel. While it offers high corrosion resistance, this material doesn't provide the hardness properties of its 400 series counterpart, so it is more workable and malleable. Instruments produced with 300 series stainless steel include **retractors, cannulas, rib spreaders,** and **suction devices.**

---

1 - **Scissors** – Surgical instruments used to cut, incise, and/or dissect tissue.

2 - **Osteotomes** – Chisel-like instruments used to cut or shave bone.

3 - **Chisels** – Wedge-shaped instruments used to cut or shape bone.

4 - **Rongeurs** – Surgical instruments used to cut or bite away at bone and tissue.

5 - **Forceps** – Surgical instruments used to grasp.

6 - **Hemostatic forceps** – Surgical instruments used to control flow of blood.

7 - **Needleholders** – Surgical instruments designed to drive suture needles to close or rejoin a wound or surgical site.

8 - **Martensitic(stainless steel)** – This metal is also known as 400 series stainless steel. It is magnetic, and may be heat-hardened.

9 - **Retractors** – Surgical instruments primarily used to move tissues and organs to keep them exposed throughout surgery.

10 - **Cannulas** – Surgical instruments with a hollow barrel (or lumen) through their center. Cannulas are often inserted for drainage.

11 - **Rib spreaders** – A retractor used to expose the chest.

12 - **Suction devices** – Surgical instruments used to extract blood from a surgical site.

13 - **Austenitic (stainless steel)** – This metal is also known as 300 series stainless steal. It is non-magnetic, cannot be heat-hardened, and is more corrosion-resistant than martensitic stainless steel.

14 - **Serrations** – Parallel grooves in the jaws of surgical instruments.

15 - **Ratchet** – The part of a surgical instrument that "locks" the handles in place.

16 - **Passivation** – A chemical process applied during instrument manufacture that provides a corrosion-resistant finish by forming a thin transparent oxide film.

This softer type of steel is called **Austenitic stainless steel**.

Stainless steel can stain, spot, and rust. A more appropriate name is, then, "stain-resistant," because stainless steel is not truly stain "less." However, proper care will ensure that a stainless instrument performs as it should, and that it lasts a long time.

Manufacturing Steps

The first step in manufacturing a surgical instrument is to forge the material to create a stamp of its rough outline from a heated bar of stainless steel. The heating and cooling process used to create an instrument is very important because good forging produces good instruments. Most high quality forgings come from mills in Germany, but forgings also come from Japan, Pakistan, France, and Sweden.

After the forging is completed, the instrument must be ground and milled. First, the excess steel surrounding the forging (called "flash") is removed. For ring-handled instruments such as scissors and hemostats, more than twenty milling operations are needed. These include the creation of the male and female halves, the cutting of precise **serrations**, and the machining of the **ratchets**.

In today's instrument manufacturing environment, there is more reliance on machines than in years' past. Presses, lathes, computer numeric controlled (CNC) milling machines, and drop hammers are now used, in comparison to the files, grindstones, and other hand tools used in the past. Despite these technical advances, surgical instrument makers must still possess a high degree of manual skill. They complete several years of training in an apprenticeship during which they learn under the guidance of a trained and experienced crafts person. Instrument makers perform hundreds of quality checks and finishing applications to every instrument during the manufacturing process to ensure its quality.

At the completion of the assembly process, instruments undergo a final heating procedure called "tempering." Depending upon the style of the instrument, a device is heated to approximately 1500°F (815.6°C), and then cooled in a controlled environment to provide its proper hardness. If the cooling process is not completely controlled, instruments could become brittle, and break easily while performing their normal function. After instruments have been tempered to ensure hardness, their corrosion resistance can be addressed.

To do so, instruments undergo polishing and **passivation**. Polishing is necessary to achieve a smooth finish, and ultimately determines the final appearance or finish of the instrument. Surgical instruments can be shiny (called mirror-finish), or they can have a matte- or satin-finish: a gray-colored surface that does not reflect light. Both finishes are widely accepted, and create a smooth surface. However, because the mirror finish is smoother, it tends to stain less frequently. Passivation uses nitric acid (HNO_3) to remove all the iron content still found on the outside layer of the instrument. The removal of this iron helps to build a protective outside layer of chromium oxide (Cr_2O_3), which is highly resistant to corrosion, and continues to build up throughout the instrument's life.

The instrument is now ready for final inspection, and it will be carefully examined. Ratchets, tips, scissor blades, serrations, box locks, and spot welds will be tested. Finally, the instrument is ready to be etched and packaged. Etching is an acid-based chemical procedure that uses stencils to apply the company name, the part number, and the country of origin. Laser etching and stamping are additional methods used for marking instruments.

As you have seen, the surgical instrument manufacturing process is lengthy and detailed, and it requires a significant amount of experience, skill, and craftsmanship. A typical manufacturing cycle from forging to finished instrument usually takes up to six weeks.

CLASSIFICATION AND OVERVIEW OF SURGICAL INSTRUMENTS

Learning Objective 2. Define basic categories of surgical instruments based upon their functions, and identify the points of inspection, anatomy (features) of, and procedures to measure the following types of instruments:

- Hemostatic Forceps
- Needleholders
- Tissue Forceps
- Dressing Forceps
- Retractors
- Scissors
- Suction Devices
- Single and Double Action Rongeurs
- Kerrison/Laminectomy Rongeurs
- Nail Nippers
- Graves and Pederson Vaginal Speculums

Surgical instruments are designed for a specific surgical purpose. Injury to the patient and destruction of or damage to the instrument can occur when the incorrect instrument is used. For example, one might incorrectly pull a pin with a needleholder instead of a pin puller or pair of pliers, and this can damage the needleholder.

To properly inspect and test surgical instruments, Central Service Technicians must know the anatomy and points of inspection of the devices, and how to measure them. This will enable them to properly and efficiently assemble instrument sets.

Many of the most common categories of surgical instruments will be discussed in this section.

Hemostatic Forceps

The primary function of hemostatic forceps is to control the flow of blood. **Figure 11.1** identifies the anatomy and points of inspection of a hemostatic forceps; **Figure 11.2** shows the correct way to measure this instrument. Some other names for hemostatic forceps are hemostats, stats, snaps, Kellys, and clamps.

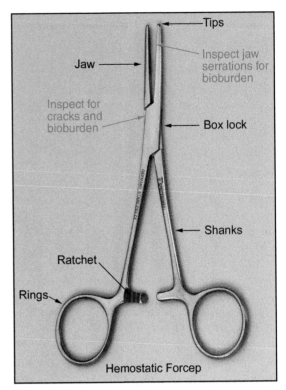

Figure 11.1

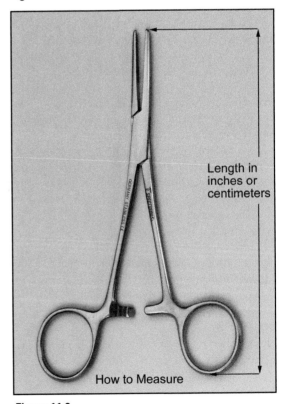

Figure 11.2

Figure 11.3 Identification of Hemostatic Forceps

Length		Jaw Pattern	Name
Inches	Cm		
3½	8.9	Full Serrations	Hartman Mosquito (see Figure 11.5)
5	12.7	Full Serrations	Halstead Mosquito (see Figure 11.5)
5½	14.0	Full Serrations	Crile Hemostat (see Figure 11.4)
5½	14.0	Partial Serrations	Kelly Hemostat (see Figure 11.4)
6¼	15.8	Full Serrations	Rochester Pean
6¼	15.8	Full Serrations with 1 x 2 Teeth	Rochester Ochsner or Kocher
6¼	15.8	Longitudinal Serrations and Cross Serrated Tip	Rochester Carmalt

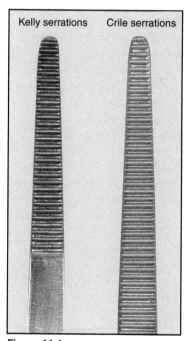

Kelly serrations   Crile serrations

Figure 11.4

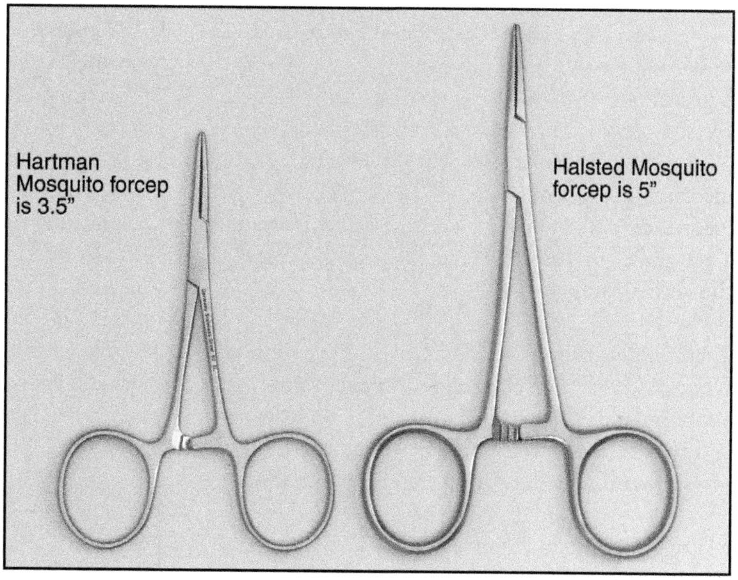

Hartman Mosquito forcep is 3.5"

Halsted Mosquito forcep is 5"

Figure 11.5

Figure 11.3 provides basic information that can help to identify several types of hemostatic forceps. Jaw features can consist of full serrations (Crile hemostat) or partial serrations (Kelly hemostat). Note: these two types of forceps are shown in **Figure 11.4**. Hemostatic forceps can also have longitudinal serrations (Rochester Carmalt), and serrations with 1x2 teeth (Kocher forceps). **Figure 11.5** identifies two common hemostatic forceps: the Hartman Mosquito 3.5," and the Halsted Mosquito 5."

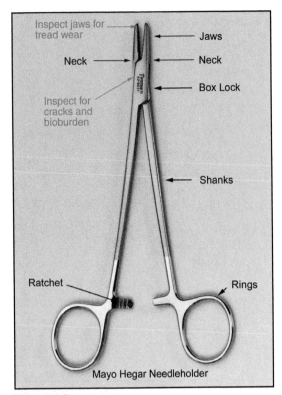

Figure 11.6

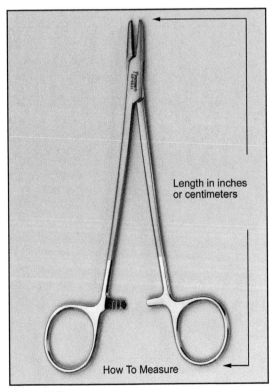

Figure 11.7

Needleholders

These instruments are designed to drive suture needles to close surgical sites. **Figure 11.6** identifies the anatomy and points of inspection of a needleholder, and **Figure 11.7** shows the correct way to measure this instrument.

Needleholder jaws (the portion that holds the needle) can be manufactured of stainless steel or tungsten carbide:

- *Stainless Steel Jaws.* There are two patterns of jaw tread: smooth or serrated. Stainless steel jaw treads cannot be repaired, re-jawed, or have the serrations replaced after they wear out. This can occur with one or two years of use, and then the needleholder must be replaced.

- *Tungsten Carbide Jaws.* The most popular needleholders in surgical use have these jaws. The key visual factor is the bright gold rings. When gold is placed on an instrument, this indicates that the working portion (jaws) is made of Tungsten Carbide. Jaws made of this metal are typically preferred because they are harder and last longer, they grip the needle more firmly, and they can be replaced.

Figure 11.8 shows needleholders with stainless steel and tungsten carbon jaws.

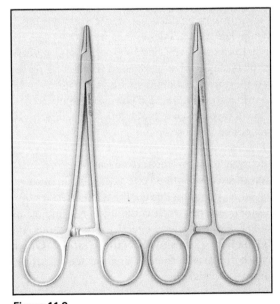

Figure 11.8

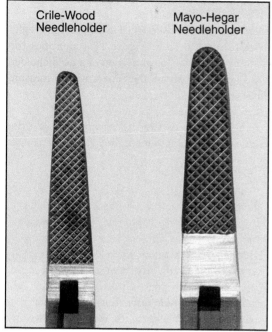

Figure 11.9

Other names for needleholders are needledrivers, Diamond Jaws, and Gold Handles. The two most common needleholder designs are Mayo-Hegar and Crile-wood, and they are shown in **Figure 11.9**. Note that the Crile-wood is narrower than the Mayo-Hegar design.

Tissue Forceps

The primary function of tissue forceps is to manipulate tissue. A design feature of this tweezer-styled forceps is the multiple-teeth configuration at the distal tips. The teeth assist in grasping tissue, and they provide a more secure grip. **Figure 11.10** identifies the anatomy and points of inspection of a tissue forceps. **Figure 11.11** shows the correct way to measure this instrument.

The most common teeth configurations for tissue forceps are one tooth on one side, and two teeth on the other. With this design, the teeth interlock one another, and the teeth configuration is indicated by 1x2. Other common teeth configurations are 2x3, 3x4, 5x6, 9x9, and 1x2 with serrations. Other names for tissue forceps are rat tooth, brown forceps, and pickups.

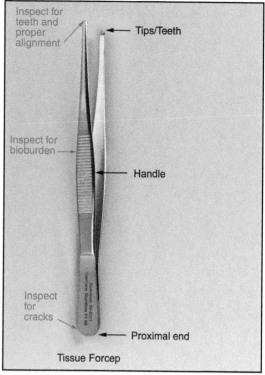

Figure 11.10 Anatomy and points of inspection of a tissue forceps

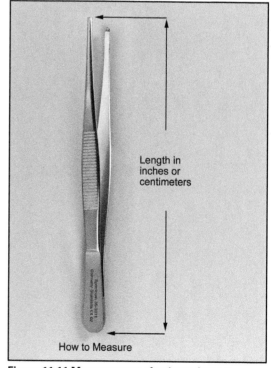

Figure 11.11 Measurement of a tissue forceps

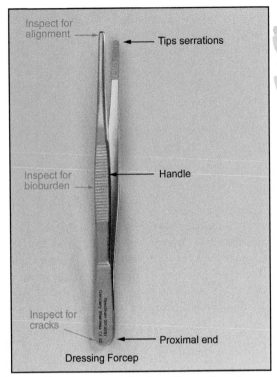

Figure 11.12 Anatomy and points of inspection of a dressing forceps

Dressing Forceps

Dressing forceps are identical to tissue forceps except they have serrations rather than teeth at the distal end. The primary function of this instrument is to manipulate tissue and to pack surgical sites. **Figure 11.12** shows the anatomy and points of inspection of a dressing forceps. **Figure 11.13** shows the correct way to measure this instrument. Other names for dressing forceps are smooth forceps and plain forceps.

Retractors

The primary function of retractors is to move tissue aside for exposure and visualization of the surgical site. Retractors can be hand-held, self-retaining, or table-mounted. Small retractors held by the surgeon's fingers retract skin and subcutaneous tissues, while larger retractors are used to retract muscle tissue and organs. Self-retaining retractors (**Figure 11.14**) are designed with a mechanical action that keeps them open to retract. To test a self-retaining retractor, simply push down on retractor lever, and let it go. If the lever springs up, the instrument is in proper working order. In

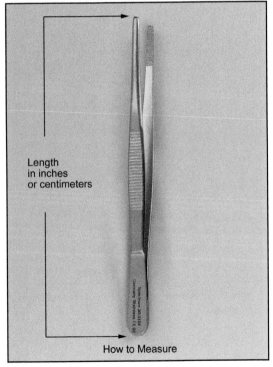

Figure 11.13 Measurement of a dressing forceps

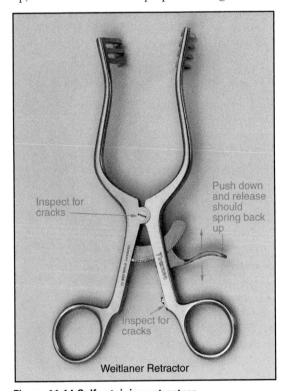

Figure 11.14 Self-retaining retractors

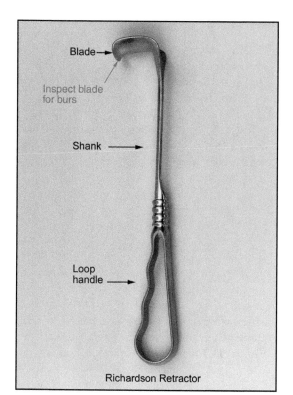

Figure 11.15 Anatomy and points of inspection of a retractor.

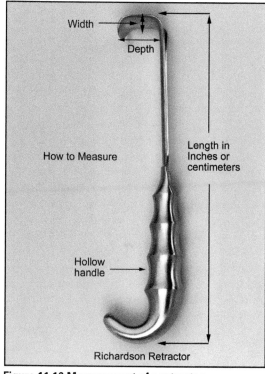

Figure 11.16 Measurement of a retractor

the event the lever remains in the down position, remove it from the instrument set, and send the instrument to the repair vendor.

Some common self-retaining retractors are Weitlaner, Gelpi, and Beckman-Adson. **Figure 11.15** shows the points of inspection of a loop handle retractor. **Figure 11.16** shows the correct way to measure a hollow handle retractor.

Scissors

The primary function of scissors is to cut tissue, suture, and other material in the surgical field. For dissection, curved scissors are primarily used because their curve allows for better visualization. The opening action of the scissors also helps to dissect and spread tissue. **Figure 11.17** shows the anatomy of and points of inspection for a scissor.

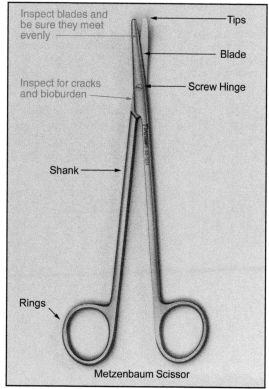

Figure 11.17 Anatomy and points of inspection of a scissors

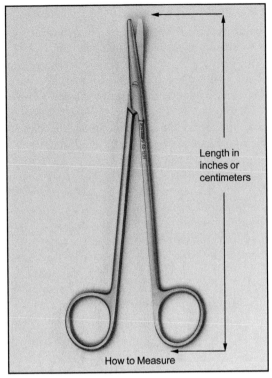

Figure 11.18 Measurement of a scissors

Figure 11.18 shows the correct way to measure this instrument. The standard Mayo scissors has a beveled blade, and is the most popular. The second most popular Mayo design is the Mayo Noble. As seen in **Figure 11.19**, it does not have a beveled blade.

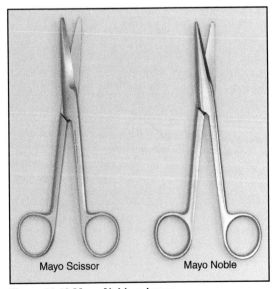

Figure 11.19 Mayo Noble scissors

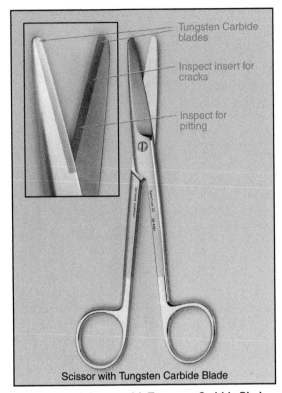

Figure 11.20 Scissors with Tungsten Carbide Blades

Surgical scissors have various blade features for specific surgical applications:

- *Tungsten Carbide Blades* – These scissors have gold rings on the handles, and tungsten carbide blade edges (see **Figure 11.20**). Scissors with these blades have a harder and stronger cutting edge, and they allow the scissors to remain sharper for a longer time than other scissors. Their primary design function is tissue dissection with blades that hold their edge longer. Always be sure a gold handled scissors is dull before it is re-sharpened to extend the life of the instrument.

- *Serrated Blades* – The design feature of a serrated blade is the prevention of tissue slippage or escape during the cutting process. Serrations are generally found on one of the blades; however, there are some scissors with dual blade serrations.

- *Microgrind or Supercut Blades* – Black rings visually identify these scissors from standard

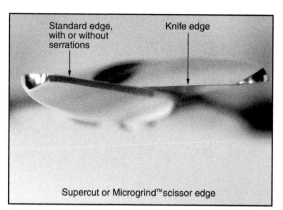

Figure 11.21 Diagram of a black-handled carbide blades scissors

Suction Devices

The primary function of suction devices is to extract (suction) blood and fluids from the surgical site. **Figure 11.22** shows the anatomy of and points of inspection for a suction device. **Figure 11.23** shows the correct way to measure this instrument. The two most common suction devices are the Baron and Frazier suction tubes. These suction devices include a metal stylet that is used during the surgical procedure to unclog the suction channel. Note: this sylet is not to be used to clean the device. The only cleaning tool for a suction device is the proper cleaning brush.

or gold-handled tungsten carbide scissors. The design of a black-handled scissors is to simulate a tissue lancing/slicing action. While all other scissors cut tissue with a crushing action, a black-handled scissors has one blade sharpened like a knife to slice tissue. The other blade is a standard design that causes a guillotine effect (see **Figure 11.21**). Black-handled scissors must be specially sharpened two to three times a year under normal use conditions.

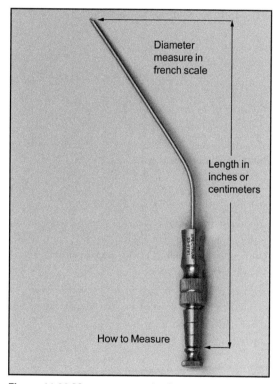

Figure 11.23 Measurement of a Suction Device

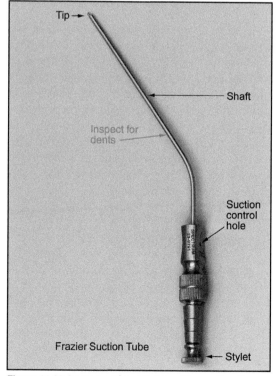

Figure 11.22 Anatomy of and Points of Inspection for a Suction Device

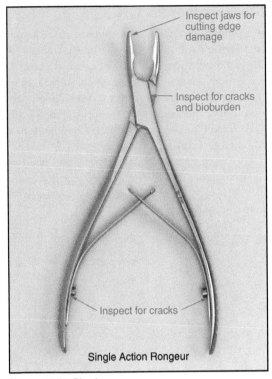

Figure 11.24 Single
Action Rongeur

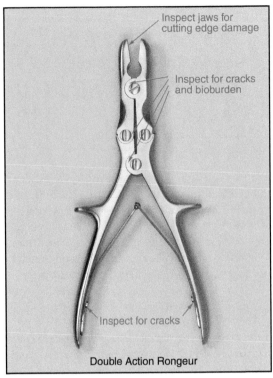

Figure 11.25 Double Action Rongeur

Single and Double Action Rongeurs

The primary function of a Rongeur is to cut or bite away at bone and tissue. The difference between a single action (**Figure 11.24**) and a double action (**Figure 11.25**) rongeur is the design of how the jaws close. With a double action instrument, the surgeon squeezes the handle, and this creates two movements for the jaw to close. This double movement reduces the amount of hand strength, so the instrument bites more with less hand strength. The main inspection point on single and double action rongeurs is the jaws. Any dents or gouges of the jaws prevent the instrument from working correctly. All rongeurs should be sharpened a minimum of two times annually.

Kerrison/Laminectomy Rongeurs

The primary function of this style of rongeur is in spine surgery to remove the disc or lamina. This instrument must be sharpened two to three times annually depending on usage. The distal portion must be inspected after every use to look for bioburden and cutting edge damage (see **Figure 11.26**). When Kerrison rongeurs are being

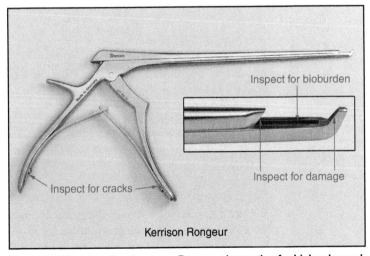

Figure 11.26 Kerrison/Laminectomy Rongeurs inspection for bioburden and cutting edge damage

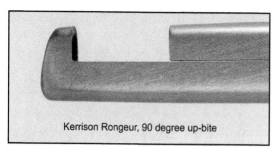

Kerrison Rongeur, 90 degree up-bite

Figure 11.27 90 Degree Rongeur

assembled on trays, it is important to identify the different bite designs: for example, the 90 degree up-bite (**Figure 11.27**), If a Kerrison rongeur is sticking in a closed position, a repair vendor will need to disassemble, polish, sharpen, and re-assemble the instrument. The polishing process will remove bioburden in the sliding track.

Nail Nippers

The primary function of nail nippers (see **Figure 11.28**) is to cut toe and finger nails and, occasionally, to trim small bone fragments. The cutting surface and edge should be inspected along with the hinge area and spring.

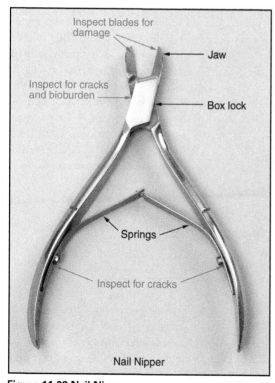

Inspect blades for damage

Jaw

Inspect for cracks and bioburden

Box lock

Springs

Inspect for cracks

Nail Nipper

Figure 11.28 Nail Nippers

Graves and Pederson Vaginal Speculums

The primary usage of these medical instruments (see **Figure 11.29**) is to expose the vaginal cavity. One important inspection point is to assure that the thumb screws are present and functioning. It is also important to inspect all sides of the blades for damage. As noted in **Figure 11.30**, a Pederson blade is narrower than that on a Graves speculum.

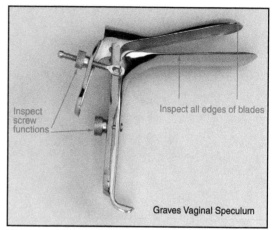

Inspect screw functions

Inspect all edges of blades

Graves Vaginal Speculum

Figure 11.29 Graves & Pederson Vaginal Speculum

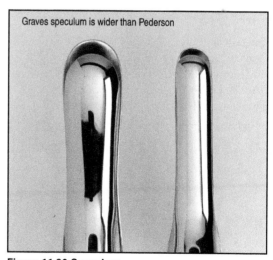

Graves speculum is wider than Pederson

Figure 11.30 Speculum

Post-Operative Care of Surgical Instruments

Within 15 minutes to 1 hour of the surgical procedure, blood can begin to dry on surgical instruments. Users should take precautions to insure that blood and soil is not allowed to dry on instruments. To prevent damage associated with dried blood, separate the rings

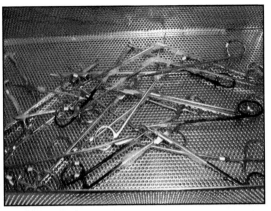

Figure 11.31

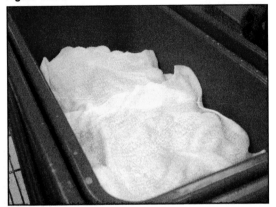

Figure 11.32

(see **Figure 11.31**) and ratchets for box lock exposure on applicable instruments, and cover them with a towel moistened with water (**Figure 11.32**). Another useful technique is to spray an enzymatic foam or detergent-based solution onto the instruments to prevent blood from drying. With either tactic, the instruments should be transported to the Central Service decontamination area as soon as possible.

SOLUTIONS THAT DAMAGE INSTRUMENTS

Learning Objective 3. Identify solutions that can damage stainless steel instruments.

Numerous solutions ranging from those typically used for housekeeping to kitchen-related cleaning purposes can damage stainless steel instruments. If the solution's container does not specifically note that its intended purpose is for use on surgical instruments, the product should not be used to do so. **Figure 11.33** identifies common solutions that should not be used to clean surgical instruments.

The use of saline as a soaking or rinsing agent accelerates the rusting and pitting of surgical

Figure 11.33: Solutions that Damage Surgical Instruments

Saline	Bleach	Surgeons' Hand Scrubs
Betadine	Iodine	Porcelain Cleaners
Peroxide	Hand Soaps	Household Lubricants
Dish Soaps	Laundry Detergents	Household Powder Cleansers
Soaking in Water	Long-Term Soaking in Rust Remover	
Soaking in Saline	Long-Term Soaking in Stain Remover	

Rusts and Stains

No steel is truly "stainless," and, in fact, all stainless steel instruments will stain. The occurrence of rust on surgical instruments is possible; however, it is very rare. Stainless steel is composed of rust-resisting alloys, and proper processing helps to control staining and rust.

"Rust" that appears on an instrument is most likely to be a stain. A pencil eraser can be used for an "eraser test" to help determine the difference between staining and rusting. After a stain is discovered, use the eraser to remove the discoloration. Then look at the metal below the discoloration to determine if there are any tiny pit marks. If pit marks are discovered, this is corrosion: the origin of the rusting. However, if the metal is smooth and clean below the stain, the source of discoloration is a stain; there is no rust.

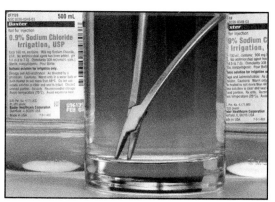

Figure 11.34

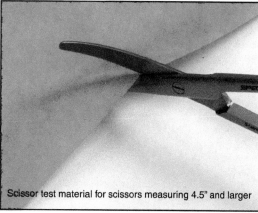

Scissor test material for scissors measuring 4.5" and larger

instruments. In many cases, the use of saline may void instrument warranties (**Figure 11.34**). Therefore, controlling instrument exposure to saline is very important. For clinical reasons, operating room personnel cannot eliminate the exposure of stainless steel instruments to saline. However, after the surgical procedures are completed, saline must be removed as an early step in the cleaning process. Operating room personnel can help by removing instruments from saline as soon as possible.

INSTRUMENT SHARPNESS TESTING AND IDENTIFICATION

Learning Objective 4. Explain procedures to test instruments for sharpness, and to identify (mark) them.

Instrument Sharpness Testing

It is essential to monitor the sharpness of surgical instruments. Figures **11.35–11.42** illustrate proper sharpness testing procedures for common surgical instruments.

Figure 11.35

Instrument: Scissors 4 ½" and larger

Test Material: Red test material

Test: Scissors must be able to cut through to the tip two to three times. The distal tips of scissors are the most crucial portion because this is where they first become dull. They must cut clean through the tips of the instrument.

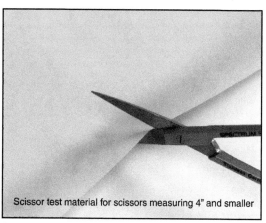

Scissor test material for scissors measuring 4" and smaller

Figure 11.36

Instrument: Scissors 4" or smaller

Test Material: Yellow test material

Test: Scissors must be able to cut through the tips two to three times. The distal tips of scissors are the most crucial portion, and must cut clean through the tips of the instrument.

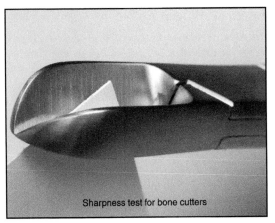

Sharpness test for bone cutters

Figure 11.37

Instrument: Bone Cutter

Test Material: Index card

Test: Cut off a piece of the index card.

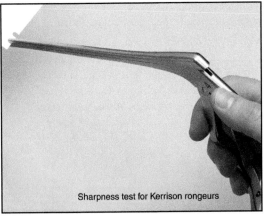

Sharpness test for Kerrison rongeurs

Figure 11.38

Instrument: Kerrison Rongeur

Test Material: Index card

Test: Properly punch a clean hole through the card.

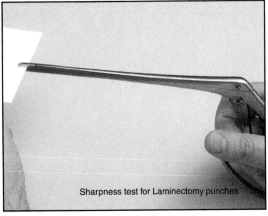

Sharpness test for Laminectomy punches

Figure 11.39

Instrument: Laminectomy Rongeur

Test Material: Index card

Test: The rongeur should make a clean bite using half of the jaw.

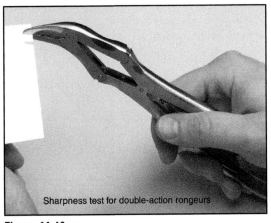

Sharpness test for double-action rongeurs

Figure 11.40

Instrument: Double Action Rongeur

Test Material: Index card

Test: The rongeur should make a clean bite through the card.

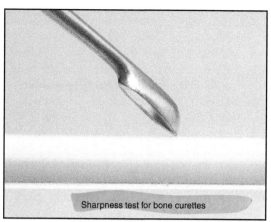
Sharpness test for bone curettes

Figure 11.41

Instrument: Bone Curette

Test Material: Plastic dowel rod

Test: Shave off pieces of the dowel rod.

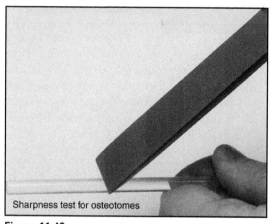
Sharpness test for osteotomes

Figure 11.42

Instrument: Chisels and Osteotomes

Test Material: Plastic dowel rod

Test: Shave off pieces of the dowel rod.

Instrument Identification Procedures

There are literally, thousands of different surgical instruments and many of them look very similar. Others are identical, but are designated for use in specific procedures. Central Service Technicians must insure that the correct instruments are placed into the proper trays. Many health care facilities use different instrument marking methods to mark instruments for faster and easier identification.

Marking surgical instruments for identification can be done several ways. One popular method is to use tape, and proper techniques for its application are important:

- Clean your fingers with alcohol to remove oils, grease, and any possible dirt.

- Wipe alcohol on the site of the instrument where the tape will be placed to remove any lubricant or moisture that might be on the instrument. Note: the site should always be the shank of the instrument, and never the rings. Tape that is applied to a rounded surface such as instrument rings will not adhere to the instrument's surface.

- As shown in **Figure 11.43**, cut the tape on an angle to allow its edge to lay flat.

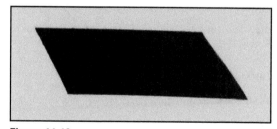

Figure 11.43

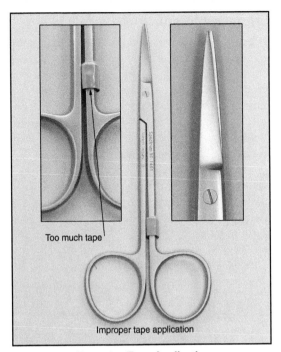

Too much tape

Improper tape application

Figure 11.44 Excessive Tape Application

• Wrap the tape one to one and one-half times around the device. Apply the tape with a firm, pulling tension. Be careful not to apply excessive tape. (See **Figure 11.44**)

• After the tape is applied, autoclave the instrument to allow the heat to help bond the tape to the instrument.

Other methods of marking instruments include:

• *Acid Base Etching* – This process can be done by the instrument repair vendor, or a kit may be purchased so the etching process can be done at the facility. Acid base etching uses a stencil, solutions, and electricity to mark stainless steel. This process is semi-permanent, and it can be buffed off during the instrument repair process.

• *Heat-Fused Nylon* – This color-coding is often referred to as "dipping," and is typically done in a repair facility. Heat fused nylon is a powder coating process that leaves a thin layer of color nylon on the instrument. Nylon coating can last years; however, once it begins to chip, all the nylon must be removed from the instrument.

• *Laser Etching* – This process is permanent and costly due to the off-site set-up charges that are incurred.

Note: surgical instruments can also be marked with an electric etching process, but this marking method should not be used because it damages the surface of the instrument. Electric etching, or engraving as it is sometimes called, damages instruments and can make them more difficult to clean.

Repair Vendors Maintain Instruments

All surgical instruments are designed to be sharpened or restored. A proactive approach to maintaining the instrument inventory is important and involves:

1. Identifying the most frequently used surgical sets.
2. Identifying the surgical service/specialty (i.e. ortho, neuro, ENT, etc.) that generates the most complaints about dull instruments.
3. Scheduling the repair vendor to:

   • Sharpen all cutting instruments. Note: all scissors must be on a sharpening schedule based upon how frequently they are used.

   • In spect all instruments for cracks.

   • Re-jaw gold-handled needleholders when necessary. Tungsten carbide insert replacements must have the exact number of teeth per square inch, and the same thickness to reduce surgeons' complaints about these instruments.

   • Service orthopedic and neurological sets a minimum of two times annually to include sharpening all cutting (osteotome) and biting (rongeur) instruments.

INSTRUMENT LUBRICATION AND TRAY ASSEMBLY

Learning Objective 5. Emphasize the importance of instrument lubrication, and review tray assembly safeguards.

Lubrication is Important

Surgical instruments with moving parts must be lubricated after each use or in accordance with manufacturer's recommendations. The use of a neutral pH lubricant extends the life of the instrument, and makes the device easier for the surgeon to use. Each Central Service workstation should have lubrication available for this purpose. Lubricants are available in spray bottle formulas. ALL lubricants must be approved for use as a surgical instrument lubricant. The point of application should be the instrument's hinged area or any working component such as a moving/sliding area.

Tray Assembly Tips

Tray organization and sterile field presentation of instruments are important concerns for effective processing, and to protect the instruments as they are processed. Recommendations include:

* Heavy instruments should be placed on the bottom or side of the tray.

* Select an instrument tray that allows adequate space for weight distribution.

* All curved instruments should be curved in same direction to protect tips from being damaged.

* Tissue and dressing forceps should be softly nested together. (see **Figure 11.45**)

* Delicate instruments should be kept in micro cases or small protective cases within the surgical tray.

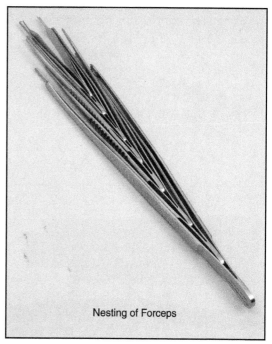

Nesting of Forceps

Figure 11.45

* The use of metal instrument holders called stringers can assist in faster sterile field assembly, and safer handling of instruments, especially sharps. (See **Figure 11.46**)

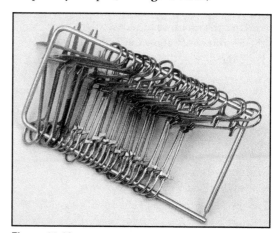

Figure 11.46

* Laser-finished instruments (typically those with a non-reflective black coating) should never have metal-to-metal contact that can damage, chip, and scratch the

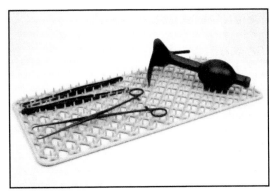

Figure 11.47

finish during decontamination or tray assembly. A silicon nipple mat (see **Figure 11.47**) can prevent metal-to-metal contact as can a foam or lint-free towel.

Gomco and Mogen Circumcision Clamps

Gomco circumcision clamps (see **Figure 11.48**) are patented medical devices. If they are used, assure that they are authentic. Intermixing parts from non-patented/disposable clamps with authentic clamp parts can have dangerous results. A facility should standardize and consistently use either reusable or disposable clamps. Mixing the components (not matching the correct-sized bell/stud with same-sized plate) will cause the clamp to malfunction.[1]

The gap of Mogen circumcision clamps (see **Figure 11.49**) should be measured each year to assure that it is between 1.5 mm to 2.5 mm. Mogen clamps, like Gomco clamps, should never be repaired or sharpened because they do not have a cutting edge.

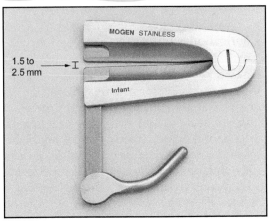

Figure 11.49

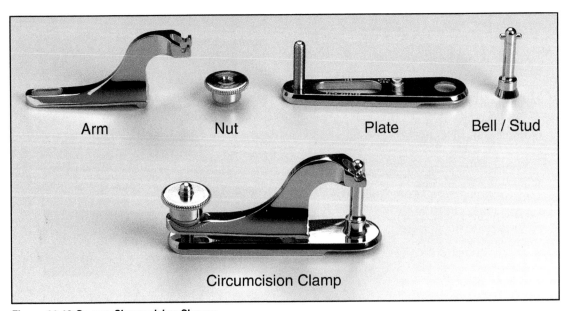

Figure 11.48 Gomco Circumcision Clamps

ENDNOTES

1. For more information and recommendations about Gomco and Mogen circumcision clamps, contact E.C.R.I.: (610) 825-6000. www.ecri.org

REFERENCES

Schultz, R. Inspecting Surgical Instruments: An Illustrated Guide., Stow, OH, RMPS Publishing. 2005.

Gregory, B. Orthopedic Surgery. St. Louis, Mo. Mosby Publishing Co., Inc. 1994.

Tighe, S. Instrumentation for the Operating Room. St. Louis, Mo. Mosby Publishing Co., Inc. 1994.

Glaser, Z. Surgical Instrument Quality. Infection Control and Sterilization Technology. May, 1997.

Storz Instruments. The Care and Handling of Surgical Instruments. St. Louis, Mo. Storz Instruments. 1991.

Reichert, M. Sterilization Technology for the Health Care Facility. Second Edition. Gathersburg, Md. Aspen Publishers. 1997.

CENTRAL SERVICE TERMS

Scissors

Osteotomes

Chisels

Rongeurs

Forceps

Hemostatic Forceps

Needleholders

Martensitic (stainless steel)

Retractors

Cannulas

Rib spreaders

Suction devices

Austenitic (stainless steel)

Serrations

Ratchet

Passivation

Chapter 12
Complex Surgical Instruments

Chapter Outline

Chapter Learning Objectives:

As a result of successfully completing this chapter, readers will be able to:

1. Provide an overview of and discuss procedures to care for and effectively process powered surgical instruments.

2. Explain basic concerns important when handling and processing endoscopic instruments.

3. Discuss detailed information about flexible endoscopes.

4. Review general processing and inspection requirements for rigid and semi-rigid endoscopes and laparoscopic instruments.

5. Identify basic protocols important at each step in the loaner instrumentation process.

POWERED SURGICAL INSTRUMENTS

Learning Objective 1. Provide an overview of and discuss procedures to care for and effectively process powered surgical instruments.

From their origin in early Greek times, surgical instruments have evolved to the complex surgical instruments used today to perform medical "miracles." Forceps, scissors, needleholders, and retractors along with numerous other simple instruments are in common use. However, they are joined by powered surgical instruments, endoscopes, and other very complex and delicate devices with circuit boards and computer chips.

Surgical techniques continually evolve, and surgical instrumentation has kept pace with the age of technology. The surgeons' needs to diagnose, treat, and/or cure disease drive the requirements for ever-increasingly sophisticated instruments to achieve these goals. While modern instrumentation has expanded the range of surgical procedures, the technology has also dramatically increased the difficulty in cleaning, decontaminating, and sterilizing these devices. Engineers and manufacturers are aware that their products are hazardous if they cannot be adequately processed to provide sterile instruments for the surgeon. Central Service Technicians must learn how to proficiently clean, disinfect, and sterilize this new generation of very costly surgical instruments as they fulfill their important responsibilities to patients and their facilities.

Overview

This section addresses the processing of instruments powered by electric motor, compressed gas (pneumatic), and battery. The size, compactness, and design complexity of these devices range from drills used on the tiniest ear bones to drills and saws used on the largest leg bones. Powered surgical instruments have greatly reduced the brute force historically required for orthopedic

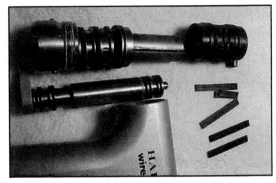

Figure 12.1

surgeries, and they have also decreased the time required to perform them. This, in turn, has significantly decreased patient pain and post-surgical healing times.

All powered surgical instruments (PSIs) are highly complex and fragile. For example, drills and saws have motorized handpieces that cannot be submerged in any fluid. Materials used to construct these instruments are varied, so the selection of cleaning and disinfection products is critical. Those chosen must be compatible with materials used and yield successful processing results. Equipment manufacturers' recommendations must be followed to prevent damage to instruments that can have an array of **lumens,** channels, attachments, and multiple moving parts that pose a severe challenge to processing tasks. **Figure 12.1** provides an example of the complexity of this instrumentation by showing some internal components of a motorized handpiece.

Powered surgical instruments become grossly soiled during use. Central Service Technicians must protect themselves during processing. By design, these instruments must be manually processed, and the potential for accidental exposure to blood and body fluids is high. In addition to personal safety concerns when cleaning powered surgical instruments, Central Service Technicians must also insure that they process each instrument and accessory in accordance with manufacturer's instructions. Manufacturers must validate (prove effective) appropriate high-level disinfection

Lumen – The interior path through a needle, tube, or surgical instrument.

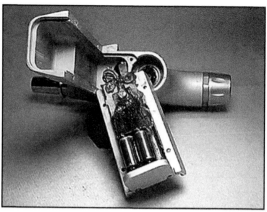

Figure 12.2

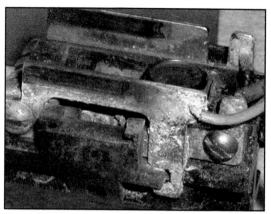

Figure 12.3

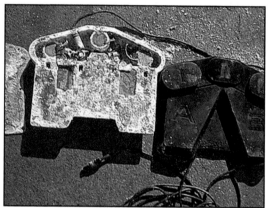

Figure 12.4

and/or sterilization methods for each of their instruments (systems). Their recommendations must always be followed to avoid instrument damage and liability for ineffective processing procedures. Failure to follow manufacturer's processing guidelines may result in instrument malfunction or inadequate sterilization, both dangerous scenarios for the patient, and improper processing may also result in instrument damage which can require costly repairs. For example, powered surgical instruments contain several working components and will be damaged if fluid (i.e. water, cleaning solution, etc.) is allowed to penetrate into the interior of the instrument. That is called fluid invasion. **Figures 12.2, 12.3, and 12.4** illustrate the type of damage that occurs when powered surgical instruments and their accessories are damaged by fluid invasion. Central Service Technicians must take special care to provide adequate cleaning and at the same time prevent fluid invasion. Specific training is required for all instruments and equipment processed to assure that they are safely handled and properly prepared for reuse.

Power Sources

Power sources for surgical instruments are of three types: electric, pneumatic (air), and battery.

Electric-Powered

Instruments powered by electricity require a cable that can be sterilized. One end attaches to the motorized handpiece on the surgical field; the other end attaches to a power unit (motor/electrical adapter) that plugs into an 110v electrical outlet. These cables require routine maintenance involving disassembly, cleaning and lubrication, and inspection for cuts and/or other damage. Central Service Technicians may require additional training and tools to perform these tasks. During processing, it is imperative that fluid does not enter the cable or hand-piece. Most manufacturers recommend connecting the cable to the handpiece during processing to help prevent damage caused by fluid invasion.

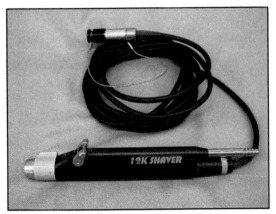

Figure 12.5

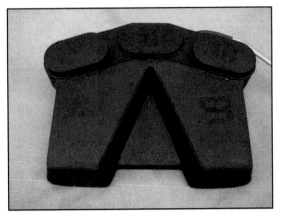

Figure 12.6

Arthroscopy shavers are an example of a frequently used electric-powered instrument.(See **Figure 12.5**)

The most common problems associated with electric power equipment are:

- Damage to electrical parts during sterilization.

- Condensation that enters the equipment when seals wear out.

- Electrical contacts become worn and affect equipment handling.

Procedures to care and handle electric-powered equipment include:

- Do not immerse the equipment in any solution including water.

- Do not use solvents or lubricants unless specified by the equipment manufacturer.

- Use a nylon bristle brush to clean the distal tip.

- Dry the equipment with a lint-free towel.

Electric powered equipment can be operated with a footswitch. (foot-controlled pedal) (See **Figure 12.6**). To clean it, follow the manufacturer's instructions, and avoid pulling on or stressing the power cord.

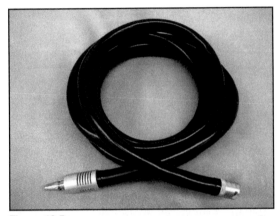

Figure 12.7

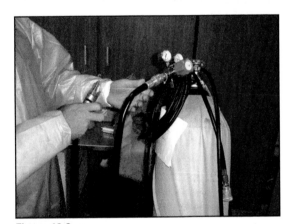

Figure 12.8

Pneumatic-Powered (Air-Powered)

Pneumatic (air)-powered instruments using compressed gas (CO_2) require a hose that can be sterilized. (See **Figure 12.7**) One end attaches to

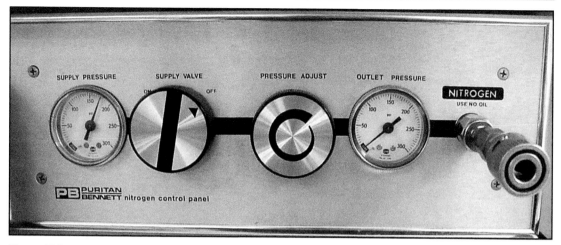

Figure 12.9

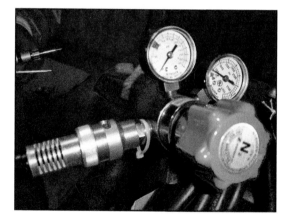

Figure 12.10

the motorized handpiece on the surgical field. The other end attaches to the source of compressed air which can come from a stand-alone cylinder (tank) with a pressure regulator (See **Figure 12.8**), or "piped in" through a wall- or column-mounted regulator panel (See Figure 12.9).

Instrument hoses must be inspected for cuts and other possible damage. They must be pressurized for proper inspection which requires an air source in the processing area. Any damage, "bubble," or "bleb" in the hose casing requires that the hose be removed from service. It is imperative that fluid does not enter the hose or handpiece during processing. Most manufacturers recommend connecting the cable to the handpiece during processing to help prevent damage caused by fluid invasion.

Care of Air Hoses

All air-powered equipment must be attached to an air hose to operate. The primary reason that air hoses fail relate to sterilization issues: the heat from sterilization breaks down the rubber component and o-rings and causes air leakage. To clean the hose, use a mild detergent; don't allow fluids to enter hose, and never use abrasives to wash the hose liner. Proper coil size for sterilization should be 9" to 12". Hoses should not be coiled tightly. Standard air hoses are 10 feet, and are operated at 100 pounds per square inch (psi). Note: for longer hose lengths, add 1 psi for every foot over ten feet.

Different types of powered instruments require different operating pressures, and a chart of these pressures should be available where the instruments are processed. Extreme care is required because testing instruments at an improper pressure can injure the operator and/or severely damage the instrument.

Nitrogen can also be used for pneumatic power, and tanks of this gas contain a regulator with two gauges. One gauge measures the pressure to the handpiece, and the second gauge measures the amount of nitrogen remaining in the tank. (See **Figure 12.10**) Central Service Technicians must be

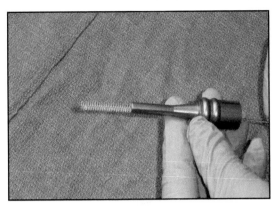

Figure 12.11

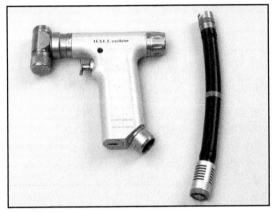

Figure 12.12

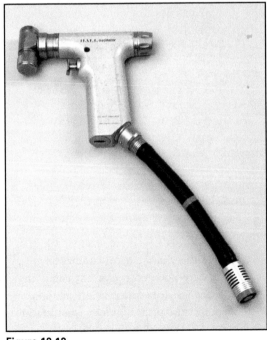

Figure 12.13

certain to follow manufacturer's instructions and test instruments using the appropriate gas.

To properly care and handle air equipment:

- Never immerse in any solution or water.
- Properly insert the cleaning brush into attachments and burr guards. (See **Figure 12.11**)
- Carefully wipe and rinse the outer case.
- Use a decontamination hose to protect inner components. (see **Figures 12.12** and **12.13**)
- Burr guards must be lubricated according to the manufacturer's instructions.

Common Reasons Why Power Equipment Must Be Repaired

- Corrosion of internal components from steam condensation.
- Corrosion of internal components from immersion in solutions such as water.
- Internal corrosion from bioburden caused by improper cleaning.
- Corrosion caused by bioburden.
- Physical damage due to mishandling. (See **Figure 12.14**)
- Lack of or improper preventive maintenance.

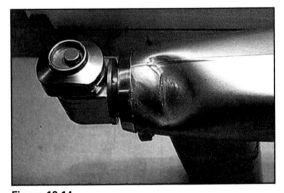

Figure 12.14

Battery-Powered

Instruments powered by battery are the least cumbersome of the three available power systems.

Example of a Battery Powered PSI and Two Styles of Batteries

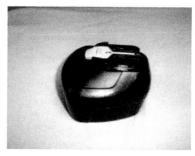

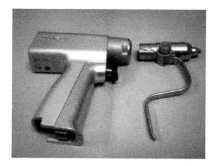

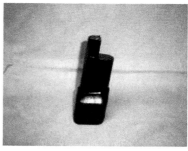

Figure 12.15

The battery is inserted into the instrument so the device is free to maneuver across the sterile field. (See **Figure 12.15**) This freedom of movement, however, comes with a price: batteries require charging, and this requires increased handling. Batteries and chargers are specific to each system, and are not interchangeable. Additional space to accommodate the chargers also creates an expense. Always check the manufacturer's instructions for battery sterilization guidelines.

A primary reason that batteries do not hold a charge relates to steam damage of the battery cells. However, they can be replaced very efficiently. The most important procedure is to carefully follow the manufacturer's recommendations for the flash sterilization of battery packs.

To properly care for and handle battery-powered instruments:

• Never immerse handpieces, attachments, or batteries in any solution including water.

• Clean surgical debris from attachments and handpieces using a nylon brush and mild detergent.

• Rinse under running water while assuring that the water does not enter the battery contact area.

• Use a decontamination battery to protect electrical components from moisture. (See **Figures 12.16, 12.17**, and **12.18**)

How to Create a Decontamination Battery

Locate a dead battery. Use instrument marking tape to make red "Xs" on the battery pack, and keep this battery in the decontamination area. When battery-powered equipment enters the Central Service department, select and insert the appropriate battery pack to protect the electrical components from moisture.

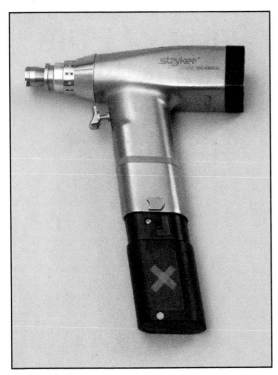

Figure 12.16

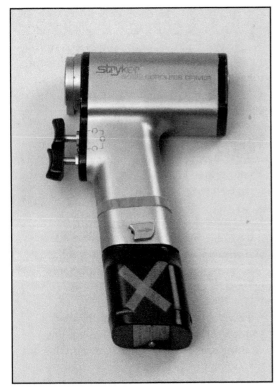

Figure 12.17

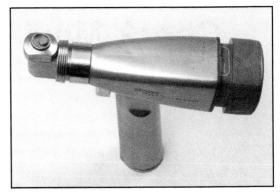

Figure 12.18

Processing Procedures

Powered surgical instruments cannot be dropped or roughly handled, and most will not tolerate submersion in any liquid. This restriction (no submersion) adds to the difficulty and potential danger involved in cleaning and disinfecting handpieces. Since they must be processed manually, testing and lubricating carries the potential to aerosolize internal debris and/or cleaning chemicals. Central Service Technicians must

Popular Powered Surgical Instruments

- Dermatome/Dermabraiders for harvesting skin grafts or reshaping skin surfaces.

- Cebatomes for removal of bone cement.

- Sternal saws for splitting the sternum to perform open-heart surgery.

- Dental drills for repair/reconstructive work on teeth and jawbones.

- Micro drills for reshaping middle ear bones or driving very small wires through bones.

- Wire drivers, drills, and saws made in the appropriate size and shape to work on the smallest facial bones to the largest bones.

- Saws designed to perform specific cutting actions such as reciprocating or oscillating.

Check Moving Parts of PSIs

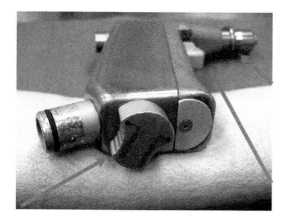
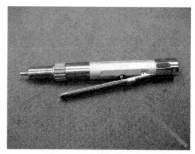
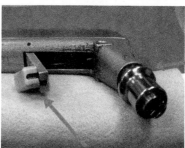

Figure 12.19

exercise great care from the time they are received until they are packaged for sterilization for their own protection as well as that of patients. Personal protective equipment should be used throughout the cleaning, disinfection, and testing processes.

Biohazardous debris is not the only danger when handling these items. By design, they hold blades and drill bits or burrs that cut bone. Devices are occasionally returned with these cutting devices still intact so Central Service Technicians must know how to safely disarm them. Many instruments have hollow channels that can be impacted with bone chips that can puncture gloves. Undivided attention and great care are necessary to provide protection against injuries.

Basic steps for manually cleaning and disinfecting powered surgical instruments are listed here to demonstrate the complexity of the process. Refer to the manufacturers' guidelines for complete details and recommendations for processing specific handpieces:

- At the point of use (and immediately after use) remove all bits, burrs, and blades from attachment devices; remove the attachment device from the handpiece, and disconnect it from the power source.

- At the point of use (including during use), remove as much tissue debris as possible with a sponge moistened with sterile water. Do not use saline as it will corrode and damage handpiece components.

- Separate simple devices (those with no internal mechanisms) that can be soaked and cleaned while other surgical instruments (examples: holding devices and burrs) are processed.

- Prevent fluid invasion by insuring that handpieces are attached to the hose during cleaning to prevent solutions from entering the motor.

- Clean the exterior with a germicidal detergent recommended by the manufacturer. Use a soft bristle brush, and pay special attention to any recessions and moving levers, switches, and/or controls. (See **Figure 12.19**) Move them several times to assure that they have been thoroughly cleaned, and that they operate smoothly.

- Clean recessions and cannulas using a stiff bristle brush of the proper diameter and length.

- Clean, rinse and inspect the hose, cable, or battery pack, and inspect it for signs of damage and/or excessive wear.

- Lubricate the handpiece with the type and amount of lubricant recommended by the equipment manufacturer.

- Dry all components with a soft, lint-free cloth.

- Some manufacturers recommend operating handpieces to assure proper functioning, and for dispersal of lubrication (if added) prior to packaging for sterilization. (See **Figure 12.20**)

- Package and sterilize the unit as recommended by the manufacturer. Special racks or positioning devices may be needed to assure that all device surfaces are properly exposed to the steam. Assure that condensation does not collect as it can damage the device.

Remember that motorized handpieces are very delicate, expensive, and require gentle care. Proper use and handling, coupled with regular preventive maintenance and service, will assure that the devices are available for use as needed.

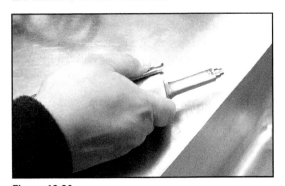

Figure 12.20

BASICS OF ENDOSCOPIC INSTRUMENTS

Learning Objective 2. Explain basic concerns important in the handling and processing of endoscopic instruments.

Flexible, rigid, and semi-rigid endoscopes (scopes) have transformed how surgery is performed. While they benefit the patient and the physician, scopes are very complicated and difficult to reprocess. Serious nosocomial infections can occur, and very expensive equipment can be damaged if the correct reprocessing protocols are not consistently utilized.

Background

The simplest form of powered surgical endoscopes began when lights were designed into rigid scopes, and batteries or electrical current were used to illuminate bulbs or fiber optic light carriers. Examples include laryngoscopes, rigid bronchoscopes, rigid esophagoscopes, sigmoidoscopes, cystoscopes, and speculums that were primarily used for diagnostic procedures. As expertise and knowledge grew, these instruments became increasingly sophisticated. Flexible fiber optic endoscopes have all but replaced the rigid originals.

The next technology leap permitted surgeons to do much more than diagnose a condition; they could perform corrective surgeries with these new minimally invasive instruments. Surgical techniques such as laparoscopy and arthroscopy came into demand as physicians and patients realized the benefit of shorter hospitalizations, less painful surgical procedures, and faster recovery times.

The flexible endoscope was introduced in the mid-1950s. A key to its development was the optical properties of coherent glass fiber bundles that enabled flexible instruments to diagnose and treat disease in ways not possible with rigid devices. This breakthrough, followed in the 1960s with similar instruments for colonoscopy, gastroscopy, and bronchoscopy, drastically changed gastroenterological and pulmonary medicine.

Technological advancements continue today in abdominal, arthroscopic, urological, otolaryngeal, and cardiac surgery. Recent endoscopic developments permit heart conditions to be treated without opening the chest and cutting the ribs.

Endoscopic procedures are a major part of nearly every hospital's practice. Lesions in the gastrointestinal tract and lungs can be directly visualized and diagnostic biopsies and therapeutic procedures can be performed without surgery or general anesthesia. In the 1980s, video endoscopes with a computer chip at the tip to transmit electronic data to a monitor began to replace fiber optic scopes so everyone in the room could observe the case (procedure) on the monitor.

Special Processing Concerns

The fiber optic light carriers and camera systems that enable surgeons to see inner body spaces/surfaces are very sensitive to pressure and bending. End connections may need to be protected from exposure to fluids during cleaning, disinfecting, and sterilizing. Most flexible endoscopes need to be "leak tested" before submersion to assure that internal electrical circuitry can protect components from fluid damage.

Endoscopes are used to view the body's internal organs, either through natural openings such as the mouth or anus or through small incisions (examples: over joints or in the abdomen or chest). Therefore, they must always be thoroughly cleaned and disinfected or sterilized between uses. Note: The decision to sterilize or high-level disinfect a scope is based upon its use according to the Spaulding Classification System.

As with other technological advances, complications can arise. Gastrointestinal endoscopies and bronchoscopy procedures can cause bleeding and perforation which are usually immediate and obvious. It is not always easy to recognize another possible complication of endoscopies: infectious transmissions. Although several studies have indicated that infection risk is low, the actual rate of disease transmission may be larger than suggested.

Studies of endoscopic procedures historically considered the scope's cost to be most significant. Today, operating costs are greatly impacted by daily activities performed in the scope's care and handling. For example, irreparable damage can be caused to an endoscope's accessory instruments by forcing them through the biopsy channel when an obstruction is encountered. This causes the accessory instrument to buckle somewhere in the scope's internal lumen.

Most healthcare processes have been reviewed in recent years in efforts to reduce operating budgets. Endoscope care including costs for supplies, chemicals, space allocation, and personnel have been part of this analysis. It is, however, important to consider how changes in operating protocols could potentially affect infection control issues and repair costs.

Endoscopic procedures greatly reduce the amount of patient trauma when physicians perform minimally invasive surgery. The patient's suffering is reduced, recovery time is shorter, and the chance of nosocomial infections is lowered. As healthcare professionals find ways to better treat patients and meet the demands of third party reimbursement agencies, advancements will continue. As technology evolves, the complexity of reprocessing and the role of the Central Service Technicians also increase.

Regulations and Guidelines

Federal regulations enable endoscope users to maximize safe care for the patient while considering the well-being of the equipment, the users, and the environment. In addition to federal laws, state and local governments may have stringent mandates. The following government agencies have rules or laws that impact the use of flexible endoscopes, and their requirements must be reflected in policy development and practice.

- Occupational Safety and Health Administration (OSHA): (http://www.osha.gov) – OSHA provides broad guidelines and specific requirements to protect employees from workplace infection.

• Department of Transportation (DOT): (http://www.dot.gov) – DOT ensures a safe, efficient, accessible, and convenient transportation system. Its laws include those relating to the transport of biohazardous materials such as minimally reprocessed endoscopes needing repair.

Other federal agencies including the Centers for Disease Control and Prevention (CDC) (http://www.cdc.gov), the Food and Drug Administration (FDA) (http:// www.fda.gov), and the Environmental Protection Agency (EPA) (http://www.epa.gov) have issued regulations applicable to endoscope processing.

Professional guidelines are suggestions developed by practitioners to represent their membership's concerns about patient protection. Accreditation bodies examine institutional polices and procedures with the expectation that professional guidelines are incorporated.

Numerous professional organizations impact endoscopy by developing professional guidelines. Several are noted in **Figure 12.21**.

Other organizations that influence endoscopy practices include:

• AAMI – Association for the Advancement of Medical Instrumentation.

• ECRI – Emergent Care and Research Institute.

• AMDR – Association of Medical Device Reprocessors. (if using third party reprocessors)

• The Joint Commission.

• OEMs – Original Equipment Manufacturers.

• Individual State Boards of Nursing.

Figure 12.21 Professional Associations With Endoscope Guidelines

Association	Guideline Topics
The Society of Gastroenterology Nurses and Associates (SGNA) - (www.sgna.org).	• Guidelines for use of high-level disinfectants and sterilants. • Safe and effective handling of glutaraldehyde solutions. • Reprocessing flexible gastrointestinal endoscopes
The American Society of Gastrointestinal Endoscopy (ASGE) – (www.asge.org).	• Infection control during gastrointestinal endoscopy. • Reprocessing of flexible gastrointestinal endoscopes.
The Association of Professionals in Infection Control and Epidemiology (APIC) (www.apic.org).	• Guidelines for infection prevention and control in flexible endoscopy.
The Association of PeriOperative Registered Nurses (AORN) – (www.aorn.org)	• Recommended practices for use and care of endoscopes.
American Society for Testing and Materials (ASTM)	• Standard practice for effectiveness of cleaning processes for reusable endoscopes

Endoscopes and the Spaulding Classification System

The reprocessing recommendations published by the CDC and FDA are based upon the Spaulding classification system which categorizes instrument disinfection needs according to its intended use, and its risk of transmitting disease. The system classifies "critical items" to be those that penetrate skin or mucous membranes, or that enter an area of the body that is normally sterile. These items (for example, biopsy forceps or angioscopes) must be sterilized. "Semi-critical items" only touch intact mucous membranes. These items (for example, flexible colonoscopes and flexible gastrointestinal endoscopes) require high-level disinfection at a minimum to destroy mycobacterium, vegetative bacteria such as methicillin-resistant staphylococcus aureus (MRSA) and vanomycin-resistant enterococcus (VRE), non-lipid and small viruses, fungi, and some (but not many) bacterial spores.

Infection Control Issues

Effective infection control policies and practices are critical to minimize or eliminate cross-contamination. The flexible endoscope is a potential nightmare for infection control. Its long, dark, and narrow lumens pose a fundamental reprocessing concern because they are not directly accessible, and are extremely difficult to clean. In addition, if channels are not thoroughly dried after reprocessing and are stored wet, they become a dark and damp medium for bacterial growth. The instrument cannot be sterilized by high temperature, and is functionally and cosmetically sensitive to the chemicals needed for cleaning, disinfecting and/or sterilizing. Human immunodeficiency virus (HIV), the Hepatitis B and C viruses, and resistant pseudomonas cause the most concern for patient-to-patient or patient-to-employee transmission, but other possibilities include candida and tuberculosis.

Other infection control-related issues include:

- The potential for inadequate education/training of employees who process the instruments.

- Time needed for adequate processing.

- Commitment of the employees including policy writers to safely reprocess the devices.

- Failure to adequately inspect scopes prior to reprocessing.

- Failure to adequately inspect reprocessing supplies and equipment.

- Failure to follow the original equipment manufacturer's (OEM's) instructions for the reprocessor's installation, filter changes, connection devices, and culture routines.

- Failure to follow directions on the labels of reprocessing chemicals.

- Use of the scope without adequate leak tests. (An unidentified hole in the scope permits contaminants to grow exponentially with each use, and cleaning chemicals can damage internal components.)

- Poor manual cleaning habits that do not effectively remove bioburden from the scope which reduce the effectiveness of disinfecting or sterilizing chemicals.

- Automated endoscope processor contamination when equipment is not used according to the manufacturer's directions.

- Improper drying and/or storing times or procedures.

The FDA requires that the labeling of endoscopes include a recommendation for at least one reprocessing method. The level of reprocessing should be based on the device's contact with the patient, and the risk for disease transmission.

Endoscope manufacturers provide manual reprocessing instructions for each endoscope model. Users should check with their endoscope and endoscope accessory manufacturers to determine whether these items can be processed in an **automatic endoscope reprocessor (AER)**. (See **Figure 12.22**) Also the manufacturer should be questioned to determine whether these items require specific steps to be taken before being reprocessed in an AER.

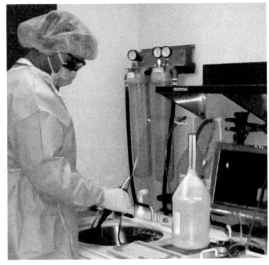

Figure 12.22

Routine use of high-level disinfection has not been shown to pose an infection risk, and has become the standard of care for flexible endoscopes. Study of infection cases have shown probable causes to include improper use and/or connection with AERs, faulty filters yielding waterborne contamination, the endoscope's design, and inadequate cleaning and/or processing.

Additional possible causes of infections related to endoscopes include:

- Failure to leak test or to test correctly.

- Failure to adequately (manually) clean all channels.

Automatic Endoscope Reprocessor (AER) – Automated equipment designed to clean, disinfect, and rinse flexible endoscopes.

- Failure to adequately flush all channels with disinfectant solution.

- Failure to fully immerse.

- Failure to adequately time the length of disinfectant contact.

- Use of disinfectant solutions after their expiration date.

- Use of a reprocessing procedure being driven by a patient diagnosis. Note: all scopes should be processed in the same manner.

- Failure to sterilize the biopsy forceps.

- Inaccessible manufacturer's instructions.

- Variations in staff training.

- Improper processing of reusable cleaning supplies.

- Use of personnel not adequately trained in proper processing procedures.

- Lack of competence reviews for processing and procedures.

- Improper storage and transport.

- Pressure from physicians to process scopes more quickly so they can perform surgeries on more patients.

- The inherent difficulty of properly processing these instruments.

- Space constraints.

- Absence of or inadequate quality control program.

- Poor water quality.

- Facility processing equipment.[1]

Meticulous manual cleaning begins immediately after use with an enzymatic detergent and proper cleaning protocols. This helps clean the endoscopes by removing organic material that may harbor microbes on the outside of the insertion tube and from the lumens of all accessible channels, and it increases the ability to properly disinfect them.

Chemicals for Endoscope Reprocessing

When selecting endoscope reprocessing chemicals, one should consider whether:

- They are effective for the intended purpose.

- Their cost is reasonable.

- They are compatible with the endoscope and the AER.

Applicable regulations and guidelines are helpful in developing facility policies and procedures for endoscope reprocessing. The facility's Infection Control Committee must be consulted for advice about the use of high-level disinfectants. These, in turn, impact protocols which should be used, and provide the foundation upon which employee performance can be assessed.

The FDA approves the use of high-level disfectants and sterilants used for critical and semi-critical medical devices based on their identified use. There are many environmental, safety, selection, and use concerns applicable to chemicals for reprocessing endoscopes that apply to other surgical instrumentation. The following discussion addresses chemical concerns specifically applicable to endoscope reprocessing.

Liquid enzymes and detergents are preferred for processing flexible endoscopes. However, if powdered detergents are used, care must be taken that all product granules are completely dissolved before immersing the instrument in the detergent solution.

Before cleaning, all channels should be irrigated with a large amount of enzyme detergent and tap water to soften, moisten, and dilute organic debris.

Selecting Enzymatic Detergents

When selecting enzymatic detergents for use with endoscopes, assure that they:

- Break down complex proteins, carbohydrates, and fats.

- Are low-foaming.

- Are effective at room temperature.

- Have a mild/neutral pH.

- Are easy to rinse.

- Are fast-acting.

- Are safe for personnel who use them.

- Are compatible with the instrument/material to be cleaned.

Several high-level disinfectant solutions including glutaraldehyde, orthophthalaldehyde (OPA), and peracetic acid solutions are approved for endoscope disinfection. Assure that the monitoring processes and strips are correct for the brand and concentration of disinfectant selected.

High-Level Disinfection Recommended

The minimum recommended practice for endoscope disinfection is high-level disinfection with a liquid sterilant/disinfectant with evidence of efficacy in clinical practice published in scientific literature. To achieve adequate high-level disinfection, all internal and external surfaces and channels must be in contact with the disinfecting agent according to the disinfectant manufacturer's labeling instructions. Prior to selecting a disinfectant, the scope's manufacturer must be consulted to ensure that the disinfectant is compatible with the instrument. In addition, if an automatic endoscope reprocessor (AER) is used, that manufacturer must also be consulted.

Glutaraldehyde

Advantages of glutaraldehyde in the endoscopy setting include:

- It is active against gram-negative and gram-positive bacteria, fungi, viruses, and spores.

- Its acidic-based concentration is compatible with most endoscope materials including metal, rubber, and plastic.

- Sterilization may be accomplished with extended exposure times.

Disadvantages of glutaraldehyde include its unstable half-life which is impacted by dilution and time. In an alkaline concentration, it can be corrosive to high-carbon metals. Glutaraldehyde also has a fixative component that, over time, can cause a sticky build-up within the endoscope's channels. Solutions with surfactants are very difficult to rinse from the endoscope, and are not advised for use with flexible endoscopes.

Potential safety hazards of glutaraldehyde include:

- Documented cases of patient chemical burns caused by ineffective rinsing that leaves residual chemicals in/on the scope.

- Reported employee inhalation and contact dermatitis irritations after use of improper processing procedures.

An acid glutaraldehyde disinfectant is available. Compared with alkaline preparations, some acid solutions are more corrosive to metal. Acid solutions of glutaraldehyde (pH to 6.3) are stable for long periods without loss of active aldehyde groups. A 2% acid glutaraldehyde product acts as a chemical sterilant, and is acceptable for high-level disinfection for endoscope reprocessing.

Ortho-Phthalaldehyde Solution (OPA)

Orthophthalaldehyde (OPA) solution is a high-level disinfectant for semi-critical devices when used/re-used according to directions at or above its minimum effective concentration (MEC) of 0.3% at 68°F (20°C) in a manual system, or 77°F (25°C) in an AER. The solution has a re-use period of up to 14 days. OPA is available commercially in a ready-to-use solution which requires no diluting or mixing. It has a life expectancy of 75 days in its original container once opened, and has an expiration date on the container.

The OPA solution's concentration during its use life must be verified with OPA Solution Test Strips prior to each use to determine that the MEC of 0.3% is present. If the solution does not pass the MEC concentration test, it must be discarded, and it should also not be used after 14 days even if the test strip indicates an acceptable MEC concentration.

Although OPA does not have an odor, the solution should be used in a well-ventilated area, and in closed containers with tight fitting lids.

Peracetic Acid

A peracetic acid formulation is available for single-use in an AER. Concentrated (35%) liquid peracetic acid is diluted with a buffer, surfactant, and anti-corrosive dry powder to its 0.2% (2000 ppm) use dilution. The labeled contact conditions for sterilization are 12 minutes at 122°F to 133°F (50°C to 56°C). During the sterilization cycle, time and temperature are automatically controlled and monitored. The cycle includes rinsing with tap water that has been passed through a 0.2-micron filtration membrane. The efficacy of this filtration process depends upon the quality of the incoming tap water. Biological and chemical indicators designed for this system are available, and should be used for quality monitoring. As well, the printout should be studied for accuracy and completeness.

Advantages to the use of peracetic acid in endoscopy include:

- The processor holds only one scope at a time, which removes the potential for compression damage.

- The scope is placed in a grooved tray to protect it from puncture while processing.

- The chemical is mixed in the machine in a consistent concentration while the processor's cycle time is dependent upon water quality, temperature, and pressure.

- Printout documentation listing cycle parameters accompanies each cycle.

- Items are sterilized for immediate use.

Disadvantages to the use of peracetic acid in endoscopy include:

- The on-going monitoring of biological parameters incurs additional expense.

- Some scopes may not be compatible with peracetic acid solutions.

- The system is not approved to sterilize water bottles or their water delivery systems. The bottle itself is not designed to allow the peracetic acid solution to flow into and out of the closed-end container in a controlled manner. Additionally, there is not a quick connect system to attach to the water delivery system, so the water bottle cannot be processed in this system. The water bottle manufacturer must be consulted for processing information; most can be sterilized in the steam sterilizer.

What About Other Disinfectants?

Some agents are not recommended by APIC for use on endoscopes and endoscopic equipment. Reasons include an incomplete anti-microbial coverage (failure to meet the definition of a high-level disinfectant), and because of toxic exposure to personnel or physical damage to equipment. For example, the combination of glutaraldehyde and iodophors, hypochlorites, quaternary ammonium chloride compounds, skin antiseptics, and phenolics do not meet all criteria necessary for endoscopic cleaning and disinfection.

Automatic Endoscope Reprocessors

Automatic endoscope reprocessors (AERs) are machines that clean, disinfect, and rinse flexible endoscopes. Their design permits the exterior of the scope and all lumens to be exposed to cleaning, disinfecting, and rinsing solutions. To facilitate the flushing of the lumens, specific tubing connections must be connected, and scopes are placed in the AER after initial cleaning and brushing. (See **Figure 12.23**)

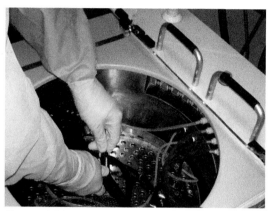

Figure 12.23

Most AERs are connected to a water filtration system specifically designed to remove bacteria from the rinse water. A typical water filtration system includes two types of filters: a 5 um particulate filter and a 0.1 um or 0.2 um bacterial filter. When properly maintained, bacterial filters reduce, but do not eliminate, the risk of patient contamination from opportunistic microorganisms sometimes found in tap water. Due to frequent use and the colonization of bacteria on their membranes, however, bacterial filters have been reported to fail. This allows bacteria to pass through the filters, and contaminate the instrument during the final water rinse. Proper maintenance and replacement of these filters are necessary to reduce the risk of filter failure.

The labels of some disinfectants require elevating their temperature above room temperature to achieve high-level disinfection. Most AERs feature a heater that conveniently and rapidly elevates the temperature to a predetermined setting. Since they are typically enclosed systems, most AERs limit staff exposure to liquid chemical sterilants and their vapors, which often increase during heating because of an increase in the disinfectant's vapor pressure. Some AERs feature audible and visual alarms that are activated when a safety fault that could jeopardize process success is detected.

The successful outcome of instrument reprocessing with a disinfectant is impacted by rinse water quality. However, this parameter is difficult to monitor and control. Water quality in different regions of the United States and other countries vary considerably. Some potable water supplies contain few, if any, microorganisms; others are significantly contaminated.

Under ideal conditions, bacterial filters can be expected to produce bacterial-free, but not sterile, rinse water. Filtered non-potable water contains viruses, endotoxins, pyrogens, and microbial debris smaller than the bacterial filter's rated size (for example, 0.1 um or 0.2 um). Filtered water may even contain bacteria suspected of penetrating through the bacterial filter's membrane. Proper maintenance of the filters and their housings is essential to minimize the likelihood of instrument recontamination during the final water rinse.

As with any medical device, AERs require periodic preventive maintenance to help ensure their safe and effective operation. Failure to perform these measures which, unfortunately,

When Can An AER Be Used?

Not all endoscopes and their accessories can be reliably reprocessed in an AER. For example, elevator-wire-channels of many duodenoscopes cannot be accessed by the AER, and must be manually reprocessed. If not specifically indicated in the AER labeling, ask AER manufacturers whether the endoscope being used has been tested with their system. Compare the reprocessing instructions provided by the instrument with that of the AER manufacturer. Resolve any conflicting recommendations, especially when they involve the use of channel connections or capping/non-capping of specific lumens or channels.

can be time-consuming and cumbersome, may result in patient injury. A few specific models with outdated and flawed designs have been responsible for patient contamination. However, modern AERs are designed to prevent the colonization of waterborne microorganisms in their internal components and plumbing lines. Although most AERs disinfect their internal components during routine endoscope reprocessing, some may require use of additional measures to prevent the growth of biofilms. Review the AER's operating manual to determine required preventive maintenance procedures.

Automatic endoscope reprocessors offer several advantages to manual reprocessing. Among other useful features, AERs automate, standardize, and simplify at least one step required for endoscope reprocessing: they reduce personnel exposure to the disinfectant and its vapors. Their use may also increase quality assurance by consistently documenting several cycle parameters, usually provides fresh and bacteria-free rinse water, and elevates the temperature of the liquid chemical sterilants if required by its label.

Other advantages of AERS include:

- Timed cleaning.

- Consistent exposure to the cleaning agent.

- Timed contact with liquid chemical disinfectants.

- Use of an air flush cycle to remove excess moisture.

- Use of copious and consistent amounts of water.

Endoscope design limitations create the need for some manual reprocessing steps. For example, manual preprocessing (cleaning) and post-processing (rinse with 70% alcohol, and follow with a forced air dry) is necessary. Refer to the AER's operating manual for information about limitations of automated cycles.

When using AERs:

- Follow the manufacturer's instructions to connect the endoscope to the AER.

- Place the valves and other removable parts in the AER, if possible.

- Attach channel cleaning connectors to all channels.

- Follow the manufacturer's instructions for using disinfectants.

- Set the machine for the recommended time.

Staff Education

Central Service Technicians working with complex medical instrumentation such as endoscopes must be thoroughly trained in proper processing protocols. Their competency should be reviewed annually using a competency checklist such as the sample illustrated in **Figure 12.24**.

Department-wide education is the key to effective infection control in endoscopy, and should be updated with each new piece of equipment and with each change in the chemical or process that is employed. Training and education should be addressed from a unit-specific standpoint and should include:

- Standard precautions.

- Regulatory requirements.

- Procedures for reprocessing:

- Equipment, accessories, and AERs.

- Cleaning, rinsing, disinfecting, drying, and storing.

Competency Verification Checklist for Manual Endoscope Cleaning and Reprocessing with a Failed Leak Test*

Employee Name/Title: _____

Department/Date: _____

Validator: _____

Task	Compliant w/Policy	Needs Assistance	Correction Plan	Initials
Skills Evaluation				
- Wears Protective Covering, gloves, gown, and splash shield				
Pre-Cleaning				
- Wipes Insertion Tube with Enzyme Cleaner				
- Suctions Enzyme Cleaner through Scope				
- Clears Air/Water Channels				
Leakage Test				
- Attaches Water Resistant Cap				
- Detaches All Removable Parts				
-Insuflates Scope Prior to Submerrsion				
- Observes Scope for at Least 60 Seconds				
- Angulates Scope in all Directions				
- Identifies Leak				
- Deflates and Covers Area of Leak with Tape				
- Reinflates and Keeps Inflated for Remainder of Scope Cleaning and External Disinfection				
Cleaning				
- Soaks, Scrubs, Brushes, and Rinses all Removed Parts				
- Immerses and Cleans Exterior of Scope				
- Brushes Entire Suction/Biopsy Channel System				
- Rinses all Removable Parts Under Running Water and Removes Residual Detergent				
Disinfecting				
- Places Scope in a Disinfecting Solution According to Protocol				
Rinsing				
- Rinses all External Surfaces and all Removable Parts				
Drying				
-Decompresses Scope				
- Wipes External Surfaces with Alcohol				
Hazard Identification				
- Notifies Repair Facility that Scope is Only Externally Disinfected				
- Sends Scope Immediately for Repair per Policy				

Employee Signature: _____

Validator's Signature: _____

* Reprinted with Permission from Integrated Medical Services (IMS)

Figure 12.24 Sample Competency Checklist

- Leak testing.

- Mechanisms of disease transmissions.

- Maintenance of safe work environments.

- Safe handling of liquid chemical disinfectants and sterilants.

- Procedures for waste management.

Continuous quality improvement (CQI) for endoscope processing is measured by monitors and indicators including:

- Annual competency reviews.

- Minimum effective chemical concentrations.

- Biological monitors.

- Equipment repair patterns.

- Preventive maintenance schedules.

- Identified infections.

CLOSE LOOK AT FLEXIBLE ENDOSCOPES

Learning Objective 3. Discuss detailed information about flexible endoscopes.

Flexible endoscopes are appropriately named:

- The term, "flexible," means capable of bending which is necessary to gain access to internal body organs.

- The term, "endo," means inside; a flexible endoscope can visualize inside the body.

Flexible endoscopes are long and complex instruments used to visualize abnormalities and pathologies inside the body, to perform diagnostic tests, and/or to obtain tissue specimens for biopsy.

Scope Components

Endoscopes are comprised of a head with controls and a flexible shaft with a maneuverable tip. Hundreds of special fiber optic fibers are arranged around one or more lumens. A series of lenses and mirrors along with coils or springs and cables run the length of the instrument to control the tip's movement. An imaging cable is also usually included.

Components are assembled within an impervious material covering (one that does not allow anything to pass through it) to produce an instrument that can bend gently (but not sharply at right angles) to maneuver inside the body. Note: Care must be taken to avoid breaking any fibers by bending the endoscope at sharp angles or by dropping it. Endoscope lengths range from a typical esophagogastroduodenoscope (about 36" long) to colonoscopes (usually 60" or longer).

Some flexible endoscopes are only used to visualize internal organs, and do not have internal channels. Others may consist of two or three systems. For example, a mechanical system angles and bends the scope to maneuver it. An optical system transmits images from the distal tip for viewing. Some scopes also have additional systems (channels) for instrument insertion, irrigation and suctioning. (See **Figure 12.25**)

The largest operating channel is the instrument (biopsy) channel which is 1.2-4.2 mm in diameter. It allows the passage of fine, flexible accessory instruments (for example, biopsy forceps or diagnostic brushes for scrapings) from a port in the scope's head through the tip, and into the field of view within the body. It is also used for suctioning. Other channels transmit air to stretch the organ being examined for better viewing or water to clean the distal lens if it is soiled with bile, secretions, blood, feces, or other materials.

Endoscopes require several connector devices:

- The light guide connector attaches to a light source.

- The suction connector suctions fluid matter from the body.

- The water container connector provides water to clean the scope's lens.

Endoscope Channels

Instrument Channel

Optical Channel

Air/Water Channel*

Suction Channel

*Some Flexible Scopes have separate Air and Water Channels

Figure 12.25

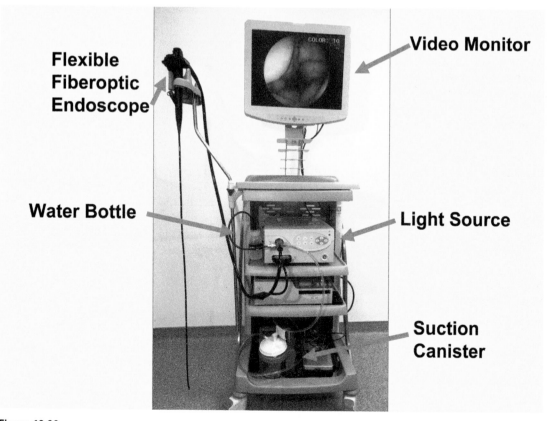

Flexible Fiberoptic Endoscope

Video Monitor

Water Bottle

Light Source

Suction Canister

Figure 12.26

• The venting connector allows the penetration of ethylene oxide gas during scope sterilization. This must be in place during sterilization to prevent rupturing the bending sheath.

Images travel through the endoscope to the eyepiece or monitor for viewing. **Figure 12.26** provides an illustration of a common Flexible Fiberoptic Endoscope equipment set up. Biopsies are taken by threading a flexible biopsy instrument through the biopsy channel to obtain a tissue specimen. (See **Figure 12.27**) This tissue is then brought up the channel for removal. Other accessory pieces such as cytology brushes, snares, and electrodes pass through this channel.

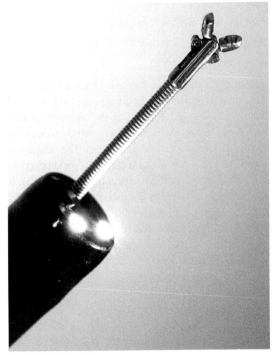

Figure 12.27

The scope's control section contains the fiber bundle and/or image-conducting cable, control wires for the distal tip movement and, usually, several other channels. The endoscope head is connected to a light source (and to a computer-driven monitor if it is a videoscope) by a universal cord.

Types of Flexible Endoscopes

There are a variety of flexible endoscopes in use today.

Bronchoscope

Bronchoscopy involves the direct visualization of the tracheobronchial tree, and involves:

• Diagnosis to secure uncontaminated secretion for culture, to take a biopsy, or to find the cause of a cough or hemoptysis (spitting up blood).

• Treatment to remove a foreign body, to excise a small tumor, to apply a medication, to aspirate the bronchi, or to provide an airway during a tracheotomy.

Tiny forceps inserted through the bronchoscope are manipulated for a tissue biopsy. The diameter of a flexible scope is small enough to reach into the bronchi of upper, middle, and lower lobes for examination and/or biopsy.

The set-up for flexible bronchoscopy includes the following:

• Fiber optic light source.

• Flexible bronchoscope.

• Flexible biopsy forceps.

• Flexible cytology brush (optional); if used, slides and alcohol are necessary to collect a specimen.

• S uction unit.

The bronchial endoscope is passed through a "bite block" positioned between the patient's upper and lower jaws/teeth to protect it from the usually severe and costly damage that occurs when a patient bites it forcefully. (This block may be unnecessary for patients that do not have teeth.)

Cystoscope/Ureteroscope

A flexible cystoscope is used to visualize the urethra and bladder. A ureteroscope is passed through the urethra and bladder to the urethra and kidneys to look for obstructions such as kidney stones. It can also be used for patients who cannot assume a lithotomic position (patients are on their back with hips and knees flexed, and thighs apart) such as those with spinal cord injuries or severe arthritis. Flexible cystoscopy may be accomplished with the use of a local anesthetic.

The following instruments are required:

- Cystoscope/Ureteroscope.
- Light source.
- Biopsy forceps.
- Snares/guide wires.
- Electrosurgical unit and accessories.
- Water feed supply.

Note: These procedures are performed on a special type of operating table which allows for fluid drainage/collection, and for x-ray imaging.

Gastroscope/Esophagoscope

Gastroscopy is performed by a gastroscope, and involves the visual inspection of the upper digestive tract (including esophagus, stomach, and duodenum) with aspiration of contents and biopsy, if necessary. Esophagoscopy is the direct visualization of the esophagus and the cardia of the stomach, and removal of tissue or secretions for study.

Instrumentation includes:

- Flexible gastroscope.
- Flexible light source.
- Flexible biopsy forceps.
- Electro-surgical unit and accessories.
- Suction unit.
- Air and water feed supply.

Colonoscope/Sigmoidscope

Colonoscopy involves the visual inspection of the entire large intestine with a colonoscope. Sigmoidoscopy involves the visual inspection of the lower part of the large intestine with a sigmoidoscope. These scopes are passed into the

colon through the anus or ostomy (or stoma). They are important diagnostic tools, and may be used for biopsy and removal of polyps, and to control bleeding ulcers.

The following instruments are required:

- Colonoscope.
- Light source.
- Biopsy forceps.
- Snares.
- Electrosurgical unit and accessories.
- Suction unit.
- Air and water feed supply.

Cleaning and Processing

When cleaning a flexible endoscope, it is important to remember its design: a head with controls and a flexible shaft through which other tubes pass. Commonly used accessories are also complex medical devices. The scope and instruments/accessories offer the potential for organic debris and for microorganisms to hide. The manufacturer of the accessory pieces must be consulted for processing instructions. Some tightly-coiled metal instruments such as biopsy forceps present a real cleaning challenge. (See **Figure 12.28**) They require steam sterilization

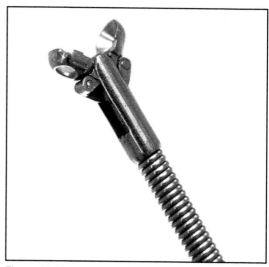

Figure 12.28

since other methods are not effective due to the tightly coiled design.

Background

Sterilization is not mandated for flexible scopes since they do not break the mucosal barrier. Polymeric (non-heat stable) materials are most commonly used in scope construction. Most scopes can be completely immersed in liquid. However, prior to immersion cleaning, a leak test is typically suggested by the manufacturer; see below. Consult with the scope's manufacturer and the hospital's Infection Control Committee, and follow the SGNA recommendations for proper disinfection or sterilization protocols.

As with all other medical devices, endoscopes must be thoroughly cleaned prior to disinfection, or the chemical germicide will be ineffective. Use of an AER does not replace the need to manually clean the endoscope (including its internal channels).

Those who reprocess endoscopes should follow Standard Precautions. They should wear personal protective equipment including gloves, gowns, facemasks or shields, and hair covering. (See **Figure 12.29**) Endoscopes should be reprocessed in a large, well-ventilated area to help protect personnel from chemical vapors. An appropriate enzymatic detergent is typically recommended for scope processing since it is more effective for lumened instruments.

It is important to keep current on information about enzymatic cleaners. New challenges

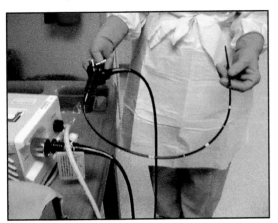

Figure 12.29

develop every day. For example, Olean (Olestra) was introduced in 1998, and was marketed as a substitute in fat-free foods. Unfortunately, the human body does not digest this ingredient. When a patient eats a food containing this substance before an endoscopic procedure, the chemical leaves an orange/pink oily substance that coats the insertion tubes, internal channels of the scope, and the biopsy forceps. This residue does not break down with routine cleaning agents. Note: There is a synthetic lipid remover (SLR) available for this substance.

Manual cleaning is the most important step in processing flexible endoscopes. As with all medical devices, the processing procedure begins at the point of use to prevent blood or protein material including patient debris from drying on the instrument and later being carried into reprocessing solutions. Also, organisms can grow and multiply dramatically within a short time after a procedure is completed. Suction channels should be rinsed with clean water to remove as much blood and tissue debris as possible at the point of use to rinse away as much soil as possible before it has a chance to dry.

Cleaning should be performed with soft, lint-free cloths or sponges and brushes specifically designed for use with the scope. Effective cleaning reduces disinfection failures by reducing the presence of organic soil that harbors microorganisms and prevents the penetration of germicides.

Cleaning accessories may be disposable or reusable. If reusable, they must be thoroughly cleaned after each use, and they must be sterilized or disinfected according to the manufacturer's recommendations. Use of ultrasonic cleaners is often recommended to process accessories, especially those with a tight metal-coiled design.

Lubrication may result in extensive damage if not done correctly. Ultrasonic cleaning will damage some instrument accessories unless recommended by the manufacturer. Note: some ultrasonic equipment has been designed to process delicate, lumened instruments. However, it is crucial to consult with the instrument's manufacturer to assess whether this process will be harmful.

Six basic steps are required to clean and reprocess endoscopes:

- Pre-cleaning.

- Leak testing.

- Cleaning.

- High-level disinfecting/sterilizing.

- Drying.

- Storing.

Pre-Cleaning

Pre-cleaning is the removal of gross debris from the endoscope's external surfaces and internal channels. The insertion tube should be wiped with an enzymatic detergent solution formulated for endoscopes applied by a soft, lint-free cloth. Suction the solution through the endoscope until the solution is visibly clean by alternately suctioning the solution and air. Finish with water. Clear the air and water channels according to the manufacturer's instructions.

Leak Testing

A **leak test** is necessary to ensure that the flexible covering and the internal channels of the endoscope are watertight. Leak testing involves submerging the endoscope, and forcing air through it. If bubbles appear, there is a leak.

A crack or a leak in the scope covering can occur, for example, if an accessory such as a forceps nicks the inner lumen. Reprocessing solutions will leak into the internal parts of the instrument, and damage its mechanical and electrical components. These small defects may not be seen, but can substantially damage the scope. Leak testing is, therefore, mandatory before further cleaning.

It is necessary to consult the manufacturer's instructions for the proper leak testing procedures

> **Leak test (endoscope)** – *An endoscope processing procedure that ensures the device's flexible covering and internal channels are watertight.*

for the specific endoscope. However, basic steps for leak testing a scope include:

- Visually inspect the scope for tears, holes, and joints that may leak. Pay close attention to the seams and body joints. If any tears or holes are found, the scope cannot be submerged, and the scope will need to be repaired. Submerging a scope with a hole or tear can cause fluid invasion.

- Remove all valves and attachments from the endoscope.

- Attach the leak tester to the EtO venting connector (fiber optic scope), or to the leak tester connector of the water-resistant cap (on videoscopes), and pressurize the scope before placing the scope in water. Always pressurize the scope before placing it in the water for leak testing because water can invade the scope's interior in a few seconds. When the interior of the scope is pressurized with air, one can see and/or feel the bending rubber expand. A continuous stream of bubbles from the interior of the scope indicates a leak.

- The most common area for leaks is the bending rubber at the distal tip of the insertion tube; always check this area first. With only the distal end of the insertion tube submerged in water, ungulate the distal tip in all directions to assure that any small holes sealed by the bending rubber will open. The control knobs of the endoscope must be out of the water for this step because the rubber o-rings between the control knobs are not designed to operate under water with excessive pressure. When manipulated to the maximum position, they may leak, and allow fluid to pass them into the scope's interior.

- Completely submerge the scope under water.

- Observe the control knobs. Bubbles will appear if an o-ring is damaged.

- Observe for holes in the scope's internal channels. If there are holes, air bubbles will exit a channel opening at the valve ports, the air and water inlets, the suction port of the light guide connector, the biopsy port, or the channel opening(s) at the insertion tube's distal tip. Air trapped in the channels may take a few minutes to clear, and may falsely appear to be a leak. Flushing the channels with water can clear this air. Note: A continuous stream of bubbles indicates a leak.

- Observe the insertion and light guide tubes. Examine the entire length of both tubes for bubbles. If either tube is buckled anywhere, the chance of holes being formed is increased.

- Remove the scope from the water and drain.

- Release pressure. Verify deflation of the scope by observing the bending rubber, or hearing the sound of air being released.

- Disconnect the leak tester from the scope. Never disconnect the leak tester under water; water could enter the leak tester connector, and invade the scope's interior.

A pinpoint hole in the delicate rubber sheath that covers the distal bending section of the endoscope can fog the operator's view because fluid may leak through the hole into the optical system. This problem can be prevented (and expensive repairs can be avoided) if this part of the instrument is carefully inspected between procedures, and repaired before the damage becomes serious.

If the endoscope has passed the leak test, it is watertight, and reprocessing may proceed. As with any disinfection or sterilization process, the scope must first be thoroughly cleaned.

Cleaning

Steps for cleaning endoscopes include:

- Detach all removable parts; soak and scrub, or brush them to remove all debris.

- Immerse the endoscope in an enzymatic detergent solution, and thoroughly clean its exterior. All accessible channels (for example, the suction and air/water valves, biopsy port openings, and all other channel openings)

should be brushed to remove particulate matter. Be sure to use the correct-sized brush for the lumen's opening. An enzymatic detergent must be suctioned or pumped through all channels to remove dislodged material. Crevices and lumens likely to harbor contaminated organic material should be given special attention. Channel irrigators and some automated endoscope washers/disinfectors may be useful in this step.

- Thoroughly brush the entire biopsy/suction channel system until there is no debris visible on the brush. To assure that the channel is being cleaned, the brush must be cleaned and rinsed each time it is placed in the scope.

- The tip of the endoscope must be wiped or brushed to remove any debris or tissue lodged in or around the air and water nozzle. When cleaning the endoscopic retrograde cholangio-pancreatography endoscope, the distal tip must be brushed with the elevator in both up and down positions to ensure that no matter is lodged in that movable part.

- Attach cleaning adapters to the endoscope, and cover the biopsy port.

High-Level Disinfection and Liquid Chemical Sterilization

As with cleaning, manual high-level disinfection involves immersing the instrument in a basin containing the appropriate solution for the time recommended by the solution's manufacturer. Other steps include:

- Immerse the endoscope in disinfectant which is in a basin large enough for the endoscope. Do not coil it too tightly.

- Use the cleaning adapters to fill all channels (including air, water, suction/biopsy, elevator, and auxiliary water) with disinfectant until no bubbles are seen exiting the channels.

- Place all valves and removable parts in the disinfectant. To prevent damage to the endoscope, do not soak accessory equipment such as forceps with the endoscope.

• Cover with a tight lid to minimize exposure to chemical vapors.

• Check the disinfectant's label instructions to determine the correct immersion time, and set a timer for that time.

• When immersion is complete, purge the endoscope's channels with air to remove the disinfectant.

After disinfection, the scope must be thoroughly rinsed to remove all traces of the disinfectant from the internal channels. Filtered water is preferred for this rinse to prevent reintroduction of waterborne organisms into the high-level disinfected endoscope.

Proper rinse procedures include:

• Thoroughly rinse the exterior surface and lumens of the endoscope with water.

• Flush all channels with copious amounts of water.

• Thoroughly rinse all valves and other removable parts.

Reprocessing an Endoscope with Failed Leak Test:Medium-to-Small Hole

A scope that fails a leak test should be immediately shipped to a service technician or manufacturer for repair. Each manufacturer provides information about procedures for reprocessing a flexible endoscope with an identified leak. OSHA mandates that medical equipment should be decontaminated to the maximum extent possible before transportation. When decontamination is impractical, the equipment should be labeled as 'biohazardous." When a leak of any size/type is identified, there is an increased risk of fluid invasion when the endoscope is submerged. In other words, there is no such thing as a "minor" leak; all leaks can cause major (costly) repairs.

Follow the basic steps recommended by most scope manufacturers to reprocess an endoscope that has failed a leak test including:

• Completely depressurize the scope.

• Occlude (shut) the site of the leak with waterproof tape.

• Re-pressurize the scope; leave the leak tester attached and pressurized throughout the remaining steps of reprocessing to minimize fluid invasion.

• Clean the scope externally with enzymatic cleaner. The scope can be wiped down, and the internal channels can be brushed and flushed with small amounts of solution using an all-channel irrigator.

• Rinse the scope externally with large amounts of water.

• If the scope passes the leak test, manually soak it for the time recommended for high-level disinfection. Rinse again.

• Depressurize the scope.

• If unable to seal the leak with electrical tape to complete the disinfection process, contain the scope in a clear plastic bag, and label the bag as "biohazardous" for transportation to a service center. Include information to the repair service that alerts the technicians and the courier service that the scope is a biohazard. Place all papers associated with the device outside of the bag.

If neither sterilization nor high-level disinfection is an option, the endoscope should be considered contaminated, and then it should be identified and shipped as a biohazard. It is important to check with the shipper for additional guidelines.

When the scope is returned from repair, it must be completely reprocessed according to the facility's protocols prior to patient use.

Cleaning Reusable Brushes and Accessories

Cleaning organic matter from the spiral-wound configuration of reusable brushes as part of the cleaning/sterilizing process is very difficult (if not impossible). Therefore, brushes should be thoroughly cleaned by use of ultrasonic cleaning and steam sterilization. Endoscopic accessories that enter sterile tissue should be sterilized between uses if they are designed as reusable, or they should be discarded if they are disposable.

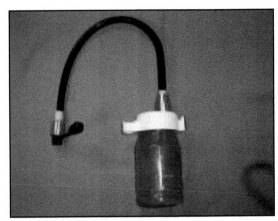

Figure 12.30

The endoscope's reusable parts that were removed and placed in detergent before cleaning must also be cleaned, rinsed, disinfected, and rinsed again prior to drying and storage. Some of these parts may be heat stable; if so, they should be packaged, steam sterilized, and then properly stored in their package.

An endoscope processing log should be maintained to document the date, time, scope's serial number, effectiveness of the disinfectant, and name of the Central Service Technician who performed the processing. AER printouts should also be filed.

Drying

Regardless of whether the endoscope is processed manually or with an AER, a final drying step is needed. After rinsing, the endoscope should be irrigated with 70% isopropyl alcohol, followed by forced-air drying. Note: alcohol is used since it evaporates quickly, and facilitates drying of the endoscope. Drying the exterior of the endo-

Water Bottle Precautions

The water in an endoscope's water bottle is sprayed through the water channel to the patient's internal organs. (See **Figure 12.30**) For this reason, it must be properly cared for. The water bottle should be sterilized at least once a day (ideally after each use). Only sterile water should be used to fill it, and water should never be stored in the water bottle overnight.

scope, and purging the remaining water from the channels help prepare it for storage by minimizing the moisture necessary for bacterial growth.[2]

Ethylene Oxide Sterilization

Some flexible scopes may be sterilized using Ethylene Oxide gas. Review and follow manufacturer's instructions for sterilization. Flexible scopes that are ethylene oxide sterilized may require a venting cap during sterilization. (See **Figure 12.31**) Follow manufacturer's instructions carefully to avoid damaging the scope.

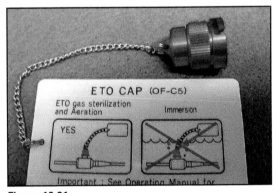

Figure 12.31

Storing

Storage is the final step in reprocessing. If flexible endoscopes are not stored properly, bacteria could grow even though the scope has previously received high-level disinfection or sterilization. As well, it is important to minimize the collection/retention

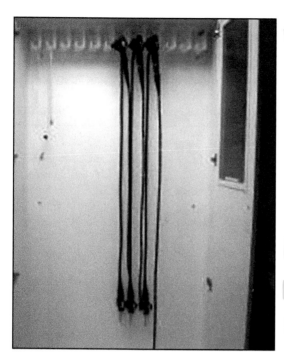

Figure 12.32

of moisture.

Before storing, the scope should be completely dry both internally and externally. Dry endoscopes should be stored in a manner to prevent recontamination or damage from sharp, jagged edges. They should be stored (a) with the insertion tube hanging vertically (not coiled), (b) with the weight of the control body supported and angulation locks off and (c) in a dry, dust-free cabinet with good ventilation. (See **Figure 12.32**) Endoscopes should be stored without removable parts such as control valves, distal hoods, and caps in place. The water-resistant cap should be removed from the video scopes while they are in storage.

Storage concerns include the potential for physical damage to the endoscope. This most often occurs from damage to the fiberoptics by tightly coiling the instrument. Storing scopes in a moist environment or exposing them to damage by storage in a high-traffic area are two additional potential problems.

If there is residual moisture, or if the endoscope is stored in a wet area, airborne microbes or those transferred from the hands of healthcare workers may begin to proliferate. Storage cabinets should be cleaned daily with a hospital-approved disinfectant.

Flexible endoscopes must always be carefully carried, or they can easily be broken. If carried improperly, they can become damaged if they are struck against walls, doorways, carts, and other fixtures. To prevent this, scopes should always be carried loosely coiled while holding the distal tip securely.

Endoscopic Accessories

Endoscopic accessories are of two types: diagnostic and therapeutic.

Diagnostic Accessories

- **Biopsy Forceps.** This consists of two distally-located cups or jaws that open or close when a control located at the proximal end is manipulated. Jaws can have smooth or serrated edges. When the edges are open, they expose a sharp spike that grasps the tissue seized between the jaws when they close to prevent tissue slippage.

- **Brush for Cytology.** This consists of a plastic tube that encloses a wire with a short brush at its distal end. When the brush is inserted in the lumen of the gut through the endoscope's biopsy channel, it becomes exposed when the examiner pushes it through the plastic tube. The brush is retracted into the plastic sheath, which is inserted through the biopsy channel beyond the end of the scope. The operator visualizes the tip, and extends the brush through the plastic sheath. The brush's bristles are rubbed against the mucosal surface, and become coated with exfoliated cellular material.

- **Cannulas for Opacification.** These small plastic (silicone) catheter-type devices have markings located at the tip (three black bands), which are separated by two white bands.

- **Measuring Device.** This flexible, rod-like accessory is marked at its distal end with a series of spaced bands.

Therapeutic Accessories

- Electro Coagulating ("hot biopsy") Forceps. This is similar to a biopsy forceps, but has a mechanism to directing electrosurgical current to lesions so the small polyps can be transected without bleeding.

- Polypectomy Snares. This accessory consists of a pre-formed, oval or hexagonal wire loop (when opened) inside a plastic tubular sheath. The loop can be rotatable or non-rotatable, and is manipulated over the polyp, and closed around its base like a noose. Electro-surgical current then burns the polyp free.

- Polyp Retriever. This consists of finger-like metal prongs inside a tubular plastic sheath. The prongs spread apart spontaneously when they are extruded from the sheath's distal end. The polyp retriever grasps tissue specimens for retrieval after they have been transected or cut free.

- Foreign Body Forceps. This accessory secures and extracts foreign bodies from the respiratory or digestive tracts. It is a modified version of biopsy forceps in which the jaws are spoon- or claw-shaped or serrated.

- Electrodes for Electrocoagulation or Electrodesiccation. This ball-tipped electrode is located at the distal end of a plastic cannula, and is used for electrocoagulation of bleeding points, and electrodesiccation of polypoid growths.

- Injection Needle. This accessory is used for injection sclerosis of esophageal varices (stretched veins), and for injection of India ink (or other marking dyes) in the layer of loose connective tissue under a mucous membrane to designate the site from which a suspicious lesion was removed. It is a small (25 gauge), specially designed and retractable injection needle attached to flexible tubing which is approximately 1.8 mm in diameter.

- Laser Probe. This accessory is made of specially-constructed fiber optic quartz glass bundles which transmit a laser beam, when passed through an endoscope. When connected to a laser unit, these fiber optic bundles help control bleeding from gastrointestinal lesions.

CLOSE LOOK AT RIGID AND SEMI-RIGID ENDOSCOPES

Learning Objective 4. Review general processing and inspection requirements for rigid and semi-rigid endoscopes and laparoscope instruments.

The technology and design of rigid and semi-rigid endoscopes is constantly evolving, and a wide variety and range of sizes are available as they become useful in more specialties and procedures. (See **Figure 12.33**) For example, laparoscope usage was limited to gynecology (GYN) surgeons who diagnosed endometriosis or ligated fallopian tubes for birth control. GYN procedures have now expanded the use of these scopes, and they are also now used by general surgeons to remove gallbladders or repair hernias, and by ENT surgeons to remove sinus polyps. As well, orthopedic surgeons repair knee, wrist, and ankle joints, neurosurgeons release carpal tunnels or perform discectomies, and cardiovascular surgeons repair hearts.

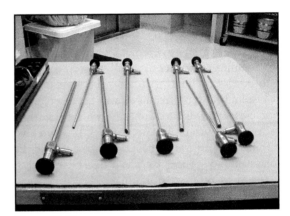

Figure 12.33

New technology will continue to evolve, and the instruments will become more complex and smaller. As diameters decrease, fibers are also becoming smaller and more fragile. This fragility results in easier fracturing or misalignment of the smaller glass rods if they are not handled properly, and results in expensive and time-consuming repairs. Video cameras are being used with scopes to allow easier visualization and recording of the procedures as they are projected to a video monitor. These scopes, cameras, and cables are extremely fragile, and require gentle care.

The optical element for rigid endoscope systems is called a telescope. It is an integral part of the system, and provides the image and light through two distinct systems. This element is the most expensive and fragile part of the system. In rigid endoscopic devices, the optical lens train transfers the image to the user's eye or a video monitor. The lens train is comprised of precisely aligned lenses, spacers, and mirrors. Visualization occurs as light is transferred from a light source through the glass fibers distributed around the lens train. Rigid rod lens optics provide the best endoscopic images.

Reprocessing Procedures

The complex structure of rigid and semi-rigid endoscopes requires intricate cleaning methods. Soaking in an enzymatic solution, scrupulous hand cleaning with brushing, and rinsing with copious amounts of water are very important. Few scope lenses can be placed in an ultrasonic cleaner because they can be loosened or fractured. However, accessory instruments such as graspers, scissors, and dissectors with internal moving parts and channels can benefit from an irrigating ultrasonic machine for enhanced cleaning. The accessory items in these sets that can be disassembled for cleaning must be taken apart for cleaning, disinfection, and/or sterilization. For example, the Verres Needle used for insufflation of the peritoneal cavity should be disassembled. (See **Figure 12.34**) Operating scissors, by contrast, may not permit disassembly for cleaning. Instruments with internal moving

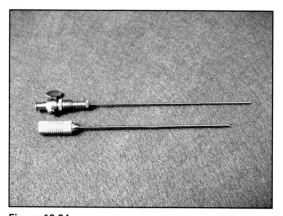

Figure 12.34

parts pose a great challenge as they are prepared for sterilization. Manufacturers are becoming more aware of the processing difficulty these items pose, and are slowly making design changes.

Rigid telescopes consist of an eyepiece with glass ocular lens, fiber optic light bundles, and a metal shaft containing the lens train, fragile glass fibers, and objective lens. Always clean each telescope separately.

Telescopes should be placed in perforated and protected telescope cases. Handle the scope by the heavy eyepiece end, but support the distal end as you do so. Avoid touching the ocular or objective lens. Do not bend the telescope shaft, or drop or strike it against any hard surface. Do not allow the scope to be struck by other objects or instruments. Never place the scope near the edge of a counter or table from which it may fall.

Inappropriate and/or incomplete reprocessing can cause infections in patients and/or medical personnel. Special concerns must be addressed because rigid/semi-rigid scopes are very difficult to clean. Proper care and handling of all endoscopic instrumentation requires complete disassembly and meticulous cleaning. Do not loosen or remove the eyepiece unless recommended by the manufacturer because damage and fluid invasion can result.

Steps in reprocessing rigid scopes are basically the same as that discussed earlier for the flexible counterparts:

- Clean.
- Inspect.
- High-level disinfect.
- Sterilize.
- Inspect.

Disconnect the light cable from the telescope, and remove the light cable adapter. All residual organic matter, blood, and irrigation solution must be removed prior to any sterilization or disinfection process. Manually clean scopes using soft brushes, soft cotton cloths, and a mild protein-dissolving enzymatic detergent and water solution.

Detergents alone are not recommended as they contain high concentrations of surfactants that can leave a film on the telescope. Warm water (100°F to 120°F; 37.8°C to 48.9°C) is best for cleaning. Copious rinsing is essential since disinfection solutions work only on contact, and they can harden organic material (which appears to be "corrosion") on instruments. Dry with a soft, clean towel.

Do not use disinfectant solutions that contain long-life surfactants because these solutions can leave residues that provide a conductive pathway for electrical currents. Note: Electro-surgical problems have occurred during some procedures when disinfection solutions containing surfactants have been used. Surfactants lower the surface tension of a solution to less than that of water. Then the solution can penetrate into small cracks and crevices which water cannot enter, and this helps the disinfection process. However, these solutions are more difficult to rinse off, and the eventual build-up of residue can result in electro-surgical malfunctions.

Clean the lenses and fiber optic inlet post with a cotton-tipped applicator dipped in 70% isopropyl alcohol to remove any residue or film that remains after cleaning.

Basic guidelines designed to enhance cleaning, disinfection, and sterilization of rigid and semi-rigid endoscopes include:

- Follow the manufacturer's recommendations for selection of cleaning, disinfection, and sterilization products. Failure to do so could result in damage to the instruments/ lenses because of material incompatibility.

- Never soak these instruments during cleaning or high-level disinfection in a metal soak pan. Chemical reactions between dissimilar metals can result in damage.

- Instruments may need to be soaked in a vertical position to prevent air pockets, and to allow enzymatic detergent and disinfection solutions to access all internal channels.

- Utilize "flush ports" when available to circulate, under pressure, enzymatic detergent through

channels. Rinse with distilled water, and follow with a compressed air flush to prevent retaining liquids that might dilute disinfection/ sterilization solutions.

- Lenses must never be placed an ultrasonic cleaner. Other components may be cleaned utilizing an ultrasonic cleaner that is designed for use with laparoscopic instruments.

- Gently brush clean the exterior of instruments and accessible lumens/channels with the appropriate size, type, and length of brush.

- Thoroughly rinse with distilled water, and "rough dry" using a soft, lint-free cloth.

- Inspect the instruments for cleanliness, missing parts, and visible damage. Pay special attention to insulated sheaths and electrical cables. (Shock or burn to the patient or operator is possible if they are not intact.) Test moving components to assure they are functional.

- Instruments must be thoroughly air-dried before storage or packaging for sterilization.

- Remember that these instruments are very fragile, and they must be handled with extreme care.

Inspection Requirements

Before and after every endoscopic procedure, all surfaces of telescopes must be carefully inspected for any scratches, dents, protrusions, evidence of burns at the distal tip, or other irregularities that may have occurred during the procedure.

Lens Inspection

Avoid touching the ocular or the objective lenses of the telescope, because fingerprints and debris will impair the view. Debris can also act as an abrasive, and scratch the lens.

Examine the non-video scope for optical clarity by looking through the lens while viewing a non-glare white paper with writing on it. The paper should be held approximately three inches from the distal tip. Move the tip of the scope progressively closer to the printed paper until it is about 1/4" away. The image should be crisp and clear with minimal distortion. If the image is discolored or hazy, it may be due to improper cleaning, disinfectant residue, a cracked or broken lens, moisture within the shaft, or external shaft damage that has broken some fibers. Clean the outside of the proximal and distal lenses with a lint-free applicator saturated with 70% isopropyl alcohol. Repeat the inspection process. Do not use the scope if visibility remains cloudy or distorted after cleaning.

Inspect the optical fibers surrounding the lens train at the tip of the scope by holding the light post toward a moderately bright light (such as an overhead light, window, or x-ray light box), and look at the distal tip. The light carriers should be apparent as white areas at the perimeter of the lens. Black dots, irregular or shadowed areas may indicate broken or damaged fibers that will cause a loss of light transfer. Directing the tip of the scope toward a bright light, and observing the light post will provide the same information.

Check the eyepiece seal for any visible signs of damage. Assemble the telescope into the desired instrument by aligning the locking pin with the notch on the instrument. Check for proper alignment of the telescope in the instrument by visually confirming a clear view. Note: One cannot see through a video orthoscope for a manual inspection; a light source is needed.

High-Level Disinfection And Sterilization

High-level disinfection is recommended only for telescopes that come into contact with mucous membranes. Sterilization is recommended for telescopes to be used in any laparoscopic, arthroscopic, OB/GYN, plastic, reconstructive, or aesthetic surgery procedures.

Be sure the scope is clean and dry prior to sterilization. Check with the scope's manufacturer to determine how the scope should be disinfected or sterilized.. Scopes may be sterilized in ethylene oxide following the manufacturer's requirements. Autoclavable scopes are now available; however, most manufacturers still recommend low temperature sterilization to prolong the life of the lens.

Selecting Repair Providers

Due to the complexity and volume of endoscopic instrument usage today, many hospitals do not have the expertise and/or equipment required to maintain this technology. Facility administrators have turned to the manufacturer, third party, or independent repair services to provide some or all required maintenance.

When evaluating repair facilities, the following procedures can be helpful:

- Compile a list of service suppliers.
- Obtain references from other facilities that have used their services.
- Question both service suppliers, and those who have used them:
  - How well do suppliers respond to fast turn-around needs?
  - What warranties do suppliers offer?
  - Does repaired equipment still experience unscheduled downtime after service?
  - Are repair parts readily available?
  - Are new or used parts installed?
  - Are service and/or support personnel available to answer questions during surgical procedures?
  - Does the service supplier offer user training programs as needed?
  - Does the service supplier maintain adequate liability and shipping insurance?
  - Are on-site inspection visits unrestricted?

When any service is provided, both the provider and the recipient should be concerned about the quality of the service.

Laparoscopic Instruments

Laparoscopic instruments along with a scope, camera, light source, and insuflator are used to perform surgeries with several small holes versus large incisions. Some units conduct electricity to the working distal tip, and are typically insulated with a black material. Non-electric units do not have the black insulation coating.

Laparoscopic insulation is very susceptible to pin holes, cracks, tears, and overall loosening. These defects must be discovered as the instruments are assembled because the electricity that escapes through insulation failures can cause burns, infections, and extended patient recovery times.

To inspect the insulation, locate the metal collar at distal tip (See **Figure 12.35**). The insulation should fit tightly against the collar, and this union should be tight and snug with no spaces visible. Next grip the insulation, and try to slide it back. If the insulation slides (moves), the instrument needs repair. Finally, visually check the instrument shaft looking for cuts, cracks, and nicks to the insulation, and inspect the insulated handle for chips or cracks.

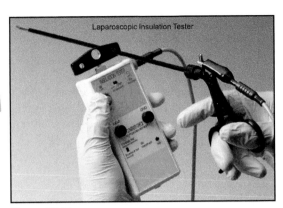

Laparoscopic Insulation Tester

Figure 12.36

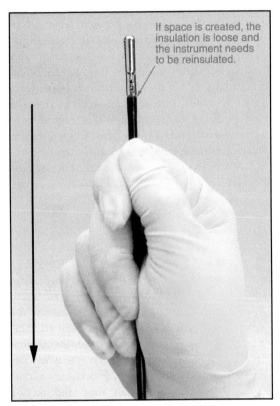

If space is created, the insulation is loose and the instrument needs to be reinsulated.

Figure 12.35

Electronic testing devices (See **Figure 12.36**) can detect microscopic holes in the shaft of a laparoscopic instrument. Electronic testing should be done prior to set assembly on the clean side of sterile processing. The electronic testing device can also be used to test electric cables and forceps, electrodes, and insulated bayonet forceps.

Laparoscopic hooks and spatulas are used to cut and/or cauterize. They must be inspected for insulation failure in the shaft and at the distal tip. Those which are cannulated (have a hollow barrel) will require a brush for proper cleaning. (See **Figure 12.37**)

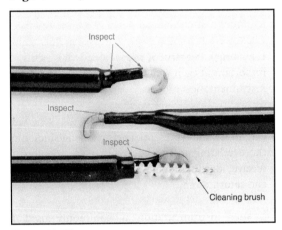

Inspect

Inspect

Inspect

Cleaning brush

Figure 12.37

Laparoscopic instrument ring handles can be designed in three styles:

- Free Handle – No ratchet or spring finger with an open and close action.

- Ratchet Handle – Similar to hemostats with various locking points on the ratchet.

- Spring Handle – Opens under slight tension, and closes by spring action.

Prior to purchase the cleaning and sterilization parameters must be carefully reviewed to determine if the required cleaning and sterilization requirements can be met with the facility's existing processing resources.

Other Specialty Instruments Create Processing Challenges

Each specialty service within the Operating Room and other areas within the facility and associated clinics typically have instrumentation which requires special care and handling. Examples include:

- Neurology – Steriotactic Biopsy systems, aneurysm clip systems, and testing electrodes.

- Cardiology – Cardiac endoscopes.

- Electro Physiology – Cables and cords.

Each instrument must also be processed following the manufacturer's recommendations.

LOANER INSTRUMENTATION

Learning Objective 5. Identify basic protocols important at each step in the loaner instrumentation process.

Loaner instrumentation comes in many sizes and variations, and represents a new challenge including those relating to procedures that are required to receive, decontaminate, assemble, sterilize, store, and return them.

Loaner instrumentation is commonly used in orthopedic and neuro-surgical procedures, and they are often delivered in numerous trays with many instruments in each tray. Each instrument is different, and requires special attention during

Loaner instrumentation – Instruments or sets borrowed from a vendor for emergency or scheduled surgical procedures that will be returned to the vendor following use.

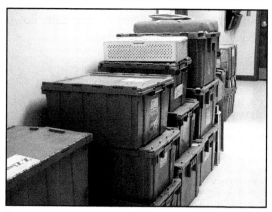

Figure 12.38

the cleaning process. These instruments can be a challenge to clean, and they can create new concerns as surgical volume increases.

Large facilities can receive up to one hundred loaner trays daily. Those trays are shipped into the facility before the procedure is scheduled and returned after the procedure. (See **Figure 12.38**) In some cases, vendor sales representatives may hand deliver the loaner trays to the facility. This influx of temporary instrumentation poses challenges with storage space, additional washer and sterilizer loads, and the labor requirements to process and wrap these trays. Central Service Managers must develop and implement policies and procedures to ensure the safety of the staff and patients as handling and processing procedures are developed.

Receipt and Inventory Procedures

Loaner instruments should be considered contaminated and handled accordingly. From the time they are received, facility staff accept responsibility for them, and must ensure that every device is cleaned, disinfected, and sterilized according to the manufacturer's written instructions. Inventorying the instruments and sets when they arrive is an important step. Procedures include confirming that the correct item and number of items are delivered, and that the equipment functions correctly. When the vendor or courier delivers the instrumentation, Central Service Technicians wearing proper protective attire should check loaner instruments for accuracy and completeness (See **Figure 12.39**)

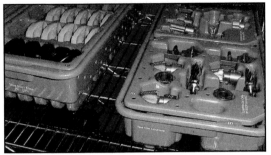

Figure 12.39

An inventory control sheet provides valuable information to protect the facility and the vendor. The Central Service Technician should log receipt of loaner instrumentation and implants with information including:

- Date.

- Time.

- Signature of delivery person.

- Initials of receiving person.

- Doctor's name.

- Patient's last name.

- Number of trays.

- Number of implants.

- Perform an inventory control check to verify the types and numbers of instruments and implants.

- Perform a quality assurance check by visually inspecting instruments and implants for damage.

The inventory control sheet should follow the instrument set/s through the entire process.

Decontamination

The decontamination process is the most critical step in processing loaner instrumentation. As stressed throughout this manual, one can clean without sterilization, but one cannot sterilize without cleaning. The manufacturer's instructions for cleaning and disinfecting the products must always be followed.

Each manufacturer has specific instructions about the type of enzymatic detergent, temperature, and mechanical cleaning method to be used. These instructions must be consistently used to ensure that proper disinfection has taken place. Remember that, even if trays are received still intact from a previous sterilization process, the trays must be considered contaminated and processed accordingly. (See **Figure 12.40**)

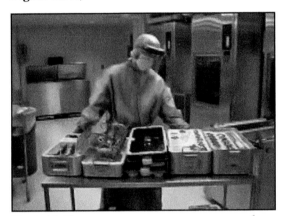

Figure 12.40

Inspection and Assembly

After cleaning and disinfection, Central Service Technicians must inspect each device for cleanliness and functionality and then assemble, and prepare the loaner instrumentation for sterilization. Each instrument should be examined for residual bioburden, and for any defects that might cause it to function improperly. (See **Figure 12.41**) Defective instruments should be documented and reported to the appropriate supervisor and operating room personnel immediately to prevent delays in scheduled surgical procedures.

Loaner instruments without defects should be prepared for sterilization. Using the techniques

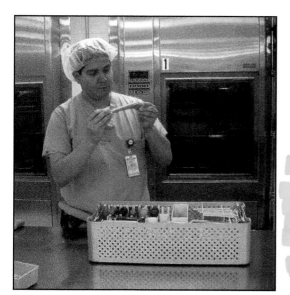

Figure 12.41

discussed in this manual, chemical indicators/integrators should be placed in each layer of the instrument set, and the instruments should be wrapped using the appropriate wrap weight and sterilization tape. Placing these sets in another container system will potentially lead to sterilization failure.

Each manufacturer establishes the specific criteria for their instrument sterilization. That criteria is based on the complexity and configuration of the instruments and in some cases is also based on European models, which consider times required to kill the **prion** that causes Creutzfeldt-Jakob disease (CJD).

Vendors may create cycle time constraints and require sterilization standards that are different from those used in the facility. Facilities must follow the manufacturer's sterilization standards. When

---

Prion – Virus-like infectious agents that cause a variety of neurodegenerative diseases in humans and animals, including scrapie in sheep and goats, bovine spongiform encephalopathy (BSE) in cattle, and Creutzfeldt-Jakob disease (CJD) in humans. Prions are thought to differ from viruses by containing only protein and not DNA or RNA. They are extremely resistant to inactivation by heat and disinfecting agents. (AAMI ST35R/DS/2002).

---

complex instruments are introduced to a facility, the vendor should visit the facility and provide on-site cleaning and sterilization instructions to ensure that Central Service personnel have properly prepared the instrumentation for the sterilization cycle. Facility personnel must follow those instructions to insure patient safety.

Handling and Storage

After the loaner instruments have been sterilized, they should be moved to a department area with low traffic flow, and away from the direct airflow of cooling vents. This will prevent inadvertent touching and condensation from cool air blowing on them. Care should be used when handling and moving the trays after the cooling process has taken place. These trays are often heavy, and their packaging may be easily compromised (torn) if not handled properly. Loaner trays should be handled as little as possible, and should never be slid across a surface. They should always be lifted and set on storage shelves or case carts for use in the operating room. Use of transport trays is recommended to avoid damaging the processed trays. (See **Figure 12.42**)

After the trays have been used in the surgical suite, they must be reprocessed. One exception: they will not need to be sterilized unless they are needed for immediate reuse. However, all instrument trays must be decontaminated before they are shipped out of the facility. Typically, trays are decontaminated, and are then stored in a separate room for vendors to pick up. The appropriate location is often a

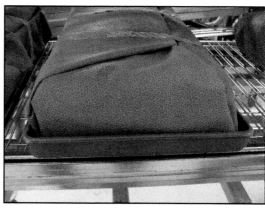

Figure 12.42

---

concern because storage space is usually limited. Vendors should obtain their instruments as soon as possible after the devices are decontaminated. An exit inventory of all instruments is recommended to help ensure that any missing or damaged instrumentation is identified in a timely fashion.

As technology advances, surgical instruments and equipment will become more complex. Central Service Technicians will continue to be challenged with keeping abreast of new technologies and standards to insure that patients are provided with safe and functional instruments for their treatment and care.

ENDNOTES

1. A study by McCracken (Journal of Infection Control and Sterilization Technology, 1995) reviewed 241 G.I. inspected endoscopes at 80 facilities. The results disclosed:

- *38 facilities had patient-ready scopes with at least one channel visually encrusted with dried debris.*
- *26 scopes had severely scratched channels.*
- *Only 3 out of 56 facilities that dried scopes between patients were successful.*

Also, Kaczmarek, et.al. (American Journal of Medicine, March, 1992) reported that an inspection of endoscopes at 22 hospitals and 4 ambulatory care centers showed 23.9% of bacterial cultures from internal channels of 71 patient-ready gastrointestinal scopes grew 100,000 or more bacterial colonies.

2. The American Society of Testing and Materials (ASTM) has incorporated this recommendation in its ASTM Standard F1518-94.

OTHER RESOURCES

For Flexible Scopes:

Goldstine, S. "Processing Flexible Endoscopes." Infection Control Today. March, 1998.

Reprocessing of Flexible Gastrointestinal Endoscopes. "Position Statement." Society of Gastroenterology Nurses & Associates. December. 1995.

Infection Prevention & Control in Flexible Endoscopy, "Part I Cleaning: The Vital First Step." Infection Control Rounds, Vol. 3 No 1. April, 2001.

Muscarella, L. "Automatic Flexible Endoscope Reprocessors." Gastrointestinal Endoscopy Clinics of North America. Vol. 10, No; 2. April, 2000.

For Rigid and Semi-Rigid Scopes:

Care and Handling Instruction Manuals: Olympus America, Inc. Two Corporate Center Drive Melville, NY 11747-3157 (800) 548-5515

Circon Corporation 6500 Hollister Avenue Santa Barbara, CA 93117-3019 (888) 524-7266

Karl Storz Endoscopy-America, Inc. 600 Corporate Pointe Culver City, CA 90203-7600 (800) 421-0837

The Difficulty of Reprocessing Reusable Rigid Laparoscopic Forceps and Other Endoscopic Accessories: Are Disposables the Answer? Health Device, Vol. 23, Nos. 1-2, pp. 57-58. 1994.

Descoteaux, J; Poulin, E; Julein, M; and Guidoin, R. Residual Organic Debris on Processed Surgical Instruments. AORN Journal, Vol. 62, No.1, pp. 23-24. 1995.

CENTRAL SERVICE TERMS

Lumen

Wire drivers (pneumatic-powered surgical equipment)

Oscillating saws (pneumatic-powered surgical equipment)

Sagittal saws (pneumatic-powered surgical equipment)

Drills (pneumatic-powered surgical equipment)

Reciprocating saws (pneumatic-powered surgical equipment)

Automatic Endoscope Reprocessor (AER)

Leak test (endoscope)

Loaner instrumentation

Prion

Chapter 13
Sterile Packaging and Storage

Chapter Outline

Chapter Leaning Objectives:

As a result of successfully completing this chapter, readers will be able to:

1. Explain the basic objectives of the packaging process, and review basic selection factors for materials to be used with specific sterilization methods.

2. Provide an overview of reusable packaging materials.

3. Provide an overview of disposable packaging materials.

4. Discuss basic package closure methods.

5. Review basic procedures to prepare pack contents for packaging.

6. Explain basic packaging procedures for peel pouches and flat wrapping materials.

7. Review general packaging concepts:
   - Package labeling
   - Special concerns
   - Sterility maintenance

8. Provide basic information about sterile packaging, storage, and transport.

Reusable Sterilization Packaging Materials

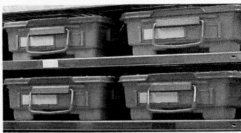

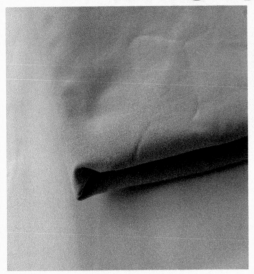

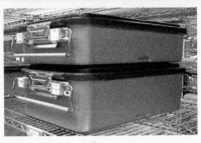

Woven Textiles   **Rigid Sterilization Containers**

Figure 13.1

Once Items have been cleaned, inspected, and assembled, they are ready for sterilization. In order to maintain their sterility after sterilization, items must be packaged. That packaging helps maintain the integrity (sterility) of the sterile items until they are opened and used.

OVERVIEW OF STERILE PACKAGING PROCESS

Learning Objective 1. Explain the basic objectives of the packaging process, and review basic selection factors for materials to be used with alternative sterilization methods.

We can draw some comparisons between food packaging and sterile packaging. Both types of packaging must protect items and keep them safe until they are used. Both can be compromised in a way that affects the package's contents and makes them unsafe for use. Sterile packaging is designed with tamper-evident seals so users can tell if the package has been opened and re-sealed, and many

food products use these **tamper-evident seals** on their packaging for the same reason. Finally, there are several packaging options for food products and sterile items, and not all types of packaging are appropriate for all items and processes. For example, soup could not be packaged in aluminum foil, carried to work and heated in a microwave oven. Sterile item packaging must also consider the sterilization process that will be used.

Central Service Technicians must be familiar with the various packaging materials available for sterilization, and they must be able to select the packaging which is most appropriate for the item

Seals (tamper-evident) – Sealing methods for sterile packaging that allow users to determine if the packaging has been opened. Tamper-evident seals allow users to determine if packages have been opened (contaminated) and help them identify packages that are not safe for patient use.

Disposable Sterilization Packaging Materials

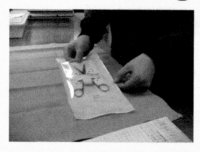

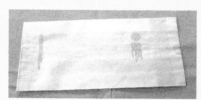

Pouches

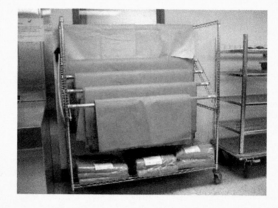

Nonwoven Wrap

Figure 13.2

and sterilization process to be used. They must be able to apply the selected packaging in a manner to insure success of the sterilization success, and to protect the item during the storage and handling that follows sterilization.

There are two basic categories of sterility packaging: reusable and disposable. These are shown, respectively, in **Figures 13.1** and **13.2**, and both will be discussed at length in this chapter.

Objectives of Packaging Process

There are three primary objectives for both basic categories of packaging materials:

- They must allow penetration of the chosen sterilant, and must be compatible with any other requirements of the specific sterilization process (such as drying).

- They must be able to maintain the sterility of the package contents until it is opened.

- They must create a package that can be opened aseptically (without contaminating the contents) by the user.

- The contents of a sterilized package must be sterile at the moment of use.

The U.S. Food and Drug Administration (FDA) classifies sterilization packaging as Class II Medical Devices (those presenting a potential risk). The consequences of using a non-sterile item during a surgical procedure can be life-threatening. In addition to selecting and applying the appropriate packaging material, Central Service Technicians must also be able to construct packages that allow the sterilization process to be successful and protect the package contents from contamination.

Selecting Packaging Material

The first step in the packaging process is to select the appropriate type of packaging material and method. Different types of packaging are needed for alternative sterilization methods, and styles of packaging may vary based on package contents. Much research has been conducted to devise suitable packaging materials, and there is a wide variety of packaging materials and methods available to the healthcare market.

Understanding the packaging requirements and options for each sterilization method can help Central Service Technicians make good packaging choices. Typically, packaging materials have already been selected, purchased, and are in use in the Central Service department. However, since there is no single packaging material for all situations, Central Service Technicians must still select the material that is best suited for the sterilization process to be used.

Only materials specifically designed for sterilization packaging and approved by the FDA are acceptable. In addition, there are other special concerns based on the sterilization method that will be used: basic selection factors are listed below.

• Packaging used for steam sterilization must be capable of withstanding high temperatures of 250°F – 275°F (121°C – 135°C). The packaging must allow air removal and steam penetration to the contents to be sterilized, and must permit drying of the contents and packaging material.

• Packaging choices for ethylene oxide sterilization allow adequate penetration of the gas sterilant and removal of the gas residue. (aeration)

• Packaging choices for dry heat sterilization must be able to tolerate 2-3 hours exposure time and a temperature of 320°F – 400°F (160°C – 204°C) without melting, burning, or otherwise being destroyed.

• Packaging choices for gas plasma sterilization must be able to tolerate a deep vacuum draw without absorbing the sterilant, interrupting the cycle, or damaging the contents.

In addition to selecting the appropriate packaging material, Central Service Technicians must also understand how to apply (use) sterilization packaging appropriately to achieve the desired results: sterilant penetration, barrier effectiveness, and aseptic opening.

REUSABLE PACKAGING MATERIALS

Learning Objective 2. Provide an overview of reusable packaging materials.

Reusable Fabric Materials

Before the early 1980's, woven textiles were the reusable packaging material of choice. However, new technologies have increased the choices for sterilization packaging. The standards for manufacturing today's packaging materials have been based on penetration and microbial barrier capability measurements for a minimum of 140 thread count (thread per square inch) muslin.

Muslin, Type 140 cotton, calico, and barrier cloth are common names for fabrics made of 100% unbleached, loosely woven cotton fibers. Muslin wrappers are most generally made of two-ply (double thickness) fabric fastened together as one wrap.

Other woven fabrics used in sterilization are:

• Duck cloth.

• Twills.

• Barrier cloth.

• Treated barrier fabrics.

Note: Canvas was once used as sterilization packaging, but it is not recommended because of its tight weave that makes steam penetration and drying difficult.

Muslin – *Broad term describing a wide variety of plain-weave cotton or cotton/polyester fabrics having approximately 140 threads per square inch.*

Superheating – *The condition that arises when steam is at a temperature which exceeds that of saturated steam at the same pressure.*

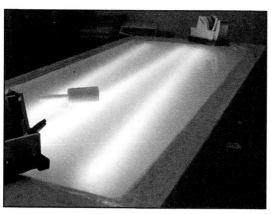

Figure 13.3

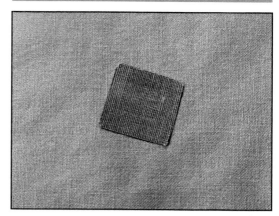

Figure 13.4

Textile packaging is still the packaging method of choice for some healthcare facilities. The selection of reusable textiles is often impacted by costs and/ or the environment (the desire to reduce the waste generated by disposable packaging materials). Some facilities contract with off-site companies to pick-up used textile wraps and then launder, inspect, and return them to the facility for reuse.

Textile packaging requires more labor because it must be laundered and inspected to insure that there are no tears or punctures from previous use. That inspection is performed using a light table (See **Figure 13.3**) that has a light source built into the tabletop to help spot small holes and punctures. As the wrap is passed over the lighted table top, light shines through small holes and punctures making them easier to identify. Textile packaging must also be checked and de-linted as needed to minimize the risk of lint entering the sterile pack and ultimately the sterile field.

If holes or punctures are discovered, the linen wrap must be repaired using a heat-sealed patch designed to cover the hole. (See **Figure 13.4**) The size of the surface area covered by heat-sealed patches on reusable fabrics should be considered before the fabric is reused. Reusable materials with heat-sealed patches can be effectively sterilized. However, the limit (the percent of exposed area that can be patched) depends on the method of sterilizing, positioning in the sterilizer, the number of layers of patched fabric, and the type of fabric patch. Some patching materials are not totally steam penetrable; they are surface-sterilized only.

Although the steam entering through unpatched areas may be sufficient to sterilize the pack contents, excessive use of non- or semi-permeable patches may hinder the sterilization process. A facility's Infection Control Committee should investigate the use of patched wraps to establish an "accept/ reject" standard for the total surface area of patch that is permitted for use within the facility.

All linen packaging materials should be held at room temperature (64°F to 72°F; 18°C to 22°C) and at a relative humidity ranging from 35% to 70% for a minimum of two hours prior to sterilization. This will permit adequate steam/ sterilant penetration, and prevent **superheating** of the fabric during sterilization.

Historically, linen packs have been limited to a size of 12" (height) x 12" (width) x 20" (length), and they were not to weigh more than 12 pounds. Maximum density must not exceed 7.2 pounds per cubic foot because higher densities may reduce sterilant access to all contents. The density of the pack is determined by calculating the volume (cubic inches) of the pack, and the volume is then divided by 1,728 (12" x 12" x 12": one cubic foot) to yield the cubic feet of the pack. The weight of the pack divided by the cubic feet of the pack equals density in pounds per cubic foot. (See **Figure 13.5**)

Linens should be securely applied without compressing package contents. (Note: wrapping techniques are discussed later in this chapter.) Contents must be packaged with sufficient spacing to enable steam and gasses to reach all surfaces.

Figure 13.5 Standard for Preparations of Fabric Packs:

CALCULATION OF PACK DENSITY

Maximum Dimensions	12"W x 12"H x 20"L
Maximum Weight	12 lbs.
Maximum Density Permitted	7.2 pounds per cubic foot

FORMULA FOR COMPUTING PACK DENSITY:

Step #1: $\dfrac{\text{DIMENSIONS OF PACK (in inches)}}{1728 \text{ (number of cubic inches in a a cubic foot)}}$ = VOLUME OF PACK IN CUBIC FEET

Step #2: $\dfrac{\text{WEIGHT OF PACK}}{\text{CUBIC FEET OF PACK}}$ = DENSITY (pounds per cubic foot)

APPLICATIONS OF FORMULA:

Application #1: Using a standard 12" x 12" x 20" pack weighing 12 pounds

Step #1: $\dfrac{12 \times 12 \times 20}{1728}$ = $\dfrac{2880}{1728}$ = 1.666 cubic feet

Step #2: $\dfrac{12 \text{ pounds}}{1.666 \text{ cubic feet}}$ = 7.2 pounds per cubic foot (acceptable pack density)

Tight packaging will not allow for fiber swelling (expansion), and the steam or vapor will not penetrate the material. It is possible to wrap even a small pack so tightly that its density will be too great for adequate sterilant penetration.

Rigid Container Systems

Rigid container systems are box-like structures with sealable and removable lids. (See **Figure 13.6**) They are made of anodized aluminum, stainless steel, plastic or a combination of these materials. Rigid containers have lids and filters that allow sterilant penetration while providing a microbial barrier. Filters may be disposable (a synthetic spunbond product) (See **Figure 13.8**) or reusable (with ceramic filters or a valve system).

Rigid containers consist of an inner basket to hold the instruments, and an outer container that acts as a protective barrier. Both the inner basket and outer container have handles for ease of carrying. **Figure 13.7** identifies the common components of a rigid sterilization container system's outer container.

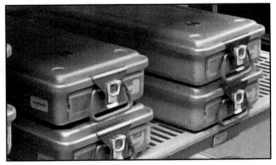

Figure 13.6

Examples of Disposable Rigid Sterilization Container Filters

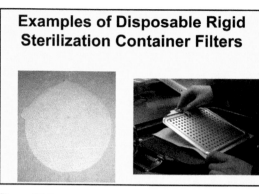

Figure 13.8

Some manufacturers of rigid container systems recommend that times for instrument sterilization, drying, and aeration be extended when using their containers. It is important to consult the specific container manufacturer's recommendations before using a rigid container system.

Rigid containers are regulated by the FDA, and containers are required to have a **510k (certification)** that they will perform as an effective packaging material.

Advantages and Disadvantages

There are several advantages of rigid sterilization containers. They:

- Provide an excellent barrier to microorganisms.
- Are easy-to-use.
- Eliminate torn wrappers.
- Protect instruments from damage during processing, storage, and transport.

Rigid container system – *Instrument containers that hold medical devices during sterilization and also protect devices from contamination during storage and transport.*

510k (certification) – *A package of information submitted to and approved by the Food and Drug Administration relating to a device having "substantial equivalence" to one or more legally marketed "predicate" (base of comparison) devices.*

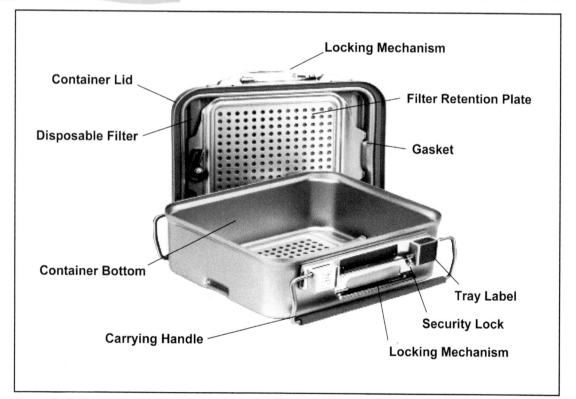

Figure 13.7

There are also potential disadvantages to the use of these systems:

• Safety concerns linked to ergonomics. A large (12" by 23" by 6") empty container weighs approximately 8-9 pounds. This requires Central Service Technicians to use good body mechanics when lifting and moving containers. Note: loaded instrument baskets must be added to this base weight, and employees should be able to comfortably carry a container or instrument set at waist height.

• Additional cycle time may be required to thoroughly dry the container. Sterilization efficacy is also impacted as a container's weight increases because of excess condensation. The "wet pack syndrome" has been noted and discussed for many years. While it is difficult to generalize about solutions, it is known that heavier sets, and those with greater metal mass, are more likely to experience this problem, especially when instruments are not properly disbursed in the container.

• Plastic containers may require longer dry times because they lack metal which produces heat by conduction to help drying.

• Additional space may be needed to store those containers that are larger than traditional wrapped containers.

• Additional labor may be required since the containers must be cleaned between uses. This may also affect washer loads if a mechanical washer is used.

• Latching mechanisms on containers create potential problems. When latches and welds break, the containers cannot be used. Also, sharp edges can injure employees.

• Filter retention plates may become dislodged and contaminate instruments. Note: some

Wet pack – Containers with moisture (inadequate drying) after the sterilization process is completed.

manufacturers have addressed this potential problem by modifying or changing the design of the container's filter retention plate.

Cleaning and Inspection Procedures for Rigid Containers

To clean a rigid sterilization container, first remove its disposable filters or release its filter protector/holder. Valve-type closures must be cleaned according to the manufacturer's written instructions. Likewise, interior baskets must be removed and cleaned. Process chemical indicators and disposable labels and locks must be removed, and dividers/pins may need removal if they interfere with the cleaning process.

Instructions provided by the container's manufacturer for cleaning and rinsing should be followed. Particular attention should be given to the type of detergent used. For example, some containers cannot be exposed to certain chemicals such as high alkaline solutions. The container should be inspected for cleanliness and damage before assembly. The use of appropriate cleaning methods along with standardized packaging and loading will improve the effectiveness of the sterilization process.

It is important to inspect all container system components to help assure their proper function. Prior to each use, the gasket must be inspected to assure that there are no debris, cuts, or tears. (See **Figure 13.9**) The inspection should also focus on the top and bottom valve or filter mechanism and the latching mechanism. For example, rivets should be checked to assure that they are secured. If

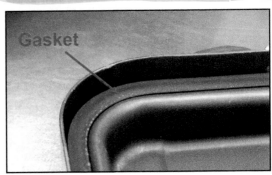

Gasket

Figure 13.9

loosened, they can provide a hole that can become a pathway for entry of bacteria.

As noted earlier, the weight of instruments placed in the container is an important concern. The number of instruments placed in the tray must not exceed the quantity that can be effectively sterilized and dried. Rigid containers should be carried by their handles (not by the lid) to avoid breaking the container's seal.

DISPOSABLE PACKAGING MATERIALS

Learning Objective 3. Provide an overview of disposable packaging materials.

Disposable (non-woven) materials were introduced as "engineered fabrics" in the 1940s, and they have made their way into our everyday life. Coffee filters, teabags, vacuum cleaner bags, and disposable diapers are all examples of "engineered fabrics," which are also referred to as disposable non-woven materials. These materials are used in both disposable flat wraps and in rigid container filters. Before using, both disposable flat wraps and rigid container filters should be inspected for tears or holes that may have occurred during transport and handling. These materials are a popular choice for sterilization packaging because they have excellent barrier effectiveness, and they can be discarded after use. There are three types of disposable packaging materials in common use: paper, polyolefin plastic, disposable nonwoven wraps. Please note: For dry heat sterilization, aluminum foil, glass and metal can also be used however, their use is much less common because dry heat sterilization is not used as widely as other sterilization methods.

Papers are commonly used as sterilization packaging materials. It is important to insure that the paper packaging is intended for use as sterilization

---

Papers (kraft-type) – A medical grade paper packaging material used for numerous sterilization applications.

SMS (spunbond-meltblown-spunbond) – A non-woven packaging material which is the most popular flat wrap.

---

packaging, and that it has been approved by the FDA. Note: papers which contain cellulose cannot be used in gas plasma sterilizers because cellulose absorbs the sterilant and reduces penetration. As this occurs, the contents being sterilized may not have exposure to the proper amount of the sterilant.

Kraft-type papers (medical grade) are generally smooth-surfaced, and they are available in sizes to accommodate many medical devices and porous or soft-good items. Pouches of medical grade papers specially formulated for sterilization are also available. **Figure 13.10** is an example of a Kraft-type paper pouch.

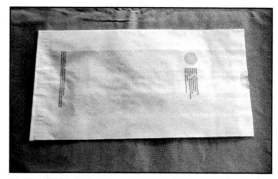

Figure 13.10

One non-woven packaging material, **SMS (spunbond-meltblown-spunbond)**, is the most popular flat wrap. It is made by a process in which polyolefin layers (synthetic materials that are softened by heat and hardened by cooling) are exposed to high heat, and are pressure-bonded together to form sheets. Flat wrapping products

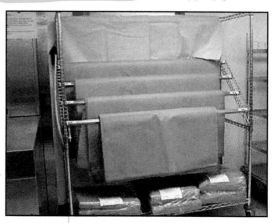

Figure 13.11

are constructed of non-woven SMS fabrics for sterilization wrapping, and they are designed as single-use disposable products: they must never be reused. These materials are available in a range of weights and a wide variety of sizes. (See **Figure 13.11**) Flat wraps are also available as single sheet or double sheet wraps that are bonded together.

Paper-plastic and spunbond polyolefin-plastic combinations (called peel packs or peel-open pouches) are the most commonly used packaging materials for small instruments, light-weight items. (See **Figure 13.12**) They are called peel-pouches because, after they are sealed, they must be peeled open for aseptic opening.

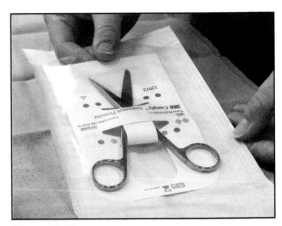

Figure 13.12

There are two basic types of combination peel-pouches:

- Paper/plastic combinations – These are typically acceptable for use with the steam and ethylene oxide sterilization processes. They are not compatible with dry heat or gas plasma sterilization. As suggested by their name, they have a paper side and a plastic side. The plastic side allows visibility of the package contents, and the paper side allows sterilant penetration.

- Spunbond polyolefin-plastic combinations – These are used for gas plasma sterilization. (Sometimes referred to as Tyvek® pouches) Like paper-plastic combinations, they have a plastic side so package contents are visible. The other side is composed of a polyolefin that contains no cellulosic materials and is, therefore, compatible with gas plasma sterilization processes.

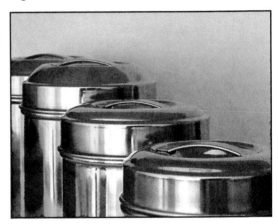

Figure 13.13

Note: Be careful when selecting peel-pouches. Paper/plastic combinations are not compatible with gas plasma sterilization and Spunbond-polyolefin combinations will melt in high temperature processes such as steam.

Aluminum foil and borosilicate (Pyrex®) glass or solid (nonperforated) metal containers are for use with dry heat sterilization processes only. **Figure 13.13** is an example of solid metal containers that may be used in dry heat sterilization.

The use of each packaging material has advantages and disadvantages. Central Service Technicians

must insure that they select the type of packaging most suitable for the item(s) being packaged and the type of sterilization selected. Then they can begin preparing the package contents for packaging and the sterilization process to follow.

METHODS OF PACKAGE CLOSURE

Learning Objective 4. Discuss basic package closure methods.

Overview

The purpose of a package closure (seal) is to seal the package securely, maintain the sterile integrity of the contact area during transport and storage, and prevent resealing if the package is opened or if the seal is compromised.

Only approved methods of closure should be used to seal a sterile package. There are several types of package closures, and Central Service Technicians must insure that they use the method that is appropriate for the packaging used.

Do Not Use!

Several package closure methods are never appropriate:

- Do not use safety pins, staples, or other sharp objects to seal packages. Punctures create holes that allow contamination. Even the smallest space (hole) is large enough to allow bacteria to pass through.

- Do not use paperclips or binding clips; they can be removed and replaced without evidence of barrier compromise.

- Do not use tapes which are not designed specifically to withstand the rigors of sterilization.

Acceptable Closure Methods

Several methods of package closure are acceptable for use:

- Tapes designated as "indicator tapes" are considered best practice because they are made specifically to withstand sterilization, and they will change color after being exposed to the sterilization process. They do not, however, provide proof that adequate sterilization of package contents has occurred. Indicator tapes or indicator stickers which change color after exposure should be used on every package to avoid mixing processed and unprocessed packages. **Figure 13.14** provides examples of indicator tapes. The package on the left shows how the indicator tape used to seal the package looks before steam sterilization and the package on the right shows how the specially designed indicator tape turns color during a sterilization process.

- Rubber bands or similar closures are only acceptable if the manufacturer of the wrapper material explicitly recommends their use. If recommended, care is needed to select the proper-sized bands that allow a snug fit without creating excessive wrinkles or folds in the fabric that may reduce the effectiveness of sterilant penetration. If bands are used, the

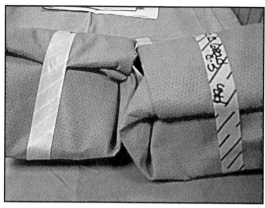

Figure 13.14

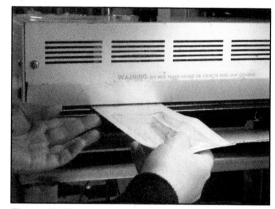

Figure 13.15

label or indicator stickers should be placed in such a way that any attempt to remove the band will damage the band and reveal the compromised status of the pack. Note: Rubber band applications are designed for specific packaging methods and should only be used as recommended by the specific manufacturer.

- Heat seals are used for paper-plastic or plastic-to-plastic seals. The package is placed inside the jaws of the heat sealer (See **Figure 13.15**), and the two sides are fused together. Be sure to follow the instructions of the heat sealer and the packaging manufacturers to insure appropriate exposure times and temperatures. Inadequate exposure times or temperatures may cause inadequate seals, and those that exceed recommendations may cause package damage. Central Service Technicians should use extra caution when operating heat sealers to avoid burns which can be severe.

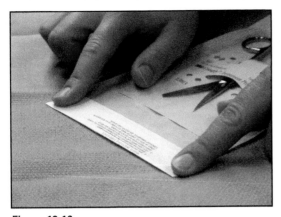

Figure 13.16

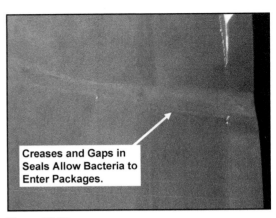

Creases and Gaps in Seals Allow Bacteria to Enter Packages.

Figure 13.17

Tamper Evident Seals for Rigid Sterilization Containers

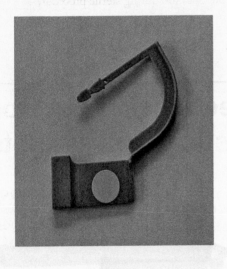

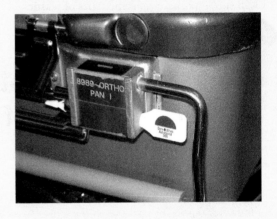

Figure 13.18

• Self-Adhesive Seals. Some paper plastic and polyolefin-plastic packages contain self-adhesive seals that do not require heat. An adhesive portion is covered with a removable strip at one end of the self-adhesive sterilization pouch. When it is removed, that portion of the seal should be carefully folded over the opening of the package. **Figure 13.16** shows a Central Service Technician sealing a self-adhesive sterilization pouch.

Care must be taken to avoid gaps, wrinkles, or creases which compromise the seal integrity for both heat seal and self-seal closure systems. **Figure 13.17** provides an example of a crease in a heat seal. This seal is unacceptable because it has a gap that will allow bacteria to enter the package.

• Sealing tape is sometimes used to secure pouch openings. Care is needed to ensure that the seal is secure without compromising gaps.

Proper taping technique includes the folding of corners up so the side edges of the top corners are parallel to the bottom edge of the pouch. Assure that the plastic is folded onto the plastic (not paper-to-paper) so steriliant access is not impeded. Then fold the open bottom edge over the folded corners. Seal with tape overlapping the edge of the pouch by about ¼ inch. Observe carefully to ensure that there are no gaps, creases, or wrinkles, and that the tape has completely covered the pouch's open edge, and is securely attached to the plastic.

• Rigid Container Seals are designed to break when the seal on the container has been broken. The most common types are plastic components that lock in place and must be broken to open the container. Small bands that tighten as they react to the heat during sterilization can also are placed on certain types of rigid containers and these will break when the seal of the container is broken. **Figure 13.18** shows examples of some types of plastic seals that are used to seal rigid containers.

Central Service Technicians must use closure methods that are specifically designed for the packaging material that is chosen. They must also check the seals on all packages before dispensing them to user units. Any seals which appear to have been opened should not be issued or used.

PREPARATION OF PACK CONTENTS

Learning Objective 5. Review basic procedures to prepare pack contents for packaging.

After instruments and devices are decontaminated, cleaned, dried, and inspected, those requiring sterilization must be properly arranged, assembled and, finally, packaged (wrapped) for sterilization. Items may be wrapped separately or as a group. They can also be placed in trays, basins, or containers specifically designed for sterilant access and aseptic presentation during sterile procedures.

Protectors can protect packaging from the sharp points of some instruments.

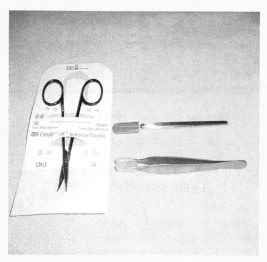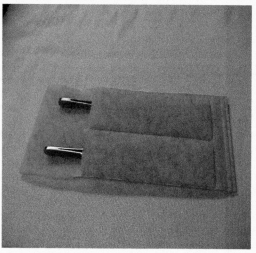

Figure 13.19

Before Packaging

Before packaging, instruments must be carefully inspected to ensure cleanliness, proper functioning, and alignment. Organic material such as blood or other fluids will interfere with sterilization and optimal functioning. There should be no corrosion, rust, pitting, burrs, nicks, cracks, or chipped plated surfaces on the instruments. Cutting edges must be sharp. Moving parts must move freely without sticking or stiffness. The manufacturer's instructions for some instruments may require lubrication after cleaning or prior to sterilization and these instructions must be incorporated into departmental procedures. Instruments that need repair should be taken out of service for replacement or repair. The continued use of broken or excessively worn instruments could put patients and/or facility personnel at risk.

Delicate and sharp instruments should be protected while being handled, and when being assembled for sterilization. Sharp points may be protected with special holders, commercially available tip guards, or foam sleeves (See **Figure 13.19**). Suppliers of protective coverings should be consulted to assure that coverings are permeable to the sterilant to be used. For example, latex tubing should never be used to protect instrument tips, as it will prevent steam and ethylene oxide penetration to the instrument.

Multi-part instruments should be disassembled prior to sterilization with all parts in easy access for aseptic assembly after the pack is opened. Instruments that open (such as scissors and hemostats) should be kept in unlocked, open positions to enable the sterilant to reach all parts. Use a cuffed towel to keep these instruments open. Placing one finger ring under the cuff, and the other over it prevents closure during pack handling and loading of the sterilizer. There are also devices that can be purchased to help keep instruments open during the sterilization cycle. **Figure 13.20** shows examples of reusable holders that can be used to hold hinged instruments open for sterilization.

Instrument Sets

Most instruments are prepared in groups called sets, trays, or kits. Smaller sets used for smaller procedures such as suturing, wound irrigation, or cut downs (accessing deep veins for intravenous fluid delivery) are often called procedure (or procedural or floor) trays. Items such as empty syringes, gauze (appropriate when included in tray assembly instructions), towels, and other non-instrument items are usually included as required by procedure instructions. These packs are designed to be used in patient care areas such as nursing units and the emergency room, and they are often designed to include all (or most of) the items needed for a minor procedure. This set-up helps avoid delays which result when staff must locate necessary items such as gauze and syringes. It is important to include only those items within trays that have documented sterilization instructions from their specific manufacturer. Do not sterilize items within these trays without written instructions from the manufacturer.

Requirements for pack contents are identified by users. Packs for the same procedure should be kept uniform, if possible. If doctor preference or unique situations require additional or alternate devices, it is usually best to package the individual items separately. These are then added or substituted aseptically when the two packs are opened. It is also recommended that procedures requiring the same basic instruments utilize a basic pack. For example, the same instruments required for a laparotomy (opening the abdomen) are required for pelvic area, abdominal access, and gynecological procedures. The special instruments needed for the specific procedures are then wrapped in separate smaller supplied packs (for example, "urological instruments," "intestinal instruments," or "abdominal hysterectomy instruments.") This saves time, helps with storage space, and facilitates inventory control.

Content requirements for basic and specialty packs must be specified on the Instrument Tray Packing List (count sheet) which is specific to the pack being assembled. The list should be in plain view whenever a pack is assembled, and it should then be referenced by Central Service personnel with instrument assembly responsibilities. To avoid errors, one should never rely on his/her memory to assemble trays. The list specifies which and how many of each item should be included. It should also, at a minimum, identify the specific pack to

Reusable holders can help keep ring-handled instruments open.

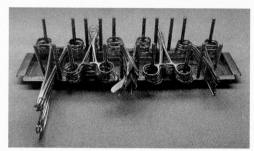
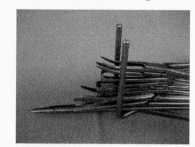
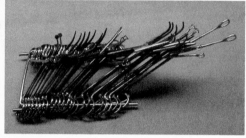

Figure 13.20

be assembled and the requesting department. It should also note instrument descriptions, vendor's names, catalogue numbers, and quantities required. In most healthcare facilities, the person responsible for pack preparation initials the label. This provides individual accountability and a mechanism for facilitating problem identification and corrections.

Assembly Procedures

For larger packs, instruments are usually placed on a stainless steel, heat-tolerant plastic or anodized aluminum tray with a perforated or mesh bottom to facilitate sterilant penetration/release and drying. (See **Figure 13.21**) Tray liners are often used to absorb moisture, and to provide cushioning to minimize instrument wear and tear. Surgical (Huck) towels or other absorbent materials may also be used in the pack when greater absorbency is required, or if instruments must be separated to prevent damage. All wrapped items should have a sterility indicator to verify that it has been exposed to the sterilization process. Peel pouches should not

be used inside instrument trays as it is not possible to ensure correct positioning for sterilization.

Gauze squares should never be used as additional packaging (wicking) material in trays or packs. Surgery staff must count gauze sponges during procedures, and their counts must be exact. The introduction of additional sponges into the

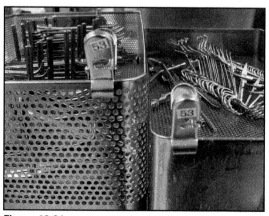

Figure 13.21

operating room as packaging material may cause confusion, and affect the sponge counts.

Basin sets should be assembled in a way that allows moisture to drain from them during sterilization. Therefore, all items that will hold water must be placed in the same direction to facilitate drainage. When more than one basin is sterilized, wicking material such as a surgical towel or specially-designed **wicking materials** can be used to facilitate drying.

Moisture is a concern when preparing packs for steam sterilization because, when steam contacts metal, it is immediately cooled when heat transfers to the metal. As this occurs, the steam condenses and forms droplets on the metal. Wicking materials help to absorb the moisture and facilitate drying during the dry cycle. However, if packs are too dense, the excessive amount of metal may result in the condensation of too much moisture, and a wet pack will be created. To avoid this problem, additional absorbent materials may be added, or very dense packs can be divided into two separate packs. Note: Creating two packs may be preferable if the pack's weight is too heavy for easy handling by the Central Service Technician. To reduce the possibility of wet packs, the ANSI/ AAMI Standard (ST 79:2006) states that the weight of wrapped basin sets should not exceed seven (7) pounds. While there is no set weight limit for instrument trays, Central Service Technicians should consult manufacturers' instructions and sterilizer instructions for guidance. Excessive weight from the metal mass is less likely to permit adequate cooling before condensation, and may result in a wet package interior. When a wet pack occurs, the package must be considered contaminated.

Instruments of the same type should be arranged together to facilitate their location during an emergency. Those with ringed finger access may be grouped together on racks, tray pins, or stringers to

---

Wicking material – *An approved absorbent material that allows for air removal, steam penetration and facilitates drying.*

---

assure that instruments with locks are maintained in the open position. The order or arrangement in the pack should be determined by Central Service managers and user department personnel. When possible, instruments should be presented in their order of use. Heavier items must be placed at the bottom or end of the pack to avoid damage to more delicate devices.

There may be sterilant penetration or pack balance concerns that prevent the "perfect pack" arrangement requested by the user department. Central Service managers should inform user department personnel about pack limitations. The ultimate goal must always be to create a pack that can be successfully sterilized.

Surgical Supplies

Numerous non-instrument surgical supplies such as cotton balls and dressings may be required by users. Most of these items are available as commercially sterilized products, and it is often more cost effective to purchase them pre-sterilized. However, if the facility chooses to process them internally, these and similar items should be wrapped individually or in usable quantities. Do not use canisters or other containers with non-filtered lids (for example, large quantities of sponges, cotton balls, or cotton-tipped applicators) because the sterilant cannot enter the closed containers, and it is not appropriate for the lid to be propped open in the sterilizer. Note: if the lid is not closed, the contents can be contaminated as soon as the sterilizer door is opened. To ensure that the sterilant contacts all surfaces of syringes, plungers should be removed from their barrels, and the devices should be placed on their sides. Stylets and needles should be arranged in a similar manner. Also, plugs in a closed system should be removed for all methods of sterilization EXCEPT dry heat, for which items can be pre-assembled because of the conduction heating process.

Powered Surgical Instruments

Follow the manufacturer's instructions for preparing powered surgical instruments for sterilization. This includes the correct level of disassembly and lubrication. If they have not been purchased pre-sterilized and ready for use, disposable components

---

(i.e. blades, burrs, etc. that have been purchased unsterile) should be included in the pack. Place trigger handles in the safety position, and turn power switches off before packing.

Powered surgical instruments often use a sterilization container supplied by the manufacturer. Extended or special sterilization conditions may be required, and details about these procedures should be supplied by the instrument's manufacturer. After items are inspected, disassembled (if necessary), and placed in a container according to the manufacturer's instructions and accepted work practices, the pack is ready to be packaged for sterilization.

BASIC PACKAGING PROCEDURES

Learning Objective 6. Explain basic packaging procedures for peel pouches and flat wrapping materials.

Clearly written and illustrated procedures for preparation of items to be packaged should be readily available and should be used by all personnel each time packaging procedures are performed. Many packs have unique characteristics that may require special configurations and preparations.

When defining general packaging procedures, the following information should be included:

- Name of the device or multiple devices to be packaged.

- Essential steps for preparation and inspection, and for assembly and disassembly of device(s) according to the manufacturer's written directions and/or specifications.

- Sterilization method used for processing the item(s).

- Type(s) and size(s) of package(s) to be used.

- Correct placement of items in the package.

- Type and placement of internal and/or external chemical process indicator(s) in accordance with the facility's policies.

In addition to general packaging considerations, Central Service Technicians should also follow packaging protocols for the specific type of packaging being used.

Can't write on plastic side may bleed in package

Peel Pouches

Peel pouches are usually used for smaller, lightweight items. They are also useful when it is important to see the contents of the package, such as when a description of the contents is difficult to view on the label. Peel pouches are available on rolls that allow Central Service Technicians to cut off the length desired for each package, and they are also available in precut sizes. Foam inserts or tip protectors help to protect a pouch's contents from damage, and prevent the tips from penetrating the package. If foam inserts or tip protectors are used, assure that the material is appropriate for the type of sterilization to be used, and that it is non-toxic and free of non-fast dyes. Items should be placed into the pouch so the end of the item to be grasped during presentation (example: finger rings of an instrument) will be presented first when the package is opened at the point of use. (Note: this is the chevron end for pre-made pouches.) **Figure 13.22** illustrates the Chevron end of a pre-made pouch. It is designed in a manner that makes it easier to open. Easier opening reduces the risk of product contamination during aseptic opening.

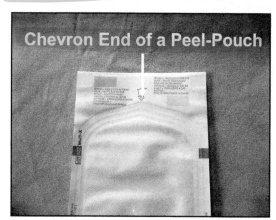

Chevron End of a Peel-Pouch

Figure 13.22

Pouches must be sized and applied properly to allow for adequate air removal, sterilant penetration, and drying. Trapped air acts as a barrier to heat and moisture, so it is important to remove as much air

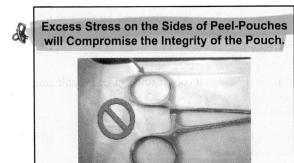

Excess Stress on the Sides of Peel-Pouches will Compromise the Integrity of the Pouch.

Figure 13.23

as possible before sealing. Also, pouches should not be filled too full. Stretching film-paper pouches may cause the paper to tear or the seals to rupture during sterilization or handling. To allow space for package contraction and proper circulation, leave about one inch of space between the items in the pouch and the sealed edges. **Figure 13.23** illustrates an unacceptable size pouch/item combination. Note how the ring handles of the instrument place stress on the sides of the pouch. That stress compromises the package's barrier and will most likely rupture the side seams of the package during the harsh air removal and heat up of the steam sterilization process. Pouches should not, however, be too large because movement of the pack may result in the contents sliding from end to end or side to side. That excessive movement of their contents could break seals or puncture the pouch's paper side.

Observe pouch contents for moisture after sterilization and again prior to storage. You've learned that steam condenses on a metal's surface when heat is transferred to the metal. The rate of transfer increases as the size and weight of the metal increases because there is a greater metal-to-heat ratio. The retained moisture then forms water droplets on the contents, which may compromise the seal's integrity or the barrier protection capability of the pouch material. This, in turn, contaminates the contents. Prevention of condensation is only possible when sterilizers with heated dry cycle capabilities are used. However, limiting pouch contents to small items can usually reduce the problem.

Paper-plastic pouches have a plastic side to permit visibility of the contents, and a paper side that may be penetrated by air, steam, or sterilant. These pouches must only be labeled on the plastic side (for example, with a felt-tip permanent marking pen), or on areas specifically provided by the manufacturer (for example, on fold-over paper-flap seals and paper labels on the plastic). Writing on the paper side of the pouch may cause damage to the package which may not be noticeable but which may compromise the barrier protection.

Pouches must be closed using a seal that is tamper-evident, so there is no danger of packages being opened and resealed for later use. After a sterile package is opened, it is contaminated, and may not be resealed and reused.

Heat sealing is a pouch closure method. There are several varieties of heat sealers available. The manufacturer of the sealer and/or pouch material must verify that the two are compatible. If they are not, the seal may not bond, or there may be burn-through, and both actions will compromise the seal. Multiple-band or wide-band heat sealers should be used to reduce the possibility of an incomplete seal. The manufacturer's instructions for temperature settings, applied pressure, and contact times should be written into procedures, and should always followed.

To seal paper or polyolefin to plastic, the edges must be placed well within the pre-heated jaws of the sealer. Then pressure is applied for the prescribed time, and the jaws are released. Heat seals must be observed for bubbles and creases. Seals that are not smooth and complete may allow bacterial contamination after sterilization.

Packages with self-seals are available which have an adhesive backing that the Central Service Technician can expose to "press seal" the end of the pouch. Pouch manufacturers should provide adequate directions to accomplish a secure seal. Adhesive seals must not permit the pouch to be opened and resealed. Another alternate: peel pouches may also be sealed using a fold and tape method.

In addition to single pouches, there are two popular ways that paper-plastic and polyolefin-

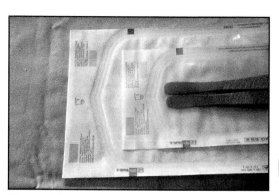

Figure 13.24

plastic packages can be used to meet specific packaging needs:

- Wrap within a pouch – Sometimes (usually to accommodate unique sterile presentation issues) it is desirable to place a single wrapped package into a pouch. The initial wrap is done as normal, and the package is secured with sterilizer-indicator tape. The wrapped item is then inserted into the pouch with the taped closure visible through the plastic. The pouch should be sealed as previously described.

- Double Pouches – While double pouching is not necessary for sterility maintenance, it may be required for aseptic presentation of multiple items or for those having more than one part. Double pouches are prepared by placing the item(s) into one paper-plastic pouch and sealing. (See **Figure 13.24**) This pouch is then placed inside another (slightly larger) pouch and end-sealed. Care is needed when selecting the appropriate sequential sizing. Never fold the inner pouch because this can interfere with air removal and sterilant penetration. "Paper side-to-paper side and plastic side-to- plastic side" is the rule for double pouching to assure sterilant penetration, drying, and content visibility.

Plastic-paper pouches and similar packages should be positioned in the sterilizer standing on edge in loading racks, or they should be placed in baskets specifically designed for these packages. They can also be held on edge by an alternate means (for example, a peel pouch rack or tray pins), and they must be properly spaced. Pouches should be loosely spaced in the basket to ensure that the sterilant can reach the breathable paper side of each pouch since the plastic side is not penetrated by air, steam, or sterilant. Arrange the pouches paper-to-plastic, paper-to-plastic in a perforated or mesh bottom tray. Lining the tray or basket with absorbent material such as a cotton towel or disposable liner made for this purpose will help remove condensate and assist drying.

Flat Wrapping Techniques

Flat wrapping procedures are primarily used for large packages, but they may also be appropriate for smaller items. They involve use of either reusable woven textiles (linens) or disposable non-woven wraps.

There are two methods of using flat wrapper packs:

- Sequential - The package is wrapped twice and is "a package within a package." The term sequential indicates that the contents have been wrapped in sequence (one after the other).

- Simultaneous – The package is only wrapped once, but it requires a special double-layered synthetic non-woven material bound on two or four sides.

There are also two techniques for wrapping packages, and both are used with the sequential and simultaneous wrap methods:

- Square Fold – This is also called the in-line or parallel fold, and it is most frequently used for larger packs and instrument trays.

- Envelope Fold – This is more commonly used for small packs and most instrument sets and individual items.

Sequential wrapping was used prior to the development of newer synthetic wrap materials. It is still used today where such materials are not purchased or where circumstances (for example, large and/or heavy packs) require extra physical protection. Examples of sequentially wrapped packages include the following:

- Double-wrapped muslin (140 count) – two double-layered wraps.

- Double-wrapped barrier cloth (280 count or above) – two single-thickness wraps.

- Double-wrapped paper – two paper wraps.

- Double-wrapped non-woven – two single non-woven wraps.

Figures 13.25 and **13.26** illustrate Sequential wrapping techniques using the Envelope and Square fold methods.

Simultaneous wrapping uses two layers of synthetic non-woven material such as SMS bound on two or four edges. Since the material is already double-layered, the contents are only wrapped once. Both methods are acceptable, although one may be more appropriate for specific situations.

Figures 13.27 and **13.28** provide examples of simultaneous wrap techniques using the Envelope and Square fold methods.

The advantage of sequential wrap is that it affords a "second chance" for sterile presentation. The disadvantages: sequential wrap requires more wrapping time and more unwrapping time.

The advantage of simultaneous wrap is lowered labor costs and increased output in the Central Service and Operating Room. The disadvantage is that the absence of the second layer removes the "second chance" aspect during aseptic opening/presentation. Regardless of the wrap method chosen, if the package appears damaged or tampered with, the contents must be reprocessed.

Choose the right-sized wrap for either method. The wrapper must be large enough to completely contain the contents without leaving excess material which could inhibit sterilant penetration and release. Wrappers must be snug, but not so tight as to impede sterilant entry or exit. If the wrapper will also be used to create a sterile field, it must be of sufficient size to extend at least 6 inches below the edge of the surface being covered.

Wrap folding must always be done in the same sequence. This allows the individuals opening sterile packages to establish a pattern which conserves time and reduces the possibility of error.

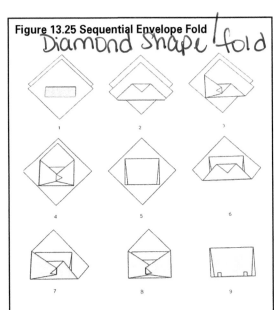

Figure 13.25 Sequential Envelope Fold

Diamond Shape fold

1. The wrap is placed on the table to form a diamond shape with the bottom corner pointing toward the front of the table. The item to be wrapped is placed in the center of the wrap, parallel with the edge of the table.

2. The lower corner is brought up to cover the contents and the tip is folded back on itself to form a tab or flap (which is used later to assist in opening the pack aseptically).

3. Fold the left corner over the contents and fold the tip back to form a tab.

4. Fold the right corner over the left fold and fold the tip back on itself to form a tab.

5. Bring the top corner down over the contents and tuck the corner under the right and left folds leaving a small tab visible for easy opening.

6. The second wrap is applied by placing the single wrapped item into the center of the remaining wrap and repeating the wrap sequence to form a package within a package. The lower corner is brought up to cover the single wrapped item and the tip is folded back on itself to form a tab or flap.

7. Fold the left corner over the single wrapped item and fold the tip back to form a tab.

8. Fold the right corner over the left fold and fold the tip back on itself to form a tab.

9. Bring the top corner down over the single wrapped item and tuck the corner under the right and left folds leaving a small tab visible for easy opening. The package is usually secured with indicator tape.

Figure 13.26 Sequential Square Fold

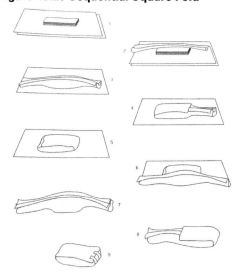

1. The edge of the wrapper is placed parallel with the edge of the table. The instrument tray or linen pack is placed square in the center of the wrapper parallel with the edge of the wrapper as shown in step 1.

2. The edge of the wrapper is folded over the top of the contents covering the lower half (step 2). The edge is then folded back over itself (back towards the technicians) to form a cuff. This will facilitate aseptic opening of the pack when used.

3. Step 3 illustrates how the upper edge of the wrap is brought down over the upper half of the contents and folded back on itself to form another cuff overlapping the original cuff to prevent a gap between the upper and lower folds.

4. The left edge of the wrapper is folded snugly over the pack and back on itself to form a cuff.

5. The right side of the wrapper is folded over the pack, overlapping the previous fold and folded back to form a cuff.

6. The second wrap is applied by placing the single wrapped item into the center of the wrap and repeating the steps performed for the first wrap to create a package within a package. The edge of the second wrapper is folded over the single wrapped item covering the lower half. The edge is then folded back over itself (back towards the technician) to form a cuff.

7. The upper edge of the wrap is brought down over the upper half of the single wrapped item and folded back on itself to form another cuff overlapping the original cuff to prevent a gap between the upper and lower folds.

8. The left edge of the wrapper is folded snugly over the pack and back on itself to form a cuff.

9. The right side of the wrapper is folded over the pack, overlapping the previous fold and folded back. The package is usually secured with indicator tape.

Figure 13.27 Simultaneous Envelope Fold

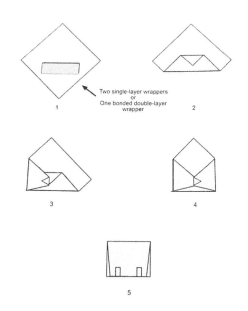

Two single-layer wrappers
or
One bonded double-layer wrapper

Note: Use only wrappers designed for use in double simultaneous wrapping.

1. The wrap is placed on the table to form a diamond shape with the bottom corner pointing toward the front of the table. The item to be wrapped is placed in the center of the wrap, parallel with the edge of the table.

2. The lower corner is brought up to cover the contents and the tip is folded back on itself to form a tab or flap (which is used later to assist in opening the pack aseptically).

3. Fold the left corner over the contents and fold the tip back to form a tab.

4. Fold the right corner over the left fold and fold the tip back on itself to form a tab.

5. Bring the top corner down over the contents and tuck the corner under the right and left folds. A small tab may be incorporated for easy opening. Secure with indicator tape.

Figure 13.28 Simultaneous Square Fold

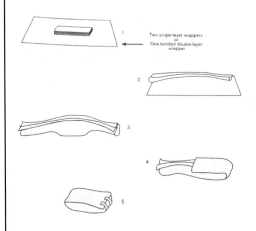

Two single-layer wrappers
or
One bonded double-layer wrapper

Note: Use only wrappers designed for use in double simultaneous wrapping.

1. The edge of the wrapper is placed parallel with the edge of the table. The instrument tray or linen pack is placed square in the center of the wrapper parallel with the edge of the wrapper as shown in step 1.

2. The edge of the wrapper is folded over the top of the contents covering the entire item (step 2). The edge is then folded back over itself (back towards the technician) to form a cuff. This will facilitate aseptic opening of the pack when used.

3. Step 3 illustrates how the upper edge of the wrap is brought down completely over the contents and folded back on itself to form another cuff overlapping the original.

4. The left edge of the wrapper is folded snugly over the pack and back on itself to form a cuff.

5. The right side of the wrapper is folded over the pack, overlapping the previous fold and folded back to form a cuff or tucked under and secured with indicator tape.

BASIC PACKAGING CONSIDERATIONS

Learning Objective 7. Review general packaging concerns:
- Packaging labeling
- Special concerns
- Sterility maintenance

In this section, we'll discuss packaging labeling, special packaging concerns, and sterility maintenance.

Package Labeling

It is essential that all packages be labeled before sterilization. The label must be complete and accurate to ensure that the correct pack is selected and opened.

Label information should include the following:

- Description of package contents.

- Initials of package assembler.

- Lot control number.

- Identification of sterilizer and cycle to be used.

- Date of sterilization (unless inherent in lot control number).

- Requesting department or the surgeon's name (special request items) may also be included on the label.

- Assigned storage location to prevent items from being misplaced.

Standardized abbreviations and terms avoid confusion. Slang terms and nicknames should not be used. Labeling is necessary for the end user, and also for sterilization processing, quality assurance, stock rotation, and inventory control purposes. Central Service Technicians with the responsibility for labeling packages must use clear, legible handwriting and accurate descriptions. Confusion caused by an illegible or inaccurate package label can compromise patient safety because items may be misplaced, or the label may be misread and incorrectly dispensed. Either situation can cause a delay in patient care and treatment.

Labeling should be documented on label-sensitive tape or on commercially available pre-printed, adhesive labels. Do not write directly on the packaging material. For pouches, the labels should not be placed on the paper or spunbond polyolefin side, as they may inhibit sterilant penetration. Felt tip pens are generally used for marking, but they should be indelible, non-bleeding, non-fading, and non-toxic.

Sterility Maintenance Covers

Protective plastic over-wraps (called dust covers or sterility maintenance covers) can be applied to packages after sterilization to protect the package from dust, moisture, and other contaminates. The plastic material should be at least 2 to 3 mils thick. Steam sterilized items must be thoroughly cooled and dried, and EtO sterilized items must be aerated before they are over-wrapped in plastic. The seal of the dust cover should be secured with either a heat seal or security-tape sealing process. The over-wrap should be clearly marked as a "dust cover" or "protective over-wrap" to prevent its use as a part of the sterile field. Protective over-wraps are not to be placed in the sterilizer, and they should be placed over pre-sterilized items only.

Special Packaging Concerns

Several basic packaging concerns require special mention:

- All packaging materials should be held at room temperature (67°F to 72°F; 18°C to 22°C) and at a relative humidity ranging from 35% to 70% for a minimum of two hours before sterilization. This will permit adequate steam/sterilant penetration, and prevent superheating of the fabric during sterilization.

- Sterilizer manufacturers generally recommend that wrapped pans of instruments should not exceed 16 pounds in weight. Limiting the number, weight, and density of instruments in a package does assist in the drying of the set. However, there is no "magic number" for the weight of instrument sets. The weight of any wrapped or containerized instrument set should be based on the ability of personnel to use proper body mechanics when carrying a set, the design and density of individual instruments comprising a set, the distribution of the mass (density) in the set, and sterilizer load and the wrap material. ANSI/AAMI ST77 recommends a maximum weight of 25 pounds for containerized instrument sets.

- All sterilized packages, whether sterilized by the facility or purchased as sterile-ready-to-use products, should be inspected to ensure that the packaging material and/or the seals have not been compromised prior to placing into sterile storage, prior to dispensing, and prior to opening the package.

- No single packaging method or system meets all requirements for packaging and sterilization of all devices required for patient care procedures. Written policies and procedures should establish authority, responsibility, and accountability for selection and use of packaging materials. Procedures should be developed cooperatively with all user departments, and must be carefully reviewed and approved by the Infection Control and Quality Assurance/Improvement Committees.

- Packaging procedures should be performed only by the department responsible for sterilization. Other departments (examples: Operating Room, Delivery Room, Emergency Room, and X-Ray) whose personnel might prepare and package their own instruments and supplies before sending them to Central Service for sterilization should be discouraged from this practice. Often Central Service Technicians do not know about all items in the package, and it could be processed inappropriately. Also, supplying packaging materials to each of these departments is not cost-effective. If, however, a facility does allow pack preparation outside of the Central Service department, applicable personnel must receive training and know and follow appropriate policies and procedures.

Sterility Maintenance

Sterilized packages must maintain their content sterility until they are intentionally opened.

Traditionally, the sterility of a package has been thought of as "**time-related**." That is, the package was considered sterile until a specific expiration date was reached. Then the package was taken out of inventory and reprocessed. However, the Joint Commission and the Association of peri-Operative Registered Nurses (AORN) now recognize that sterility is "**event-related**."

This event-related sterility acknowledges that microbial contamination of a sterile package is caused by an event such as improper handling or transport rather than by time alone. For example, one may purchase a carton of milk at the grocery store with an expiration date that is several days away. However, if he/she forgets to put the carton of milk in the refrigerator, it will become warm and will sour. Even though the milk had an expected shelf-life, an "event" happened that caused its shelf-life to be shortened.

Event-related sterility depends on the quality of the wrapper material, handling procedures, storage and transport conditions, and the number of times the package is handled before use.

By closely controlling the environment and events to which a sterile package is exposed rather than just the time the package is in storage, the probability of package contamination can be minimized. However, expiration dates on commercial products must be adhered to as they reflect product usability or stability rather than sterility of the contents. Packages which contain dated products must be labeled with the earliest expiration date.

Sterility (time-related) – *A package is considered sterile until a specific expiration date is reached.*

Sterility (event-related) – *Items are considered sterile unless the integrity of the packaging is compromised (damaged) or suspected of being compromised (damaged) regardless of the sterilization date. This is sometimes referred to as ERS (Event-Related Sterility).*

STERILE PACKAGING, STORAGE, AND TRANSPORT

Learning Objective 8. Provide basic information about sterile packaging, storage, and transport.

After sterilization, sterile packs and instruments are stored until needed. The activities of personnel in the storage area and the environment itself impact the maintenance of pack sterility.

Storage Considerations

There must be careful inventory control of stored items to assure they will be available when needed.

Proper use of stock rotation principles is important to assure that packs with time-sensitive expiration dates are used before they must be discarded. Storage areas for sterile supplies located outside of the Central Service department must be included in the quality assurance and infection control audits conducted for the sterile storage area in the department. If satellite storage sites are used, personnel responsible for the areas should be trained about requirements for sterility maintenance.

Basic Concerns

The primary conditions that can adversely affect the ability of a sterile package to maintain its sterility until it is opened by the user at the point of use include:

- Moisture and liquid/fluid contamination.

- Dirt, dust, and debris.

- Physical damage to the package including abrasions, cuts, tears, punctures, broken seals, and the breakdown of packaging material (example: some plastics become brittle).

Storage environments should be clean, dry, and easily accessible by authorized personnel. They should also be well-lighted so package labels can be easily read. There should be no dark corners or blind spots which could lead to improper product identification and misplaced or forgotten inventory. Adequate lighting is also critical to personnel safety.

Storage Areas Must Be Kept Clean

Sterile storage areas must be kept clean. All storage units should be cleaned routinely with a hospital-approved germicidal agent. Housekeeping procedures should specify the concentrations and specific details for cleaning these areas.

Cleaning tasks for sterile storage shelves should be scheduled on a by-section basis, moving into areas where supply packages have been removed. Shelving units should be damp-dusted routinely. Care is needed to avoid excess handling of supplies, and surfaces must be dry before supplies are returned to the cleaned shelves.

Cleaning should begin in Sterile Storage and move from there to assembly, and it should be completed in the decontamination room. Flow of cleaning tasks should be from the cleanest area to the dirtiest area.

Work surfaces should be made of easy-to-clean smooth and durable material. There should be no exposed light fixtures, pipes, or ducts that can collect and shed dust. Decontamination, preparation, and packing areas should be physically separated. If this is not possible, extra care is required so air and traffic always flows from clean to dirty areas, and no pass-through traffic should be permitted.

Air supply to the storage areas should be as clean and dust-free as possible, and this usually requires filtration. The room should be under positive air pressure to reduce airborne contamination from air outside the storage area. Storage temperatures should be between 64°F to 75°F (18°C to 24°C) with less than 75% relative humidity. Very dry air can affect seals, and can cause plastic materials to become brittle. Excessive humidity can cause tapes and labels to lose their adhesion, loosen seals, or affect package content identification. Moisture can also condense on the packaging material and seep or "wick" through it while carrying microorganisms to compromise pack sterility (wet packs). Moisture also provides an excellent opportunity for fungal growth through the packages. It is important to keep packs at least 2 inches away from exterior walls, windows, and window seals where condensation can form on interior surfaces of exterior walls.

Sterile packages should not be stored near or under sinks, exposed water pipes, sewage lines, or air conditioning drains. Packs should be kept 8-10 inches above the floor to prevent contamination from floor cleaning agents, spills, and inadvertent shoves and kicks.

There should be at least 8-10 inches between the highest package and the ceiling to allow for proper air circulation. Note: fire codes may specify 18 inches distance from sprinkler heads. Spacing must also be planned and maintained to prevent packages from being touched, bumped, or leaned upon when the room is cleaned, or when personnel are storing or retrieving packs.

The storage area(s) should be located away from areas with heavy traffic, and access to these areas should be restricted. Authorized individuals entering a storage area must follow hand hygiene policies, wear proper attire, be in good health, and maintain good personal hygiene.

All Central Service personnel should maintain a high level of personal hygiene including clean hair, body, nails (no artificial nails), and clothing at all times. Central Service Technicians should frequently wash their hands or use waterless hand sanitizers according to department policies. Fingernails should be short to reduce the microbial load under the nails, and to minimize the potential for rupturing packages and pouches that will contaminate them.

Stored items should be arranged so that packages are not crushed, inappropriately stacked, bent, or compressed. If the air inside the package is forced out, it can potentially rupture closures and seams in the process. Additionally, by forcing the air out of the pack, a void is created. When the source of compression is released (the weight on its top is removed), a slight suction can be created by the void. This can potentially establish conditions for the packs to "suck in" contaminated air.

In open shelf storage systems, items are placed on shelves that are not enclosed. Shelves usually have open racks to prevent dust accumulation. Open shelving is convenient and less expensive than closed (enclosed) shelving. However, packages are more vulnerable to physical hazards (usually accidental) and environmental challenges including from cleaning solutions and microorganisms. For added protection, many facilities devote some or all of their storage space to closed shelving units to protect sterile packages from microbial, environmental, and physical challenges from the outside environment. Closed shelving is usually reserved for expensive or delicate items. Doors should be opened slowly when accessing the packs to minimize air rushing into the unit that may contaminate packs.

Sterile storage areas are also used to store pre-sterilized products from outside vendors. Products are delivered at the receiving dock, typically in shipping containers made of corrugated cardboard (although other forms exist). These outer shipping containers should be removed in the receiving or an adjacent "break-out" area. They have been exposed to the environmental challenges of land, air, and/or sea transportation, and they may be very dirty, insect-infested, and contaminated with microorganisms including fungus and bacterial spores.

After externally purchased sterile items have been removed from their shipping containers, they must be placed in clean transport containers for transfer to the sterile storage area. A covered or enclosed cart with solid bottom shelves should be used. Written procedures should be in place to maintain the cleanliness and sterility of vendor-purchased sterile products, and to prevent their damage during break-down and transport. Sterile storage areas and procedures for their upkeep should be addressed in sterile storage and quality assurance inspections.

Sterile Stock Arrangement

The logical arrangement of stock improves efficiency, decreases staff injuries, and facilitates appropriate stock rotation.

Sterile items should be arranged so they are easy to locate. This may best be accomplished by organizing them alphabetically by name, functionality or specialty (related items are shelved together), or numerically based on stock codes. Shelves should bear the label designating where packs should be stored and pertinent information for reorders. For safety

reasons, heavier items should be placed on lower and middle shelves. Lighter and less cumbersome items can be placed on higher shelves.

Sterile packages should be arranged and maintained to allow stock rotation on a **First In, First Out (FIFO)** system. This ensures that the oldest items are used first. The longer an item has been in storage, the longer it has been exposed to the environment and physical abuses, and the more likely it is to have been compromised. Practicing a FIFO inventory control system prevents a "neglected packs syndrome" where hard-to-reach packs may remain in storage much longer than others, and are more likely to be damaged. It is important to note that items with expiration dates should be used in the order of their expiration dates with the items that will expire soonest being used first.

The goal of a stock arrangement system is to provide minimal pack handling while allowing FIFO rotation. Many facilities use a left-to-right system: the newest item is placed on the left, and the older items move forward to the right. The pack on the far right is the first to be picked-up for use. Other facilities place the new packs in from the back of the shelf, and pick up the oldest from the front of the shelf. Remember, packs must be lifted correctly to avoid any damage to the pack.

Another stock arrangement method involves lining up the packs from left to right with the oldest on the far left. A colored sliding shelf divider containing the words "use this first" printed on the right side is moved up against the next pack on the right (now the oldest pack). When that package is removed, the marker is again moved to the right, next to what is now the oldest package. As new packs are stored, they are placed to the left of the divider, so the oldest will always be at the far left of the shelf. When the last (and oldest) pack on the right is removed, the divider is placed in the original position to the left of the first pack on the left side of the shelf (the oldest pack), and the

> **First In, First Out** – *A stock rotation system in which the oldest product (that which has been in storage the longest) is used first; often abbreviated "FIFO."*

cycle is repeated. The advantages of this method include less work for personnel, and fewer traumas to the sterile packages. A disadvantage: the system requires several narrow shelves instead of one wide (large capacity) shelf.

Transport Considerations

Transportation of sterile packages from receiving to the Central Service department or later to the site of use should be done in covered or enclosed carts. Shelves should be of solid bottom construction. As the cart wheels turn, they pick up dirt and dust and sling it upward onto the underside of the solid shelves. This emphasizes the need to wash both the top and the bottom of cart shelves.

Policies and procedures are required to maintain cleanliness, and to ensure that the carts are properly maintained. Damaged doors that do not close securely can allow air to enter as the cart moves. This "wind" effect can force dirty air under pressure against the packs to potentially contaminate them.

The importance of avoiding contact with sterile packages cannot be over-emphasized. This includes bumping into, leaning on, backing into, touching when counting, and excessively rearranging the packages. When a package is moved or handled, it should not be "cradled." Any sterile items that are dropped to the floor should be considered contaminated and removed even if no damage is apparent. The jarring and compression on landing can force dust and airborne microorganisms into the package. The floor could be wet, sharp edges of trays could puncture through the wrap, and dirt could be carried onto the storage shelf to contaminate the next pack placed in that position. **Figure 13.29** provides an example of a wrap that has been compromised (torn) by sharp tray edges.

Central Service Technicians and end users must be trained to recognize any signs of sterility compromise. A log of sterile pack contamination events should be maintained and analyzed to implement preventive actions.

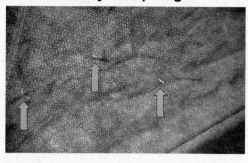

Sterile Packaging that has been Torn by Sharp Edges

Figure 13.29

When removing the package from the shelf, its front should be lifted from underneath with one hand. The other hand should be placed midway under the package, and the unit should then be lifted off the shelf. Packages should not be dragged or pushed against any surface because this causes friction or abrasion which can potentially cause a pressure cut or snag and compromise sterility. Shelf liners help to create a cushion between the hard surface of the shelf and bottom of the packages. These are recommended if the facility is experiencing tearing on pack bottoms. This is usually a greater concern with heavy packs, procedure sets and, especially, instrument trays. The edges of the metal trays and weight of the instruments increase the adverse impact of the friction. Burrs or sharp edges on the shelves themselves may also contribute to sterile pack damage.

When packs are removed from storage, they must be carefully observed for expiration date, tears, abrasion, tracks, fuzzy ("worn") areas, punctures, compromised seals, dirt, and evidence of moisture. The sterilization process indicator must be checked to ensure that the package was subjected to the sterilization process. If any of these adverse conditions are noted, the pack should be considered contaminated. If the contents are reusable, they should be removed from the package for reprocessing. If the contents are disposable, they should be discarded. Single-use wrap should not be reused after it has been sterilized.

REFERENCES

1. *Association for the Advancement of Medical Instrumentation. 2006 ANSI/AAMI ST 79:2006, Comprehensive guide to steam sterilization and sterility assurance in healthcare facilities.*

2. *Association of peri-Operating Room Nurses. Recommended Practices for Cleaning and Caring for Surgical Instruments and Powered Equipment. In: 2002 Standards, Recommended Practices, and Guidelines. Denver, Co. 2002. (267-75).*

3. *American Society for Hospital Central Service Personnel. American Hospital Association. Chapter 6: Preparation and Packaging for Sterilization. In: Training Manual for Central Service Technicians, 4th ed. Jossey-Bass/AHA Press Series, (114-39).*

4. *Shimkus, J. Abuzz about Fuzz. Materials Management in Health Care 7(5). May, 1998.*

5. *Beezhold, D. Medical Glove Safety. The Guthrie Journal 69(1): Winter, 2000. (1-5). Online: www.guthrie.org.*

6. *Occupational Safety and Health Administration OSHA Technical Information Bulletin: Potential for Allergy to Natural Rubber Latex Gloves and Other Natural Rubber Products. April, 1999 (2-5). http://www.osha-slc.gov/html/hotfoias/tib/TIB19990412.html.*

7. *Reese, D, et al. 2001 Sep. Latex Allergy Literature Review: Evidence for Making Military Treatment Facilities Latex Safe. Military Medicine 166(9) Sept, 2001 (764-770).*

8. *Association of Operating Room Nurses. Recommended Practices for Selection and Use of Packaging Systems. In: 2002 Standards, Recommended Practices, and Guidelines. Denver, Co. 2002. (287-92)*

9. *Ritual and Romance: CDC Draft Bans Brushes, Nails. 2002 February. Hospital Infection Control 29(2). Feb, 2002. (22-23).*

10. *Joint Commission on Accreditation of Healthcare Organizations (JCAHO). 1998. Infection Control, Standard IC.4. In: Accreditation Manual for Hospitals. Chicago: JCAHO, 75-7.*

CENTRAL SERVICE TERMS

Seals (temper-evident)

Muslin

Superheating

Rigid container system

510k (certification)

Wet pack

Papers (kraft-type)

Spunbond-meltblown-spunbond

Wicking material

Sterility (time-related)

Sterility (event-related)

First In, First Out

Chapter Outline

Chapter 14

Point of Use Processing

Chapter Learning Objectives

As a result of successfully completing this chapter, readers will be able to:

1. Define the term, "flash sterilization," and review industry standards for the process.

2. Explain the need for and basic procedures to perform flash sterilization.

3. Describe quality control monitoring procedures for flash sterilizers.

4. Review concerns about point-of-use processing of heat-sensitive medical devices.

5. Discuss the use of oxidative agents for low-temperature point of use processing.

Point of use processing occurs immediately before an item is used, and/or close to a patient care area such as a sub-sterile room in the operating room. Items that are processed at point of use are usually done so without external packaging (unwrapped), and are transported a short distance for immediate use. While these processes are safe, the unwrapped condition of the items increases the risk of contamination during after-processing transport, so strict handling guidelines must be followed.

Point of use processing is generally done with a steam sterilization process *(flash sterilization)* or with oxidizing chemicals. In both cases, careful attention must be paid to protocols for item preparation and handling.

The primary reason for using point of use processing is speed: items can be processed quickly to best meet patient needs. This chapter will examine the use of flash sterilization and oxidizing chemistries for point of use preparation of items.

— Autoclave

FLASH STERILIZATION STANDARDS

Learning Objective 1. Define the term, "flash sterilization," and review industry standards for the process.

Flash sterilization is done every day in our country's hospitals and surgery centers. Several important facts must be understood to ensure that flash sterilization is performed safely. Note: A detailed overview of the principles of steam sterilization is covered in Chapter 15.

Several agencies and organizations have established standards, guidelines, and recommendations for flash sterilization, and these will now be discussed.

Association for the Advancement of Medical Instrumentation

The Association for the Advancement of Medical Instrumentation (AAMI) recently published its American National Standard 79. It states that flash sterilization should only be considered when:

- Work practices ensure proper cleaning and decontamination, inspection, and placement of instruments in trays or containment devices recommended for flash sterilization.

- The area's physical layout provides for direct delivery of sterilized items to the point of use.

- Procedures are developed, followed, and audited to ensure aseptic handling and personnel safety during transport to point of use.

- The item is used immediately after flash sterilization.

While AAMI standards are not laws, they are recognized nationally as standards for best practices, and are recognized in a court of law as professional standards.

Association of peri-Operative Registered Nurses

The Association of peri-Operative Registered Nurses (AORN) publishes its "Recommended Practices and Guidelines," which are based on the AAMI standard (see above) and best peri-operative practices.[2] AAMI committee members who represent AORN ensure that the AAMI recommended practices are feasible for the operating suite environment. These standards indicate that:

- Flash sterilization should only be used in selected clinical situations, and in a controlled manner.

- The use of flash sterilization should be minimized.

- Flash sterilization should only be done when there is insufficient time to process by the preferred wrapped or container method.

Point of Use Processing – That which occurs when a medical device is processed immediately before use, and/or close to the patient are area.

Flash sterilization – The process by which unwrapped instruments are sterilized for immediate use when an emergency situation arises. Always wet.

• Flash sterilization should not be used as a substitute for an adequate instrument inventory.

Further, flash sterilization should only be performed if:

• The device manufacturer's instructions are available and followed.

• All devices and all lumens are thoroughly cleaned.

• Placement of the instruments in the container or tray allows for steam penetration.

• There is a procedure for aseptic transfer to the sterile field.

• Documentation and monitoring results are maintained to allow tracking of processed items to individual patients.

The Joint Commission

The Joint Commission has the following expectations for the practice of flash sterilization:

• It is used only for unanticipated situations.

• It is not a routine practice for turnover instruments (needed for immediate use).

• There is a plan to ensure that the daily case schedule does not require the same instrumentation multiple times, and that there is sufficient time for appropriate instrumentation reprocessing.

• The instrument inventory is increased, if necessary, to avoid the need for flash sterilization when possible.

• A plan is identified for improving or decreasing the use of flash sterilization.

• Attention is paid to the frequency of flash sterilization use.

• Documentation is detailed and adequate to track instruments to the patient for which they are used.[3]

The Joint Commission requires healthcare facilities to "document what they do" and "do what they document." Operating rooms can be cited by The Joint Commission for improper flash sterilization when facility personnel do not follow their own written policies and procedures. The Joint Commission expects each hospital's clinical and practice settings to follow the recommended standards and guidelines established by AAMI and AORN. It also looks for written policies and procedures used by hospitals for flash sterilization to determine whether actual practice follows what is written.

The Joint Commission concerns also address the monitoring of actual practices Are quality control checks done every month, quarter, or year? How frequently does the policy state that quality control checks will be done? What are the consequences if the facility is not compliant in quality control processes?

Originally, flash sterilization was intended for use only in an emergency (example: when a one-of-a-kind instrument was contaminated or dropped from the sterile field). Flash cycles were designed to process one instrument at a time, and were originally cleared by the FDA for processing single items. In fact, it is strongly recommended that large trays and/or multiple trays NOT be flash sterilized because:

• Large trays require longer heat-up time.

• Larger loads increase total cycle time.

• Use of large or multiple trays increases instrument cooling time.

• Full trays frequently need an increased exposure time when porous or complex instruments are included.

FLASH STERILIZATION PROCEDURES

Learning Objective 2. Explain the need for and basic procedures to perform flash sterilization.

Several workplace and workflow issues impact current flash sterilization practices. For example, operating room managers try to control costs, which can yield insufficient equipment inventories. Busy operating room schedules may not allow sufficient time for a wrapped sterilization method.

Also, there is often a lack of space in the operative suite for proper decontamination.

Need for Flash Sterilization

Operating rooms run on tight schedules and, to accommodate each surgeon, procedures are often scheduled in back-to-back blocks. The same type of procedure requiring the same type of instrument set may be scheduled immediately after the previous procedure. Many operating rooms do not have sufficient instrument sets to accommodate this type of scheduling. Facilities may be reluctant to purchase multiple instrument sets for specific procedures due to budgetary constraints.

These inventory and time constraints can make it very difficult for instruments to be processed with a wrapped method. However, The Joint Commission and some state health departments indicate that these are not acceptable reasons to overuse flash sterilization.

Many hospital operating rooms were built decades ago, and they do not include a separate decontamination room in the operating suite. Even when their areas are renovated, the extra space for a proper decontamination room is typically not available. Unless a facility is new and has planned for decontamination facilities for operating rooms, the resources needed to properly decontaminate items for flash sterilization are generally unavailable.

IUS – Immediate use Sterilization.

Additional issues also impact the frequent use of flash sterilization. Most facilities have at least one surgeon using personal specialized instruments who does not want facility personnel to reprocess them. He/she may operate in several hospitals, and have only one set of instruments which cannot be left at a facility for wrapped processing. These personal instruments are then brought to the facility without having been processed and sterilized. Even if they are delivered in a "sterile package," the handling and care of the instrumentation was not monitored by hospital staff, so it must be decontaminated and sterilized to assure sterility.

Always wet, not wrapped

Flash Sterilization Cycles

Flash sterilization can be accomplished with three types of cycles: gravity displacement, pre-vacuum, and Express. Gravity cycles are traditionally called "flash" cycles, and they may be pre-programmed into the control systems of steam sterilizers. Pre-vacuum cycles were added to sterilizers used in operating rooms when more complex operating room instrumentation (examples: orthopedic and neurology instruments and power equipment) were manufactured to permit gravity and pre-vacuum flash sterilization. The Express Cycle is a limited application cycle for a single instrument wrapped in a single-layer wrap.

Note: Express cycles are not available on all steam sterilizers. Users should not attempt a single wrap Express process unless their sterilizer is designed to perform that function.

Flash Sterilization of Implants

According to the Food and Drug Administration, an implantable device is one that is placed into a surgically-or naturally-formed body cavity with the intention of remaining there for a period of 30 days or more. A few examples include cranial aneurysm clips, hip and breast prostheses, plates, and screws.

AORN standards do not recognize flash sterilization for implants because the process increases the risk of surgical site infection: a leading cause of healthcare facility-associated infections. Instead, it suggests careful planning, inventory management, and cooperation with suppliers.

AAMI also specifies that implantable medical devices should not be flash sterilized. If they are, and they are then placed into a patient before biological indicator results are known, documentation must be completed for premature release of implantable devices. Also, an Exception Form for Premature Release of Implantable Devices must be completed.

Regardless of the type of cycle used, all steam sterilization cycles proceed through the same phases: conditioning, exposure, and exhaust and/or drying. In the conditioning phase, steam enters the chamber as air is removed through the drain. Pressure increases inside as the chamber reaches the sterilizing temperature. The exposure phase (for example, 3, 4, or 10 minutes) begins when the thermocouple senses the constant pre-set cycle temperature. During the exhaust phase, filtered air enters, steam is removed from the chamber, and the pressure inside the chamber returns to atmospheric pressure. There is typically only one minute of drying time programmed into flash cycles. While this assists in removing steam from the chamber, it is not sufficient to completely dry the device(s) being sterilized.

The gravity displacement cycle uses gravity in the conditioning and exhaust phases to displace the air, and to replace it with steam. Both **porous** and non-porous items can be flash sterilized in a gravity displacement sterilizer if the appropriate times and temperatures are used for each. Gravity flash sterilizers were the only type available for operating room use for many years, and they are still in common use.

If the flash sterilization load consists of a single instrument comprised of metal and without lumens, a three-minute cycle at 270°F (132°C) should be used. If the load includes complex or lumened instruments, mixed materials (example: rubber and plastic), or multiple instruments, a 10-minute cycle at 270°F (132°C) should be used. Gravity flash cycles have abbreviated cycle times, so strict adherence to the sterilizer's and instrument manufacturer's instructions is necessary. Gravity flash cycles do not typically include drying time.

Unlike gravity flash cycles, pre-vacuum flash cycles are standard sterilization cycles with a limited drying time. The typical pre-set pre-vacuum flash cycle drying time (usually one minute) helps decrease steam in the chamber, but it does not dry the instruments. The limited drying time makes the

Porous – *Possessing or full of pores (minute openings).*

processed item unsuitable for storage, and it defines the pre-vacuum cycle as a flash cycle. During a pre-vacuum flash cycle, air and steam are mechanically injected and removed during the conditioning and exhaust phases. Both non-porous and porous items within wraps, pouches, or containers can be sterilized in pre-vacuum cycles if the appropriate times and temperatures are used for each. A pre-vacuum load that consists of mixed materials or items with lumens must be processed for four minutes at 270°F (132°C).

Complex medical devices may require longer exposure times. However, the exposure times should never be less than the minimum recommended flash exposure time. Cycle parameters cited in the AAMI standard, in AORN Recommended Practices, and in sterilizer manufacturers' operating instructions, provide minimum exposure requirements. The manufacturers of these more complex medical devices must provide recommended cycle and exposure times for flash sterilization. If these are not included in the operator's manual, the information should be requested in writing from the manufacturer. Additional cycles can be programmed into many sterilizer control systems for any medical devices requiring different exposure times.

The Express cycle has a limited application. This cycle should only be used for simple, all-metal, non-porous instruments without lumens that are not constructed of mixed materials. A reusable or disposable single-layer wrap is the only recommended packaging to be used, and it protects sterile goods during transfer to the point of use after sterilization.

The Express cycle is preset by the manufacturer for four minutes at 270°F (132°C) with three minutes of drying time, and a total cycle time of 12 minutes. Express cycles are abbreviated pre-vacuum cycles. They feature two mechanical steam pulses and vacuum pulls in contrast with four pulses and pulls for a standard pre-vacuum, and this is the reason for their limited processing capabilities. The Express cycle is a just-in-time process with no shelf life. The recommended procedure is to handle the instruments as though no wrapper exists. The operator should wear sterile gloves and use sterile towels to hold the tray. He/she should place the wrapped tray on a sterile impervious surface (one that liquids cannot pass through), and the tray should not be placed on a working sterile field while opening it. Even though this cycle has a short drying time, the single wrapper may still be damp, and an aseptic technique is important.

Decontamination in the Operating Room

All contaminated instruments must be properly decontaminated prior to sterilization regardless of whether the sterilization process occurs in a flash sterilizer in the operating room, or in a wrapped container in the Central Service department. The decontamination area in the operating room should have the same environmental considerations as if it was in Central Service. For example, it should be designated only for instrument decontamination. Inappropriate areas for operating room decontamination include scrub sinks, sinks in sub-sterile rooms, and hand washing sinks. The walls, floors, and work surfaces should be of non-shedding construction material that can withstand frequent chemical cleaning and disinfection. Proper lighting is needed so staff can effectively inspect instruments for cleanliness and function before sterilization. The ventilation system should provide at least 10 air exchanges per hour. It should maintain negative air pressure in the decontamination area and positive air pressure in the clean prep and pack areas so "dirty" air cannot flow to clean spaces. Temperature in the decontamination area should be between 60°- 65°F (16-18°C), and relative humidity should be between 30 and 60 percent. Both values should be recorded daily.

Ideally, the decontamination and preparation areas should be physically separated to permit negative pressure airflow. The pass-through window and all doors should remain closed. However, since it is frequently not possible to have separate areas for dirty and clean activities in the operating room, spatial separation is acceptable if there is good environmental control. The areas for decontamination and preparation should have a definitive workflow pattern from "dirty" to "clean." Decontamination should be

performed when no one else is in the room, and clean inspection and preparation should not be done at the same time as decontamination tasks. In this case, the room should be divided into separate clean and decontamination areas. Air should flow from the clean side of the room to the soiled side, and should then be exhausted from there. Soiled-side drawers and cupboards and clean-side surfaces should be appropriately labeled. In this environment, the staff must work to maintain the separation of clean and dirty areas.

Preparing Staff and Instruments

Operating room staff must practice safe handling techniques for contaminated instruments and safely transport them to the decontamination area without risking exposure to other people and surfaces. The proper cleaning solutions should be available for decontamination, and the appropriate containers for flash sterilization are also needed. Each nurse and Central Service Technician should know how to prepare an item for flash sterilization, and practice the appropriate technique for aseptic transfer of a flash sterilized item to the sterile field.

Simple techniques can protect staff and the environment from the contaminated instrument before it is decontaminated and flash sterilized. For example, contaminated instruments should always be contained or covered during transport to the decontamination area.

The same personal protective equipment (PPE) required in the Central Service department is needed for operating room personnel. This will protect them from injuries and/or exposure to cleaning solution splashes and aerosols, and from pathogens that may be present. All PPE must properly fit the employees who wear it.

Pre-cleaning is the most important part of the decontamination process, and yet this activity is often performed carelessly. Up to 99 percent of the microorganisms on an instrument can be removed with thorough cleaning. Items must be pre-cleaned to remove any debris on the instruments' surfaces that could prevent effective sterilization.

Instruments can be cleaned with manual methods or with the use of a mechanical method such as an ultrasonic cleaner or an automated washer-disinfector. To properly decontaminate dirty instruments, they must be opened and disassembled to the smallest part. Then soil and debris can be washed away from the jaws, box locks, crevices, and other challenging areas.

The selection of the appropriate enzymatic presoaks and detergents allows effective cleaning and protection of surgical instruments. Manufacturers must always be consulted for recommendations about the cleaning chemistries to be used for their devices. Also, detergents and enzymatic solutions must be correctly diluted to be effective. Caution: never use saline, environmental germicide, or a betadine-impregnated scrub brush to pre-clean instruments. Anything that contains sodium (salt) will cause pitting and corrosion, and can damage the surfaces of the surgical instrumentation. All detergent residue and soil must be thoroughly rinsed from surfaces, and special rinses with distilled, demineralized, or deionized water may be needed. Manufacturer's instructions should include procedures for proper disassembly, cleaning, and rinsing of each device.

Wire brushes and sharp instruments should never be used to clean or remove dried and caked debris (bioburden) from instruments. However, the internal surfaces of lumens and channels of microscopic/endoscopic devices should be manually brushed with recommended cleaning tools.

All instruments must be appropriately prepared to ensure that they are actually sterilized during a flash sterilization cycle. The first step is to inspect the instruments for cleanliness and function; make sure that scissors are still sharp, that clamps are not sprung, and that box locks are clean. Instruments must be opened or disassembled, and must be positioned in the tray to allow for proper air removal because its presence inhibits steam contact and sterilization. Concave and broad-surfaced instruments should be positioned standing on their edges.

Instruments with lumens must be flushed with sterile or distilled water before flash sterilization.

Moisture inside lumened instruments helps to create steam inside as it moves air out which, in turn, allows the inner surfaces to be contacted by sterilant. Do not use tap water for flushing the lumens because of the possible presence of pyrogens (substances that can cause fever in a patient) in the water. Debris from dead microorganisms in tap water can be pyrogenic.

If trays are used for flash sterilization, they should be perforated or mesh-bottomed to ensure good circulation of the steam in the sterilizer's chamber. If rigid containers are used, they should be specifically designed for flash sterilization, and the manufacturer's validated guidelines must be followed. Before purchasing a rigid container system for flash sterilization, perform product testing of the containers during the trial period with a biological indicator using the recommended flash sterilization cycles. Instrumentation that will be routinely sterilized in the container should be part of the product testing protocol. Exposure times may be longer than the usual recommended times, but not shorter. AAMI guidelines should be followed to validate container products.

Transport After Processing

Sterile trays of instruments must be moved to the point of use without contamination, and policies and procedures are needed to audit this practice. There are several options for transfer to the sterile field. Every staff member must perform transfer techniques in the most aseptic manner possible to protect the sterilized items en route. The person with transportation responsibilities must be alert to all sources of potential contamination. There should be no nonsterile obstacles located in the path of transport, nor should there be areas of high aerosolization such as a scrub sink area. The path of transport should not pass any staff member who is not wearing a mask or appropriate head covering.

Sterile towels or a sterile flat metal tray can be placed over the instruments using aseptic technique to provide protection from environmental contamination during transport. However, the tray should not be placed directly into the sterile field. The scrubbed person should carefully remove the item from the tray with a sterile clamp or his/her

Biological Integrators, internal strips are placed in items to be sterilized.

sterile gloved hand, being careful not to receive a burn or to contaminate the sterile item.

In addition, scrubbed personnel should transport flash sterilized items only in restricted areas which should be cleared of people and activities that might cause contamination of the transporter and/or the sterile item.

QUALITY CONTROLS FOR FLASH STERILIZATION

Learning Objective 3. Describe quality control monitoring procedures for flash sterilizers.

Quality control monitoring procedures are needed for flash sterilizers in the operating room for the same reasons that process quality controls are needed in the Central Service department.

Chemical Monitoring

Chemical indicators (CIs) should be placed in each tray among the instrument(s) with every cycle. The CI responds to a chemical or physical change to one or more physical conditions in the chamber, and it indicates exposure to the appropriate parameters for sterilization. However, a chemical indicator does not verify that sterilization was achieved. It only confirms that one or more of the physical parameters were present. **Class 5 integrators** are a good choice for sterility assurance monitoring because they monitor all the critical parameters of the sterilization cycle (time, temperature, and the presence of steam (moisture), and they correlate to the outcome of a biological indicator. Class 5 chemical integrators are correlated to the biological kill of Geobacillus Stearothermophilus, the microorganism used to monitor steam sterilization cycle efficacy. Chemical indicators must be accurately read at the completion of each cycle to ensure that the specific parameters for that specific indicator were met.

Class 5 (chemical integrators) – Integrating indicators designed to react to all critical parameters over a specified range of sterilization cycles.

Biological Monitoring

Conventional biological indicators (BIs) are strips that have been populated with a standardized viable population of bacterial spores. The bacterial spores on the strip have been shown to be resistant to a specific mode of sterilization (for example, steam, peracetic acid, gas plasma, or ethylene oxide). After the biological indicator is run in a cycle, it must be incubated for a specific length of time as required by the BI manufacturer to determine if any organisms survived the sterilization cycle. Conventional BIs can be purchased in two forms: within a process challenge device or as self-contained (naked) BIs without the extra challenge of the process challenge pack.

An enzyme-based, early-readout BI shares the same characteristics of the conventional BI with one exception: the readout is based on an enzyme activity with a florescence that is read as positive or negative.

The BI manufacturer's instructions should be followed for activating and incubating the product. The incubation temperature for Geobacillus stearothermophilus is 122-140°F (50-60°C). If the media on the strip does not change color after incubation, it indicates that a successful sterilization cycle occurred. The rapid-readout BI used for flash sterilization is incubated for a period of time according to the manufacturer (either one or three hours) depending on the product.

A "control BI" is incubated with the processed BIs. The control, an unsterilized or processed spore strip, should always be positive (it should grow spores and change color) after incubation. It confirms that the spores on the indicators were alive and viable for testing.

For routine monitoring, AAMI recommends that a biological test be done at least weekly, preferably every day that the sterilizer is used. Each cycle used (gravity, pre-vacuum, and/or Express) should be routinely and individually tested. Every type of tray (open, rigid container, protective organizing case, or single-wrap pack for the Express cycle) should be tested separately, and with each cycle in which they are used.

Biological testing or Attest – Test pack w/ BI vial + integrator. Done daily.

every test is only ran every 24 hrs.

Only the shortest exposure time for each temperature and tray combination is tested.

The frequency of routine BI testing must be stated in the facility's policies and procedures. BI tests should be conducted in accordance with their manufacturer's instructions for use. Biological testing for flash sterilization in an empty chamber is actually a more rigorous biological challenge to sterilizer performance than a loaded chamber. Performing the test in an empty chamber minimizes heat-up time, because there is little metal mass to absorb the heat, and this minimizes the ability of the process to kill microorganisms. The empty sterilizer climbs to temperature quickly, and the killing time is not extended by the extra time taken to heat-up a tray of instruments. If organisms are killed at the lower exposure time under these conditions, they will be killed at the higher exposure times for flash sterilization.

For the test cycle, the BI should be placed in a perforated or mesh bottom surgical instrument tray, on the lower shelf of the sterilizer, and directly over the drain. This is normally the coldest part of the chamber. It is not acceptable to place this tray on the chamber floor.

A control BI is incubated along with the test BI after the cycle is run. If the test BI is positive for growth, this is a failing result. The sterilizer must be taken out of service immediately. In addition, all items that were processed in that sterilizer since the last passing test must be considered non-sterile. The failure must be reported to the Central Service supervisor, and necessary policies and procedures should be followed to begin the investigative process. This is why documentation of all flash sterilization cycles is so important: all flash-sterilized items must be traceable to a patient.

Failure investigation procedures should include:

- Checking mechanical and chemical monitors.

- Requesting a sterilizer check by a qualified service technician.

- Requesting the lab to test for bacillus growth.

- Notifying the Infection Control department and physicians.

- Re-testing the sterilizer after maintenance or repair.

- Completing all appropriate documentation.

Residual Air Removal Test

The Residual Air Removal Test, more frequently known as the Bowie-Dick Test, is required for sterilizers with a pre-vacuum cycle. This test must be run every day before the pre-vacuum cycles are used. The test is performed on pre-vacuum cycles only, and it checks the efficiency of the sterilizer's air removal system during the pre-vacuum cycle to detect inadequate air removal or air leaks in the chamber.

Hospital staff can build their own Residual Air Removal Tests according to AAMI instructions, and commercial test packs are also available. Always follow the manufacturer's instructions for use and interpretation of the results. Routine monitoring using the test should be performed every day after a warm-up cycle, and before running the first cycle of the day. It is important to have a warm chamber to avoid the risk of an air-removal test failure.

There are many commercially-prepared Bowie Dick tests on the market today, and most hospitals use them. However, many tests are difficult to read because they employ shades of black or gray, which can make it hard for Central Service staff to differentiate between "pass" and "fail." There is technology available that is easier to read and interpret because it uses a distinct yellow-to-blue color change, and it also provides diagnostic information. In addition to detecting a chamber leak, it can indicate failures from wet or superheated steam, or the presence of non-condensable gases in the steam line.

For air Removal test. Done daily.

Daily routine Bowie-Dick test procedures follow:

- Precondition (warm up) the sterilizer according to the sterilizer manufacturer's recommendations.

- Place a Bowie-Dick test pack by itself in an empty chamber on the bottom shelf over the drain.

- Set the sterilizer for a 3.5 minute exposure at 273°F (134°C). Note: exposure time should never exceed four minutes, and no drying time is necessary.

Cycle Monitoring and Record Keeping

Real-time assessment of a sterilization cycle must be completed and documented after every cycle before instruments are removed from the chamber. Cycles should be physically monitored before, during, and after every cycle. This is critical because the sterilizer's mechanical indicators show the system's real-time status, and they provide the earliest evidence of malfunctions. Cycle data are shown on gauges and display screens, circle graphs, and computer printouts, and are considered legal documentation.

As part of the facility's policies and procedures, it is important to assure that everyone understands how to read all the information provided by the sterilizer. For example, staff should know that the steam pressure on the chamber and jacket gauges must be equal during the exposure phase of the cycle: both should be at least 27 **pounds per square inch gauge (psig)** for a 270°F (132°C) setting.

To monitor the cycle, it is important to:

- Confirm that the previously run cycle was completed satisfactorily before using the sterilizer.

- Select the correct sterilization cycle and parameters for the item to be sterilized.

- Assure that the cycle is properly completed before removing items for use.

Pounds per square inch gauge (psig) – *A measure of ambient air pressure; the pressure that a gas would exert on the walls of a one-cubic foot container.*

AAMI has long recommended that thorough documentation be kept for each flash sterilization cycle. Central Service personnel generally do an excellent job of recording the terminal sterilization cycle data in their department. However, some surgical departments have been slow to recognize the importance of documentation for flash sterilization cycles, nor do they implement a routine quality assurance process to document it. In fact, documentation is necessary for epidemiological tracking, for tracing sterilization cycles to individual patients, and for the on-going assessment of items that have been flash-sterilized.

The documentation for each flash cycle should include the:

- Patient's name.

- Contents of the flash sterilization load.

- Type of sterilization cycle used.

- Cycle parameters.

- Reason for flash sterilization.

- Signature of the staff person responsible for release of the flash sterilization load for patient use.

There is no national recommendation for how long to maintain cycle records. State and local statutes can provide guidance if they exist, but many do not address this issue. In the end, each facility must assure that it has policies and procedures in place that address record retention. Pediatric facilities should consider keeping records through a patient's age of majority, in case that patient files a case when he/she is of legal age.

The following stakeholders should be involved in writing record-keeping policies because they can provide input for a hospital's infection control program and its liability concerns.

- Risk Management department personnel.

- Central Service and Operating Room managers.

- Infection Control department representatives.

- Facility administrators.
- The facility's attorney.
- The facility's insurance carrier.

Staff Education for Flash Sterilization

The education of staff about the correct use of flash sterilization is a critical aspect of a hospital's flash sterilization practices. This education should be based on the facility's clearly defined policies and procedures. Testing should be conducted and documented to assure that all staff members understand the written flash sterilization procedures. An annual education review is important, and the actual practice of flash sterilization in the Operating Room should be audited by a periodic quality assurance monitoring process as required by the policy.

POINT OF USE PROCESSING CONCERNS FOR HEAT-SENSITIVE DEVICES

Learning Objective 4. Review concerns about point-of-use processing of heat-sensitive medical devices.

The demand for less invasive surgical procedures is changing the nature of healthcare, and the trend from traditional "open" surgical operations to minimally invasive surgery (MIS) has been dramatic. Today, more than 20 million people annually undergo rigid and flexible endoscopic procedures, and the rate of change from traditional surgical operations to less invasive techniques for operative and diagnostic procedures is expected to increase.

The demand for MIS techniques has led to the development of more sophisticated, delicate, complex, and heat-sensitive medical devices. Reprocessing them presents many challenges for healthcare providers, including the risk of transmitting infection if they are not effectively decontaminated.

In addition to reprocessing challenges, the budgetary constraints that yield a typically limited inventory of expensive MIS devices must be balanced with the demand for surgical productivity and quick case turnover. As the number of daily procedures continues to rise without an increase in device inventory to match increased need, there is more use of and damage to the scopes, and repair costs increase as well. Tight budgets can also lead to staffing issues. As people work harder to accomplish "more with less," shortcuts are often taken, and steps may be skipped during reprocessing to save time. As pressures mount on the staff to keep up with an increasing patient load and to keep operating costs down, the demand for highly efficient reprocessing methods increases.

Selection of Processing System for Heat-Sensitive Devices

The selection of an appropriate reprocessing system or method for heat-sensitive devices depends on the:

- Resistance of microorganisms to the microbicidal process.
- Intended use of the device (for example, endoscopic procedures that only contact intact mucous membranes or open surgical procedures that invade the vascular system or a sterile body cavity).
- Device design such as complexity or delicacy that affects cleaning and reprocessing.
- Compatibility of the device's design and component materials with the reprocessing method.
- Time required for reprocessing.
- Method's ease of use.
- Safety of the process for patients, healthcare workers, and devices.
- Ability to monitor the process.
- Level of exposure to hazards caused by the process.
- Overall process costs.

In today's world of antibiotic-resistant organisms and life-threatening infections, healthcare professionals often prefer to sterilize devices instead of disinfecting them. The primary method of sterilization over the years has been steam, which has generally been used for stainless steel instruments. However, this is not typically an option for MIS devices because of the high temperatures needed for sterilization. Note: manufacturers are now developing instrumentation that can withstand the high steam sterilization temperatures because it is still viewed as the optimal method.

Ethylene oxide (EtO) has also been used for years to sterilize heat-sensitive devices, but its popularity continues to decline because of the long cycle times required for sterilization and aeration. Gas plasma sterilization methods continue to be tested and proven effective and compatible with more types of device designs and materials. However, the gas plasma process requires additional preparation time to thoroughly dry pre-cleaned devices before they can be prepared and wrapped for sterilization.

The selection of a disinfection or sterilization method is based on the intended use of a device. AORN and the Centers for Disease Control and Prevention (CDC) have developed recommendations based on Dr. E. H. Spaulding's classification of medical devices.[4] Items used for patient care are divided into three categories based on the degree of risk of infection:

- **Critical devices** – Instruments or objects introduced directly into the bloodstream or other normally sterile areas of the body.

Critical devices (Spaulding medical device classification system) – Instruments or objects introduced directly into the bloodstream or other normally sterile areas of the body.

Semi-critical devices (Spaulding medical device classification system) – Those which come in contact with non-intact skin or mucous membranes.

Non-critical devices (Spaulding medical device classification system) – Those that contact intact skin.

Examples are surgical instruments, cardiac catheters, and needles. Critical devices should undergo a sterilization procedure before each use that is recommended by the device's original equipment manufacturer.

- **Semi-critical devices** – These come in contact with non-intact skin or mucous membranes, where the risk of infection is less than with critical devices. Examples are non-invasive endoscopes, endotracheal tubes, anesthesia breathing circuits, and cystoscopes. Although these items come in contact with intact mucous membranes, they do not ordinarily penetrate body surfaces. It is desirable, but not absolutely essential, to sterilize many of these items. They should receive a minimum of high-level disinfection which should be expected to kill vegetative (growing) microorganisms, most fungal spores, tubercle bacilli, small or non-lipid viruses, and medium-sized or lipid viruses.

- **Non-critical devices** – These contact intact skin, and include blood pressure cuffs, crutches, bed boards, and other medical accessories. The risk of infection is low with these devices so they only require intermediate or low level disinfection or cleaning.

Reprocessing Options

The desire for faster turnover times to reprocess heat-sensitive devices led to the expanded use of high-level disinfection. While high-level disinfection kills most microorganisms, bacterial spores will not be eliminated without longer exposure times. Disinfectant manufacturers must include immersion times on label instructions, and times can vary depending on the type and temperature of disinfectant and the microorganisms to be killed. There is controversy about instrument soaking times in and proper temperatures of disinfection solutions, and this presents challenges to healthcare professionals.

One researcher has stated that the ideal disinfectant would:

- Provide high efficacy (high-level disinfection and sporicidal activity).

- Exhibit rapid activity.

- Assure material compatibility.

- Be non-toxic.

- Be non-staining.

- Provide monitoring capability.

- Be easy-to-use.

- Allow prolonged reuse.

- Provide long shelf life without loss of activity.

- Assure unrestricted disposal.[5]

There has been a dramatic shift from manual to automated processing. This removes much of the "human factor" and variability from the process, ensures a validated process with predictable outcomes, and helps to reduce instrument damage and repair costs. It also frees the staff to care for patients or to assume other tasks. Although these benefits are valued by all healthcare facilities, they can be critical for those operating with minimum staffing.

When selecting disinfection and/or sterilization methods, three priorities to consider are:

- Safety of the chemicals and the process for the patients, healthcare staff, instruments, and environment.

- Efficacy of the chemistries and the process, including the ability to prevent biofilm formation in an automatic reprocessor.

- Efficiency of the process. (Consider this factor after the first two priorities are addressed.).

OXIDATION PROCESSES FOR LOW-TEMPERATURE STERILIZATION

Learning Objective 5. Discuss the use of oxidative agents for low-temperature point of use processing.

The use of oxidative processes has increased for low-temperature processing as the technology gains acceptance and credibility. As decision-

makers gain a greater understanding of their benefits, reprocessing systems and methods using these compounds will continue to be developed and more widely used.

Background

Healthcare professionals must understand the chemistry, mode of action, efficacy, indications for use, process monitoring, and environmental safety of oxidative processes to best use them in healthcare environments. Oxidative processes are considered safe for patients, healthcare workers, instruments, and the environment, and they also discourage biofilm build-up.

Oxidation occurs when a **molecule, atom,** or **ion** loses an **electron. Oxidizing agents** remove electrons from another substance and, in the process, are also reduced. They do one of three things during a reaction: contribute oxygen, extract hydrogen, or extract electrons. Many persons associate the term, "oxidation," with "rusting." Rust can result from oxidation (iron forms iron oxide), but not all materials that interact with oxygen result in rust.

Oxidative chemistries include peroxygen compounds that contain an additional atom of oxygen bound to oxygen. They use oxidative reactions to interrupt cell functions of

Oxidation – *The process by which a molecule, atom, or ion loses an electron. The act or process of oxidizing, chemical breakdown of nutrients for energy.*

Molecule – *The smallest quantity of matter that can exist in a free state and retain all of its properties.*

Atom – *The fundamental unit of a chemical element.*

Ion – *An electronically-charged particle that is formed by the loss or gain of one or more electrons.*

Electron – *A negatively-charged particle that moves around the nucleus (central core) of an atom.*

Oxidizing agent – *A material that removes electrons from another substance.*

macromolecules (proteins, carbohydrates, lipids, and nucleic acids) within the microorganism. After these reactions occur, the microorganism dies. The mechanism of action is non-specific, but it involves the loss of the macromolecule structure and function.

Oxidative chemistries exhibit excellent cleaning, disinfecting, and sterilizing properties, and they are generally non-toxic. A simple example is hydrogen peroxide. When hydrogen peroxide breaks down it is converted into oxygen and water Hydrogen peroxide is a very good oxidative agent, and it can achieve either high-level disinfection or sterilization.

Peracetic acid (PA) is a liquid oxidizing agent that is an effective biocide (killer of microorganisms) at low temperatures. Its chemical formula is acetic acid (vinegar) plus an extra oxygen atom. This extra oxygen atom is highly reactive, and it interacts with most cell components to cause cell death. At relatively low concentrations (less than 1%), PA is an effective germicidal agent, and it is more potent than hydrogen peroxide. It is a weak acid that is germicidal in higher concentrations in the alkaline pH range. Combined with proper buffers and anti-corrosives, PA can safely disinfect or sterilize flexible scopes and other medical devices. It is sporicidal, tuberculocidal, fungicidal, virucidal, and bactericidal. It can be used for sterilization or high-level disinfection, depending on the exposure time, formulation, and labeled use.

In addition to its broad spectrum of antimicrobial activity, PA is highly water-soluble and free-rinsing. As with the other oxidizing agents, it is environmentally friendly, and its by-products (acetic acid, water, and oxygen) are not harmful. Unlike other oxidative chemistries, it is also very effective (superior to glutaraldehyde) in the presence of organic matter at low temperatures. Peracetic acid is also an effective agent against the formation of biofilm.

In several studies that compare alternative germicides, PA was found to be the most active against bacterial spores. When compared to a variety of disinfectants and sterilants, it was the most effective against a wide range of bacteria, mycobacteria, viruses, yeasts and fungi. Studies also show PA is more effective than hydrogen peroxide, formaldehyde, and glutaraldehyde.[6]

PA has traditionally been used in healthcare settings to sterilize rooms, equipment, hemodialyzers, and medical, surgical, and dental instruments. It has been used in a liquid chemical sterile processing system since 1988, and this system is in wide use

Ethylene Oxide and Oxidizing Technologies in Sterile Processing: What's the Difference?

In Chapter 16, you'll learn that ethylene oxide (EtO) is typically the sterilant of choice for heat sensitive items that cannot be reprocessed with steam. Why is EtO used in the Central Service department and peracetic acid (PA) used for this purpose for point of use processing in the operating room?

EtO and other processes used for low temperature sterilization are gas/vapor technologies used for terminal loads of wrapped items that can be stored for future use. PA technology involves a liquid, and processing is done immediately before use on unwrapped items such as rigid and flexible endoscopes and their parts and accessories. Since the processed items are wet, they cannot be stored for future use.

Oxidative chemistries – *A class of compounds that contain an additional atom of oxygen bound to oxygen and that uses oxidation to interrupt cell function.*

Macromolecules – *Large molecules (proteins, carbohydrates, lipids, and nucleic acids) within a microorganism.*

Peracetic acid (PA) – *A liquid oxidizing agent that is an effective biocide at low temperatures. It is increasingly used in a sterilization system that processes immersible diagnostic and surgical instruments, primarily flexible and rigid scopes. Items must be used immediately after sterilization because they are wet, and no method exists to store them.*

Ozone has also been used as a disinfectant and sterilant. It is a broad spectrum antimicrobial agent created with oxygen, water, and electricity. It is a very reactive oxidative gas that quickly and effectively deactivates microorganisms by denaturing cell membranes. Since oxygen and low humidity water vapor are the by-products of this process, it is environmentally friendly. However, because it is a rapid oxidizing agent, ozone can be harsh on some materials used in flexible endoscopes. For this reason, it is not in common use as an agent in point of use processing systems.

today. It allows healthcare workers to sterilize surgical and diagnostic instruments between patient procedures near the site of patient use. It is used for heat-sensitive devices that previously required high-level disinfection because of the inability to tolerate the high temperatures of steam sterilization.

Liquid Chemical Sterile Processing System

A liquid chemical sterile processing system using a tabletop microprocessor-controlled unit, a single-use cup of PA-based sterilant, and a variety of device trays and containers was patented and introduced in the late 1980's. The processor is automated and creates, monitors, and maintains the following conditions and functions. Criteria for sterilization are:

- Proper concentration level of buffers.

- Adequate dilution of sterilizing ingredient.

- Proper processing temperature (122°F - 133°F; 50°C – 56°C).

- Exposure time to the sterilant (12 minutes).

- Constant fluid circulation during sterilization and rinse cycles.

- Sterile filtration of incoming tap water by a verifiable sterile filtration membrane.

- Four sterile water rinses.

The processor has push button operation and an internal self-diagnostic and monitoring system that produces a printed strip to provide critical information during each cycle. The cycle will cancel if the microprocessor detects any unmet process parameter.

The active ingredient of the sterilant is 35% peracetic acid. The sterilant container also contains other ingredients in powdered form that buffer the sterilant to a nearly neutral pH, and contain corrosion inhibitors that protect the devices being sterilized. The sterilant and buffers are packaged separately in a single-use container to ensure safe handling. Single-use packaging of the sterilant and the automated creation of the proper dilution within the system ensures the optimal concentration of the sterilant with every cycle. The sterilant concentrate is not intended for reuse or for use in a manual open-pan sterilization system.

The processor accepts interchangeable trays and containers that hold many types of rigid or flexible devices, and ensures that the instruments are correctly positioned for processing. Cleaned and rinsed devices that have been correctly leak-tested are placed in the appropriate tray or container that is positioned in the processor. Several criteria must be met to place medical devices in the sterile processing system's trays and containers for processing:

- The device must easily fit into the tray or container.

- The device must be immersible.

- The device must withstand temperatures of up to 133°F (56°C).

- All device surfaces must come into contact with the use dilution.

Note: not all devices can be processed in this system even if they meet these criteria. Devices must be tested and validated by the manufacturer of this sterile processing system to assure successful sterile processing.

Devices with channels such as flexible endoscopes are attached to specific trays with special connectors that allow fluid to flow through the internal channels. A sterilant cup is placed in the processor. A cup cutter in the bottom of the sterilant compartment penetrates the bottom part of the outer cup to release the buffers during processing. An aspirator probe is inserted into the top of the sterilant cup, and the tubing is positioned appropriately so that the PA can be aspirated (removed by suction) from the cup during the process. The processor lid is then closed, the system is activated by pushing the start button, and microprocessor controls the processing.

The buffers mix with water to form the chemical protection system. The active ingredient (PA) is then brought into solution. The sterilant (PA and buffers) is automatically mixed with sterile water that is created by filtration within the processor to form the use dilution within the processor's chamber. The use dilution concentration of the PA is 0.2% with a pH of approximately 6.4. Sterilization takes place between 122°F - 133°F (50°C – 56°C) which is safe for most heat-sensitive devices.

The use dilution comes in contact with all accessible external and internal instrument surfaces. Exposure to the use dilution lasts for 12 minutes, and is followed by four sterile water rinses to remove any sterilant residue. The by-products of acetic acid (vinegar, water, and oxygen) are safely disposed of in the normal sanitary sewer system. The entire sterile processing cycle is completed in approximately 30 minutes. The sterilized devices are then removed from the system for immediate use. Processing trays and containers are available that incorporate tortuous (winding or crooked) pathways to protect sterile instruments from contamination during transport.

Process Monitoring

The sterilization process for the PA system just described is standardized with a microprocessor that continually detects and monitors various process parameters throughout every cycle. Process monitoring involves several dimensions.

Operator Observation and Interaction

Operators must understand how to observe and interact properly with any automated processing system to assure its optimal operation. With this system, the first step is to examine the sterilant container closely before placing it in the sterile processing unit. The appearance of the cup and packaging box should be checked prior to use to determine if the container has been compromised, is wet, has turned a bright yellow color, and/or has a strong vinegar-like odor (or feels light weight). The expiration date must be verified so that outdated chemicals are not used. The bottom part of the cup that contains the buffer powders should not be hardened. Note: sterilant boxes should be stored upright.

After placing the sterilant cup in the system, the aspirator probe must be properly positioned, and the tubing must be inspected for kinks that would prevent aspiration of the PA to form the use (proper) dilution. The operator should look through the system's window lid to confirm the presence of the use dilution and constant solution flow. At the end of the cycle, the sterilant cup should be checked to note the complete aspiration of the active ingredient. If fluid is noted in the cup, appropriate disposal methods must be employed according to the instructions, and the devices must be processed again if the chemical indicator has not turned to the appropriate color.

Parametric Monitoring

During the sterilization phase of the process, the system continually monitors and verifies the three critical process parameters including concentration (175 or greater), temperature (122°F - 133°F; 50°C -56°C) and exposure time (12 minutes). The sterilizer will cancel the process if these parameters are not met. Process parameters must be checked by the operator on the printout at the end of the cycle. Any "fault" messages or cycle cancellations will be documented on the printout. The sterile processing printouts provide an audit trail, and they can also be used to record the biological and chemical monitoring results.

Steris System 1 | chemical liquid Sterilizer – PA
Sterilant - low
temperature

Chemical Monitoring

Chemical indicators monitor the presence of the minimum necessary concentration of the active ingredient during the sterilization process. However, a chemical indicator does not guarantee load sterility; it only shows that an adequate amount of the active ingredient was present for sterilization to be achieved. The manufacturer recommends that a chemical indicator be included with each sterile processing cycle to verify the presence of the active ingredient. The single use chemical indicator strip is read (according to manufacturer's instructions), recorded, and then discarded.

Biological Monitoring

Biological monitoring consists of a test challenge compared to a control culture obtained from a live spore strip of Geobacillus stearothermophilus. The frequency of the testing will be determined by the healthcare facility's internal policy; however, a chemical indicator should be run with all biological testing. After appropriate incubation, the test challenge is compared with the control, and the results are recorded.

Diagnostic Cycle

The diagnostic cycle should be run every day the processor is used. The first phase of the diagnostic cycle tests the electrical, mechanical, pneumatic, and hydraulic systems. The second phase verifies the integrity of the sterile filter membrane. A failed diagnostic cycle prevents any attempt to use the sterilizer until the fault is corrected, and a successful diagnostic cycle is passed. Sterilant is not used when running a diagnostic cycle.

No Environmental Monitoring Needed

The operation of the sterile processing system being described requires no special air monitoring or engineering controls beyond the standard ventilation of 10 air exchanges/hour. Testing has shown that all ingredients of the PA-based sterilant fall well below airborne permissible limits to eliminate the need for monitoring.[7]

Toxicity and Residues

Toxicity evaluation of this system's sterilant concentrate and use dilution (sterilant concentrate mixed with water) was undertaken to determine the safety risks, if any, associated with human contact. The sterilant concentrate was found to be caustic to skin and eyes, but only moderately toxic if orally ingested. The sterilant concentrate package was designed to prevent operator exposure to the concentrate.

The use dilution underwent acute (short-term) oral and dermal (skin) toxicity testing and ocular (eye) irritation testing. The use dilution has a nearly neutral pH, is nontoxic by oral or dermal administration, and has no caustic effect to the skin. The amount of sterilant residue which may remain on medical devices after processing also was studied. After replicate sterilization cycles and exposures to use dilution and the sterile rinses, extracts were taken for study. No evidence was found that the cycles resulted in any cumulative increase in residue, and PA could not be detected.[8]

Limitations of Process

There are limitations with the liquid chemical sterilization process described above:

- Devices must be totally immersible so not all complex devices can be placed in the system.

- Devices must be able to withstand a temperature range of 122°F - 133°F (50°C 56°C) which can exclude some devices.

- Items are processed immediately before intended use so there is no shelf life for processed items.

- Items must fit easily in the sterilization containers and trays with no pinching or bending that would restrict flow.

- The sterilant must make contact with all internal and external surfaces of the device.

- Not all devices have been validated by the system's manufacturer for processing in this system.

High-Level Disinfection Using Oxidizing Chemistries

Several manufacturers have recently released automatic endoscope reprocessors into the healthcare marketplace that utilize a high-level disinfectant with a mechanical process. These reprocessors represent a new generation technology because traditional high-level disinfection has essentially involved a soaking process. They are economical, easy-to-use high-level disinfection systems that incorporate safety for staff and patients as a priority. The new technology includes such features as:

- Minimal requirements for attaching tubing to endoscope ports and channels.

- Oxidizing chemistry generated within the processor itself to avoid employee exposure to chemicals.

- Process indicators to verify that an effective dose of high-level disinfectant solution was generated within the chamber during the cycle.

- A method for actuating suction valves for complete high level disinfection solution.

- A printer to document every cycle and verify critical process parameters.

- Single or dual scope reprocessing capabilities.

- Optional wash phases to supplement manual cleaning.

- Real-time cycle status and audible alarms.

- A barcode scanner for positive identification on cycle printout.

- Automated thermal and chemical self-decontamination cycles to help prevent biofilm from forming in the processor.

Oxidizing compounds continue to be applied for new disinfection and sterilization technologies, and this underscores their safety and value for infection control and human health.

ENDNOTES

1. *ANSI/AAMI. Comprehensive Guide to Steam Sterilization and Sterility Assurance in Healthcare Facilities. American National Standard ST 79. Association for the Advancement of Medical Instrumentation. Arlington, VA. 2006.*

2. *AORN Recommended Practices and Guidelines. Recommended Practices for Sterilization in peri-Operative Practice Settings. Association of periOperative Nurses. Denver, CO. 2006.*

3. *The Joint Commission, Accreditation Manual for Hospitals, Joint Commission, Oakbrook Terrace, IL, The Joint Commission, 2006.*

4. *ANSI/AAMI ST79:2006, "Comprehensive Guide to Steam Sterilization and Sterility in Healthcare Facilities".*

5. *Rutala, W. and Weber, D. Disinfection and Sterilization in Health Care Facilities: What Clinicians Need to Know. Healthcare Epidemiology. Sept. 2004.*

6. *Rahl, R. Choosing Between Dialdehydes and Peracetic Acid Chemistries for Endoscope Reprocessing. EndoNurse, Vol. 4, No. 3. June/July, 2004. (pp 36-38).*

7. *Springthorpe, S. Disinfection of Surfaces and Equipment. Journal of Canadian Dental Association 66. 2000. (pp.558-560)*

8. *Stein, Barry L., MD, Lamoureux, Esther, MD, Miller, Mark, MD, Vasilevsky, Carol-Ann, MD, Julien, Lynne, RN, Gordon, Philip H. MD, "Glutaraldehyde-induced Colitis," Canadian Journal of Surgery, April 2001; 44(2): 113-116.*

REFERENCES

Flash Sterilization. Steris Video Library. Steris Corporation. 2001.

Alfa, M, DeGagne, P, and Olson, N. Comparison of Liquid Chemical Sterilization with Peracetic Acid and Ethylene Oxide Sterilization for Long Narrow Lumens, American Journal of Infection Control Vol. 26. 1988. (pp 469-77)

Surgery in Transition. Surgical Services Management Vol. 4, No 1. January 1998. (p. 56)

Hewitt, A. Infection Control Challenges with Endoscopic Instruments. Endo Nurse. Oct/Nov, 2002.

Rutala, W. and Weber, D. Disinfection and Sterilization in Health Care Facilities: What Clinicians Need to Know. Healthcare Epidemiology. Sept, 2004.

Bierman, S. Biofilm: Secret Refuge of the Microbial World. Infection Control Today Vol. 7, No.12. 2005.

Dix, K., Chemical Sterilants Revolutionize Decontamination. Infection Control Today Vol. 7, No.12. 2003.

Fukunaga, K. and Khatibi, A. Glutaraldehyde Colitis: A Complication of Screening Flexible Sigmoidoscopy in the Primary Care Setting. Annals of Internal Medicine Vol. 133, No. 4. 2000. (p 315)

McDonnell, G. Peroxygens and Other Forms of Oxygen: Their Use for Effective Cleaning, Disinfection and Sterilization. PacifiChem 2005. USA Symposium # 50: Biocides Old and New: Where Chemistry and Microbiology Meet. Honolulu, Hawaii, December 15-20, 2005.

Momba, M., et al. An Overview of Biofilm Formation in Distribution Systems and its Impact on the Deterioration of Water Quality. Water SA Vol. 26, No.1. 2000. (pp. 59-66)

Nelson, D. Recent Advances in Epidemiology and Prevention of Gastrointestinal Endoscopy Related Infections. Current Options in Infectious Diseases Vol. 18, No.4. 2005. (pp. 326-330)

Pollick, M. WiseGEEK 2006. http//www.WiseGEEK.com.

Rahl, R. Choosing Between Dialdehydes and Peracetic Acid Chemistries for Endoscope Reprocessing. EndoNurse Vol. 4, No.3. June/July, 2004. (pp. 36-38)

Shuster, L. ACG: Glutaraldehyde-Induced Colitis in Patient Undergoing Routine Screening Colonoscopy, October, 2003. (http://www.pslgroup.com/dg/221452.htm)

Rook, T. and McDonnell, G. Efficacy of Biocides Against a Pseudomonas aeruginosa Biofilm within a Simulated Device Lumen, Presented at the 101st. American Society of Microbiology General Meeting. Orlando, FL, May 20-24, 2001.

Customer Technical Information Bulletin. User Vapor Exposure and the Steris Process. Steris Corporation, 1997.

Technical Briefs. Disposal of Steris 20 Use Dilution. Toxicity of Liquid Chemical Sterilants and Disinfectants at their Use Dilution. Steris Corporation, 1997.

CENTRAL SERVICE TERMS

Point of use processing

Flash sterilization

Porous

Class 5 (chemical integrators)

Pounds per square inch gauge (psig)

Critical devices (Spaulding medical device classification system)

Semi-critical devices (Spaulding medical device classification system)

Non-critical devices (Spaulding medical device classification system)

Oxidation

Molecule

Atom

Ion

Electron

Oxidizing agent

Oxidative chemistries

Macromolecules

Peracetic acid (PA)

Chapter Outline

FACTORS THAT IMPACT STERILIZATION

- Important Factors for Sterilization
- Methods of Heat Transfer associated with high temperature sterilization

ADVANTAGES OF STEAM STERILIZATION

ANATOMY OF A STEAM STERILIZER

- Components of Steam Sterilizers

TYPES OF STEAM STERILIZERS

- Table Top Sterilizers
- Gravity Air Displacement Sterilizers
- Dynamic Air Removal Sterilizers
- Steam-Flush Pressure-Pulse Sterilizers
- Special Purpose Sterilizers (Flash)
- Special Purpose Sterilizers (Instrument Washer Sterilizers)

STEAM STERILIZER CYCLE PHASES

- Conditioning
- Exposure
- Exhaust
- Drying

CONDITIONS NECESSARY FOR EFFECTIVE STEAM STERILIZATION

- Contact
- Temperature
- Time
- Moisture

BASIC WORK PRACTICES FOR STEAM STERILIZATION

- Preparing Devices and Packs for Steam Sterilization
- Loading a Sterilizer
- Unloading a Sterilizer
- Controlling Wet Packs
- Cleaning and Maintaining Sterilizers

DRY HEAT STERILIZATION

- When Dry Heat is Appropriate
- Advantages and Disadvantages
- Types of Hot-Air Convection Sterilizers
- Dry Heat Sterilization Procedures

Chapter 15
High Temperature Sterilization

QUALITY CONTROL CONCERNS

- Need for Quality Control
- Chemical Indicators
- Sterilization Load Control Information
- Physical (Mechanical) Monitoring
- Biological Indicators
- Details About Process Control Devices
- Bowie Dick Tests
- Validation and Verification

SPECIAL HIGH TEMPERATURE STERILIZATION CONCERNS

- D-Values and Sterilization Effectiveness
- Creutzfeldt - Jakob Disease (CJD)
- Solutions

ENDNOTES

CENTRAL SERVICE TERMS

Chapter Learning Objectives:

As a result of successfully completing this chapter, readers will be able to:

1. Discuss factors that impact the effectiveness of sterilization and the methods of heat transfer associated with high temperature sterilization.

2. Discuss the advantages of steam sterilization.

3. Explain the anatomy of a steam sterilizer and identify the function of each major component.
   - Sizes of steam sterilizers
   - Components of Steam Sterilizers

4. Provide basic information about the types of steam sterilizers.
   - Table Top
   - Gravity Air Displacement
   - Dynamic Air Removal
   - Steam-Flush Pressure-Pulse
   - Special Purpose Sterilizers (Flash)
   - Special Purpose Sterilizer (Instrument Washer Sterilizer)

5. Provide basic information about the phases in a steam sterilizer cycle:
   - Conditioning
   - Exposure
   - Exhaust
   - Drying

6 Describe the conditions necessary for an effective steam sterilization process:
   - Contact
   - Temperature
   - Time
   - Moisture

7. Explain basic work practices for steam sterilization:
   - Preparing devices and packs for steam sterilization
   - Loading a sterilizer
   - Unloading a sterilizer
   - Controlling wet packs
   - Cleaning and maintaining sterilizers

8. Explain the basics of dry heat sterilization:
   - When dry heat is appropriate
   - Advantages and disadvantages

   - Types of hot-air convection sterilizers
   - Dry heat sterilization procedures

9. Explain the need for quality control and review sterilization process indicators that help assure quality control:
   - Need for quality control
   - Chemical indicators
   - Sterilization load control information
   - Physical and mechanical monitoring
   - Biological indicators
   - Process challenge devices
   - Bowie-Dick tests
   - Validation and Verification processes

10. Review the basics of three special high temperature sterilization concerns:
    - D-values and sterilization effectiveness
    - Creutzfeldt-Jakob disease (CJD)
    - Solutions

High temperature (thermal) sterilization is the sterilization process of choice in healthcare facilities, and is achieved by subjecting items being processed to thermal energy from moist heat (steam) or dry heat. High temperature sterilization has long been recognized as an effective way to kill microorganisms. Steam sterilization is the most frequently used sterilant for devices not adversely affected by moisture or heat because of its successful record of safety, effectiveness, reliability, and low cost. In fact, other methods are only used when the object being reprocessed cannot withstand the heat and/or moisture required for steam sterilization. By contrast, dry heat sterilization is seldom used because of the required lengthy exposure times. The proper use of both dry and moist heat methods are discussed in this chapter.

As with all sterilization methods, devices to be processed must first be thoroughly cleaned, decontaminated, and properly prepared. Cleaning involves the removal of all visible soil, and decontamination kills most, but not all, microorganisms. Sterilization is required to kill any remaining microorganisms.

Bioburden – *The number of microorganisms on a contaminated object; also called bioload, or microbial load.*

FACTORS THAT IMPACT STERILIZATION

Learning Objective 1. Discuss factors that impact the effectiveness of sterilization and methods of heat transfer associated with high temperature sterilization processes.

The success of every sterilization process is not guaranteed. Several factors and conditions impact the effectiveness of sterilization, and they are the introductory topics in this chapter.

Important Factors for Sterilization

The effectiveness of all sterilization methods can be affected by several factors:

- The type of microorganisms present. Some microorganisms are more resistant to the sterilization process than others.

- The number of microorganisms (**bioburden**) present. More microorganisms on a medical device make the sterilization process more difficult.

Methods of Heat Transfer Associated with High Temperature Sterilization

Heat Transmission

High temperature sterilization depends upon the transfer of heat: an energy exchange between the sterilizing agent and the object being sterilized. Heat transfer can be accomplished three ways.

Type of Heat Transfer	Description	Sterilization Method
Conduction (solids)	Transmission of heat from one part to another part of a material. Example: transfer of heat from one end of a metal bar to the other end of the bar. (**Figure 15.1** illustrates conduction heating.)	Dry heat
Convection (liquids and gases)	Transfer of heat from one point (or one molecule) to another as the liquid or gas circulates. (**Figure 15.2** illustrates the transfer of energy from steam to an object and the condensation that occurs when the steam loses some of its heat in the process.)	Steam
Radiation	Transfer of heat from one object to another without warming the space between the objects (Example: from the sun to the earth).	Radiation (not used in hospitals)

Disengage — Shut down!

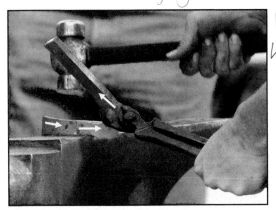

Figure 15.1 Conduction Heating

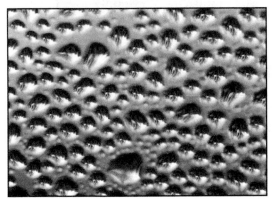

Figure 15.2 Condensation from the Heat Transfer of Steam

- The amount and type of soil present. Soil acts as a shield to protect microorganisms.

- The amount of protection the medical device provides. Microorganisms can be protected by cracks and crevices of the device and by its design.

The last three factors above are influenced by cleaning, a process that is absolutely essential as a first step in processing. As you have learned in earlier chapters, "You can clean without sterilizing, but you can never sterilize without cleaning."

The following pages will examine the two types of high temperature sterilization processes used by hospitals, Steam and Dry Heat.

ADVANTAGES OF STEAM STERILIZATION

Learning Objective 2. Discuss the advantages of steam sterilization.

Steam sterilization is the most commonly used type of sterilization in healthcare facilities. It has a long history as the sterilant of choice for a wide variety of items. Steam sterilization has long been preferred because:

- It is low cost. *= Electricity + Water*

- Sterilization cycles are fast. *= steam*

- It is a relatively simple technology. *= ETO*

- It leaves no chemical residues or by-products behind.

Steam sterilizers date back to the early days of formalized healthcare. Prior to steam sterilization boiling water was commonly used to kill bacteria. Scientists recognized the need to increase temperatures beyond the boiling point to kill greater numbers of heat resistant bacteria. **Figure 15.3** is an illustration of the first pressure steam sterilizer (autoclave) that was developed in 1880 by Charles Chamberlain, a colleague of Louis Pasteur. It resembled a pressure cooker and was able to use pressurized steam to reach temperatures of 120°C and higher. Although it looks primitive by today's standards, it was the first generation of the steam sterilizers used today.

Today's steam sterilizers come in many sizes, and they offer several cycle selections that allow Central

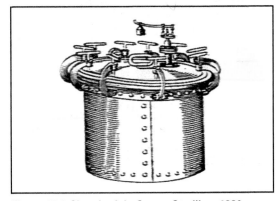

Figure 15.3 Chamberlain Steam Sterilizer 1880

Service Technicians to customize sterilization cycles to the specific items being sterilized. This chapter will explore commonly used steam sterilizers, sterilization cycles, and good work practices for preparing items for steam sterilization and using steam sterilization processes.

ANATOMY OF A STEAM STERILIZER

Learning Objective 3. Explain the anatomy of a steam sterilizer and identify the function of each major component.
- Jacket
- Door, Gasket, and Chamber Drain
- Thermostatic Trap
- Gauges and Controls

Steam sterilizer come in many sizes and offer several cycle choices from small Table top sterilizers that are used primarily in clinic and dental settings (See **Figure 15.4**) to mid-sized (See **Figure 15.5**) and large units (See **Figure 15.6**) designed to sterilize large quantities of items.

Just as doctors must understand the anatomy of patients, a Central Service Technician must understand the anatomy of a sterilizer to better understand how it operates.

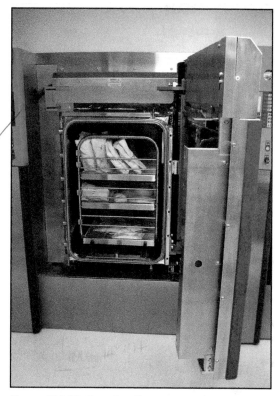

Figure 15.5 Medium Sterilizer

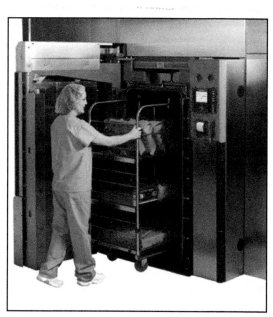

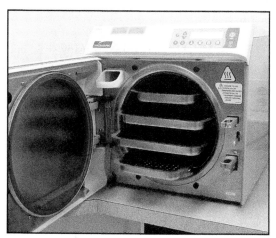

Figure 15.4 Table Top Sterilizer

Figure 15.6 Large Steam Sterilizer

Components of Steam Sterilizers

Jacket

Sterile Processing Departments in hospitals typically use jacket sterilizers, and the illustration in **Figure 15.7** shows a cutaway diagram of a steam sterilizer and illustrates how steam from an external source enters the jacket. In most hospitals, steam is supplied to the sterilizers from a main steam line; the units themselves do not generate the steam. Smaller sterilizers in clinics and dental practices usually manufacture their own steam or get their steam from an independent generator.

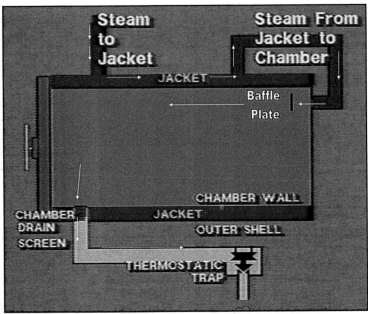

Figure 15.7 Sterilizer Jacket

The interior chamber walls of the sterilizer are heated by steam in the metal jacket to help minimize the amount of condensation that occurs when hot steam contacts the chamber walls as a cycle begins. The jacket surrounds the sides, top, and bottom of the vessel, and steam circulates in this space to preheat the walls.

The outside of the jacket is covered with insulation (See **Figure 15.8**) to help prevent condensation from forming on the jacket's outer and inner walls. This insulation also provides a safety feature: personnel working behind the sterilizer will not be burned. The outer shell is typically located behind a wall, and is not readily visible to the sterilizer technician.

Door, Gasket, and Chamber Drain

The door is the weakest part on a steam sterilizer. It has a safety locking mechanism that automatically activates when chamber pressure is applied, and it can only be unlocked when pressure is exhausted. The door can be tightened, but not loosened, while the chamber is under pressure.

The door gasket is designed to maintain a tight seal that prevents steam from escaping from the chamber, and air from entering the chamber. (See **Figure 15.9**)

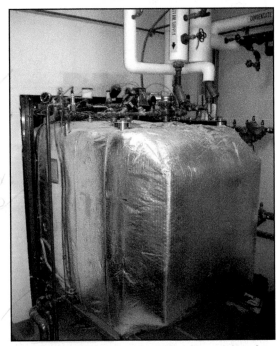

Figure 15.8 Insulation surrounding the exterior of a steam sterilizer.

The chamber drain is located at the front or center of the floor of most types of steam sterilizers and must be cleaned at least daily. (See **Figure 15.10**)

If Clogged you'll get wet packs wet instruments ect.

Thermostatic Trap

As seen in **Figure 15.11**, the thermostatic trap is located in the drain line. The drain and the area surrounding it are the coolest place in the sterilizer. A sensor in the trap measures steam temperature, and automatically controls the flow of air and condensate from the sterilizing chamber.

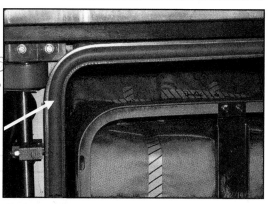

Figure 15.9 Door Gasket

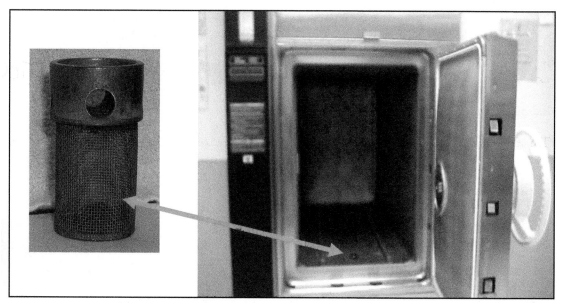

Figure 15.10 Chamber Drain

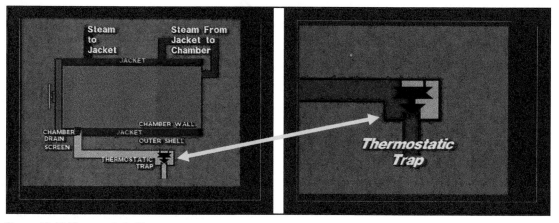

Figure 15.11 Thermostatic Trap

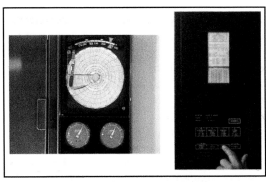

Figure 15.12 Gauges, Controls, and Monitors Provide a Visual and Written Record of Sterilizer Cycles

Gauges and Controls (Monitors)

The sterilizer's gauges and/or controls (monitors) provide a visual and written record of sterilization conditions. (See **Figure 15.12**) Central Service Technicians must check them throughout the sterilization cycle to assure that necessary parameters are met.

A simple printout from a steam sterilization cycle usually contains the following information:

• Date and time the cycle began.

• Selected cycle parameters and activities such as type of cycle, sterilization temperature, and dry times.

• A written record of actual cycle activities (i.e. temperatures, exposure times, pressures).

Older steam sterilizers have round charts that record sterilization activities. Charts are changed daily, and the time listed on the chart is the chart's location. The date is noted, and the pens are checked daily to assure they are recording.

Charts or printouts should be initialed by the Central Service Technicians responsible for cycle monitoring and, if all sterilization parameters were met, the load may be released. If any steam sterilization parameter was unmet, the supervisor should be notified immediately, and the sterilization load should not be released.

TYPES OF STEAM STERILIZERS

Learning Objective 4. Provide basic information about the types of steam sterilizers.
- Table Top
- Gravity Air Displacement
- Dynamic Air Removal
- Steam Flush and Pressure Pulse
- Special Purpose Sterilizer (Flash)
- Special Purpose Sterilizer (Instrument Washer Sterilizer)

There are several types of steam sterilizers available today. Healthcare facilities usually purchase sterilizers that will meet their specific needs (i.e. chamber size, style, and available cycle options).

Table Top Sterilizers — Dentist Offices

Table top sterilizers are a type of gravity air displacement sterilizer frequently used in clinics and dentists' offices. They are relatively simple, and are essentially horizontal pressure cookers. Water is poured into the sterilizer either through a port (See **Figure 15.13**) or the bottom of the chamber, and is electrically heated until it turns to steam. The steam rises to the chamber's top and, as more steam is produced, air is forced out through the drain near the bottom of the chamber, and the steam enters the drain. Then a thermally-operated valve closes which causes the steam to build-up pressure until the operating temperature (normally 121°C [250°F]) is reached. The timer can than be activated. At the end of the cycle, the relief valve is opened to allow the steam to escape.

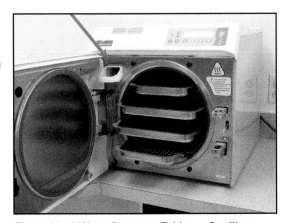

Figure 15.13 Water Port on a Tabletop Sterilizer

Normally, the steam passes through the water reservoir where it condenses back to water, and does not enter into the room. After the gauge pressure has dropped to zero, the door can be opened, and devices can be removed after they have cooled. Note: packages should cool first since steam may still be escaping, and may cause wet packs if articles are placed on a cool table or shelf.

As with all sterilizers, Central Service Technicians should carefully review the sterilizer manufacturer's operator's manual for specific operating instructions.

are Flash Sterilizer, Bowie Dick Test done

Gravity Air Displacement Sterilizers

Small-to-medium sized gravity air displacement sterilizers are used in hospitals, outpatient clinics, and Central Service and/or sub-sterile rooms. These units create steam in the presence of air. Hot air is introduced which rises to the top forcing cooler air to the bottom of the chamber and out the drain, while dynamic air removal units eliminate air during the preconditioning phase with pressure and vacuum pulses. While their operation appears simple, many mistakes can be (and frequently are) made. Therefore, a thorough knowledge of sterilization theory and practice is essential for those operating these units. These sterilizers have sophisticated automatic controls such as temperature-indicating charts and printouts (for recordkeeping). They also feature carriage loading tracks, and an in-house steam supply and drain.

Gravity air displacement sterilizers can be used to sterilize liquids. Note: Sterilization of solutions is discussed later in this chapter. This requires special procedures using a slow exhaust cycle with the potential for personal injury. The sterilizer manufacturer's written instructions must be strictly followed. Current FDA requirements specify "Not for Patient Use" labeling for the liquid cycle.

Dynamic Air Removal Sterilizers

Dynamic air removal sterilizers are very similar in construction to gravity air displacement sterilizers

except that a vacuum pump or water ejector removes the air during the preconditioning phase prior to reaching the exposure temperature. This reduces the total cycle time, and adds a level of sterility assurance by providing a series of pulses where a vacuum is drawn followed by pressure pulses during a preconditioning phase. During the cycle complete phase, filtered air is admitted.

Dynamic air removal sterilizers usually operate at higher temperatures (270°F–275°F [132°C–135°C]) than gravity sterilizers. The pre-conditioning phase increases the speed of operation, and reduces the chance of air pockets in the chamber during the cycle. To assure the actual removal of air in these sterilizers, the integrity of the sterilizers should be checked daily by processing a Bowie-Dick (or Daily Air Removal) test. Additionally, some manufacturers provide an automatic cycle (Vacuum Leak Test) to test the vacuum tightness of the chamber. Note: Bowie-Dick tests are discussed later in this chapter.

No Vacuum or Bowie-Dick Test

Steam-Flush Pressure-Pulse Sterilizers

Steam-flush pressure-pulse (SFPP) sterilizers use a repeated sequence of a steam flush and a pressure pulse to remove air from the sterilizing chamber and processed materials. Air removal occurs above atmospheric pressure; no vacuum is required. Vacuum pulsing is not used because a series of steam pressure pulses force air out the drain in a manner similar to that of air removal systems. Like a pre-vacuum sterilizer, this process rapidly removes air from the sterilizer's chamber and wrapped items. Unlike the pre-vacuum sterilizer, the steam-flush pressure-pulse process is not susceptible to air leaks, so Bowie-Dick type testing is not required with this process.

Special Purpose Pressure Sterilizers (Flash)

Flash sterilizers and instrument washers – sterilizers are examples of special purpose pressure sterilizers.

→ Final Processing – wrapped, in containers.

in SPD Departments. Flash + terminal sterilization

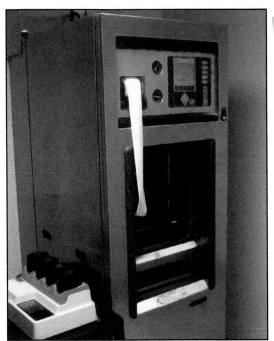

Figure 15.14 Flash Sterilizer

[handwritten: ✗ nonporous - not being able to absorbe.]

Flash Sterilizers

Flash sterilizers (See **Figure 15.14**) are often found in operating rooms or surgical suite sub-

sterile rooms, Labor and Delivery and Special Procedures areas that perform invasive procedures. Their intended use is for the emergency sterilization of instruments when there is not time for terminal sterilization. (A detailed discussion of Flash Sterilization was included in Chapter 14.)

Instrument Washer-Sterilizers

Instrument washer sterilizers (IWSs) (See **Figure 15.15**) may be found in the Central Service decontamination area, adjacent to operating rooms, or in clinics and surgery centers. They are combination units that wash and sterilize instruments. Their most frequent use is to decontaminate instruments placed into the sterilizer prior to cleaning. An IWS usually floods the chamber with cold water to prevent proteins from setting on the instruments. The machine goes through a mechanical cycle to wash away particulate matter. The water is then drained, one or more rinses are flushed through the chamber, and a sterilization cycle then occurs. NOTE: An IWS decontaminates instruments to ensure the safety of the personnel, but it does not provide a terminal sterilization cycle for immediate patient use.

Minimum Cycle Times For Gravity-Displacement Steam Sterilization Cycles*				
Item	Exposure time at 250°F (121°C)	Exposure time at 270°F (132° C)	Exposure time at 275°F (135°C)	Drying times
Unwrapped nonporous items e.g. instruments		3 minutes	3 minutes	0-1 minutes
Unwrapped nonporous items e.g. instruments		10 minutes *[handwritten: ex: lumens]*	10 minutes	0-1 minutes
*This table represents the variation in sterilizer manufacturers' recommendations for exposure at different temperatures. Consult the manufacturer's recommendations for the specific sterilizer that is used.				

Flash sterilizer – A sterilizer that uses higher temperatures for shorter exposure times to handle emergency sterilization of dropped instruments.

Instrument washer sterilizer (IWS) – Combination units that wash and sterilize instruments to insure the safety of processing personnel..

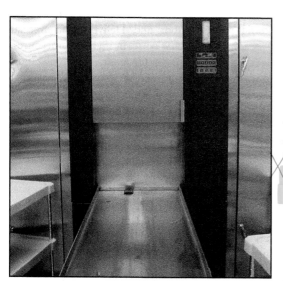

Figure 15.15 Instrument Washer-Sterilizer

STEAM STERILIZER CYCLE PHASES

Learning Objective 5. Provide basic information about the phases of a steam sterilizer cycle.
• Conditioning
• Exposure
• Exhaust
• Drying

Along with understanding the types of steam sterilizers used in the healthcare facility, Central Service Technicians must also understand how those machines function.

To begin, Central Service Technicians should be familiar with two basic sterilization cycles: **Flash Sterilization** and **Terminal Sterilization**. Flash sterilization involves sterilizing an item that is not packaged. The equipment to do so is called a "flash sterilizer," and is located in the Surgery, Labor and Delivery, Special Procedures, as well as other departments performing invasive procedures. (A detailed discussion of flash sterilization was

Flash Sterilization – *The process of sterilizing an item that is not packaged.* (unwrapped)

Terminal Sterilization – *The process of sterilizing an item that is packaged.* (wrapped)

must be dry.

covered in Chapter 14.) By contrast, "terminal sterilization" refers to sterilizing an item that is packaged. Terminal sterilization, is most often performed in the Central Service department and may be performed in other departments.

The following discussion will focus on the basic components of a steam sterilization cycle.

A saturated steam sterilization cycle has at least three, and possibly four, phases:

• Conditioning.

• Exposure.

• Exhaust.

• Drying (in most instances).

In order to be successful, steam sterilization relies on the removal of air from the sterilizer chamber so that steam can enter and make direct contact with the items being sterilized. Steam sterilizers are often defined by the method by which that air is removed. Air can leave the sterilizer chamber passively (through a natural displacement process where steam displaces the air in the chamber) or actively (through the use of a mechanical air removal system). These methods of air removal identify the basic types of saturated steam sterilizers used in healthcare settings today:

• Gravity air displacement sterilizers ("gravity") (passive air removal).

• Pre-vacuum steam sterilizers ("pre-vac") (active air removal).

• Steam Flush Pressure – Pulse (SFPP) (active air removal).

Conditioning

At the beginning of the sterilization cycle, the sterilizer's door is closed and the machine is started. The door's gasket forms and maintains a tight seal to prevent steam from escaping, or air from entering. Steam enters at the upper back portion of the sterilizer, and strikes a baffle plate to prevent the steam from directly hitting the load. As steam enters, air is displaced through the drain.

Exposure

As steam continues to enter the sterilizer's chamber that is now a closed space, the pressure begins to rise as does the steam temperature. After the desired temperature is reached, the sterilizer's control system begins timing the cycle's exposure phase. The cycles selected are typically the standard sterilization time and temperatures because they have been shown by scientific validation to kill all microorganisms.

Exhaust

At the end of the exposure phase, the chamber's drain is opened, and the steam is removed through the discharge line. This creates a slight chamber vacuum,

and sterile, filtered air is gradually re-introduced into the chamber through a special filter. The chamber gradually returns to atmospheric temperature (normal chamber temperature), and steam and water are discharged through the discharge line. The discharge line empties to a drain funnel that has chorgrill or wadded wire which causes steam to condense to water that will drain out of the sterilizer. Sterilizer drain systems have a space of approximately 2 – 3 inches between the discharge line and drain funnel to the floor drain that helps prevent a drain back-up into the sterilizer.

The diagrams below provide illustrations of the process.

Figure 15.16 shows (in red), steam entering the chamber, and air is being displaced (in green) down the chamber's drain.

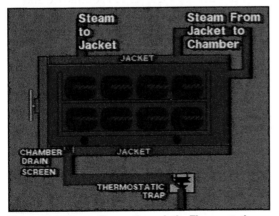

Figure 15.16 Steam Enters the Chamber

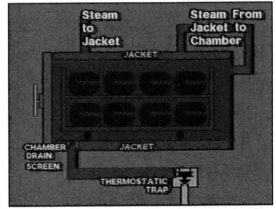

Figure 15.18 Closed Thermostatic Trap

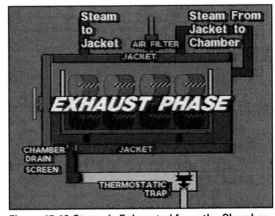

Figure 15.17 Steam Passes through the Thermostatic

Figure 15.19 Steam is Exhausted from the Chamber

Figure 15.17 shows (in red), steam that has passed the chamber drain screen, and is going past the thermostatic trap.

Figure 15.18 shows (in red), the thermostatic trap being closed after the desired temperature is reached.

Figure 15.19 shows (in red) steam being exhausted from the sterilizer.

Drying

Drying begins at the conclusion of exhaust phase if packaged items are in the load. Otherwise, the load contents will be wet and considered contaminated. The drying process uses the heat of the chamber walls as well as heated, filtered fresh air to re-vaporize any liquid water, and to remove it from the load and chamber. At the end of this dry time, the end-of-the-cycle signal sounds, and the door may be opened.

FoR Point-of-use only

Flash sterilization cycles have a minimal drying time and in some cases no drying time at all.

Not Steril Storage.

Always follow operating manual instructions that discuss mechanical monitors to assure that sterilization parameters are met.

CONDITIONS NECESSARY FOR EFFECTIVE STEAM STERILIZATION

Learning Objective 6. Describe the conditions necessary for an effective steam sterilization process:
- Contact
- Time
- Temperature
- Moisture

No matter what type of steam sterilization is used, there are some requirements that are universal to the steam sterilization process.

Steam sterilization requires four conditions: contact, temperature, time, and moisture. These conditions are discussed in order of their importance.

Contact

The most frequent reason for sterilization failure is the lack of contact between steam and the microorganisms on the entire surface of the device being sterilized. This failure may be related to human error or mechanical malfunction. Frequent causes of steam contact failure include:

- **Failure to adequately clean the object being sterilized.** Any coating of soil such as protein or oils can protect the microorganisms from direct steam contact.

- **Packages wrapped too tightly.** Air and steam do not mix readily. Air is heavier than steam, and it is displaced to the sterilizer's bottom or dynamically removed by means of a mechanical air removal system, before it is forced out through the drain. This must occur before the steam can enter, fill all spaces, and sufficiently raise the temperature for effective sterilization. If packs are wrapped too tightly, air becomes trapped and cannot escape. It then forms cool air pockets within the packages, and prevents temperatures from rising to a level sufficient for sterilization.

- **Loads that are too crowded.** Packs must be arranged with adequate spacing on the cart. If they are packed too tightly, air may be entrapped and steam may not be able to penetrate into all areas.

- **Containers that are positioned incorrectly.** Basins and other items that can hold water must be positioned so that air can be removed and water (condensed steam) can flow out. When sterilizing bottles, or other airtight containers, tops must be removed, and containers should be placed on their sides. If the containers are placed upright, air cannot be displaced, and will be trapped in them.

- **Clogged drain strainer.** Most sterilizers have a small drain strainer at the bottom of the chamber to keep lint, tape (the most frequent cause of clogged drain strainers), and other small objects from entering the exhaust line.

• Other mechanical malfunctions. Other problems such as defective steam traps, clogged exhaust lines and similar mechanical malfunctions can occur, and cannot be repaired by a Central Service Technician. A qualified service representative is needed to make repairs as specified in the sterilizer manufacturer's service manual.

Most sterilization failures are caused by human error, and can be prevented by Central Service Technicians who know how to avoid these problems.

Temperature

In order to be effective, steam sterilization must take place at specific temperatures. These temperatures are needed to kill heat resistant bacteria. The two most commonly encountered temperatures for steam sterilization are 250°F (121°C) and 270°F - 275°F (132.2°C - 134°C).

Time —4 min.

The steam sterilization process can only be effective if all items within the load are exposed to the elevated temperatures and steam contact (moisture) for an adequate amount of time. Inadequate sterilization exposure times can lead to failure of the sterilization process.

A certain amount of time is needed to kill microorganisms, and some microorganisms are harder to kill than others. However, the higher the temperature, the less time that is required to kill any specific organism.

Time and Temperature Relationship

Steam sterilization cycles are based upon the time-temperature relationship required to destroy bacterial spores. As water is heated, its temperature rises, and the volume of the water increases slightly. When boiling begins, the volume increases greatly, and the temperature remains constant. As boiling continues, all of the water changes to steam, the volume continues to increase and, with continued heating, the temperature rises. If this heating is done in a closed vessel, the steam generated will be at a much higher temperature because the volume is fixed; it cannot increase.

Moisture

Dry saturated steam is mandatory for effective steam sterilization. **Saturated steam** is like a fog because it holds many tiny water droplets in suspension. The moisture content of saturated steam should possess a relative humidity (r.h.) of 97% to 100%. Said another way, ideally steam should consist (by weight) of two-three parts of saturated water and 97-98 parts of dry, saturated steam.

Saturated steam is similar to air with 100% relative humidity. When saturated steam cools, water condenses as a liquid. Saturated steam has another important property which is important to understand for the operation of steam sterilizers. The pressure exerted by saturated steam is constant for a given temperature, and varies in direct proportion to that temperature; in other words, the higher the temperature, the higher the pressure, and the reverse is also true. Examples: to increase the temperature of steam, pressure must be increased; to decrease the temperature of steam, pressure must be decreased. The pressure involved in this relationship is absolute pressure exerted by the steam.

Figures 15.20 and **15.21** show this time and temperature relationship. This data represents the minimum sterilizer cycles recommended by the Association for Advancement of Medical Instrumentation (AAMI), and are used because of their history of producing efficient productivity with few errors.[1]

Central Service Technicians are concerned about the temperature and pressure within the

Saturated steam – *Steam that contains the maximum amount of water vapor.*

Gauge pressure (steam sterilizer) – *Absolute pressure (-) atmospheric pressure (14.7 psi at sea level); also called "overpressure."*

Absolute pressure (steam sterilizer) – *Gauge pressure (psi)(machine produced) + atmosphere pressure (14.7 psi at sea level).*

sterilizer's chamber during operation, and this concern also relates to moisture. The pressure indicated on the gauge is the **gauge pressure**, not the **absolute pressure**. The gauge pressure is the absolute pressure minus the atmospheric (barometric) pressure.

Figure 15.20 Gravity Air Displacement — Flash Steeilizer

Item	Exposure Time at 250°F (121°C)	Exposure Time at 270°F (132°C)	Exposure Time at 275°F (135°C)	Drying Times
Wrapped Instruments	30 minutes	15 minutes		15-30 minutes
			10 minutes	30 minutes
Textile Packs	30 minutes	25 minutes		15 minutes
			10 minutes	30 minutes
Wrapped Utensils	30 minutes	15 minutes		15-30 minutes
			10 minutes	30 minutes
Unwrapped Nonporous Items (e.g., instruments) (Flash cycle)		3 minutes	3 minutes	0-1 minute
Unwrapped Nonporous and Porous Items in Mixed Load (Flash cycle)		10 minutes	10 minutes	0-1 minute

Figure 15.21 Dynamic Air Removal Teeminal Steeilizer

Item	Exposure Time at at 270°F (132°C)	Exposure Time at 275°F (135°C)	Drying Times
Wrapped Instruments	4 minutes		20-30 minutes
		3 minutes	16 minutes
Textile Packs	4 minutes		5-20 minutes
		3 minutes	3 minutes
Wrapped Utensils	4 minutes		20 minutes
		3 minutes	16 minutes
Unwrapped Instruments (Flash cycle)	3 minutes	3 minutes	N/A
Unwrapped Nonporous and Porous Items in Mixed Load (Flash cycle)	3 minutes	3 minutes	N/A

A Review: Absolute Pressure and Gauge Pressure

Gauge pressure = absolute pressure (psi) + atmospheric pressure (14.7 psi) at sea level

Absolute pressure = gauge pressure (psi) + atmospheric pressure (14.7 psi) at sea level

The atmospheric room pressure at sea level is 14.7 pounds per square inch (psi) at room temperature. While the pressure gauges on sterilizers at sea level are set at zero, in reality the pressure is 14.7 pounds per square inch (absolute pressure). After the sterilizer's door is closed and the sterilization cycle is started, steam is injected into the chamber. Then the temperature rises as does the pressure in the compartment.

The pressure inside the sterilizer increases until it equals about one atmosphere (15 psi) of "overpressure" (gauge pressure) which is equivalent to 250°F (121°C). High-speed sterilizers use a higher temperature of 275°F (135°C), and requires a total pressure of about 45 psi which, at sea level, is a gauge pressure of approximately 30 psi.

The gauge pressure at sea level is always 15 psi lower than the absolute pressure. If the pressure exceeds the temperature, the steam contains air. If the pressure is lower than indicated on the steam table, **superheat** is indicated. This means the steam is "dry," and it will be inefficient at thermal transfer. Superheated steam is a poor sterilant that is about the same thermally and biologically as hot air, and is a fairly common problem, especially in vacuum sterilizers.

If the steam is not saturated (less than 97-100% relative humidity), two problems will develop, either or both of which will interfere with the effectiveness of sterilization:

Superheated (steam) – "Dry" steam; the condition of steam when its temperature is too high relative to its pressure in a steam table.

Steam Table

| Temperature | | Absolute Pressure | Gauge Pressure (lbs/in^2) | |
F	C	(psia)	Sea Level	One Mile Altitude
212	100	14.696	0	2.7
220	104	17.186	2.5	5
225	107	18.912	4	7
230	110	20.779	6	9
235	113	22.800	8	11
240	115.5	24.968	10	13
245	118	27.312	13	15
250	121	29.825	15	18
255	125	32.532	18	20.5
260	127	35.427	21	23
265	129	38.537	24	26.5
270	132	41.856	27	30
275	135	45.426	31	33
280	138	49.200	35	37
285	140.5	53.249	39	41

Figure 15.22 Steam Table

- Items in the sterilizer will remain dry, and microorganisms cannot be killed as readily as under wet conditions.

- Items in the sterilizer will remain "cool" much longer, especially if they are wrapped. (To understand this, think about baking a turkey in an oven with dry heat. It may take hours for the center to become cooked compared to one placed in a pressure cooker with saturated steam.) Saturated steam is a much better "carrier" of thermal energy than is dry air.

Use a Steam Table

Our discussion to this point relates to sterilizers located at or near sea level. However, some healthcare facilities are located at much higher elevations. Example: Denver, CO, is one mile above sea level, and the barometric pressure is about 12 psi rather than 15 psi. The readings on a sterilizer's gauge in Denver must, therefore, be three psi higher than the gauge pressure of a sterilizer operating at sea level to produce the same operating temperature in the sterilizer's chamber. The last column of the steam table in **Figure 15.22** shows the gauge pressures needed to saturate the steam at an altitude of one mile for various operating temperatures.

Another moisture concern is the reprocessing of linen. Linen packs sometimes become ultra-dry or dehydrated during storage or in the sterilization cycle. Then they must be re-laundered before being resterilized to prevent the dehydrated linen from drawing too much moisture from the sterilizing steam, and causing the temperature to rise excessively. Note: this is another example of superheat discussed above. Sometimes the linen may be scorched or charred by the extreme heat. Therefore, "expired" packs cannot just be sent through the sterilizer a second time and then be re-dated. They must first be disassembled, and the linen must be relaundered to restore moisture.

BASIC WORK PRACTICES FOR STEAM STERILIZATION

Learning Objective 7. Explain basic work practices for steam sterilization:
- Preparing devices and packs for steam sterilization
- Loading a sterilizer
- Unloading a sterilizer
- Controlling wet packs
- Cleaning and maintaining sterilizers

Preparing Devices and Packs for Steam Sterilization

Medical devices must be properly prepared before sterilization to assure that steam will come into contact with all surfaces. Central Service Technicians must understand what they are doing, and why they are doing it. This section provides sterilization preparation guidance for processing some common medical devices. As noted earlier, all devices should be thoroughly cleaned before sterilization, including those that are new and repaired since they may have manufacturing oils and other debris or contamination on their surfaces.

Effective sterilization requires that the sterilizing agent be in contact with all surfaces for the prescribed time. Air removal, steam penetration, and condensate drainage are enhanced by proper positioning, and by the use of perforated or mesh-bottomed trays or baskets. (See **Figure 15.23**) Instrument sets should be prepared in trays large enough to equally distribute the mass,

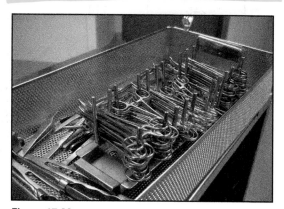

Figure 15.23

and the configuration of instrument sets should be evaluated to help ensure they remain dry.

Only non-linting material should be used in the sterilization trays, since lint can cause foreign-body reactions, and carry microorganisms into the surgical site.

Stoppers and tubes must be removed from drainage bottles, and rubber tubing should be removed from the shanks of hemostats and clamps. Instruments must be dried, and carefully inspected for cleanliness and damage before packaging. If a rigid sterilization container system is used, the basket(s) placed in the container system must be large enough to allow proper instrument arrangement. Woven mesh-bottom trays or baskets are generally used, and nothing can be placed outside of the basket.

Basic procedures to prepare devices for sterilization include:

- They should be positioned to allow the sterilant to come into contact with all surfaces.

- All jointed instruments should be in the open or unlocked position with ratchets unengaged. Racks, pins, stringers, or other specifically-designed devices can be used to hold the instruments in the open position. (See **Figure 15.24**)

- Instruments with more than one part or with sliding pieces or removable parts should be dissembled unless the device manufacturer provides documented evidence that the item can be successfully sterilized in its assembled state.(See **Figure 15.25**)

- Instruments should not be held together with rubber bands (See **Figure 15.26**).

- Items with concaved and/or broad, flat surfaces that will retain water should be placed on edge, so all water or condensate can drain.

- Heavy instruments should be arranged so they will not damage more delicate items. Lighter instruments should be positioned to protect instrument tips, and to prevent damage from changes in position during sterilization.

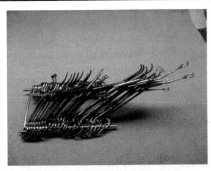

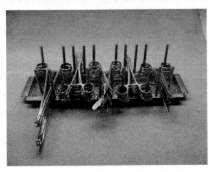

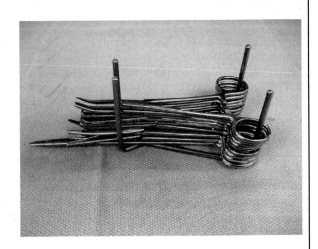

Figure 15.24 Examples of Devices Designed to Hold Jointed Instruments Open

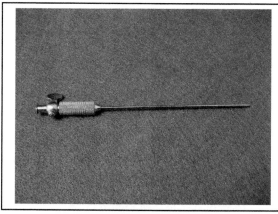
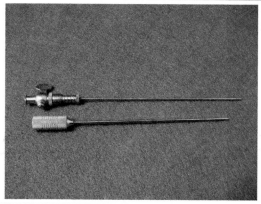

Figure 15.25 Multi-part Instruments Must be Disassembled

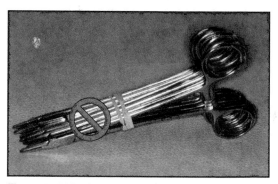

Figure 15.26 Do Not Use Rubber Bands to Hold Instruments Together.

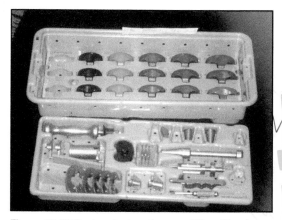

Figure 15.27 Review Instructions and Test Plastic Organizing Cases

• Complex instruments such as air-powered instruments, endoscopes, and instruments with lumens or channels should be prepared and sterilized following the device manufacturer's written instructions.

✓• Central Service Technicians must test and evaluate the effectiveness of sterilization and the drying of protective organizing cases such as loaner trays during each sterilizer cycle. (See **Figure 15.27**) Before preparing and sterilizing multi-part sets or complex instruments, specific written instructions to do so must be reviewed.

✓• Assembly Technicians should check to ensure instruments are clean and function properly. (Note: Instrument inspection is addressed in Chapters 11 and 12.)

✓ With the exception of lumens, ensure instruments are dry as the added moisture will change the dry steam concentration in the sterilizer and can cause wet load.

Catheters, Tubing, Rubber, and Other Goods

Rubber is used in some medical products, but several environmental factors can reduce its life. Examples include heat, light, and direct contact with substances such as acids, solvents, petroleum products, ether, and hot metal. *Difficult to clean*

Rubber catheters, tubing, and drains are very difficult to clean and sterilize because of rubber's rough molecular structure. In many facilities, these items are replaced with single-use disposable items. If using reusable catheters, tubings and drains, follow the manufacturers recommendations for cleaning and sterilization.

Standards are different today

Wood and cork cannot be sterilized by any hospital sterilization method.

Oils and powders cannot be sterilized by steam. Information regarding the dry heat sterilization of oils and powders will be covered later in this chapter.

When challenged with sterilizing items, it is important for Central Service Technicians to remember that no item should be sterilized without written instructions from the manufacturer.

Paper/Plastic Pouches

Paper/plastic pouches should be used for small, lightweight, low-profile items such as one or two clamps or microsurgical scissors. To double-package an item, use two sequentially-sized pouches so the sealed inner pouch will fit inside the other pouch without folding. Pouches should be positioned so that plastic faces plastic, and paper faces paper. Paper/plastic pouches should not be used within wrapped sets or containers.

Small perforated metal cages or boxes should be used instead of paper/plastic pouches to contain small items in sets. The use of paper/plastic pouches within wrapped sets or containers is discouraged since the pouches cannot be positioned to ensure adequate air removal, steam contact, and drying. AAMI ST79:2006 (8.3.4) states that "It is inadvisable to use paper-plastic pouches within wrapped sets or containment devices because the pouches cannot be positioned to ensure adequate air removal, steam contact, and drying."

Figure 15.28 shows an example of a perforated metal container that can be used to hold small items.

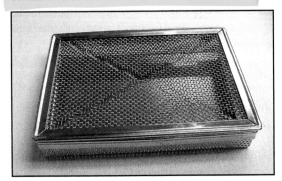

Figure 15.28

Textile Packs — 2,4,6,12 PKS

Textile products and wrappers should be made of materials that will allow adequate air removal and steam penetration/evacuation (or drying) when the package has been properly assembled. The textile product manufacturer should be consulted for recommendations about pack size and density that have been validated with hospital steam sterilization cycles.

A linen pack is prepared with clean and preconditioned textiles. Tightly woven, liquid-resistant textile items in the pack can be separated from absorbent, less dense fabrics to allow adequate air removal and steam penetration/evacuation.

Basins and Basin Sets

Graduated nested basins should differ in diameter by a least one inch. Basin sets should be prepared so that all basins are placed in the same direction. Non-linting absorbent material should separate nested basins during processing. They should be assembled to permit air removal, steam penetration, and steam removal during the sterilization and drying processes. The weight of wrapped basin sets should not exceed 7 pounds, and the total number of basin sets that can be processed per load should be determined to help ensure dry sets. Separating basins with absorbent material enhances adequate air removal and passage of steam to all surfaces, and facilitates drying.

Glass Syringes and Medicine Glasses

The size of the syringe depends on the magnitude of the area to be injected. Unless otherwise specified, all syringes should have Luer-Lok (locking) tips. **Figure 15.29** illustrates disassembly. The barrel and plunger are wrapped separately to protect the glass components from breakage, and to assure that the sterilant will contact all surfaces to promote complete sterilization (See **Figures 15.30** and **15.31**). Medicine glasses should be wrapped in a protective product to protect from breakage (do not use gauze sponges).

The use of some non-absorbent tray liners such as plastic/silicone-fingered organizing mats can cause condensates to pool. Drying should be evaluated by

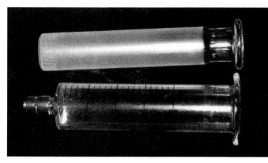

Figure 15.29 Glass Syringe Disassembled for Steam Sterilization. (Glass syringe and barrel.)

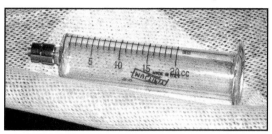

Figure 15.30 Glass Syringe Preparation for Steam Sterilization. (Barrel and syringe separated to allow for total steam contact.)

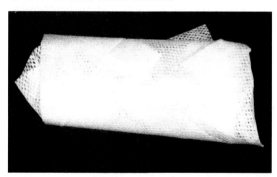

Figure 15.31 Syringe packaged in non-linting absorbent material to allow for total steam contact and to prevent breakage. Should breakage occur, the glass pieces will be contained

controlled and random sampling: opening selected sets at the completion of the drying/cooling time.

Lumens and Other Instruments

Lumens are moistened with distilled or de-mineralized water so air can be more easily displaced, and to allow steam to contact all inner surfaces. (See **Figure 15.32**) They should be moistened no more than two hours prior to wrapping and sterilization. Central Service Technicians

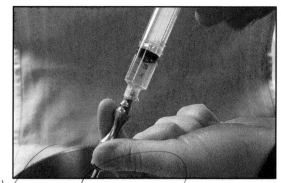

Figure 15.32 Moistening a Lumen

should consult and follow manufacturer's specific recommendations for lumen preparation.

Instruments with concave and/or broad, flat surfaces should be placed on edge during processing. Then pools of water will completely drain off or re-vaporize when the cycle ends.

Manufacturers of complex instruments are best able to specify packaging requirements and sterilization methods, including the cycle times required based on configuration of the specific devices.

Containment devices including protective organizing baskets, trays, or cases should not be used without consulting the containment device manufacturer or conducting specific testing, because the devices can affect the dynamics of sterilization and drying.

Tray liners or other non-linting absorbent material can alleviate drying problems. Absorbent material wicks condensate away from instruments, and dispenses the moisture over a greater surface area for more efficient drying. However, too much or the incorrect type of absorbent material can impede air removal and sterilant penetration, and interfere with proper drying.

Loading a Sterilizer

To assure full steam contact and removal of air, the sterilizer must be properly loaded to allow adequate air circulation and drainage of the condensate. Similar items requiring the same cycle parameters should be grouped together. Cart shelf liners, if used, should be made of a non-linting, absorbent material. The material selected should also dry in the same time selected for the rest of the load. Configuration of the load should ensure adequate air removal, penetration of steam into each package, and steam evacuation. Items capable of holding water, such as solid-bottomed pans, basins, and trays, should be positioned in the same direction. Then, if water is present, it will drain out and allow rapid, even distribution of steam throughout the load with the least amount of interference. Placing metal items below textile items enables condensate to drain out without wetting other items in the load. Sterilizers differ in design and operating characteristics, so the specific sterilizer manufacturer's written instructions should always be carefully followed.

Basic procedures for loading a sterilizer include:

- Allow for proper steam circulation and avoid overloading. Packages must be placed for efficient air removal, steam penetration, and evacuation. Remember that there must be minimal resistance, because steam is passive, and will not actively penetrate tight spaces.

- Use an absorbent shelf cover to line the sterilizer cart's shelf, particularly when disposable wraps and rigid containers are used. (See **Figure 15.33**) This will absorb moisture, and prevent it from dripping onto items on a lower shelf. Non-woven dispensable wraps should not be used since they do not absorb moisture.

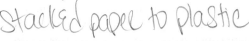

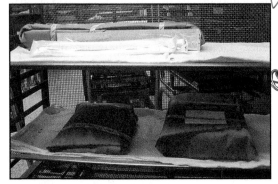

Figure 15.33 Absorbent Shelf Covers can Help Absorb Moisture.

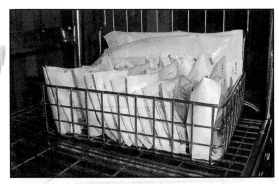

Figure 15.34 Place Small Items in Baskets.

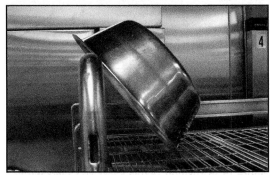

Figure 15.35 Place Items with Solid Bottoms on Edge.

- Solid containers must be positioned so air can get out, and steam can get in. Non-perforated (solid) containers should be placed on their edge.

- Small items should be loosely placed in wire baskets. (See **Figure 15.34**)

- Allow visible space between packs to allow steam circulation and drying.

- When combining loads, place hard goods on the bottom to prevent condensation from dripping onto lower packs.

- Packages must not touch chamber walls.

- Basin sets should stand on edge. They should be tilted for drainage so, if water is present, it will run out. **Figure 15.35** uses an unwrapped basin to illustrate how basins should be positioned for adequate drainage.

- Position textile packs so the layers within them are perpendicular to the shelf. **Figure 15.36** uses two unwrapped

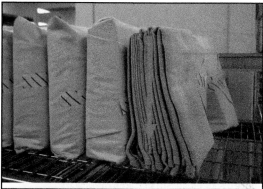

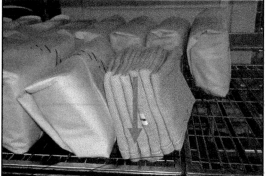

Figure 15.36 Position Textile Packs so Layers within them are Perpendicular to the Shelf.

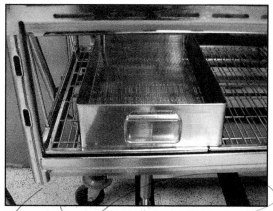

Figure 15.37 Lay Trays with Perforated Bottoms Flat.

• Surgical instrument trays with perforated bottoms should sit flat on the shelf to maintain even instrument distribution, and to facilitate proper drainage. Standing these instrument sets on their edge permits moisture to collect at the standing edge. **Figure 15.37** uses an unwrapped perforated instrument tray to illustrate how perforated instrument trays should be placed on the sterilizer rack.

towel packs to illustrate how they should be placed on the sterilizer rack to facilitate the sterilization process.

• Stand paper/plastic peel pouches on edge using a basket or rack. Placing them "plastic side down" may cause moisture to remain inside, and placing them "plastic side up" may cause water to stand on top of the plastic. Place them so that the sterilization pouches are placed paper-to-plastic, for air and steam circulation.

• When possible, sterilize textiles and hard goods in separate loads. If this is not possible, textiles should be placed on top shelves, and hard goods below (not the reverse) to avoid condensate run-off from the hard goods to the textiles below.

• Other than lumens, the items in the package must be completely dry. If items are wet going into the sterilizer, they will be wet coming out!

Unloading a Sterilizer

When sterilization is completed, the sterilizer's door must be properly opened to maintain sterility because, when the sterilization cycle is completed, packages will be very warm. They may also still contain some steam vapor. If packages were touched at this point, the vapor present might carry microorganisms from one's hand through the packaging material, and contaminate the item. Packaging materials are only effective contamination barriers when the packages are dry.

The load contents should be visibly free of any liquid. Droplets of water on the outside of packages or on the rails of carts are signals that every item in the load should be visually inspected. Caution: do not touch items during the visual inspection.

Wet items should be considered contaminated, even if they have not been touched. The unfiltered air that entered the sterilizer when the door was opened carried microorganisms that could penetrate a wet package.

To unload a sterilizer:

- Crack the door, and wait ten minutes (if a vacuum unit) or 25 to 30 minutes (if a gravity sterilizer) to assure proper evaporation and drying.

- Do not unload packages before they are cool. Placing hot or warm packages on cold surfaces will cause condensation to occur beneath and/or between them. If warm packages are placed in plastic dust covers, condensate will be trapped until opened, and the moisture may also damage the items protected by the dust cover.

- Handle the sterile packages as little as possible.

Items should not be moved or touched until they have cooled to room temperature, which is usually 30 to 60 minutes; however some heavier trays may take several hours to cool. During this time, they should be left in the sterilizer with the door open, or on the cart that has been removed from the sterilizer chamber, and moved to a suitable location. Cool-down should occur in an area free of traffic, and without strong warm or cool air currents. Avoid, for example, areas close to air conditioning vents.

Controlling Wet Packs

Wet packs may occur when a steam sterilization process is used. Packages are considered wet when moisture in the form of dampness, droplets, or puddles of water are found on or within a package after a completed sterilization cycle. **Figure 15.38** is an example of a very visible wet pack. Some wet packs are not as obviously wet, but must still be

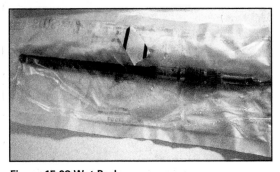

Figure 15.38 Wet Pack

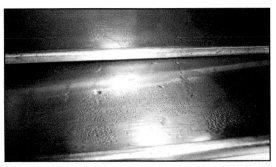

Figure 15.39 Internal Moisture on a Tray

considered wet packs. **Figure 15.39** provides an example of condensation (wetness) on the inside of a tray.

A wet pack is considered contaminated, and must be completely re-packaged and reprocessed. When doing so, all textiles and process indicators in the tray or pack must be replaced.

Causes of Wet Packs

Packs that were improperly prepared or loaded incorrectly for sterilization most frequently become wet packs. Moisture on the outside of a package may result from condensation dripping from a sterilizing shelf or cart rail above the items, or metal items loaded on a higher shelf may drip condensate onto items on a lower shelf. While these are typical sources of exterior wetness, the problem can also occur when condensation blows through the steam lines into the chamber.

Moisture found inside a package often results from metal items positioned in a way that allows water to pool or trap steam that later turns to water. Instrument and basin sets that are too dense or overloaded, and that lack absorbent materials to absorb moisture, can create wet packs. Linen packs also retain moisture if they are tightly wrapped. Instrument sets and other packages may be properly assembled, but improperly loaded. A device's design or construction material may require an extended dry time (follow the manufacturer's recommendations). Note increasing drying times to decrease wet loads may in fact increase the problems, with many products, including most disposable wraps, increasing the dry time increased the chance of a wet load.

The **Figure 15.40** shows internal moisture on instruments within a tray. The tray's plastic construction and the plastic material used to construct the devices require a longer dry cycle. Moisture can form and remain within the packages that have been improperly loaded in the sterilizer. Internal moisture can wick its way to the outside of the pack, and provide a pathway for microorganisms to enter.

The occurrence of all wet packs must be documented including those packs with internal wetness found by personnel in the user department. Note: these should be immediately returned for examination by Central Service personnel. Documentation will likely show patterns that suggest root cause. Perhaps, for example, only the heaviest instrument sets, specialty devices, packages prepared by another department, or processed by a specific Central Service Technician are involved. Identifying the root cause of the wet packs is crucial to preventing additional wet packs.

External moisture on packs is usually noticed immediately when the packs are removed from the sterilizer. Internal wetness will not be noticed until the packs are opened for use unless the moisture wicks through the wrap.

Packages should not be checked for wetness until they are thoroughly cooled since vapor normally re-vaporizes during cooling.

Assembling Instrument Sets

Only surgical instrument trays that have multiple perforations or a mesh bottom should be used. The tray should be of adequate size to ensure an even distribution of metal mass and to prevent overcrowding which can have a negative impact on sterilization and drying processes.

To resolve wet packs that occur from use of specific trays, line the tray with a lint-free absorbent surgical towel or its disposable equivalent before arranging instruments. Moisture will dry more readily from absorbent materials than from droplets or pools on solid metal surfaces. Water-repellent textile or non-woven disposable wrappers or thick super absorbent textiles should not be used. They may cause pooling or trap moisture that makes it difficult or impossible to dry. Also, some foam products hold condensate. As with all products used in sterilization, follow the manufacturer's instructions. Note: tray liners or surgical towels should not be used with rigid sterilization container systems unless approved by the manufacturer of the rigid sterilization container.

All instruments should be open and evenly distributed throughout the tray. Instruments with multiple parts should be disassembled for proper steam contact to avoid trapping steam that can condense. The position of the heavy handles of some instruments like orthopedic chisels and gauges may need to be altered for proper mass distribution.

Wrapping Instrument Sets

Before applying flat wrappers, an absorbent product should be placed between the bottom of the tray and the wrapper. This is particularly helpful when

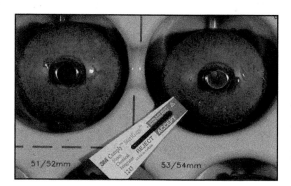

Figure 15.40 Internal Moisture on Instruments.

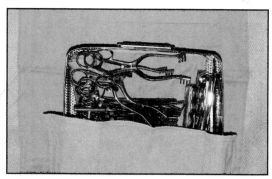

Figure 15.41 Using Absorbent Towels to Prevent Wet Packs.

using non-woven disposable wrappers because excess moisture will usually dry more readily from the textile, and prevent pooling inside the wrapper. A towel may be placed on top of the set before wrapping, if necessary, and can help to prevent torn wrappers. (See **Figure 15.41**)

Cleaning and Maintaining Sterilizers

The sterilizer manufacturer's written recommendations for sterilizer maintenance must always be followed. The following general cleaning and maintenance guidelines are illustrative of manufacturer's recommendations:

- Cool the chamber before performing any cleaning or maintenance procedure. Note:

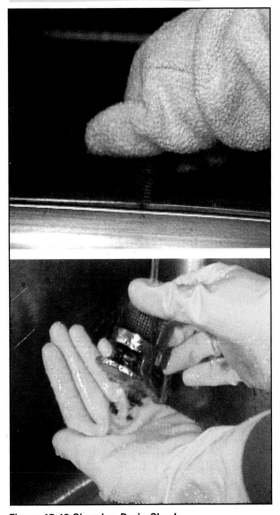

Figure 15.42 Chamber Drain Check

The chamber drain strainer may be checked when the sterilizer is hot, but be sure to wear protective gloves to avoid burns.

- The screen strainer (See **Figure 15.42**) should be removed at least daily, and cleaned thoroughly under running water using a non abrasive brush and a mild detergent. This procedure may be necessary more frequently depending upon the types of loads processed. If debris is allowed to build-up, it may be necessary to soak the strainer before cleaning. The **Figure 15.43** shows an improperly maintained strainer that is clogged, and will not properly remove air and steam. The inside of the chamber should be cleaned with a mild detergent using a long-handled mop used only for this purpose.

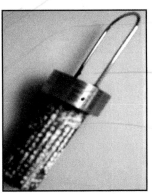

Figure 15.43 Clogged Steam Sterilizer Strainer

The following steps should be used to clean the sterilizer's interior:

- Turn off steam.

- Allow chamber walls to cool before cleaning.

- Always use caution; wear long protective gloves when cleaning the chamber's drain screen and drain.

- Check your operator's manual for frequency of cleaning. (Cleaning is typically done at least weekly.)

- The door gasket (See **Figure 15.44**) should be inspected, and wiped clean daily with a clean, damp, lint-free cloth. During the inspection, look for defects or signs of wear or deterioration, especially if the unit has a vacuum cycle.

- Carriages, carts, and loading baskets should be routinely cleaned with a mild detergent

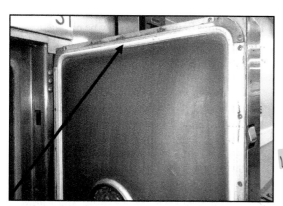

Figure 15.44 Door Gasket

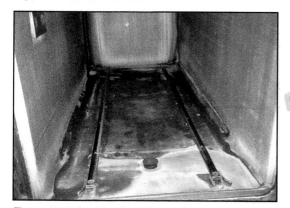

Figure 15.45 Residue Build Up on Chamber Interior

solution, and should be checked for rough areas using a lint-free cloth. Casters, rollers, and other moving parts should be cleaned and checked to ensure they move freely.

✔ Problems with residue build-up on the chamber's interior can affect the cycle's drying ability. (See **Figure 15.45**) Clean with non-abrasive and non-linting products. Also, rinse detergent and residue from chamber thoroughly to avoid deposits on devices during sterilization.

• Follow the manufacturer's instructions about the need, if any, and method to clean and flush the chamber's drain. This is important because air and steam will not pass efficiently if the drain line is blocked.

• Strong abrasives or steel wool should never be used on the sterilizer because they can scratch the surface, and allow corrosion to develop. While sterilizer chambers are made

of corrosion-resistant materials, some steam boiler water treatment chemicals can attack the chamber if the surface is damaged.

• Inspect recording devices including paper charts and printer paper daily.

DRY HEAT STERILIZATION

Learning Objective 8. Explain the basics of dry heat sterilization:
- When dry heat is appropriate.
- Advantages and disadvantages of dry heat sterilization.
- Types of hot-air convection sterilizers.
- Dry heat sterilization procedures.

Dry heat is the least used and least understood sterilizing agent. Steam and low temperature sterilization processes are routinely used, but some items cannot be sterilized with these methods. As a sterilant, dry heat functions differently from moist heat and, as is true with other sterilization methods, items must be thoroughly cleaned and correctly prepared for sterilization to be effective.

When Dry Heat is Appropriate

Dry heat is a relatively slow-acting sterilizing agent, and generally requires higher temperatures than other sterilization methods. However, one of its advantages is its ability to penetrate a variety of materials, including oils, petrolatum jelly, and closed containers not permeable to steam.

The rate of microbiological destruction associated with dry heat sterilization is influenced by temperature, time, uniformity of the heating during sterilization, permeability of the packaging material, and the bio-burden associated with the product.

Dry heat should only be used when direct contact of the material or substance with saturated steam is impractical or unattainable. Metal instruments represent the ideal for dry heat sterilization because of the heat-conducting properties of metal. However, the maximum temperature used must be restricted to a safe range beyond which the temper of the metal may be affected. For heat-stable items such as glassware, a higher temperature can be used for a shorter period of time. When sterilizing powders, the temperature must be maintained below the point at which the substance may undergo physical or chemical change. Dry heat cannot be used with fabrics or rubber since it will deteriorate these materials.

Dry Heat Uses Conduction

Dry heat sterilization is accomplished by **conduction**: heat is absorbed by an item's exterior surface and passed inward to the next layer. Eventually, the entire item reaches the proper temperature needed for sterilization. Death of microorganisms occurs by oxidation: the slow burning-up process of coagulating protein in the cells. Unlike steam sterilization, there is no moisture present, and this slows heat penetration significantly.

Advantages and Disadvantages of Dry Heat Sterilization

As with all sterilization methods, dry heat has advantages and disadvantages.

Advantages include:

• Dry heat can sterilize items such as powders and oils that cannot be sterilized with other methods.

• Dry heat will not erode the surface of glass as is possible with steam under some circumstances.

• Dry heat does not have a corrosive or rusting effect on metals including sharp instruments.

• Since dry heat uses conduction, it will reach all surfaces of items that cannot be disassembled.

Conduction – *A heat transfer method in which heat is absorbed by an item's exterior surface, and passed inward to the next layer.*

Convection – *The process of heat transfer by the circulation of currents from one area to another.*

Possible disadvantages are:

• Dry heat is difficult to control within narrow limits, except in a specially designed sterilizer.

• Dry heat penetrates materials slowly and unevenly.

• Dry heat requires long exposure times to achieve sterility.

• High temperatures required during dry heat sterilization can damage some materials.

• There are limited packaging materials that may be used with dry heat sterilization.

• Dry heat is not suitable to sterilize fabrics and rubber goods.

Types of Hot-Air Convection Sterilizers

Most dry heat sterilizers used in healthcare facilities are small table-top models, although they are usually placed on a counter top for stability. As can be seen in the photo in **Figure 15.46**, these styles of table-top units have small chambers. Note: Dry heat sterilization can only be performed using a dry heat sterilizer. Other heated chambers should not be used.

There are two types of hot-air convection sterilizers: those which employ gravity convection currents, and those which generate mechanical **convection** currents: (See **Figure 15.47**)

• Gravity Convection Sterilizers. As air within the chamber is heated, it rises and displaces cooler air that descends into the

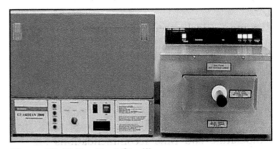

Figure 15.46 Dry Heat Sterilizers

Types of Dry Heat Sterilizers

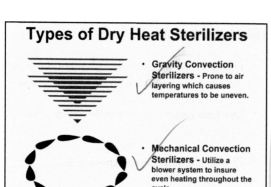

- **Gravity Convection Sterilizers** - Prone to air layering which causes temperatures to be uneven.

- **Mechanical Convection Sterilizers** - Utilize a blower system to insure even heating throughout the cycle.

Figure 15.47

Figure 15.48 Alternative Time and Temperature Recommendations for Dry Heat Sterilization

Temperature	Time
356°F (180°C)	30 minutes
340°F (170°C)	1 hour
320°F (160°C)	2 hours
300°F (150°C)	2 ½ hours
285°F (140°C)	3 hours
250°F (121°C)	6 hours; preferably overnight

lower part of the chamber. This circulation pattern causes inconsistent temperatures within the chamber. Since dry-heat sterilization requires that a given temperature be reached and maintained for a specific period of time, it is difficult to monitor the sterilization process in a gravity convection oven because the air in each layer varies in temperature.

- **Mechanical Convection Sterilizers.** These ovens contain a blower that actively forces heated air throughout all areas of the chamber. This flow creates uniform temperatures, and the equal transfer of heat throughout the load to make these ovens more efficient than their gravity convection counterparts.

Dry Heat Sterilization Procedures

Always follow the manufacturer's recommendations for preparing, packaging, and loading dry heat sterilizers, and use the facility's procedures that specify temperature and time set points, loading, patterns, and other operating parameters. The exposure times vary depending on the types of items being sterilized, how these items are packaged, and the depth of any substance being sterilized in containers.

The most widely used temperature for dry heat sterilization is a minimum of 320°F (160°C) for, preferably, two hours. Note: this requirement refers to the actual load temperature, and does not consider any appreciable time lag characteristic of a specific load after the sterilizer has reached this temperature. **Figure 15.48** indicates alternative temperature and time recommendations for dry heat sterilization.

To prepare items for dry heat sterilization, begin by checking the manufacturer's written recommendations. Here are some basic procedures:

- **Oils and Powders.** The quantity of a liquid or powder to be sterilized should be limited to that required for a single-use application, and should not exceed one ounce. Preferably, the depth of the oil in the container should not exceed one-quarter inch, because the greater the volume, the more time will be needed to heat and sterilize the oil. Only a heat-resistant glass jar or petri dish can be used. The required sterilization temperature should be based upon the manufacturer's recommendations.

- **Impregnated gauze strips.** Gauze strips should be placed in a stainless steel container, and covered with petroleum jelly or other oil based liquid. The depth of the layer should not exceed one-half inch.

4.5" inches.

- **Glass Syringes.** The syringe must be thoroughly dry. Syringes may be sterilized fully assembled (for example, with the plunger in the barrel).

- **Needles.** Needles must be thoroughly dry, and may be fully assembled (for example, stylets in place). Assure that the needle can withstand the high heat to which it will be exposed.

must be dry, may be

• Instruments. Instruments must be thoroughly dry. The ratchets and box locks may be closed, and screws may be tightened, if necessary.

assembled

Hot-air convection sterilizers should be loaded in a manner that allows the hot air to circulate freely. The chamber must never be overloaded, and ample space (about a hand's width between packages) must be allowed between each item. Packages should not touch the chamber's walls to prevent hot spots which could cause muslin to char, and all loads should be standardized for the type of containers and items being sterilized.

Central Service Technicians should use insulated handles or heavy gloves when removing items and packs from the sterilizer since they will be hot, and it is best to allow the items to cool before removing them.

Packaging Materials for Dry Heat Sterilization

Only packaging material designed to withstand dry heat temperatures should be used to assure that it does not melt or is not damaged to compromise the aseptic presentation of sterilized items. As well, only tape and package labels (for example, process indicators, and product identification and expiration labels) designed for dry heat sterilization should be used.

There are only a few types of packaging materials suitable for use in hot-air convection sterilizers:

• Heat-resistant glass such as petri dishes, test tubes, and small jars.

• Stainless steel trays and/or pans with lids.

• Cotton muslin, if the chamber temperature does not exceed 400°F (240°C).

• Aluminum foil.

• Nylon films.

• Certain sterilization containers. (Consult the container's manufacturer for written recommendations).

STERILIZATION QUALITY CONTROL

Learning Objective 9. Explain the need for quality control and review sterilization process indicators that help assure quality control:
• Need for quality control
• Chemical indicators
• Sterilization load control information
• Physical and mechanical monitors
• Biological indicators
• Bowie-Dick tests
• Validation and Verification processes

Need for Quality Control

Sterile processing requires a control system with continuous quality improvement procedures to assure that sterilization parameters are being met. Since it is difficult to prove an item's sterility without contaminating it, conditions that can prove sterility has occurred must be monitored. These monitoring protocols are an important part of the Central Service Department's quality assurance systems. Several control measures must be used to assure that the conditions within the sterilizers are adequate to achieve sterilization. These are basically the same for the steam and dry heat sterilization, but there are a few differences, and these will be noted.

Sterilization **process indicators** help to confirm that packages have been properly exposed to the sterilization process, and can be the first sign of a processing error. They are designed to respond with either a chemical or physical change to one or more sterilization conditions.

Process indicators – Devices intended for use with individual units (for example, packs or containers) to demonstrate that the unit has been exposed to the sterilization process, and to distinguish between processed and unprocessed units. Source: ANSI/AAMI ST60.

Chemical indicators (CIs) – Systems that reveal a change in one or more predefined process parameters on the basis of a chemical or physical change that results from exposure to a process. Source: AAMI TIR No. 24: 1999.

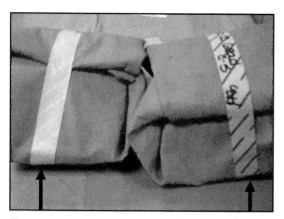

Figure 15.49 External Chemical Indicator Tape. Before Processing (left). After Processing (right).

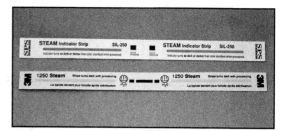

Figure 15.50 Examples of Internal Chemical Indicators

There are two types of process indicators: internal and external depending upon whether they are placed on the inside (internal) or outside (external) of the package prior to sterilization.

Some **chemical indicators (CIs)** are often the first performance test the user sees upon opening a sterile package. They provide instant results, and are visual evidence of the successful completion of the sterilization process. External process indicators including tape, load cards, or labels on the outside of the packages are also examined before the items are issued and/or used to ensure that proper processing has occurred. External CIs should be used on the outside of each package to be sterilized. For example, **Figure 15.49** illustrates external indicator tape. The package on the left has not been processed, and the package on the right has. Note the color change in the stripes on the tape.

Chemical indicators (CIs) can help to identify the reason for potential sterilization failures. They are impregnated with a dye that changes color in the presence of temperature or the sterilant, and they can detect problems with incorrect packaging, loading of, or malfunctions with the sterilizer. CIs are an integral part of the sterilization quality assurance program and are used in conjunction with physical monitors and biological indicators to demonstrate the efficacy of the sterilization process.

After sterilization, process indicators are examined by the Central Service Technician to assure complete exposure. If there has been, the chemical indicator will have changed color. By contrast, an incomplete color change may provide the first sign that part or all of a load has not been properly sterilized. While chemical indicators do not verify sterility, they can detect certain equipment malfunctions such as air leaks, wet steam, and inadequate temperature, and they may assist in the identification of certain procedural errors.

Chemical Indicators

Internal Chemical Indicators (CIs) (See **Figure 15.50**) should be used to routinely monitor each package, tray, or rigid sterilization container to detect problems due to improper processing that render the packaging contents unfit for use. The CI should be placed in the area of the package, tray, or container considered to be least accessible to steam penetration. Note: this location is not necessary at the center of the package, tray, or container. Improper loading techniques could be identified when some CIs remain unchanged in one load, while the remainder in the load do change. Failure of chemical indicators can also show problems caused by the sterilizer, by packaging, and/or from pack density.

If the interpretation of the CI in a package, tray, or container suggests inadequate steam processing, the contents cannot be used. It should be returned to sterile processing for analysis. Note: It is possible to have one or more unacceptable indicators in a load because of improper packaging or loading with the remainder of the load acceptable.

Some facilities use chemical integrators that consist of thermo (heat)-sensitive paint applied to a cardboard strip or a dye which moves along a window. When exposed to hot steam, the paint gradually changes color. These special devices react

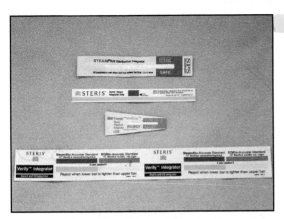

Figure 15.51 Examples of Internal Chemical Integrators

to several sterilization parameters rather than to just one. **Figure 15.51** shows some chemical integrators in common use.

Each of the five classes of chemical indicators is designed to monitor one or more specific sterilization parameters:

• (Class 1) – Processing indicators used with individual packs to demonstrate that they have been exposed to the sterilization process, and to distinguish between processed and unprocessed packs. Class 1 indicators monitor internal and external sterilization conditions.

• (Class 2) – Indicators such as Bowie-Dick tests. Note: these are discussed later in this chapter.

• (Class 3) – Single-parameter indicators that react to one of the critical parameters of sterilization, and indicate exposure to a sterilization cycle at a stated value of that parameter.

• (Class 4) – Multi-parameter indicators that react to two or more critical sterilization parameters, and that indicate exposure to a sterilization cycle at stated values of those parameters.

• (Class 5) – Integrating indicators designed to react to all critical parameters over a specified range of sterilization cycles. Their performance has been correlated to the performance of a BI under the labeled conditions of use.

Sterilization Load Control Numbers

All items to be sterilized should be labeled with a **load control number** that identifies:

• Sterilizer identification number – Example: S-1.

• Sterilization Cycle number – Example: Assume fifth load of the day – (L-5) .

• Date sterilized – Example 5-3-07.

Note the Load Control Number above: S-1 L-5 5-3-07. (See **Figure 15.52**)

Some facilities choose to use a different way of identifying the date sterilized and use a **Julian Date** on their packages. The Julian Date is number of the day in the year. For example, January 1st is day # 001 and December 31 is day # 365.

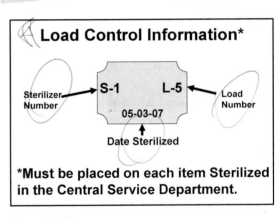

Load Control Information*

Sterilizer Number → S-1   L-5 ← Load Number

05-03-07

↑ Date Sterilized

***Must be placed on each item Sterilized in the Central Service Department.**

Figure 15.52

Load control information is usually applied to each package using labeling applicator gun to place an identification sticker containing the load information. (See **Figure 15.53**)

Load control number – Label information on sterilization packages, trays, or containers that identifies the sterilizer, cycle run, and date of sterilization.

Julian Date – The Julian day or Julian day number (JDN) is the number of days that have elapsed since January 1st.

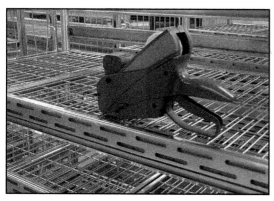

Figure 15.53 Example of a Label Applicator Gun for Load Control Information

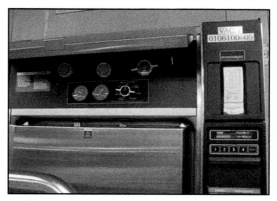

Figure 15.54 Physical (Mechanical) Monitors

All packages sterilized by the Central Service Department should have a load control sticker.

Load identification helps to retrieve items during recalls and to trace problems such as a positive chemical indicator.

The following information is recorded and maintained for each sterilization cycle:

• Date and time of the sterilizer load control number (sometimes called the lot number) which includes sterilizer information.

• Specific items sterilized including quantity, department, and item description (examples: minor pan 1 OR, towel pack 10 CS, or sternal saw 1 CVOR).

• Exposure time and temperature.

• Sterilizer operator identification.

• Results of biological testing (if applicable).

• Response of the CI placed in the BI test pack, if applicable.

• Results of Bowie-Dick testing, if performed.

This documentation ensures that cycle parameters were monitored and met, and helps personnel determine whether, and to what extent, if any, recalls are necessary. Note: a recall is initiated for a positive BI or non-responsive CI, wet packs, or other sterility problems. Knowing the contents of the load enables personnel to decide how critical a recall will be, and where to go to reclaim the packages. This documentation can be compiled manually in a sterilization log book or there are computer software programs available to compile and maintain these records.

Physical (Mechanical) Monitoring

Physical monitors include time, temperature, and pressure recorders, displays, digital printouts, and gauges. At the beginning of the sterilization cycle, the recording chart is checked to assure that it is marked with the correct date and time, and that it identifies the sterilizer and cycle. (See **Figure 15.54**) During and at the end of the cycle, and before items are removed from the sterilizer, the operator should review the record to assure that all cycle parameters were met. He/she then initials the chart to show that it was monitored, and that all sterilization parameters were met.

Physical monitors are needed to detect equipment malfunctions as soon as possible, so appropriate corrective actions can be taken if there are failures.

In some, typically table-top, sterilizers recording devices are unavailable. Then the operator should periodically monitor the time and temperature gauges during the cycle to verify and document that cycle parameters have been met.

If records indicate any malfunction or questionable operation, the department head or designee must be notified immediately. The cycle should be terminated according to the sterilizer manufacturer's

[handwritten: 270°F - 275°F]
[handwritten: 3, 4, 10 min.]

instructions. The load should be considered non-sterile, the sterilizer should be removed from service, and it should not be re-used until the problem is corrected. Quality monitoring is then needed to assure that the sterilizer is working.

After a major repair (one such as chamber weld repairs outside the scope of normal maintenance) to a dynamic-air-removal sterilizer, three consecutive Bowie-Dick test cycles should be run immediately after the other, and the test sheets should be examined. Note: Bowie-Dick tests are discussed later in this chapter. Three consecutive test cycles with a BI test pack should be run immediately after the other in an otherwise empty chamber following major repair of any type of steam sterilizer. Test results should be analyzed and confirmed to be satisfactory before the sterilizer is returned to service.

After a major repair to a dry heat sterilizer, three consecutive test cycles with a process challenge device (PCD; previously known as a BI challenge test pack) should be run immediately after the other in an otherwise empty chamber. Satisfactory results are necessary before the sterilizer can be returned to service.

Biological Indicators

Biological indicators (BIs) are also used to challenge the sterilization process. They are the only sterilization process monitoring devices that provide a direct measure of process lethality. They are intended to demonstrate whether all required conditions including air removal and steam presentation were adequate to achieve sterilization.

Biological indicators are **spores** in or on a carrier, usually (as in the case of self-contained BIs) accompanied by incubation media. A PCD may be prepared in the hospital or purchased as a commercially disposable, pre-assembled challenge test pack with the BI within each PCD pack. **Figure 15.55** shows some biological indicators in common use.

Spores are used for BIs since they are the most resistant to the sterilization method being used.

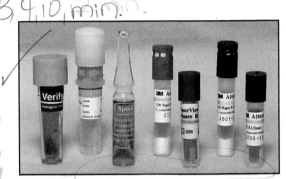

Figure 15.55 Examples of Biological Indicators

For steam sterilization, BIs consist of Geobacillus stearothermophilus (formerly named Bacillus stearothermophilus). For dry heat testing, Bacillus atrophaeus (formerly known as Bacilus subtilis) is used.

Biological indicators are placed in the load which is then sterilized. They are then incubated to determine whether microorganisms grow. If the spores are killed by the sterilization process, it is considered a negative result which is desired since it demonstrates the sterilizer's operating efficiently. Specific procedures for BI procedures vary depending upon the manufacturer used, and the recommendations of the manufacturer must be strictly followed.

[handwritten: BI - Vial Strip that Contains Spore]

A negative BI result does not "prove" that all items in the load are sterile, or that were all exposed to adequate sterilization conditions. Instead, it shows that all conditions required for sterilization were met. Central Service Technicians must follow proper preparing, packaging, and loading procedures to best assure that proper sterilization parameters will be attained.

BI process challenge devices should be used for routine sterilizer efficacy monitoring at least weekly (but preferably every day) that the sterilizer is used, and with every implant.

PCDs should also be used for sterilizer qualification testing after sterilizer installation, relocation,

Spore – A microorganism with a thick wall surrounding it that enables the organism to survive in adverse conditions including high temperatures.

[handwritten: machine validation.]

malfunction, major repair, and sterilization process failures. If a sterilizer is designed to be used for multiple types of cycles, then each sterilization mode should be tested.

A hospital-prepared PCD consists of 16 clean, preconditioned, re-usable huck or absorbent surgical towels that are in good condition. The size of each towel is approximately 16" x 26" (41cm x 66 cm). Each towel is folded lengthwise into thirds, and then folded widthwise in the middle. After folding, the towels are placed on top of each other, with the folds opposite each other, to form a stack that is approximately 9" wide, 9" long, and 6" high (23 cm x 23 cm x 15 cm). One or more BIs is/are placed between the eighth and ninth towels in the approximate geometric center of the pack. Chemical indicators are placed adjacent to them, and the pack is then taped. The pack should weigh approximately 3 pounds, and should be approximately 6" high. Note: a wrapper is not used for this test pack.

The PCD is run in a fully-loaded chamber in the area of the chamber and load that is least favorable to sterilization (in other words, the area representing the greatest challenge to the BI), which is typically called the "cold point" in the manufacturer's instruction manual. This area varies with sterilizer design, but is normally in front or the center bottom section of the sterilizer, near the drain, as seen in **Figure 15.56**.

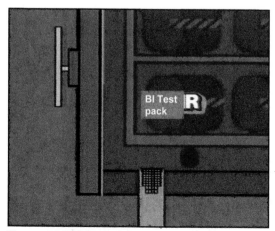

Figure 15.56 BI Process Challenge Device (PCD) Placement

Details about Process Devices

This section discusses implants, PCDs for table top sterilizers, PCDs for dry heat sterilization, control tests, procedures for PCD testing, and protocols for positive BI results.

Implants

ANSI/AAMI ST79:2006 recommends that every load containing implantable devices should be monitored with a PCD and quarantined until the results of the BI testing are available. An implantable device should not be released before the BI results are known, and this should be documented. As with all cycles, the sterilizer operator should review the sterilizer chart/printout, and the results of other indicators used to monitor the sterilization process.

PCDs for Table Top Steam Sterilizers

A representative of the same type of package or tray routinely processed through the sterilizer should serve as the PCD for qualification testing and routine biological monitoring of table top steam sterilizers. The package or tray considered to be the most difficult to sterilize should be selected from those most frequently processed. The package or tray selected should contain the items normally present during routine sterilization.

PCDs for Dry Heat Sterilization

As with table top sterilizers, the package or tray chosen as a PCD for a dry heat sterilization process should be that considered the most difficult to sterilize. Only one BI needs to be used inside a PCD to achieve a microbial challenge. Characteristics to consider when selecting PCDs include multiple layers of dressing materials, large metal masses, and mixed packs incorporating both characteristics.

There are no universally-accepted, standardized PCDs for dry heat sterilizers. Therefore, it is recommended that a representative package or tray of the type to be routinely processed through the sterilizer be used as the PCD.

Control Tests

For each BI test, at least one unsterilized BI from the same lot as the BI used in the test should be incubated as a control to verify that the test spores were living at the time of the test. The control should show a growth or a positive result. The BI manufacturer should provide information about the control test, which should also show that the media can promote growth of the test spores, and that the incubator is functioning at the correct temperature. After the incubation period, the test and control results should be read and recorded. If the control (unsterilized) BI from a lot fails to grow, it should be assumed that the test BIs from that lot are non-viable (not living), or that improper incubation occurred. Therefore, the results from the test BIs should be considered invalid, and the test should be repeated. If several test BIs from the same lot are run on the same day, only one control BI from that lot must be used.

Procedures for PCD Testing

Protocols to use PCDs include:

• The PCD should be labeled with sterilizer load information before being exposed to the sterilization cycle. The test pack to be sterilized should be properly labeled and assembled with the PCD.

• The PCD should be positioned in the chamber according to the sterilizer manufacturer's written recommendations

• The sterilization cycle should be run.

• Upon completion of the sterilization cycle, the test pack should be cooled, the BI(s) should be removed, and the sterilizer load information should be documented. The BI(s) should then be incubated according to the BI manufacturer's instructions.

• A control biological indicator should be incubated at least one time per day or with each new lot used.

An acceptable process is shown by negative (failure to grow) results from all BIs in the PCD that were sterilized, and acceptable readings from physical monitors and CIs that show the sterilization cycle was correct and complete.

Protocols for Positive PCD Results

If the BI shows positive growth, the following actions are needed:

• Results should be immediately reported to the Sterile Processing supervisor who should notify the Infection Control department and all affected departments. This notification is followed by a written report that should include:

  • The time and date of the questionable sterilizer cycle.

  • A description of the sterilizer and load, with reference to the appropriate load control number.

  • The results of physical and mechanical monitoring and internal CIs (if applicable), as obtained from the user department.

  • Any other information that can help determine whether the report is valid or questionable due to human error.

• A decision must be made about a recall, and should be based on factors including whether an improperly loaded BI should require a test inspection rather than a recall. When a recall is initiated, all items processed in that sterilizer since the last negative are recalled. These devices should be considered non-sterile, retrieved, if possible, and reprocessed. Rationale: there is evidence the sterilizer was working properly for the last negative test, and no evidence about when the sterilizer began to malfunction.

If the positive result is due to sterilizer malfunction, it should be removed from service, and the malfunction should be corrected. A faulty sterilizer cannot be made operational without identifying and correcting the problem. Extending the cycle time or increasing the cycle temperature, for example, are not appropriate procedures.

Bowie-Dick Tests

A Bowie-Dick test is used to evaluate the efficacy of air removal in dynamic-air-removal steam sterilizers. (See **Figure 15.57**) A Bowie Dick test is a Class 2 chemical indicator that is not a sterility test. It is performed each day the sterilizer is used before the first load is processed. If the sterilizer is used continuously, the test may be performed at any time, but at the same time every day. It should also be performed during the sterilizer's initial installation, and after relocation, malfunction, process failures, and major repairs.

The Bowie-Dick test detects air leaks and identifies ineffective air removal with other air removal techniques that do not utilize a deep vacuum, and the presence of non-condensable gases that can enter the chamber with the steam, and inhibit proper steam penetration. These conditions are critical to detect because, if there is insufficient air removal, steam will drive the available air back into the load, air pockets will be created, and sterilization will not occur. This will result in a large volume of non-sterile supplies that could go undetected.

A specifically-designed Class 2 chemical indicator is used to conduct the test. A shortened cycle that excludes the dry cycle should first be run to heat the sterilizer.

Validation and Verification

There is a significant difference between "validation and verification." **"Validation"** is done by the device manufacturer using a documented procedure to obtain, record, and interpret the testing results required to establish that a process consistently produces a sterile product. By contrast, **"verification"** is performed by the healthcare facility to confirm that the validation undertaken by the manufacturer is applicable to the specific setting. Note: recall our earlier discussion about differences in sterilizers including steam quality, altitude of location, and even room ventilation. Central Service Technicians perform verification by documenting the procedures to obtain, record, and interpret the healthcare facility's test results. The validation provided by the medical device manufacturer provides the framework for these studies.

The verification process involves product test packs of the product (examples: textile packs, basin sets, instrument sets, and containment devices [loaner trays]) that is, or soon will be, used. As with all sterilization test practices, the product test packs must be positioned to challenge the sterilization process.

A test sample must first be prepared. The standard PCD (outlined in section 10.7.2.1 of ANSI/AAMI

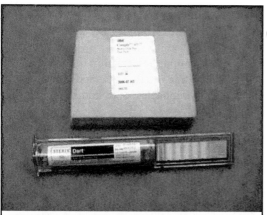

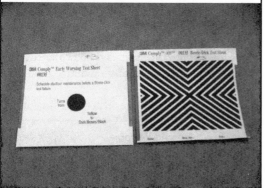

Figure 15.57 Examples of Bowie-Dick (Air Removal) Tests

Validation – Procedures used by equipment manufacturers to obtain, record, and interpret test results required to establish that a process consistently produces a sterile product.

Verification – Procedures used by healthcare facilities to confirm that the validation undertaken by the equipment manufacturer is applicable to the specific setting.

ST79:2006) presents a known challenge to the sterilization process. However, this PCD may not reflect items such as the instrument sets routinely processed in the facility. Therefore, product testing is recommended as an integral part of a complete quality assurance program to ensure the effectiveness of the sterilization process, and to avoid wet packs. The products to be tested vary depending on the types of products routinely sterilized. Basic procedures for within-facility verification include:

- For instrument sets – BIs and CIs should be placed at each end of the tray, and among instruments placed on stringers in the areas least accessible to the steam. (See **Figure 15.58**)

- For containment devices – BIs and CIs (if the latter are used) should be placed in each corner, the center, and any other areas recommended by the container manufacturer. For multi-layered instrument sets in containment devices (loaner trays), the BIs and CIs should be placed in the location determined by the product manufacturer to create the greatest sterilization challenge.

- For textile packs wrapped in woven or non-woven materials – BIs and CIs should be placed between the layers of a folded surgical gown within the pack, between multiple layers of draping material, or between layers of surgical towels.

- For basin sets wrapped in woven or non-woven materials – BIs and CIs are placed in locations within the set such as the area between nested basins where air pockets could form. Note: for this test it may be appropriate to use BIs contained in glassine envelopes rather than in ampules, since the latter could separate the basins, and permit more steam contact. Also, the ampules could break or even lift the basins, and provide an inaccurate circulation test.

- For other types of items such as bulk packages of sponges or dressings and reusable syringe sets – BIs and CIs should be placed in the area of the load that is least accessible to steam penetration.

When preparing test packs, they should be identified as "test packs" so they will not be used.

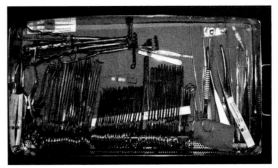

Figure 15.58 Sample Verification Set Up for Instrument Set

Test samples should be placed strategically throughout the load at the points most difficult to sterilize; in other words, those most resistant to steam penetration. After inspection and retrieval of the BIs and CIs, the sample packs used in product testing should be disassembled and inspected. The BIs and CIs should be examined to assure acceptable results, and a moisture examination should indicate that product is dry.

If test results suggest problems such as a positive BI or a wet pack, a thorough investigation is needed. Corrective actions may include changing the load configuration or item placement within the package, or servicing the sterilizer. Product use should be discontinued until the problem is resolved. The test protocol, results, and any corrective action(s) taken should be documented and maintained as part of the sterilization log or quality assurance program data.

SPECIAL HIGH TEMPERATURE STERILIZATION CONCERNS

Learning Objective 10. Review the basics of three special high temperature sterilization concerns:
- D-Values and sterilization effectiveness.
- Creutzfeldt-Jakob disease (CJD).
- Solutions.

D-Values and Sterilization Effectiveness[2]

All microbes in a given material are not generally destroyed at the same time. Death occurs in a definite relationship to time, and this rate is governed by factors including temperature, age

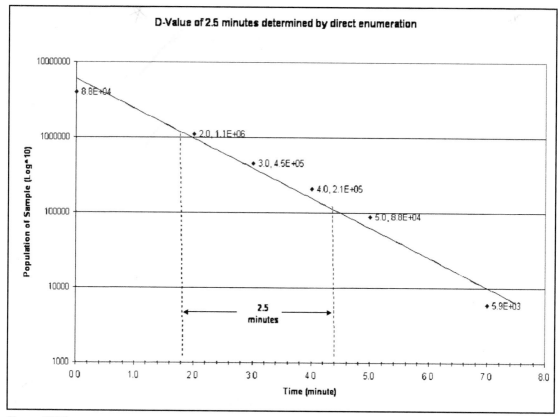

Figure 15.59

of the test culture, and environmental influences active during the growth of the test culture and during the sterilizing and recovery of the bacteria.

The "concept of logarithmic order of death" means that a given percentage of the surviving population is killed in a unit of time.

Sterilization time is measured in **D-values**: the time required to kill 90% of the microorganisms present. Each kind of microorganism has a different set of D-values which depends on the temperature. (See **Figure 15.59**)

You've learned that Geobacillus stearothermophilus (formerly Bacillus stearothermophilus) is used to challenge hospital steam sterilizers. For hospital sterilization tests, this microorganism has a

D-Value – *The amount of time required to kill 90% of the microorganisms present.*

D-value of about two minutes at 250°F (121°C), or about 20 seconds at 275°F (135°C). In other words, it would take two minutes at 250°F (121°C), or 20 seconds at 275°F (135°C) to kill 90% of the microorganisms present.

For example, if 90% of a given microbe population is killed per minute and, if the beginning population is one million cells, after one minute of a sterilizing procedure, 900,000 cells would be killed (1,000,000 [x] .90 = 900,000 microbes), and 100,000 cells would survive (1,000,000 − 900,000 [=] 100,000). After the second minute, 90,000 microbes would be killed (100,000 [x] .90 = 9,000) and 10,000 would survive (100,000 [-] 90,000 = 10,000). After the third minute, there would theoretically be 1,000 survivors (10,000 [x] .90 = 9,000 organisms killed; 10,000 [-] 9,000 = 1,000 survivors).

This illustrates why an item that has over 10^6 contamination cannot be sterilized in one cycle of the sterilizer (which is set to kill only 10^6 microbes).

Creutzfeldt-Jakob Disease (CJD)

It is rare that Central Service Technicians in the United States receive instrumentation exposed to Creutzfeldt-Jakob disease (CJD) but, when they do, they must know and apply proper processing procedures.

This section considers reprocessing concerns for instruments and medical devices that have been exposed to patients known or suspected to have CJD. The processing of this instrumentation requires a shift from the use of standard precautions where all items are processed in the same manner.

CJD is caused by abnormal forms of normal proteins called **prions**. These are transmissible pathogenic agents that are smaller than viruses, and are extremely resistant to inactivation by heat and disinfecting agents. The incubation period can be many years long, and fatality is almost certain within several months after initial onset of the symptoms.

CJD is named after the German psychiatrists who first described the disease in the 1920s. It, along with other similar diseases, is classified as a "transmissible spongiform encephalopathie"(TSE). These diseases are appropriately named because:

- They can be spread from one person to another. (They are transmissible.)

- They cause the brain to degenerate. (Under a microscope, infected tissue has a sponge-like appearance).

- They affect the brain. ("Encephalopathy" refers to disease of the brain.)

The CJD death rate in the United States is approximately one case in a million persons annually.

CJD has a relatively long incubation time (up to 30 years) during which the disease is unnoticed. Therefore, patients with CJD who have brain, spinal, or eye surgery for another purpose may contaminate instruments with the infectious agents. This makes plans and policies for control of CJD very important.

Prions are most frequently found in the brain, dura mater (the tough membrane that encases the nerves of the spinal cord), and eyes. They are also detected less frequently in cerebrospinal fluid, and the spleen, lymph nodes, kidney, and liver. They are seldom (but could be) located in blood, urine, skin, muscle, bone, adrenal gland, heart, feces, peripheral nerves, nasal mucous, gingival, saliva, sputum, and tears. When a suspected CJD patient undergoes a procedure, the facility's plans and policies must include notification of all personnel involved with that patient.

The guidelines outlined below should be followed for instruments used for brain biopsies on patients in whom no specific lesion has been demonstrated (for example, by magnetic resonance imaging (MRI) or computerized tomography (CT) scans). Alternatively, instruments used for such patients could be disposable, or the instruments could be quarantined until the pathology of the brain biopsy is reviewed, and CJD is excluded. These recommendations apply to devices and equipment contaminated with high-risk tissues such as brain, spinal cord, and eye tissue from high-risk patients (those known or suspected to have CJD):

- The use of proper cleaning procedures is an important tactic to inactivate prions. Surfaces contaminated by infected material should be disinfected with a solution of sodium hydroxide. Keep the surface wet at room temperature for one hour of contact time. Then rinse three times with water, and clean according to established routines. Note: Because this solution is caustic, it is important to carefully follow recommendations of applicable Material Data Safety Sheets for proper handling/disposing.

- Devices such as surgical instruments that are constructed to enable cleaning procedures to result in effective tissue removal can be cleaned, and then steam sterilized at:

Prions – Virus-like infectious agents that cause a variety of neurodegenerative diseases of humans and animals, including Creutzfeldt-Jakob disease (CJD) in humans.

another name *mad cow disease.*

- 275°F – 278°F (135°C – 137°C) for 18 minutes in a prevacuum or porous load unit.

- 270°F (132°C) for one hour in a gravity displacement unit.

- 250°F (121°C) for four and one-half hours in a gravity displacement unit

- Devices that are impossible or difficult to clean must be incinerated.

- Devices should be kept moist until cleaned and decontaminated to minimize the drying of tissues and body fluids on the object.

- Flash sterilization cannot be used to reprocess these devices.

- Contaminated items that have been in contact with high-risk tissue, and have not been processed according to these recommendations (for example, medical devices used for brain biopsy prior to diagnosis) should be recalled and appropriately reprocessed.

- A tracking system, if used, may be helpful to recall devices used on high-risk tissue and high-risk patients. The system should permit identification of the patient on which the devices were used, the date they were used, the procedure performed, and the surgeon's name. Facilities that do not have a commercially available or automated tracking system should create a manual system.

- Environmental (non-critical) surfaces contaminated with high-risk tissues (for example, laboratory surfaces that have come in contact with the brain tissue of a person infected with CJD) should be cleaned with a detergent, and then spot-decontaminated with 5,000 ppm sodium hypochlorite. Note: this concentration usually results from a 1/10 dilution of household bleach. However, the label should be checked for the amount of sodium hypochlorite present;

concentrations in U.S. products can range from 3% to over 6% sodium hypochlorite.

- Non-critical equipment contaminated with high-risk tissue should be cleaned, and then disinfected with 5,000 ppm hypochlorite or in NaOH (Sodium Hydroxide) depending on material compatibility. All contaminated surfaces must be exposed to the disinfectant.

- Equipment that requires special prion reprocessing must be tagged after use. Clinicians and Central Service Technicians should be thoroughly trained on the proper tagging of equipment and on special prion reprocessing protocols.

- The use of power drills or saws that are likely to contact high-risk tissue should be avoided. These items are, by their very nature and design, difficult to clean, and too expensive to discard.

The following recommendations apply to devices and equipment contaminated with low-risk tissues such as cerebrospinal fluid, kidney, liver, spleen, lung, and lymph node tissue from high-risk patients:

- Devices can be cleaned and disinfected or sterilized using conventional protocols of high-level disinfection, thermal sterilization, or chemical sterilization.

- Endoscopes (except neurosurgical endoscopes) are likely to be contaminated only with low-risk materials so standard cleaning and high-level disinfection processing protocols are adequate.

- Environmental surfaces contaminated with low-risk tissues or fluids require only standard disinfection using disinfectants recommended by OSHA for decontaminating blood-contaminated surfaces (for example, 500 to 5,000 ppm sodium hypochlorite).

Please note: Additional information about CJD can be found at: http://www.cdc.gov/ncidod/dvrd/cjd/qa_cjd_infection_control.htm#reprocessed

Solutions

There are two types of sterile solutions: **parenteral** and **external solutions**. Parenteral solutions are administered to patients intravenously (in other words, as intravenous fluids). External solutions are normally used for irrigating, topical application, and surgical use, and are given orally or by inhalation. External solutions are further defined as any aqueous medium in which water serves as the solvent for one or more solutes (chemical compounds).

Note: ANSI/AAMI ST79:2006 (section 8.5.7) states; "Primarily for personnel safety reasons, in-hospital preparation and sterilization of parenteral and irrigation is discouraged. When solutions are processed in the hospital, (i.e. in emergency situations), processing should be performed only by trained personnel…"

Both types of sterile solutions should be prepared with the same high standards of quality and purity. Preparing solutions for patient use is regulated, and preparation of solutions by Central Service Technicians should be done according to procedures that have been thoroughly reviewed by the facility's Risk Management and Infection Control personnel.

There are several types of water that can be used as a base for solutions. Basics of each type as they apply to solutions must be understood.

Water

Water, like other chemical substances, can be in the form of a gas, a liquid, or a solid. The solid form is ice; the gaseous form is water vapor. Water is always present in the air, and sometimes there is much water vapor in the air. On a hot or humid day, 1/20 of the weight of the air may be vapor.

The liquid form is the most familiar: that which comprises rain, rivers, lakes, and oceans. Water makes up the largest part of the weight of plants, animals, humans, and microorganisms.

The parts played in nature by water in its various forms are known as the **hydrologic cycle**. Water on the earth evaporates with the heat of the sun. It is then collected as water vapor in the clouds, and falls when it reaches a temperature at which the air is too cool to hold it. It is reabsorbed by plants and is collected in rivers, lakes, oceans, and in the soil, and the cycle then repeats.

Early in the 1900s, water pollution became a concern because of diseases such as typhoid fever and cholera. Measures were taken to test and treat water so that it would be safe for human use. In the 1950-60s, another problem — the introduction of detergent pollution into water systems—led to the killing of plants, fish, and algae. This was caused, in part, by phosphates in the detergents and these, along with pesticides and weed killers, cannot be removed successfully from all water systems. Rather, they pass into ground water, and eventually poison wells and other systems.

Lack of knowledge about the hydrologic cycle has resulted in death, destruction, and extinction of many species of plant and animal life. There have been some improvements since the 1970 United States Water Quality Improvement Act in the U.S., but the goal of safe water has not been attained.

Central Service Technicians must know basic information about water to make better use of it:

• Tap water. This water comes from the local water supply, and its quality varies both with the source and the local authority responsible for it. It may contain microorganisms including

---

Parenteral solutions – *Solutions that are administered to patients intravenously.* patient IV's

External solutions – *Solutions that are normally used for irrigating, topical application, and surgical use that are given orally or by inhalation.*

Hydrologic cycle – *The continual movement of water from the atmosphere to the earth and back to the atmosphere.*

Reverse osmosis – *A water treatment process in which dissolved impurities are separated from water by forcing the water through a molecular filter membrane.* special

---

Aeromonas or Aeruginosa and Pseudomonas aeruginosa. Regular microbial monitoring is essential for all water supplies; freedom from enterobacteria is essential for all water used to formulate products, wash food, or process items. The microbial count of tap water will be reflected in the softened and deionized water prepared from it.

• Softened water. This is usually prepared either by a base-exchange method using sodium zeolite, by a lime-soda ash process, or by the addition of sodium hexametaphosphate. When chemical beds are used, they must be treated regularly to inhibit microbial colonization. Bacillus spp. and Staphylococcus aureus may be introduced where brine is used to regenerate chemical beds.

• Deionized or demineralized water. An ion is an electrical charge, and there are two types of charges: anionic (negative) and cationic (positive). Deionized water is prepared by passing tap water through synthetic anion- or cation-exchange resin beds to remove ions. Any bacteria in the water source will be present in the deionized water. Beds which are not regenerated frequently with alkaline or acid solutions rapidly become contaminated.

• Distilled water. This process involves evaporation of raw water by boiling, followed by immediate condensation of the liberated steam or water vapor. The quality or purity of the condensate produced by this process can vary greatly, and still conform to the basic characteristics of distilled water. Distilled water demands unusual quality when it is to be used in critical applications. In the preparation of irrigation or injectable infusions, distilled water must be substantially free from mineral, metallic, and organic impurities. Above all, distilled water must be free from pyrogenic (fever-causing) bacterial waste.

When distilled water leaves the still, it is free from microorganisms. Any contamination that then occurs results from a fault in the cooling system or in storage or distribution. Distilled water should be sterilized as soon as possible (but no more than four hours) after distillation.

• Reverse osmosis water. The **reverse osmosis** process uses a molecular filter to retain salts, remove bacteria, and pyrogens. Water may, however, become contaminated whether in a storage vessel or the distribution system. NOTE: If microorganisms colonize a storage vessel, the vessel acts as a microbial reservoir, and contaminates all water passing through it. Therefore, it is important that the contents of all storage vessels be tested regularly. Reservoirs of microorganisms also build-up in pumps, water meters, and unused sections of pipelines and tubings. Monitoring the quality of water within the system of choice is essential to its quality.

Purified Water. Purified water is obtained by distillation, exchange treatment, reverse osmosis, or other suitable process. It is prepared from water complying with the regulations of the federal Environmental Protection Agency (EPA) applicable to drinking water. CAUTION: Do not use purified water in preparations intended for parenteral administration because sterile water must be used for injection.

The United States Pharmacopeia National Formulary (USP-NF) states packaging requirements for purified water. These include a pH between 5.0 and 7.0, and specific limits for chloride, sulfate, ammonia, calcium, carbon dioxide, heavy metals, and total solid residue limits. The bacteriological purity must comply with the federal EPA regulations for drinking water with respect to bacteriological purity. If water is to be processed for injection, inhalation or irrigation, it is important to follow applicable EPA, FDA, and/or USP-NF regulations.

Drinking water

Flasking Technique

The flasking technique can be used to produce sterile distilled water and isotonic solutions in the Central Service Department. Borosilicate glass containers are filled with freshly distilled water or other aqueous solution and sterilized at 250°F to 254°F (121° C - 123° C) for an appropriate time depending on container size. Special flask closures are used to allow air and vapor to escape during sterilization. (Typically 3% to 5% of the fluid is evaporated.) The closures automatically form a hermetic seal when the temperature drops after the sterilization exposure.

A special sterilizer cycle must be used to safely process liquids with the flasking technique. After sterilization, pressure in the sterilizer must be exhausted slowly to prevent a violent boiling over that may blow out the stopper, cause fluid loss, and create a serious potential hazard to those handling the flasks. Great care must be taken to ensure that flask contents have cooled sufficiently to allow for safe handling after the liquid sterilization process. Only specially trained personnel should be permitted to work with flask sterilization if it is used in a facility.

ENDNOTES

1. *ANSI/AAMI ST79: 2006, Comprehensive Guide to Steam Sterilization and Sterility Assurance in Healthcare Facilities.*

2. *Adapted from – Appendix A: Bacterial Growth Curve. Central Service Technical Manual. Sixth Edition. Chicago, IL., International Association of Healthcare Central Service Materiel Management. 2003. (See pp. 387-388).*

3. *Adopted from: Appendix C: Creutzfeldt-Jakob Disease (CJD). Appendix C in: Central Service Technical Manual. Sixth Edition. Chicago, IL., International Association of Healthcare Materiel Management. 2003. (See pp. 391-401). See also: Creutzfeldt-Jakob Disease. Self-Study Lesson 55. Chicago, Il., International Association of Healthcare Central Service Materiel Management. December, 2000.*

CENTRAL SERVICE TERMS

Bioburden

Exposure time (steam sterilization)

Heat-up time (steam sterilization)

Saturated steam

Gauge pressure (steam sterilizer)

Absolute pressure (steam sterilizer)

Superheat (steam)

Flash Sterilization

Terminal Sterilization

Flash sterilizer

Instrument washer sterilizer (IWS)

Conduction

Convection

Process indicators

Chemical indicators (CIs)

Load control number

Spore

Validation

Verification

D-Value

Prions

Parenteral solutions

External solutions

Hydrologic cycle

Reverse osmosis

Chapter 16

Low Temperature Sterilization

Chapter Learning Objectives

As a result of successfully completing this chapter, readers will be able to:

1. Discuss basic requirements important for any type of low temperature sterilization system.

2. Explain specific requirements for the three low temperature sterilization methods: ethylene oxide, hydrogen peroxide (gas plasma), and ozone.

3. Review (compare) important parameters of the three low temperature sterilization methods commonly used by health care facilities.

The reprocessing of heat- and moisture-sensitive items is important because synthetic materials are often used in today's complex and expensive medical devices. Ethylene oxide (EtO), hydrogen peroxide (H₂O₂), and ozone (O₃), are the terminal low temperature sterilization methods commonly used in healthcare settings.

All chemicals used to sterilize items have toxic properties, and Central Service Technicians must be trained about how to use them safely and effectively. Each sterilization method has advantages and limitations, and it is the responsibility of sterilization professionals to know when and how to safely use the low temperature sterilization methods that are available.

EtO been around since 1968

BASIC STERILIZATION REQUIRE-MENTS

Learning Objective 1. Discuss basic requirements important for any type of low temperature sterilization system.

Eight basic requirements are important for any type of low temperature sterilization system, and these are discussed in this section. To be effective in the hospital environment, the sterilization system must satisfy all requirements; failure to meet even one requirement may pose a significant risk to the patients or the healthcare workers.

Effectiveness

To be legally marketed in the United States, the Food and Drug Administration (FDA) requires that each sterilant be rigorously tested against the broad range of microorganisms encountered in today's healthcare environment. Each low temperature sterilization method discussed in this chapter uses different sterilizing agents, and each has significantly different processing protocols. However, when processed in accordance with the product's labeling, each has the capability of providing the minimum (10-6) required **sterility assurance level (SAL).**

on crest test →7

Safety

There should be no toxic sterilant residuals remaining on packaging or devices after the sterilization process is completed. As well, the equipment used for low temperature sterilization should provide a safe environment around the sterilizer. These factors must be addressed to avoid safety risks to patients and healthcare workers. All of the low temperature sterilizing agents discussed in this chapter present some safety risks because they are toxic. In fact, if they were not toxic, they would not be able to kill the microorganisms! While each presents different types of safety risks, each is safe if used properly.

Monitoring

The Occupational Safety and Health Administration (OSHA) established specific guidelines for the use of ethylene oxide (EtO) sterilization based primarily upon data developed in the 1980's. OSHA has established **permissible exposure limits (PELs)** for all low temperature sterilants. They are expressed as an 8-hour **time weighted average (TWA)**: the total allowable worker exposure during an 8-hour period.

The National Institute for Occupational Safety and Health (NIOSH) has developed documentation for Immediately Dangerous To Life Or Health

Sterility assurance level (SAL) – The probability of a viable microorganism being present on a product unit after sterilization. Abbreviated "SAL."

on cert. exam)

Permissible exposure limits (PELs) – Limits developed by OSHA to indicate the maximum airborne concentration of a contaminant to which an employee may be exposed over the duration specified by the type of PEL assigned to that contaminant. Abbreviated as "PEL."

Time weighted average (8-hour) – The employee's average airborne exposure in any 8-hour work shift of a 40-hour work week which should not be exceeded. Abbreviated as "TWA."

Alkylation – The process by which Ethylene Oxide destroys microorganisms, resulting in the inability of the cell to normally metabolize, reproduce, or both.

Oxidation – The act or process of oxidizing: the chemical breakdown of nutrients for energy.

Figure 16.1 Toxicity Standards for Low Temperature Sterilants

Sterilant	OSHA – PEL 8-Hour TWA Limit	NIOSH IDLH Limit
Ethylene Oxide (EtO)	1.0 ppm*	800 ppm*
Hydrogen Peroxide (H_2O_2)	1.0 ppm	75 ppm
Ozone (O_3)	0.1 ppm	10 ppm
*ppm = parts per million		

(IDLHs) concentrations that mandate toxicity standards for low temperature sterilants. These are identified in **Figure 16.1** which compares the standards established by OSHA and NIOSH for each sterilant. Hospitals are required to follow OSHA regulations.

Quality Assurance

The low temperature sterilization process should be capable of being reliably monitored with readily available physical, chemical, and biological indicators. The complex sterilization processes that are used, along with concerns that some critical parameters cannot be measured directly, and cannot be controlled, dictate that the process be monitored.

Process monitoring consists of the "4 R's": Run, Read, Record, and Retain, No single monitoring product provides all the information necessary to ensure effective sterilization. Therefore, recommended practices state that available information from physical, chemical, and biological indictors should be used to assess the process before releasing a load. It is absolutely essential that Central Service Technicians can read and interpret physical monitoring information and chemical indicator color changes, and know how to handle, use, and interpret the results of biological indicators.

Penetration

Many modern medical devices and instruments are significantly more complex than their counterparts of just a few years ago. Not only must the sterilant penetrate through packaging material (in some cases, multiple layers), it must also reach narrow lumens, and between tightly-matted surfaces. If the sterilant cannot penetrate to the most difficult-to-access site where microorganisms may be harbored, the sterilization process will not be effective.

The properties of a chemical sterilant affect its ability to penetrate effectively. Some chemicals such as EtO that inactivate microbes by a process called "**alkylation**," seek out specific proteins in microbes with which to react. This allows the chemical to penetrate through packaging and materials to reach remote surfaces where the microbes are located. Other chemicals that inactivate microbes do so by a less specific process called "**oxidation**." They react easily, and may be depleted before all surfaces to be sterilized are reached. Note: this is one reason why it is important to place monitoring devices at difficult locations where sterilization must take place.

Material Compatibility

There should be no changes in the functionality of the devices being sterilized after repeated sterilization cycles. Material used for packaging must:

- Be permeable to the sterilant.

- Allow the release of residual gasses during aeration.

- Provide a barrier to dust and liquids as well as microorganisms.

- Resist tearing and puncturing.

- Allow easy, aseptic opening without contamination.

- Contain no toxic ingredients or non-fast dyes.

- Have proven seal integrity.

Adaptability

The process should be compatible with or easily modified to meet existing healthcare practices.

Approval

The sterilization system must be cleared by or registered with the appropriate regulatory agencies.

ETHYLENE OXIDE

Learning Objective 2. Explain specific requirements for the three low temperature sterilization methods: ethylene oxide.

Background

Ethylene oxide (EtO) has been the primary sterilant of choice for items that cannot tolerate steam sterilization since the 1960s. It has an exceptional ability to penetrate products and compatibility with numerous materials that provide broad sterilization applications.

Figure 16.2 reviews how the four process parameters of EtO sterilization are controlled or monitored.

EtO evaporates very easily, even at below-room temperatures. This makes it easy to obtain and maintain EtO in the vapor state to spread out and fill all spaces within the sterilization chamber.

EtO kills microorganisms by reacting (combining) with specific molecules, mainly those containing genetic material or with specific protein structures. During the alkylation process, EtO contacts the target molecule in the presence of moisture. It combines chemically with the molecule, and alters its size and shape. When molecules lose their size and shape, they are unable to perform necessary functions, and this leads to the organism's death. This process is called alkylation.

Figure 16.2 Control of Ethylene Oxide Process Parameters

Parameter	Overview	Control (Monitoring) Method	Comment
Time	The longer the exposure time, the more time that sterilization can take place. Short exposure times hinder sterilization of the entire load.	Easy to measure and monitor on printout	Need to read data log print out or graph
Temperature	Higher temperatures create faster reaction rates. Colder cycle temperatures require longer exposure times for the same sterilization level.	Easy to measure and monitor on printout	Need to read data log print out or graph
Concentration of EtO	EtO is generally available in a greater concentration than that needed for a normal load.	Indirectly measured by pressure gauge	Pressure reading may not be from EtO
Relative humidity (r.h.)	35% relative humidity conditions where microbes are destroyed is considered optimal. Higher r.h. conditions are commonly used because of variations in packaging and loads.	Indirectly measured by a pressure gauge or, in newest equipment, by a direct r.h. sensor	Low r.h. is a common cause of cycle failures

The ability of EtO to fill spaces, and to only react with specific molecules, are the reasons this sterilant does not have the same lumen restrictions as other sterilant vapors. Other chemicals may be used up by reacting with multiple materials, decomposing before all surfaces to be sterilized are reached, or may be absorbed into certain materials rather than being spread throughout the load.

EtO is a small-sized molecule that can penetrate through plastics (polymers), so it can reach and sterilize areas that other chemical sterilants cannot. While this is useful, it is also the reason that long **aeration** periods are necessary before items can be safely handled or used: EtO must migrate out of the materials it penetrates. The amount of EtO that remains inside materials after sterilization is called the **residual**. This remaining EtO must be removed from medical devices and packaging before they can be safely handled or used.

When the exposure cycle ends, one or more vacuum pulses remove EtO from the chamber before the door is opened. The aeration process then removes residuals from materials in the load as warm air is circulated through the chamber. As individual EtO molecules migrate to the surface of the materials they have penetrated, they are swept away by the moving air. The more loosely packages are arranged in the chamber, the better the air can circulate around them to remove the residuals. Also, the warmer the temperature, the faster residuals migrate to the surface for removal.

EtO should not be used to sterilize liquids, because it will combine with liquids and may produce harmful chemical by-products.

Small amounts of moisture, if any, that remain on items placed in the EtO sterilizer will be changed into a vapor during the preconditioning phase as the moisture is heated, and a vacuum is pulled.

Aeration – A process in which a device is actively subjected to moving air. Example: items being sterilized with ethylene oxide gas.

Residual (EtO) – The amount of EtO that remains inside materials after they are sterilized.

Excessively wet items should be avoided because EtO does not penetrate through a water layer, and will not sterilize the surface under the water.

Leather items should not be sterilized in EtO because chemicals that may have been used in the tanning process will combine with EtO to form chlorhydrin. This chemical can cause negative health effects. Leather items potentially contaminated with chlorhydrin should be discarded because this chemical is more toxic than EtO, and is not removed by aeration.

For fire safety reasons, EtO used in healthcare facilities is often supplied in large tanks as a mixture diluted with an inert gas to render it nonflammable and non-explosive. Alternatively, EtO is also available in small cartridges with enough EtO to sterilize a single load. (See **Figure 16.3**)

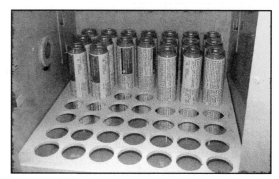

Figure 16.3

Improvements in equipment using 100% EtO, and the escalating costs of gas blends have resulted in a shift from gas blends to 100% EtO systems.

Mixed EtO Blends and 100% EtO Systems Each Have Advantages

Mixed blend EtO chambers can hold a large volume of material to be sterilized, while 100% EtO systems are used in chambers of less than 10 cubic feet. Mixed EtO blends come in large tanks that require connections to the sterilizer and, in turn, create an EtO exposure potential when a tank is connected or disconnected. Therefore, trained hospital personnel using proper procedures are required when tanks are changed.

By contrast, 100% EtO is provided in individual dose cartridges that are placed inside the chamber. A vacuum is used to puncture the cartridge, and eliminates many exposure concerns. Mixed EtO systems operate under pressure, while 100% EtO systems operate under a vacuum. If a leak develops in a 100% system, the vacuum will pull room air into the chamber rather than allow EtO to be released. The gas blended with EtO in mixed blends adds additional costs that are not part of the 100% EtO system. The result: the cost of 100% EtO per cubic foot of sterilizing capacity is significantly less than the mixed blend EtO systems.

Effectiveness

As you've learned, EtO is a very effective alkylating agent, and a good sterilant against a wide range of microorganisms. It reacts specifically with genetic and certain protein structures essential to the living cell, and destroys the cells' ability to metabolize or reproduce. It vaporizes easily, and can permeate throughout a wide range of materials to reach recessed areas and matted surfaces.

EtO – Colorless + Odorless

Safety

To minimize the risks associated with the use of EtO, employees should be instructed about:

- Hazards of EtO.
- Procedures to reduce employee exposure.
- Principles of EtO monitoring, and the interpretation of results.
- The use of protective equipment.
- Applicable OSHA standards.
- Material safety data sheets (MSDSs).
- EtO emergency plans.
- Processing procedures.
- Storage and handling of EtO gas containers.

The recommendations of the sterilizer's manufacturer and the EtO supplier should be followed and incorporated into training provided to address EtO risks.

✗ on cert. exam

Ethylene oxide is a toxic gas. EtO sterilizers should be located in a well-ventilated area with a room air exchange rate of at least 10 changes per hour. Ventilation systems and exhaust lines including floor drains should be periodically checked by qualified personnel to assure that they are working properly.

The use of EtO creates special safety concerns for patients. Ethylene oxide residues could remain on a sterilized device that is subsequently used on a patient. These residues are toxic, and should be reduced to safe levels by mechanical aeration. Minimum general recommendations for product aeration are 8 hours at 140°F (60°C), and 12 hours at 122°F (50°C). The rate of aeration is dependent upon many factors including the nature of the materials used to construct the device. Therefore, the manufacturer of the medical device must provide recommendations for appropriate aeration times and temperatures. Some types of devices have been found to require significantly longer aeration periods than the minimum recommendations just noted. The facility, through its safety committee, must establish a written emergency plan in case of an EtO leak or spill.

Loading the EtO Sterilizer

The sterilizer must be properly loaded for effective sterilization. Overloading impedes proper air removal, load humidification, sterilant penetration, and degassing (removal of residuals). As with steam sterilization, items must be properly spaced.

When possible, metal carts or baskets should be used. Since metal does not absorb EtO, operator exposure is reduced if loads are transferred to a separate chamber for aeration. Items should be arranged to avoid contact with chamber walls. Pouches should be placed on edge in wire baskets. Stacking one package on another should be avoided.

Unloading the EtO Sterilizer

It is preferable that processed loads be completely aerated before items are removed for transfer. If this is not done, it is a "must" that correct load transfer procedures be followed. EtO sterilizers with built-in aerators provide a safer environment because they eliminate the need to transfer the load into another chamber.

For sterilization cycles without in-chamber aeration, there are two times when the load can be removed. For a load processed in a sterilizer without a purge cycle, the sterilizer's door must be opened 6 inches for 15 minutes before the load is removed. Carts containing sterilized, but not yet aerated items should be pulled (not pushed) to minimize operator exposure. The load should be immediately placed into the aerator, and the aeration cycle started. Once a load has been placed in the aerator, new loads of sterilized items should not be added to the same aerator.

For sterilizers with purge cycles, loads should be removed immediately upon completion of the cycle to prevent the buildup of EtO that can occur if the door is not opened immediately for load removal. If there is a delay in door opening, the purge cycle should be repeated before opening the door and/or transferring the load.

Process and sterilizer monitors must be used to assess the extent to which sterilization parameters are attained.

Personnel Monitoring

Personnel monitoring normally involves the use of devices affixed directly to the employee's clothing in the breathing zone (within one foot of the person's nose). (See **Figure 16.4**) One limitation of personnel monitoring devices is that sampling results are not available until after the actual sampling period has ended. Therefore, OSHA also requires that facilities using EtO sterilization have a system/procedure to immediately alert the employees in case of an emergency.

Area monitors are available that provide real-time, and continuous monitoring of airborne EtO. They can quickly detect emergencies including leaks, spills, or failures in the ventilation system. However, monitors may not provide reliable breathing-zone measurements, and may not be appropriate for STEL or TWA data.

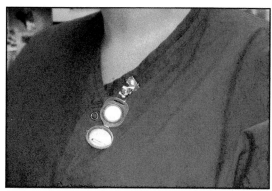

Figure 16.4

Many healthcare facilities use contracted environmental monitoring services to obtain independent monitoring data, and to perform on-site assessments. The contractor should also check the ventilation systems including room air exchanges, local exhausts, and air intakes.

To comply with OSHA regulations, the employer must inform all applicable employees about the results of personnel monitoring. These records must be kept for 30 years after the employee has completed the last EtO-related tasks.

Sterilizer Performance Monitors

An EtO sterilizer should be monitored with physical, chemical, and biological indicators. While none of these provides conclusive evidence of device sterility by itself, in combination they provide a high degree of sterility assurance.

- Physical monitors include operating pressure gauges, temperature control/measurement devices, timing recorders, and humidity sensors. Charts, tapes, and graphs detailing the measurements made by physical monitors must be carefully examined before the items are removed from the sterilizer.

- Chemical indicators (CIs) should be used on the outside of every pack to demonstrate that each pack has been processed. CIs should also be used inside every pack to measure whether some or all of the sterilization process parameters have been met. The primary advantage of an internal CI is that it may be placed inside every package to detect sterilization failures, and it can be examined as soon as the package is opened for use.

• Biological indicators (BIs) are the most accepted means for providing quality assurance for EtO sterilization. You've learned that a biological indicator is a carrier that has been inoculated with a known population of a microorganism that is highly resistant to the sterilant. The microorganism of choice for EtO is the spore of Bacillus atrophaeus (previously called Bacillus subtilis var.niger). It is assumed that killing all spores on a standardized BI indicates a successful sterilization cycle, since the BI's population and resistance exceeds that of the bioburden on items being sterilized. Note: this assumption only applies to properly cleaned, prepared, packaged, and loaded supplies. It is recommended that biological indicators be run in every EtO load.

Penetration

There is probably no better penetrating gas sterilant than EtO. It has a high vapor pressure and a low boiling point of 51.3°F (10.7°C) which means it is easily maintained in the gas phase. It is relatively stable, so it will not break down to a non-sterilizing entity as it penetrates into difficult-to-reach sites. With its solubility and diffusion properties, EtO can penetrate directly through many types of polymers.[1]

Material Compatibility

Sterilants must be compatible with the device being processed and with its packaging. EtO has excellent compatibility with nearly all of the materials used in the construction of both single-use and reusable medical devices. This is evidenced by the extensive use of EtO in the United States and other countries. However, as with all sterilization methods, follow specific device manufacturer's recommendations for the appropriate sterilization process for that specific item.

Generally-accepted EtO packaging materials are plastic film, plastic pouches, paper-plastic pouches, non-woven and paper wraps, spun-bonded polyolefin, and textiles. Aluminum foil, cellophane and nylon films should not be used. Rigid containers should be carefully evaluated for their ability to allow sterilant penetration and, particularly, for their ability to be degassed. Documentation should be requested to support the use and approval of a rigid container with any sterilant to be used.

— Steriad units —

HYDROGEN PEROXIDE (GAS PLASMA)

Learning Objective 2. Explain specific requirements for the low temperature sterilization method: hydrogen peroxide (gas plasma).

Hydrogen Peroxide (H_2O_2) is a popular low temperature sterilization method because of its short cycle times that allow faster instrument turn-around. The process uses H_2O_2 vapor and low-temperature

Figure 16.5 Control of Hydrogen Peroxide Sterilization Process Parameters

Parameter	Control (Monitoring) Method	Comment
Time	Easy to measure and monitor on printout	Need to read data log printout.
Temperature	Easy to measure and monitor on printout	Need to read data log printout.
H_2O_2 Concentration	Indirectly measured by pressure gauge	Pressure reading may not be from H_2O_2
Vacuum level	Automatically controlled by equipment	Vacuum is critical to vaporization, diffusion, and plasma generation
Plasma	Automatically controlled by equipment	

gas plasma for rapid inactivation of microorganisms, and the removal of harmful residues.

Figure 16.5 reviews the five process parameters of H_2O_2 sterilization, and how they are controlled.

Background 1

The H_2O_2 low temperature sterilization process consists of an initial deep vacuum. During this step, the load begins to warm as the vacuum evaporates any remaining water from the load. The moisture is removed from the chamber, and a second deep vacuum is pulled. The H_2O_2 sterilant is added, and it is then pulled by the vacuum to fill the space as a vapor. As the H_2O_2 diffuses and contacts surfaces, an oxidative process inactivates microorganisms. A third deep vacuum is pulled before radio frequency (RF) energy (similar to that generated by a microwave oven) is used to generate highly-charged reactive particles around the chamber's perforated metal shield. These highly-charged particles make up the plasma that recombines to form oxygen, water, and other by-products when the RF energy is turned off. Another deep vacuum is then pulled, and the H_2O injection is repeated to provide further microbial inactivation. The final deep vacuum is used with RF energy to again generate a plasma, and subsequent conversion of H_2O_2 into oxygen and water vapor.

Hydrogen peroxide is a very reactive molecule. It must be converted into a vapor, and pulled through packaging and into spaces with surfaces to be sterilized before it reacts, and is converted to water and oxygen. This is one reason why the deep vacuum is critical.

It is also a powerful oxidizer because it provides an oxygen molecule to combine with, and alter the structure of, many other molecules including those that comprise microorganisms. The property of H_2O_2 to act as a strong oxidizing chemical is why it can inactivate microorganisms quickly, and also why it has toxic properties that have resulted in OSHA establishing a PEL of 1 ppm over an 8 hour TWA.

Effectiveness 2

Hydrogen peroxide gas plasma is widely compatible with different materials. However it is not compatible with powders and stronger absorbers such as paper and linen made of cellulose, and it cannot be used to process liquids.

Hydrogen peroxide destroys microorganisms by oxidation, and H_2O_2 has been concentrated from 58% to 95% for use in the newest equipment to shorten the exposure time, and to lessen the lumen restrictions. There are still some restrictions involving the size, length, and number of lumens, and on the type of material and number of instruments per cycle.

Guidelines have been developed for lumen diameter and length to ensure adequate penetration and efficacy for the given cycle parameters. As always, recommendations of the device manufacturer should be closely followed.

Safety

— Cassette comes in a 3 closed container set.

The sterilizer is designed to allow a cassette containing concentrated H_2O_2 to be directly inserted into the machine so the operator's hands do not come in contact with any hazardous material. The cassette contains a chemical leak indicator on each side of the package that changes from yellow to red when exposed to liquid or vapor hydrogen peroxide. The leak indicator is visible through a clear plastic over-wrap to protect personnel handling the cassette. The by-products of hydrogen peroxide are ordinary oxygen and water vapor, so there should be no odors or hazardous emissions when the equipment is operating correctly.

Even though hydrogen peroxide can degrade quickly, and the highly charged particles of a plasma would be expected to speed up its breakdown, mechanical problems can lead to hydrogen peroxide residuals within the load or the release of H_2O_2 from the chamber. Chemical burns have been reported, and this emphasizes that any sterilization chemical has the potential for health risks when the equipment fails, and when the proper procedures are not followed. Central Service Technicians must be knowledgeable and safety conscious, and safety concerns must emphasize the desirability of area monitoring practices for all chemical processes.

To minimize H_2O_2 risks, employees should be instructed about:

- Hazards of H_2O_2.

- Applicable material safety data sheets (MSDSs).

- The OSHA PEL for H_2O_2 (1 ppm)

- Recommendations for changing vaporizer plates.

- Storage, handling, and disposal of H_2O_2 cassettes.

EtO monitoring everything.

Monitoring

4 H_2O_2 monitor area only

Currently, no personnel monitors are required, but sterilizer performance monitors are required. Hydrogen peroxide sterilization systems have been designed to minimize the risk of liquid or vapor phase exposure to hospital personnel. While the risk of an incidence is low, exposure can still occur. OSHA has established a PEL, and monitoring systems are available. Reported chemical burns have raised questions about operator and patient safety issues, and further discussions about area monitors are desirable. As well, employee safety problems confirm the fact that any chemical used for sterilization has the potential for health risks when equipment fails or procedures are not followed.

Hydrogen peroxide sterilizers should be monitored with physical, chemical, and biological indicators. As you've learned, none of these indicators provides conclusive evidence of device sterility by themselves. However, in combination, they provide a high degree of sterility assurance.

- Physical Monitors. Hydrogen peroxide sterilizers used today operate on a fixed automatic cycle controlled by a microprocessor. All critical parameters are monitored during the operation of the cycle, and a printed record documenting the process parameters is processed at the end of each cycle. If any process parameter does not meet established acceptable limits, the cycle will be canceled, and the printed record will indicate the reason for the malfunction. It is then necessary to repackage and reprocess the load contents.

- Chemical indicators (CIs). These should be used on the outside of every pack to demonstrate that they have been processed. Chemical indicators should also be used inside every pack to measure whether some or all of the sterilization process parameters have been met. The use of internal chemical indicators at challenging locations inside packs is especially important because of the penetration limitations of H_2O_2. You've learned that the primary advantage of a CI is that it can be placed inside every package to detect sterilization failures, and the results can be noted when the package is opened for use. Note: Some chemical indicators may be light sensitive, and will require special storage.

- Biological indicators (BIs). These are most accepted means for providing quality assurance for H_2O_2 sterilizers. The microorganism of choice for H_2O_2 is the spore of Geobacillus stearothermophilus (previously called Bacillus stearothermophilus). As noted earlier, the killing of all the spores on a standardized BI indicates of a successful sterilization cycle if supplies have been properly cleaned, prepared, packaged and loaded.

Penetration *5*

Hydrogen peroxide does not have the same inherent penetration capabilities as EtO, nor is it nearly as soluble in most materials. It has an extremely low vapor pressure, and a relatively high boiling point (above that of water), so it is more difficult to keep molecules in the gas phase. This sterilant also has relatively fragile molecules in the gas phase that break down to form non-sterilizing entities. While these properties are very desirable for aeration and process safety, they are hurdles to be overcome for sterilant penetration.

To increase the penetrating capability of H_2O_2 vapor, sterilizers have used deep vacuums, multiple pulse additions of the sterilant, and increased concentrations.

Since hydrogen peroxide degrades quickly, the highly charged particles of a plasma would be expected to hasten the breakdown of hydrogen peroxide. However, mechanical problems can lead to H_2O_2 residuals within the load.

Packaging materials can also affect the penetrating capability of sterilants. Cellulose-containing packaging materials such as paper-plastic pouches, and disposable wrappers and muslin wraps are incompatible, and should not be used with H_2O_2 processes because they absorb the peroxide, and inhibit effective penetration. Also, if the available amount of H_2O_2 is reduced because it reacts or is absorbed before reaching all surfaces at remote load locations, a sterilization failure could occur. Therefore, the chamber should not be overloaded.

Material Compatibility

In one study, more than 600 individual re-sterilizable devices from more than 125 medical device manufacturers were evaluated.[3] Approximately 95% of the devices tested could be safely sterilized with the plasma process. Devices that appeared incompatible with the process displayed cosmetic changes including the fading of colored anodized components and some plastics. Embrittlement of some adhesives as well as chemical changes in some organic and polymeric sulfides were also noted.

All manufacturers of new low temperature sterilization technologies have active device testing programs. These involve cooperative testing with device manufacturers to evaluate sterilization efficacy and material compatibility. If hospital personnel have a question about the compatibility of a device with a specific sterilization process, the device's manufacturer should be contacted because he/she is responsible for the correct reprocessing procedures for the devices. Sterile processing professionals should not sterilize items without specific instructions from the device manufacturer.

Packaging for H_2O_2 Sterilization

Devices are typically loaded into trays that have been validated specifically for the process. These trays have been tested to confirm that sterilization efficacy is achievable. Devices can also be double-wrapped in a standard non-woven polypropylene wrap, and in standard heat-sealable sterilization pouches that do not contain paper.

Since there is a limited amount of H_2O_2 for each cycle, since H_2O_2 degrades quickly, and since sufficient amounts of H_2O_2 must contact every surface to be sterilized, the chamber should not be overloaded: as load size increases, so does the amount of surface area to be sterilized.

OZONE

Learning Objective 2. Explain specific requirements for low temperature sterilization method: ozone

Ozone (O_3) is a relatively new low temperature sterilization method available to healthcare facilities. It requires no sterilant purchase or handling because the system generates the O_3 that is needed. Another advantage: aeration is not required before the load can be handled or used.

Figure 16.6 notes the four process parameters of O_3 sterilization, and how they are controlled (monitored).

Figure 16.6 Control of Ozone Sterilization Process Parameters		
Parameter	Control (Monitoring) Method	Comment
Time	Easy to measure and monitor on printout	Need to read data log printout.
Temperature	Easy to measure and monitor on printout	Need to read data log printout.
O_3 Concentration	Equipment control; detection by CIs; adequacy assessed by BI results	Necessary for sterilization
Relative humidity (r.h.)	Indirectly measured by pressure readings	Presence is critical

Background

Ozone is a powerful oxidizing agent, and the process used for sterilization is similar to that used for both the EtO and H_2O_2 processes. An initial vacuum is pulled, and moisture is added while the load is being warmed in a manner similar to the EtO process. Ozone is then generated, and allowed to diffuse through the load to kill organisms by an oxidative process. This vacuum/humidification and O_3 addition comprises the first half of the cycle. Similar to the H_2O_2 process, the first half of the cycle is repeated a second time to provide better penetration of the load.

Effectiveness

Ozone is very reactive, and has penetration limitations similar to H_2O_2. It has some restrictions relating to the size and length of lumens, and the equipment and device manufacturer's recommendations must be consistently followed.

Safety

Ozone is generated within the equipment so there is no need to handle sterilant containers. It is very reactive, and easily converts back to oxygen, so this minimizes some risks associated with the process. However, all chemicals used to achieve sterilization have potential risks.

Monitoring

Currently, no personnel monitors are required; however, OSHA has established a PEL of 0.1 ppm.

The sterilizer monitors the progress of the cycle, and O_3 production is monitored before it enters the chamber. However, physical, chemical, and biological indicators are still needed to assess the effectiveness of the process:

- Physical Monitors. Information is provided based on physical measurements collected by the sterilizer, and should be reviewed before the load is released.

- Chemical Indicators (CIs). Chemical indicators should be placed on the outside of every pack to identify packages that have gone through the process from those that have not. Chemical indicators should also be placed inside each pack to demonstrate that the sterilant has penetrated the packaging.

- Biological Indicators (BIs). The BI for O_3 sterilization contains Geobacillus stearothermophilus spores. Biological indicators demonstrate if the conditions provided by the process are able to cause microbial destruction. This remains the most valuable evidence that the process was effective.

Penetration

You've learned that O_3 is an unstable molecule, and has limited penetration for the same reasons as H_2O_2 vapor. The first half of the cycle is also repeated for these reasons and there are lumen restrictions. Recommendations of equipment and device manufacturers should be followed.

Material Compatibility

Ozone has some material restrictions because it is a strong oxidizer, and the medical device manufacturer's recommendation should be followed.

Packaging

Tyvek® packaging is recommended. Other forms of packaging should be verified as acceptable before use.

REVIEW OF LOW TEMPERATURE STERILIZATION PARAMETERS

Learning Objective 3. Review (compare) important parameters of the three alternative low temperature sterilization methods.

Low Temperature Processes – **Figure 16.7** summarizes important comparisons of the three low temperature processes discussed in this chapter.

Figure 16.7 Overview of Alternatives

Low Temperature Sterilization Process		
Ethylene Oxide	Hydrogen Peroxide/Plasma	Ozone
Sterilization Mechanism		
Alkylation	Oxidation	Oxidation
Cycle Parameters		
Time Temperature EtO Concentration Relative Humidity	Time Temperature H_2O_2 Concentration Vacuum Level Plasma	Time Temperature O_3 Concentration Relative Humidity
Cycle Phases		
Preconditioning Preheat Add moisture	Preconditioning (Preplasma) Preheat and pull vacuum to remove moisture	Preconditioning Preheat Add moisture
Exposure:	Exposure (first half):	Exposure (first half):
Add EtO, allow to penetrate load, and sterilize by alkylation	(Diffusion and Plasma) Add H_2O_2; allow to diffuse, and sterilize by oxidation. Generate plasma, and convert H_2O_2 to water and oxygen	Vacuum Humidification Inject ozone and allow to sterilize by oxidation
	Exposure (second half):	Exposure (second half):
	Repeat steps in first half	Repeat steps in first half
Aeration:		
Flush load with warm filtered air to remove residuals	Not required	Not required
Cycle Times		
1-4 hours exposure, plus 8-12 hours aeration depending upon cycle and load	28-50 minutes depending on the equipment and load	4 hours
Advantages		
Superior penetration and com- patibility	Rapid cycle times Convenient to use	No sterilant to handle No aeration
Limitations		
Long total cycle	Limited penetration, and packaging material compatibility	Limited penetration Long cycles
OSHA 8-hour TWA (in U.S.)		
1.0 ppm	1.0 ppm	0.1 ppm
Packaging		
All standard packaging	Nonwoven polypropylene or Tyvek®	Compatible with most products

ENDNOTES

1. Burgess, D. and Reich, R. Ethylene Oxide Sterilization: Scientific Principles. In: M. Reichert and J.H. Young, eds., Sterilization Technology for the Health Care Facility, Aspen Publishers, Inc., Gaithersburg, MD, 1997: 178-186.

2. Graham, G. Industrial Applications of Plasma Sterilization. The Validation Consultant. 1997. Vol. 4, No. 10; 1-22.

3. Feldman, L; and Hui, H. Compatibility of Medical Devices and Materials with Low-Temperature Hydrogen Peroxide Gas Plasma. Med. Device & Diagn. Ind., Dec. 1997; 57-62.

CENTRAL SERVICE TERMS

Sterility assurance level (SAL)

Permissible exposure limits(PELs)

Time weighted average (8-hour)

Alkylation

Oxidation

Residual (EtO)

Aeration

Chapter 17

Inventory Management

CENTRAL SERVICE TERMS

Chapter Learning Objectives:

As a result of successfully completing this chapter, readers will be able to:

1. Review the importance of effective inventory management, and explain basic inventory management concepts.

2. Explain common inventory replenishment systems:
   - Par-level systems
   - Automated supply replenishment systems
   - Exchange cart systems
   - Requisition systems
   - Case cart systems
   - STAT orders

3. Review the use of bar codes and radio frequency identification to track inventories.

4. Describe procedures for effectively distributing supplies to clinical units and the operating room.

5. Review important inventory management concepts.
   - Perpetual inventory systems
   - Alternative inventory control methods
   - Total acquisition costs
   - Inventory turnover rates and service levels
   - Inventory information systems
   - Space utilization

IMPORTANCE OF MANAGING INVENTORY

Learning Objective 1. Review the importance of effective inventory management, and explain basic inventory management concepts.

The management of **inventory** is a critical concern in every healthcare facility, and Central Service Technicians play an important role in this activity. Poorly-managed inventory can create shortages and **stock outs** that directly impact the quality of patient care, and it can also increase operating costs which can have a significant effect on the facility's budget.

What is Inventory?

The term, "inventory" has a broad meaning in healthcare facilities, and it refers to both reusable and consumable items. Let's begin our discussion of inventory by considering some key terms and concepts.

One way to think about inventory is to consider the Central Service Department. There we have three specific types of inventory. First, there are consumable items (supplies such as disposable wraps, detergents, sterility assurance test products, etc.). When the consumable inventory is used up, more supplies must be purchased to replace it. If we allow that inventory to become contaminated or if it expires (outdates), we must also spend additional money to replace the supplies that must be discarded. Therefore, we carefully follow specific guidelines for purchasing, storing, and handling our consumable inventory (supplies) to ensure that we have a safe and adequate supply.

We also have two types of reusable inventory items in the Central Service Department: less expensive items that can be cleaned and used again and again such as carts, rigid sterilization containers, etc., and more expensive reusable items that can also be used many times such as sterilizers and washers.

If we compared our Central Service Department inventories to those in the rest of the hospital, we would think of three different levels of **assets**. One type is **consumable inventory**, items that are

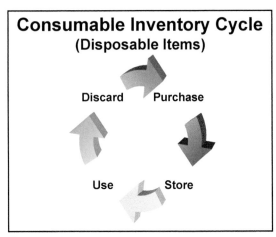

Consumable Inventory Cycle
(Disposable Items)

Discard   Purchase

Use   Store

Figure 17.1

used up and replaced. (See **Figure 17.1**) Examples include patient supplies like sutures and catheters, and operational supplies such as office supplies. Lower-cost **reusable inventory** items include wheelchairs, transport carts, etc., and higher cost equipment items would include diagnostic imaging equipment, surgical robotics systems,

Inventory Management and Central Service Technicians

As discussed in Chapter One, the scope of service (responsibilities) of Central Service Departments varies. Some departments provide supplies for the entire hospital; those in other facilities may only provide supplies for Surgery. However, all Central Service Technicians are involved in the inventory management process in some way. Case Cart Technicians work with consumable inventory supplies dispensed for each surgical procedure. Decontamination Technicians must insure that they have an adequate stock of personal protective equipment, and an adequate supply of detergents, disinfectants, cleaning brushes, and other decontamination supplies. Instrument Technicians must have replacement components for implant trays including screws, plates and pins, and they also need an adequate supply of packaging materials and chemical indicators. Central Service Technicians who operate sterilizers require quality assurance products such as biological and Bowie-Dick tests. And for some types of sterilization, they must keep an inventory of the sterilant itself.

Importance of Consumable Supplies

Lack of consumable supplies when needed can delay patient treatment and care and, in some cases, create life-threatening situations. Of lesser, but still important, concern is the customer frustration that can yield poor relationships with caregivers and user departments when needed supplies are unavailable. Inadequate supply problems encourage situations in which customers use unapproved procedures to obtain supplies and hoard (stockpile) them in non-designated supply storage areas. Since patient safety and customer satisfaction is at risk, the need for effective inventory management is evident.

Inventory – Reusable equipment and consumable items that are used to provide healthcare services for patients.

Stock outs (inventory) – The condition that occurs when reusable or consumable inventory items required to provide healthcare services to patients are not available.

Asset – Something of value that is owned by an organization or person.

Inventory (consumable) – Assets such as wrapping supplies, processing chemicals, and other items which are consumed (used up) as healthcare services are provided to patients.

Inventory (reusable) – Assets that are relatively inexpensive such as medical devices and sterilization containers that can be reused as healthcare services are provided to patients.

Equipment (capital) – Assets that are relatively expensive such as sterilizers or washers that require significant advance planning for their purchase.

Inventory (official) – Consumable products found in Central Service and other storerooms, warehouses, and satellite storage areas. Their value is usually included on the facility's balance sheet.

Inventory (unofficial) – Consumable products found in user areas such as surgical locations and labs. These items have usually been expensed to user departments and are stored in unofficial locations.

etc. In healthcare facilities, high-cost reusable items are called **capital equipment**, and their purchase must be planned well in advance when the facility's capital equipment budget is developed so money can be allocated (set aside) to purchase these items. Just as with reusable items in Central Service, these expensive purchases are not made as frequently as are the purchases of consumable items. (For example, we purchase new sterilizers for our department much less frequently than we purchase detergents and disposable wraps from our suppliers).

This chapter will focus on the management and control of consumable (disposable) inventory supplies. Hospital inventory systems and the patients they serve depend on the skills of Central Service Technicians. Inventory management involves much more than just buying items for the healthcare facility. Experienced personnel must identify exactly what items are needed, search for the best value, purchase the items, store them appropriately until they are needed, and transport them to the end user in a timely manner.

Special Inventory Management Concerns

Contemporary healthcare facilities use thousands of different types of consumable products in day-to-day operations. **"Official" inventories** are found in storerooms, warehouses, and/or satellite storerooms. **"Unofficial" inventories** are often kept in user areas (often in multiple locations; for example, the storeroom in the lab and at each laboratory work station). Note: these two types of inventories are discussed in greater detail in the next section of this chapter.

Central Service personnel are consistently challenged to maintain inventory levels so there is not "too much" or "too little" available. Excessive inventory levels result in:

• Too much cash invested in excessive stock levels.

• The potential need to borrow money to pay suppliers for the products delivered.

• More space to store supplies (and space is always at a premium in every facility!).

• Greater risk of damage, loss, obsolescence, and/or pilferage and theft.

• More time required to manage inventory levels.

At the same time, too little inventory can result in:

• Supply shortages.

• Emergency purchases (typically at greater cost than "normal" purchases).

• Negative impacts on patient care.

• Hoarding in user departments.

• Frequent handling to move inventories to point of use.

The inventory values of healthcare facilities can be very significant. Most facilities own approximately:

• $500,000 - $10 Million or more in equipment.

• $250,000 - $2 Million or more reusable inventory items.

• $500,000 - $1 Million or more in consumable supplies

Official inventories of consumable supplies are generally included on the facility's **balance sheet** as a **current asset**. Inventory locations include the Central Service, Pharmacy, and Food Services storerooms. More recently, Nursing, Cardiac Cath Lab, Radiology, and Surgery supplies have also been considered official inventory.

Unofficial inventories are those not carried on the balance sheet as a current asset, but are maintained at substantial levels in user departments for long periods prior to use. Typically, these items are expensed/allocated to the user departments upon receipt at the facility regardless of when they are actually used.

Inventory levels at most facilities typically exceed those that are required. Consider that:

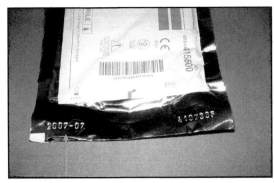

Figure 17.2

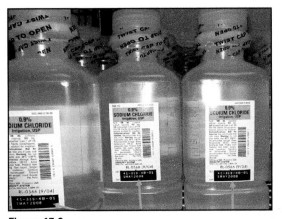

Figure 17.3

• Facilities spend approximately 30% of their operating budget on consumable supplies.

• Overall facility inventories of consumable supplies typically represent an average of 50 days' usage requirements.

• Facilities typically have a greater value of unofficial than official inventory on hand.

Maintaining sterility and integrity of items while in storage (and at all other times!) is imperative to controlling costs and to assuring patient safety. Storage locations must be maintained and kept clean. If they are not cleaned on a planned and

Balance sheet – A financial summary of what a healthcare facility owns (assets), owes (liabilities), and is worth (equity) at a specific point in time. Example: the last day of every month.

Asset (current) – An asset that is expected to be used within one year.

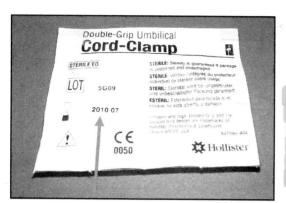

Figure 17.4

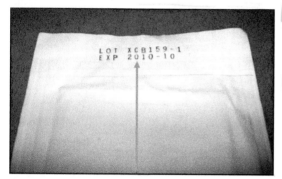

Figure 17.5

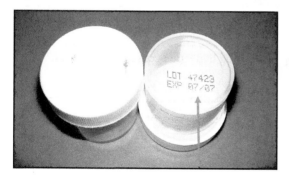

Figure 17.6

"events." These items must be discarded after the supervisor is notified so costs associated with these careless actions can be tracked.

The manufacturer's packaging may be labeled with an expiration date, or it may contain the statement, "Sterile Unless Damaged or Opened" if the manufacturer has designated that the package can be used according to event-related sterility guidelines. It is imperative that each package be inspected for damage before being dispensed and again before use.

Unfortunately, there is no established standard that specifies the package location for the expiration date, or what the marking must look like to help Central Service Technicians check each package. Everyone must assume responsibility to verify that the integrity of each package used has not been compromised, and to check package expiration dates prior to use. **Figures 17.2–17.6** show examples of different locations and methods used by manufacturers to indicate package expiration dates. As you can see, the wide variety of methods used to indicate expiration dates requires a great amount of attention to detail for Central Service Technicians.

In addition to locating and interpreting expiration dates, Central Service Technicians must also understand other information contained on package

Automated and Manual Inventory Systems

Inventory control can be accomplishing using manual or automated/computerized methods. Automated systems yield more data because more information can be monitored and stored. Instrument and equipment tracking are examples of systems that can be performed with either manual or automated procedures.

Manual systems involve processing inventory item data using a paper method. Example: when equipment is issued to a patient, information about it is recorded and stored on a paper document until a patient charge is generated, or until the item is returned, and tracking is completed. Manual methods also include information from clinical staff as they request supplies, equipment, or instruments.

frequently scheduled basis, dust accumulates which harbors invisible bio-burden. If left on packages, this will contaminate them and, when the packages are opened, these particulates become airborne and fall onto the sterile item. Clutter or overstocking in an area can create tears in packages which may (or may not) be easily visible. However, either way, sterility has been compromised. You've learned that event-related sterility means that an item is no longer considered sterile if a negative "event" has occurred. Contamination from bioburden and from package tears is an example of these unwanted

Common Package Information

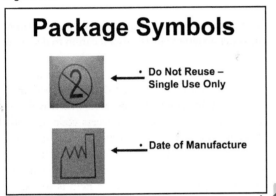

Manufacturer's Product Reference Number

REF 31145868
LOT 6188228
2009-07

Lot (Batch) Number

Identifies product to a specific production run.

Product Expiration Date

Figure 17.7

Package Symbols

• Do Not Reuse – Single Use Only

• Date of Manufacture

Figure 17.8

Carts and Totes used to Transport Sterile Items Must be Kept Clean.

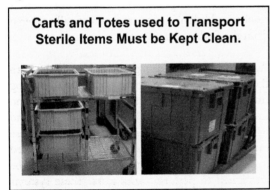

Figure 17.9

labels. **Figures 17.7** and **17.8** illustrate examples of this information.

Equipment such as carts and totes used to transport devices/supplies must be cleaned on a frequently scheduled basis. Items that are to be transported outside the facility must be contained in boxes or totes as they are transported. These totes must be cleaned daily to ensure that bio-burden is removed. (See **Figure 17.9**)

INVENTORY REPLENISHMENT SYSTEMS

Learning Objective 2. Explain common inventory replenishment systems:
- Par-level systems
- Automated supply replenishment systems
- Exchange cart systems
- Requisition systems
- Case cart systems
- STAT orders

The method(s) used to replenish needed consumable supplies in patient care units must be carefully considered and planned to best manage costs, to have items available when needed, and to minimize the supply efforts of responsible staff members. Effective systems are, to the extent possible, automatic: no intervention by the clinician is necessary to re-order.

These are several inventory replenishment systems in common use in healthcare facilities.

PAR-Level Systems

Periodic Automated Replenishment (PAR) systems establish a standard level (PAR) for each supply item stored in a specific department. This level is usually jointly determined by the user and Materiel Management staff. After these levels are set, there is typically no need for items to be ordered by clinicians. Instead, Central Service/Materiel Management (CS/MM) personnel inventory each area requiring inventory on an established basis. They check the current on hand supply and note the quantity of each item still available. The amount needed to bring the quantity of supplies to the agreed-upon standard (PAR) is determined, and automatically transmitted to the department. (See **Figure 17.10**)

Unlike exchange carts (see below), there is no need for a second cart that requires restocking, transporting, and staging. Therefore, this system is less hardware-intensive. Only supplies that are required are transported to the department, and this tactic potentially reduces the amount of inventory needed. Also, less space will be used because there are fewer carts and reduced inventory. However, this system still requires labor to transport items to track the issuing of patient items. Clinical staff scan or push a button to account for each item removed from the inventory location. PAR levels and reorder points for each item are established. An order is generated at a scheduled time for all items that are at or below their reorder point, and the order for the entire location is then placed. The supply pick list is printed in the Central Service department, and it is used to retrieve (issue) needed items from the central storage area for transport to the appropriate location. This process is repeated for all locations that utilize the automated system.

Available technology also uses information from the order generated by the user location to decrease the quantity of items available in the central location. Automated systems can be activated by a label or a button on a shelf that is scanned, or a closed supply cabinet can be used which will not open unless a user enters an access code. In both systems, the user must identify the patient to be charged for the supplies. If, instead, an item such as a box of gloves that may be used by clinicians for several patients is issued, the item is issued to the unit as a floor charge. Then, on a larger scale, when the reorder point in the central storeroom is reached, additional items are automatically ordered from the facility's suppliers.

Automated systems are generally interfaced with the materials management system for managing inventory with the admission, discharge and transfer (ADT) system for patient census, and with the patient billing system. The use of these interfaces reduces the amount of staff required to perform these functions. The staff can then be reassigned to perform other tasks. These systems do, however require staff that are knowledgeable about the interfaces, computer systems, and how to maintain them.

Automated systems are preferred when there is a need for much information and item tracking that must be frequently reviewed to determine if more instruments, equipment, or supplies are needed.

Benefits of automated systems relate to the facility's size and the number of items being monitored. Systems are expensive and significant study by the department managers and senior administrators

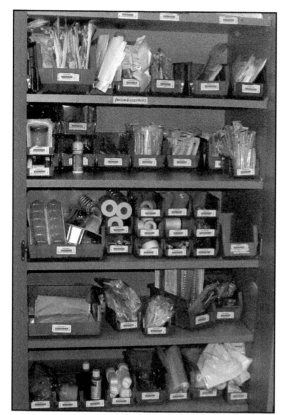

Figure 17.10

storage areas, and to inventory (count) and restock each department at its supply site(s).

Automated Supply Replenishment Systems

Automated supply replenishment systems use a computerized information system to gather and

Periodic automatic replenishment (PAR) – An inventory replenishment system in which the desired amount of products which should be on hand is established, and inventory replenishment returns the quality of products to this level; often abbreviated to "par system."

Automated supply replenishment system – Replenishment system in which items removed from inventory are automatically identified and tracked. When a reorder point is reached, item information is generated on a supply pick list in the central storeroom. Items are then issued, and transferred to the appropriate user area.

will be required to determine if a system can be cost-justified for all or some of the remote storage locations. **Figure 17.11** and **Figure 17.12** show photos of equipment used in an automated system.

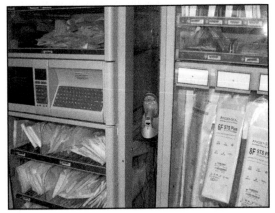

Figure 17.11

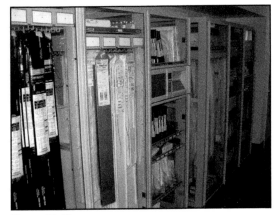

Figure 17.12

Exchange Cart Systems

An **exchange cart system** is an inventory replenishment method that involves the exchange of a freshly-loaded supply cart for an identical cart on a patient unit that has been depleted of most supplies. Supply items and quantities on the exchange cart as well as its location are determined by user unit staff and CS/Materiel Management personnel. At a pre-determined time, a full cart is brought to the unit. The partially-depleted cart is returned to the replenishment area, and remaining items are inventoried to determine the supplies and quantities that were consumed. The cart is then

replenished with the supplies needed to return the cart back to full inventory. As supplies are removed from inventory and added to the cart, they are charged to the budget of the unit which "owns" the cart. At the scheduled time, this full cart is delivered to the unit, the depleted cart is retrieved for restocking, and the cycle repeats.

A major advantage of an exchange cart system is that it is "automatic," unless there is a need to change the cart's items or quantities. Clinical staff do not need to order these items, and Materiel Management staff do not have to determine what supplies are needed.

Disadvantages associated with exchange carts include the need for duplicate inventory and carts. The system is labor- and hardware-intensive, and requires adequate space to stage the idle carts. In addition, unless the system is well-managed, numerous unused supplies will be transported back and forth each cycle. However, this system does works well for emergency medical supply carts (crash carts) which are exchanged for a newly restocked cart each time they are used (See **Figure 17.13**).

Requisition Systems

Even when par-level or exchange cart systems exist, it will still be necessary to order additional supplies because of insufficient quantities on hand, or because a specific item is not included among those routinely provided. Requisition systems exist in every facility to fill these needs.

Requisition systems require users to request needed supplies by completing a requisition. This is not an efficient use of clinical staff time and, since Central Service employees do not know what supplies are required in advance, effective inventory management becomes difficult. Requisition systems can be either manual or computer-generated, but they are usually paper-based. However, manual systems do not offer the productivity advantages of electronic order entry with computerized systems. Requisition systems that electronically requisition supplies typically eliminate the need for materiels

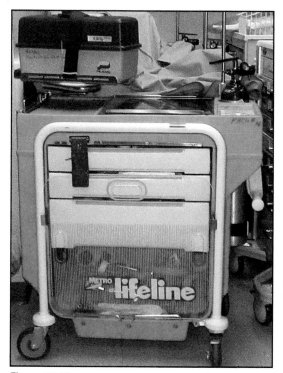

Figure 17.13

Specialty Items

Every facility has need for patient-specific and infrequently ordered specialty items that are not maintained in the routine replenishment system. Central Service Technicians must understand the requisition, ordering, tracking and replenishment processes used by their facility for these items. If a patient is scheduled for surgery and a specialty item is needed, it may need to be ordered several days prior to surgery to ensure that it is available when needed. If an item is not available when needed, the patient, physician, and clinical staff will be justifiably upset, and the patient's well-being may be endangered.

Case Cart Systems

Case cart systems are a common distribution method used to provide specific products for individual surgical procedures. Unlike other forms of distribution that service a specific unit or care group, case carts are assembled to meet the specific needs of each physician for each individual procedure (See **Figure 17.14**)

Case cart systems range from those providing disposable supplies for each surgery to comprehensive systems which provide each case's instrument, supply, equipment, and implant needs. While they are most commonly used for the Operating Room, case cart systems can be used anywhere that procedures requiring supplies and instruments are performed including cardiac catherization labs and labor/delivery units. When

management personnel to re-enter ordering information into the central inventory system. The accuracy and productivity improvements associated with automated data entry are lost when manual requisition systems are used.

Exchange cart system – An inventory system in which desired inventory items are placed on a cart which is assigned a specific location and quantity. A second, duplicate cart is maintained in another location, and exchanged once daily to ensure that sufficient supplies are available at all times.

Requisition system – A method of inventory distribution in which item needs are requested (requisitioned) by user department personnel, and removed from a central storage location for transport to the user department.

Case cart system – An inventory control system for products and equipment typically used in the operating room which involves use of a cart that is generally prepared for one special surgical case, and not used for general supply replenishment.

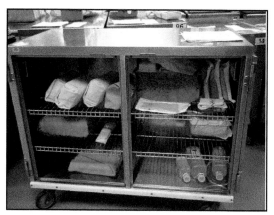

Figure 17.14

implemented correctly, these systems help to meet the needs of each physician, and still maintain an orderly system for tracking and handling supplies, instruments, and equipment.

Effective case cart systems provide many benefits to healthcare providers and patients, including more standardized infection control practices, cost reduction, and better instrument and supply tracking. Cost reductions are achieved by shifting the responsibility for cart assembly to Central Service personnel who traditionally receive lower salary/wages than do clinical staff.

Case cart systems can also provide effective control of supplies and instruments. Since a separate case cart is assembled for each individual procedure, it is easier to track what is actually used, and to identify supplies and instruments which are requested but seldom used. Quantities of supplies not being used can then be reduced which, in turn, reduces the amount of inventory that must be on hand. Close monitoring of instrument usage allows the facility to shift instruments not being used to other areas where they are needed. Monitoring can also identify instrument shortages which may be addressed with scheduling changes and/or the purchase of additional instrumentation.

Case cart systems enhance infection control practices. Since all instruments are returned to the processing area immediately after use, decontamination and sterilization processes can begin immediately. Central Service Technicians assigned to processing in a case cart system devote all their time and efforts to preparing items for reuse. Since that is their primary job function, they become specialists in cleaning, inspecting, assembling, and sterilizing complex instruments, and this expertise yields better infection control practices.

Case cart systems rely on user input to be effective. Physicians and other healthcare personnel utilizing the case cart must identify their specific needs in advance. These needs are then transferred to pick lists that Central Service staff use to assemble each cart. Care should be taken when developing requisitions to insure that products are standardized,

whenever possible. Routine follow-up is needed to adjust requisition quantities to actual usage.

Properly stocked case carts should be delivered to the user unit. Personnel assigned to the case cart area must maintain direct contact with unit employees so additional items can be supplied as needed. After the procedure is completed, used reprocessable items must be returned to the decontamination area for processing. Central Service Technicians should return unused items to stock, and then proceed with inventory replenishment and charging activities.

While case cart systems typically use carts assembled as needed for specific procedures, most systems also utilize some form of stand-by carts which remain assembled and "on stand-by" for emergency situations. These carts are used for STAT situations (for example, emergency cesarean sections) when there is no time for cart assembly. Instead, case cart personnel keep them complete and ready for use at all times.

An effective case cart system requires good communication between operating room and Central Service personnel. As cases are performed, they must be in constant communication to insure that items are correct, and that they arrive on time. Personnel in each department must be familiar with the routine duties and workflow patterns of the other. Frustration can be eliminated if, for example, surgical personnel understand the steps involved in reprocessing instruments for another case. Instead of questioning instrument turnaround times, they will understand that this time is required for cleaning, inspecting, assembling, and sterilizing according to necessary procedures.

Central Service Technicians working with case cart systems should have good medical terminology skills and a thorough understanding of surgical instruments so that they can easily communicate with their surgical counterparts. They must also remain up-to-date about new products because they serve as the link between the inventory system and the operating room.

Along with effective oral communication skills, case cart systems rely heavily on written procedures and communications. Personnel from both departments must establish procedures for product handling, outage notification, and scheduling. Even the best planned case cart system will be less-than-effective without good communication.

Case cart systems require significant input from Central Service personnel, and they require a full array of reprocessing skills and solid inventory management methods to be efficient.

STAT Orders

Emergency supply orders requiring immediate action (**STAT orders**) are a fact of life in every facility. These requests usually occur when an item is needed immediately. They can also occur for a procedure scheduled on the next day if the item is not available. These orders are time-consuming and expensive to fill, and they usually disrupt routine inventory control activities. Consider, for example, weekend and off-shift times when additional external resources such as overnight air shipments or borrowing from another facility may be required. All reasonable efforts to minimize the need for STAT requests are needed, and these include reviewing why they occur, and how they can be prevented.

Many STAT requests result from deficiencies in the daily supply and distribution system when it is not well-managed. STAT requests can become a patient safety issue if the root cause is not addressed, and routine reviews may determine if par level adjustments will help to assure appropriate inventory levels.

When STAT requests result from improper planning by clinical staff, Materiel Management/Central Service officials should assist in the planning and education efforts required to resolve the issue. While surgical staff cannot predict that

an emergency patient will require a specific non-stocked item, they may be able to plan for such a need, and assure that the item is available.

AUTOMATED INVENTORY TRACKING SYSTEMS

Learning Objective 3. Review the use of bar codes and radio frequency identification to track inventories.

There are two basic types of automated inventory tracking systems that are increasingly used in healthcare facilities. One utilizes bar codes, and the other makes use of radio frequency identification (RFID). Both of these systems must be understood by Central Service personnel.

Bar Codes

Many automated systems utilize bar code scanning which requires the user to line-up the scan indicator beam with the bar code label on the supply item (See **Figure 17.15**), and listen for the read tone. When the scanner reads the bar code the data about that specific product is recorded for use in the materiel management information system. For example, scanners in retail stores read bar codes and transfer information about each product to the cash register during a sale transaction.

Radio Frequency Identification

A new type of tracking system uses **radio frequency identification** (RFID). One example of RFID is the tags used in the retail industry that are placed on items and must be removed before walking out the

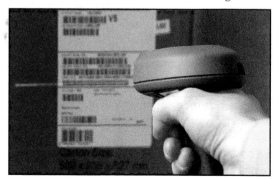

Figure 17.15

STAT order – Abbreviation for the Latin word, "Statim," which means immediately or at once.

Bar code – Numerous machine—readable rectangular bars and spaces arranged in a specific way to represent letters, numbers, and other symbols.

door to avoid sounding an alarm. Radio frequency applications are different from bar code scanning because they are not limited to line of sight. Low frequency wattage signals are transmitted to radio frequency receivers for network and software inventory applications. This technology is in its infancy, but its potential for tracking movable and other assets is significant. Signals can be transferred through walls and floors, and antennae coverage can only be determined by a technical assessment of reception capability throughout the facility. RFID applications for healthcare are being tested to track expensive supply items and moveable patient equipment.

DISTRIBUTION OF SUPPLIES

Learning Objective 4. Describe procedures for effectively distributing supplies to clinical units and the operating room.

Distribution involves moving supplies throughout the facility (generally from their storage location to the point where they are needed), and includes all clinical and non-clinical supply movements. In most facilities, most of this activity includes distributing consumable supplies from the storeroom or Central Service to clinical units, including surgery.

The goal of distribution is to move the correct items in appropriate quantities to the right places at the right times in the most cost-effective manner by the appropriate personnel.

The routine, scheduled distribution of supplies should address factors such as frequency and/or volume of use, peak activity times, and the amount of storage space available in the areas to which the supplies are distributed. With the exception of STAT orders, distribution schedules often consider:

- Day of the week – Examples: every day or three times a week on Monday-Wednesday and Friday.

- Supply type or category – Examples: medical/surgical every day, and forms and paper supplies once a week.

- Type or user area – Examples: medical and surgical units every other day, and administrative offices once a week.

- Schedule of patient activities – Examples: according to operating room schedules, and the pulmonary unit only on Tuesday.

- Physical location – Examples: "Building A" every day, and "Building F" (across town) only on Friday.

- Quantity required – Examples: twice-a-day for areas requiring large quantities but with inadequate storage, and once monthly for an off-site building with adequate storage requiring minimal supplies.

Many factors must be considered to establish the most appropriate distribution schedule. CS/Materiel Management personnel must work with user departments to establish schedules, and to revise them as workload and other factors change.

IMPORTANT INVENTORY MANAGEMENT CONCEPTS

Learning Objective 5. Review important inventory management concepts.
- Perpetual inventory systems
- Alternative inventory control methods
- Total acquisition costs
- Inventory turn rates and service levels
- Inventory information systems
- Space utilization

Perpetual Inventory Systems

A **perpetual inventory system** is frequently used to manage and control official inventories by maintaining a record about the balance on-hand of each specific item at all times. As items are ordered, received, **issued** or returned to suppliers, the transaction is documented. This allows facility personnel to know, at any time, the quantity of product which should be on hand. For example, assume ten units are ordered and arrive on day one. If there are already eight units available in the perpetual inventory system, there is balance on hand of eighteen units (10 units + 8 units = 18 units). On day two, if three units are issued, the transaction is documented to yield an on-hand balance of fifteen units (18 units - 3 units = 15 units). As additional issue and receipt transactions occur, the perpetual inventory system allows the manager to track usage. This information is used to update reorder points and quantities, and it provides the manager with real-time information to make decisions to efficiently and effectively manage inventory.

Perpetual inventories are routinely validated for accuracy by taking a physical count of the actual supplies on hand, and by then comparing that inventory quantity to the amount that should be available based upon the manual or computerized recordkeeping system. Any discrepancy between the amount that should be available (from records) and that is available (from physical count) is called a **variance**.

Radio frequency identification – A term used to describe a system in which the identity (serial number) of an item is wirelessly transmitted with radio waves; commonly abbreviated "RFID."

Distribution – The movement of supplies throughout the facility, primarily consumable supplies from the storeroom to clinical units and reprocessed supplies from Central Service to the operating room.

Perpetual inventory system – A system which keeps track of all incoming and issued supplies so that one knows, on an on-going basis, the quantity of supplies that is in storage.

Issue – The act of withdrawing supplies from storage for transfer to areas where they will be used.

Variance – The difference between the amount of a supply that should be available (from records) and the amount that is available (from physical count) when a perpetual inventory system is used.

ABC analysis – The inventory management strategy that indicates storeroom controls should first address the relatively few items with the greatest value (A items), and should lastly consider the many items with the lowest value (C items).

Examples of ABC Inventory Items

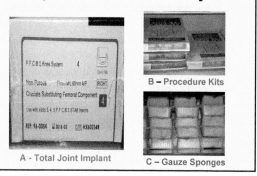

A - Total Joint Implant
B – Procedure Kits
C – Gauze Sponges

Figure 17.16

ABC Inventory Control

With thousands of items to manage, it is typically not practical to maintain detailed and accurate control over all items. Since some items have relatively little value, **ABC Analysis** allows managers to prioritize the management and control of inventory. For example, "A items" represent those with the largest annual dollar value, "B items" represent a medium dollar value of expenditures, and "C items" represent those with the smallest dollar value. "A items" represent the smallest number and percentage of the total inventory items, but the largest total dollar value, for example Hip and Knee implants. "B items" represent the mid-range proportion of number of items and value of the total inventory. "C items" represent the greatest number and percentage of items, but the lowest total dollar value, for example dressings and sponges. "A items" must be closely managed because of their financial impact. Then, control efforts should focus on the "B items," and then on the "C items." **Figure 17.16** illustrates ABC Inventory items.

Alternative Inventory Control Methods

The facility's purchasing staff must work with Central Service and other departments with official and unofficial inventories to maintain the lowest, most cost-effective inventory levels. Both must understand alternative inventory control methods, and then select/adapt those which are best for their operation. In addition to the systems discussed earlier in this chapter, these alternative methods include:

- Min/max system – The minimum/maximum inventory control method requires that the lowest quantity of each supply item which can be available before ordering be determined. (This is called the "safety stock level.") Then the largest quantity that can be available in inventory should be agreed upon. This information is then used to help determine the quantity of product to reorder. When the reorder point is reached (the minimum amount can be available in inventory), one must reorder.

- Economic order quantity system – Products are purchased in the quantity which is most economical (for example, by the case, box or dozen).

- Stockless supplies – The supplier provides a complete inventory, storage, and distribution service for the facility, and he/she delivers to user departments on a pre-scheduled basis. Note: although many facilities have some form of stockless inventory system in place, especially for office supplies and/or forms, very few have a true stockless system for medical/surgical supplies. When a stockless system is used, all responsibility for inventory is shifted from the facility to the vendor, and the facility is left without on-hand inventory. The vendor becomes responsible for the daily re-supplying of the facility. In some cases, the vendor even provides the internal distribution function, and delivers supplies directly to user areas.

- Just-in-time (JIT) system – Minimal stock is kept on-site, and most orders are delivered when needed. (Note: some medically critical items must always be available on-site.) The JIT system is based upon the Japanese "kan-ban" supply system in which the user and supplier form a close partnership and, because supplies will be delivered "just in time," the facility inventory levels and related expenses can be reduced. JIT systems shift most of the inventory away from the facility and back to the vendor, so the facility can lower its inventory level and holding costs. One caution: the vendor must manage his/her on-hand quantities to assure that supplies are available when ordered. This system generally requires more follow-up between the facility and vendor to monitor the vendor's stock and to consider acceptable substitutions.

All facilities operate some form of JIT system because it is neither possible nor cost-effective to carry an inventory of all supplies that may ever be needed, and some are acquired "just in time". Many facilities choose to extend this concept by planning supply requirements and working with vendors to schedule orders and deliveries. The more predictable this system, the less inventory the facility will need "just in case." Ordering patterns for facilities using this method are generally daily to are generally daily (five times) weekly. *In Plant supply*

- Consignment system – Items are stored at the healthcare facility. The supplier owns the inventory, and does not charge for it until it is used or lost. This method requires tight control with security measures. It is also necessary to define who is responsible for replacement in the event of a disaster such as flood, storm, or fire that damages the inventory items.

- Pick-n-pack system – Products are ordered from a vendor prepacked for a particular department (generally these items are office supplies and forms). *office supplies*

Total Acquisition Costs

Personnel in the Purchasing, Materiel Management, Central Service, and other departments must analyze **total acquisition costs** to assure that they are minimized without sacrificing quality. Acquisition costs include those related to all activities from product/service requisition to disposal: requisitioning, authorizing, ordering, receiving, storing, picking, distributing, and disposing.

Purchasing is just one of many costs related to the total cost of supplies and equipment. Other related costs of acquisition can include:

- Physical storage costs.

- Disposal of expired items.

Product Standardization Is Important

Clinical and material management staff must periodically evaluate alternative products. Product evaluations should compare equal products, and they should be quantitative and impartial. Lowest price is not the only factor to consider. Standardization of supplies, products, and services promotes low costs for acquisition, receiving, storing, distribution, and patient care services. By contrast, duplication of products and/or equipment increases the cost of materiel management and, subsequently, that of healthcare to the patients. Cost-containment efforts including utilization and product standardization should be high on the list of priorities, and they should be everyone's responsibility. Central Service personnel can be a vital part of this effort as they promote standardization and encourage less duplication. The facility's Value Analysis Committee generally reviews expensive items including those that incorporate new technology. This committee is generally comprised of senior administrators, department directors, material management representatives, finance personnel and physicians.

- Theft/pilferage.

- Obsolescence.

- Freight and delivery charges.

- Stock outs.

- Overstocks (costs of more-than-required quantities of products on hand).

When new equipment is purchased, new or different disposable supplies associated with it may be needed. Sometimes Central Service staff members aren't aware of the need for these new items until they are requested. However, that is not the appropriate time for the Central Service Manager to contact purchasing personnel to determine what item(s) are needed, and how they will be purchased and stocked. A clear process should be in place to identify what additional components will be needed any time that new equipment is planned for. That process should include identifying methods to distribute the components and educate staff about the new items and equipment.

Inventory Turnover Rates and Service Levels

The **inventory turnover rate** represents the number of times per year that inventory is purchased, consumed, and replaced.

Inventory turnover rates should be closely monitored. As they increase, there is an increased chance of stock outs; as they decrease, problems associated with excessive inventory on-hand become more likely. Facilities strive to find the best balance of inventory in order to avoid these problems. Finding the appropriate balance increases customer satisfaction and decreases operating costs.

Inventory service levels represent the percentage of items filled when an order is placed. For example, if 100 items are ordered and 92 are available, the service level is 92% (92 items available ÷ 100 items ordered), and the **inventory stock out rate** is 8% (100% - 92%). If the 8% stock out rate includes medically-necessary items, the inventory service level for these items is not desirable, even though 92% seems to be a high percentage.

Inventory service levels are an important way to measure inventory control and management; however, caution is needed. Since medically-critical items must be on hand 100% of the time, inventory investment/carrying costs can be expensive. Therefore, service levels and costs must be balanced.

Total acquisition costs – *All costs incurred by the facility to purchase a specific supply or equipment item from the point of authorization through its disposal.*

Inventory turnover rate – *The number of times per year that inventory is purchased, consumed, and replaced.*

Inventory service level – *The percentage of items filled (available) when an order is placed.*

Inventory stock out rate – *The percentage of items that cannot be filled (are not available) when an order is placed.*

Inventory Information Systems

Inventory is virtually the same as cash; without inventory one can have the equivalent value of cash on hand, in the bank, or in some other investment. Also, if inventory is lost, stolen or discarded (example: the expiration date has passed), cash will be required to purchase additional inventory. Therefore, inventory must be managed and controlled, and this occurs, in part, with use of an effective record keeping system.

Most healthcare facilities maintain a significant portion of their inventory under a perpetual inventory system, either manually or electronically. However, some facilities utilize a manual recordkeeping system to maintain on-hand quantities and to note items on order. This often involves a card system which includes the following information:

- Item description, vendor source, and unit(s) of measure.

- Information on orders placed.

- Receipt transactions.

- Issue transactions.

- Adjustments.

Manual recordkeeping systems require much time and effort to accurately maintain the transactions and the on-hand inventory levels. It is also difficult to consolidate data from these records to create meaningful inventory management reports such as for trend usage and service levels.

Facilities increasingly use computerized systems to manage and control all or part of their inventories. Numerous variations in systems and how they are used exist:

- Some materiel management specialty information systems are specifically designed for inventory management; others are one component of a broader financial management system.

- Some systems are micro- (or mini-) computer-based, while others are mainframe systems fully integrated with the facility's financial, patient care, and other systems.

- Some systems include all materiel management responsibilities; others are used only for inventory control or purchasing.

- Some systems are department-specific; others control inventories for all departments within the facility.

Benefits of a computerized system include their ability to allow inventory transactions to be processed quickly. They provide well-organized and analyzed data to help make inventory decisions helpful in adjusting order quantities and order points, tracking utilization for supply cost allocation or budget development, and calculating service levels from the vendor to the facility and then to user departments.

Stock Locator Systems

Assigning physical locations and codes for all supplies in central inventory enables department personnel to identify that area of the storeroom and/or warehouse where an item is stored. This is especially useful when storeroom personnel must fill supplementary and/or on-demand orders for staff members who come to the storeroom. In addition, when coupled with an automated materiel management system, location codes allow order picking documents to be produced in location sequence. This directs order pickers to the various stock locations through the most direct and efficient route. Stock locator systems also provide assistance when a nurse or other user department employee must obtain an item from the storeroom after hours, and locate it without anyone's help. The locator system should be both manual and electronic for ease of use. Any supply maintained in any location within the facility should have an assigned location (sometimes referred to as a bin location). A paper copy can help assist in areas that do not have automated supply cabinets. This bin location is also interfaced with the case cart system, if used, to create a path for the staff to pull the items for each preference card in sequence.

Computerized systems require a substantial investment, and will not likely eliminate staff because data entry is required for all the routine transactions associated with inventory management and control. They will, however, provide meaningful and valuable information to manage inventories.

Space Utilization

Storage space utilization is often a significant concern, especially in facilities where services have outgrown allocated space, and/or when storage areas are in high demand. Most facilities are constantly searching for additional space. An efficient storage and supply system can improve the order picking process, enhance inventory management activities, and free-up space for use by other departments for other functions. Central Service Managers must always be creative about the best ways to work within the space allocated to the department. When the space is no longer available, when the department is moved to another location, and when outputs must increase, staff must work as a team to develop new processes and work flows.

While square footage of available space is important, cubic footage (volume) should be maximized as well. For example, storeroom capacity can often be substantially increased by additional vertical storage. Storage locations should be assigned beginning with the top shelf (left side), and then moving across the shelf and then to the next shelf with this process continuing for other shelves. Be sure to leave space in between each bin location for future add-in items.

Maximum utilization of cubic footage is an important factor in the efficient use of cart space and loading of supply trucks. When placing items on shelves, make sure that the bin(s) or item(s) fill the space from front-to-back and top-to-bottom because this will make best use of available shelf space. Placing items of like size and type will assist in space utilization. If there is excessive space between the shelves (top of item to bottom of higher shelf), consider adding additional shelves to add items or increased quantities of items or the reverse: remove shelves to accommodate the space needs of bulky items.

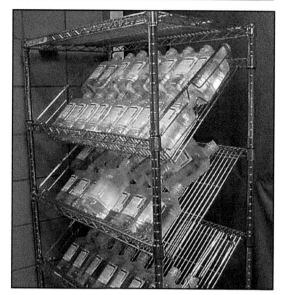

Figure 17.17

Gravity Flow Racks

As suggested by their name, gravity flow racks use gravity to allow for the efficient picking and re-supplying of fast-moving or heavy supplies. Open and accessible from the front and back, these racks have shelves that are positioned at a downward slope. This allows supplies to slide from the back over tracks or rollers to the front. (See **Figure 17.17**) As each item is removed from the front, the item behind it slides down and into the front place. Gravity flow racks allow easy and fast frontal access to a large quantity of supplies while also allowing efficient stock replenishment from behind the units to help ensure stock rotation.

The use of these racks, when combined with less accessible high-density storage for slower-moving supplies, allows Central Service personnel to balance square and cubic footage storage utilization in a cost-effective manner.

IN CONCLUSION

Inventory management is an important part of every healthcare facility. Managing inventory effectively and efficiently assists caregivers in providing quality care at lower costs, and even more importantly, it ensures that the items needed to provide care and treatment for patients are available when needed. When Central Service and Materiel Management staff work to manage and control inventory, they contribute to creating a safe environment for the patient and they increase patient satisfaction.

CENTRAL SERVICE TERMS

Inventory

Stock outs (inventory)

Assets

Inventory (consumable)

Inventory (reusable)

Equipment (capital)

Inventory (official)

Inventory (unofficial)

Balance sheet

Periodic automatic replenishment (PAR)

Automated supply replenishment systems

Exchange cart system

Requisition system

Materiel management personnel

Case cart system

STAT order

Bar code

Radio frequency identification

Distribution

Perpetual inventory system

Issue

Variance

ABC analysis

Total acquisition costs

Inventory turns

Inventory service level

Stock out rate

Chapter 18

Management of Patient Care Equipment

Chapter Learning Objectives

As a result of successfully completing this chapter, readers will be able to:

1. Discuss the responsibilities of Central Service Technicians for managing patient care equipment.

2. Identify the purposes of commonly-used patient care equipment.

3. Identify handling requirements and concerns for common patient care equipment:
   - Cleaning equipment
   - Managing inoperative equipment
   - Preparing equipment for use
   - Storing equipment
   - Tracking equipment

4. Describe the differences and explain advantages and disadvantages of purchase, lease, rent, and loan options for patient care equipment.

5. Review other basic patient care equipment concerns: maintenance and repair and outsourcing.

Along with surgical instruments and supplies, Central Service Technicians manage a large portion of the hospital's patient care equipment. Tasks include its assembly, delivery, tracking, retrieval, and decontamination. Effective handling of this equipment is an important part of their job, and managing it properly can have a significant impact on patient safety.

PATIENT CARE EQUIPMENT

Learning Objective 1. Discuss the responsibilities of Central Service Technicians for managing patient care equipment.

Patient care equipment must be readily available when it is needed. This requires that it be safe, functional, ready-to-use, and free from soil and contaminants. Central Service Technicians are responsible for insuring that these requirements are met. They must also manage equipment in a manner that minimizes costs to the healthcare facility, and an effective patient care equipment management program is essential to do so.

Importance of Responsibility

Specific guidelines should be developed for the cleaning, preparing, and tracking of patient care equipment, and they will have a dramatic impact on patient and employee safety. Equipment that has not been properly cleaned poses an infection control threat to patients and healthcare workers. That threat is magnified because the equipment may be processed by several workers during the course of preparation, storage, and distribution. If it is not properly assembled and ready for use, there may be a delay in treatment if staff must obtain necessary components such as tubing, collection devices, and pads. Also, equipment that is not accurately tracked can be "lost" within the system. This unavailability may also cause treatment delay, or add unnecessary

expense if it is then necessary to rent additional equipment to replace the "lost" equipment.

Close Look at Responsibilities

Central Service Technicians maintain the flow of the patient equipment system. They also partner with the **Biomedical and Clinical Engineering Department (Biomed).** Technicians in this department perform safety inspections and function tests on medical equipment. They are specially trained to inspect, test, and repair patient care equipment. Central Service technicians should not attempt to perform equipment testing and maintenance functions unless they have received specific training and approval to do so, nor should Biomedical Technicians clean equipment that has been used.

When any equipment item enters a healthcare facility, it must be safety-checked and tested by a Biomedical Technician before being cleared for patient use. It must also receive periodic follow-up inspections scheduled according to the equipment manufacturer's recommendations and the healthcare facility's policies. (See **Figure 18.1:** Biomedical Engineering Preventive Maintenance Sticker) Biomedical personnel maintain complete records about routine checks, repairs, and other important information for each item of patient care equipment in the facility.

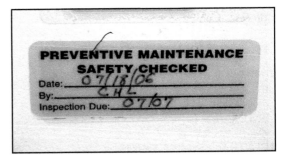

Figure 18.1: Biomedical Engineering Preventive Maintenance Sticker

---

Patient care equipment – Portable (mobile) equipment that is used to assist in the care and treatment of patients. Examples include; suction units, heat therapy units, IV infusion pumps, etc.

Biomedical/Clinical Engineering department – The hospital department responsible for performing safety inspections and function tests on medical equipment; frequently abbreviated "Biomed Department."

The Joint Commission requires that preventive maintenance (PM) standards be established for healthcare equipment.[1] Since there are many types of patient and non-patient equipment in every healthcare setting, it is difficult to generalize about necessary PM procedures. However, the following information should be recorded and maintained for each item of patient care equipment:

- Assigned equipment location.

- Ownership status (rented, leased, owned, borrowed).

- Schedule for PM.

- PM history.

- Hospital-defined PM standards.

- Repair history.

Central Service and the Biomed Department

Central Service Technicians partner with the Biomedical Department in several ways. Each time an item of patient care equipment is returned to the Central Service department for cleaning, its preventive maintenance sticker should be checked. Items due for a preventive maintenance inspection should be routed to Biomed rather than be returned to service. As a part of their routine inspection process, Central Service Technicians should also

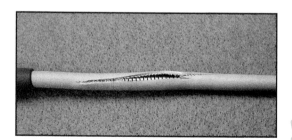

Figure 18.2

check for damaged (cracked, torn, or frayed) electrical cords (see the photo in **Figure 18.2**), cracked equipment casings, loose knobs and switches, and other signs of damage that should be corrected before the item is reused. All equipment that

appears to need repair should also be routed to Biomed personnel for inspection. Equipment-related issues can be minimized when all staff remain alert to obvious signs of the need for equipment inspection and/or repair. This, in turn, increases the level of patient and employee safety.

BASIC TYPES OF PATIENT CARE EQUIPMENT

Learning Objective 2. Identify the purposes of commonly-used patient care equipment.

Understanding the purpose of basic types of patient care equipment can improve customer service and reduce frustrations. **Figure 18.3** identifies and defines some of this equipment that typically must be handled by Central Service personnel.

Central Service Technicians must also understand requirements for cleaning, inspecting, preparing, storing, dispensing, and tracking patient care equipment. Each step in the patient care equipment process is an important component of a comprehensive patient care equipment program.

HANDLING USED (SOILED) PATIENT CARE EQUIPMENT

Learning Objective 3 Identify handling requirements and concerns for common patient care equipment:
- Cleaning equipment.
- Managing inoperative equipment.
- Preparing equipment for use.
- Storing equipment.
- Tracking equipment.

All patient care equipment dispensed for use must be considered contaminated, and handled as such, after use, regardless of its appearance. Note: patient care equipment is often not visibly soiled and may appear clean. However, it is likely to harbor microorganisms that may pose a threat to patients and staff. Central Service Technicians often make routinely-scheduled rounds to pick-up soiled equipment from user units, and transport it to

Figure 18.3 Common Patient Care Equipment

Equipment	Purpose
Airflow Regulator	Meter or gauge that controls the amount of air or gas administered.
Air Freshener	Mechanical device or scented wick/substance that eliminates odors.
Bed Check Control Unit (Bed Check Device)	Device that sounds an alarm when a patient gets out of bed.
Bili Lights (Phototherapy)	Specialty lights that treat infants with jaundice (a yellow coloring of the skin and eyes related to abnormal liver function).
Breast Pump	Mechanical device that extracts and collects milk from the breast.
Continuous Passive Motion (CPM) Device	Device that treats synovial joints (hip, knee, ankle, shoulder, elbow, wrist, and TMJ following surgery or trauma (including fracture and infection). The device moves the affected joint continuously without patient assistance.
Defibrillator	Applies a brief electroshock to restore the rhythm of the heart.
Enteral Nutrition (Infusion) Pump	Provides nutrition to patients who cannot ingest food because of recent surgery, or because various digestive organs do not function properly; also called feeding pump.
Foot Pump	Artificially stimulates the venous plantar plexus (the large vein located in the foot). It increases blood circulation in bed-ridden patients by simulating the motion of blood produced during walking.
Gastric Suction Unit	Aspirates (withdraws) gastric and intestinal contents.
Heart-Lung Machine	Pump-oxygenator that temporarily assumes the functions of the heart and lungs during open heart surgery.

Hot and Cold Therapy Devices	Reduces swelling, pain and muscle cramps, and used to treat arthritis, pyrogenic infection, and gastrointestinal cramps. Depending on the required therapy, water is cooled or heated, and then runs through a disposable pad which is wrapped around the area being treated. Smaller, "heat only" devices similar to electric heating pads are used on sore muscles.
Hypothermia Unit	Pumps heated or cooled water through a coiled pad to therapeutically raise or lower body temperature.
Infant Incubator	Creates and controls the environment of newborns.
Infusion Pump	Mechanically controls the administration of intravenous (IV) therapy fluids.
Intermittent Suction Device	Device that starts and stops suctioning at periodic intervals.
Microdrip	Intravenous adapter with a drop control that emits a drop that is 1.1 times the size of a normal drop.
Oral Suction Machine	Suctions liquids and mucus from the oral and nasal cavities.
PCA (Patient-Controlled Analgesia) Pump	Provides for automatic (self) administration of pain medication.
Respirator	Replaces or assists the breathing of a patient with respiratory problems.
Sequential Compression Unit	Limits the development of Deep Vein Thrombosis (DVT) and Peripheral Edema in immobile patients.
Suction Pump	Provides suction by altering the expansion and contraction of air within a cylinder at regular intervals. Known as "Aspirators," they use a continuous or intermittent pump and a collection container to aspirate (withdraw fluids or air from a cavity) patients with throat or lung problems, or to provide wound drainage, usually from the chest or abdominal areas.

Oral Irrigation Appliance (Waterpic)	Used for oral irrigation.
Portable Suction Unit	Mechanical suction device, powered by battery or electrical current, used in various facility locations.
Wall Suction Unit	Mechanical suction device that must be attached to a wall suction (vacuum) outlet for power.
Wound V.A.C Therapy	Provides negative pressure wound therapy by using controlled suction to close large wounds, and to promote faster healing.

the decontamination area for cleaning. In some cases, they may also make special trips to user departments to retrieve specific equipment items. In either case, the equipment should be considered contaminated and transported according to soiled item transport guidelines. (See Chapter 8.)

Disposable components such as pads, tubing, and suction canisters should be removed from each piece of equipment, and discarded at point of use. Only those items that will be cleaned and returned to use should be transported to the decontamination area.

Cleaning Patient Care Equipment

Patient care equipment should be cleaned by following the equipment manufacturer's instructions, and the healthcare facility's infection control protocols. The manufacturer's cleaning instructions are typically found in the operator's manual that accompanies the equipment when it is purchased. Alternatively, the manufacturer can be directly contacted. Whenever a new item of patient care equipment is brought into the facility, Central Service personnel should receive written instructions about procedures for cleaning and handling it. Remember that the key to equipment cleaning is attention to detail. All surfaces, including cords, switches and crevices must be thoroughly cleaned.

During the cleaning process, equipment should be inspected for obvious hazards such as cracked or frayed electrical cords, missing electrical prongs, damaged switches, or cracked and dented casings

that may indicate the equipment was dropped. All electrical equipment must have a 3-prong grounded outlet plug. (See **Figure 18.4**) Equipment with obvious damage, and equipment that is ready for routine preventive maintenance should be routed to the Biomedical Engineering Department.

Managing Inoperative Equipment

Equipment that is nonfunctioning should be identified and tagged by the user. (See **Figure 18.5**: Equipment Repair Tag.) Central Service Technicians must insure that equipment tagged for repair is routed to the Biomedical Engineering Department. If an equipment malfunction causes harm to a patient, it should not be disassembled, nor should its settings be adjusted. It should be sequestered and returned immediately to the Biomedical Department for inspection and follow-up. Since it will not have been disassembled or adjusted, Biomedical Technicians can better establish how the equipment was assembled or used, and they can recognize clues about the cause of the malfunction (such as incorrect assembly or operator error).

Preparing Equipment for Use

Patient care equipment should be prepared for use, and stored in a "ready to dispense" state. Preparation for use may include assembly, the addition of new disposable components such as tubing and pads, and a check and/or replacement of batteries in accordance with the equipment manufacturer's assembly instructions.

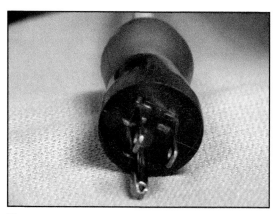

Figure 18.4 3-Pronged Plug
All electrical patient care equipment must have a 3-prong grounded plug.

Some patient care equipment requires water for operation. Central Service Technicians should become familiar with the equipment manufacturer's recommendations for the care of water reservoirs, and with specific fill procedures. Central Service Technicians should also be aware of any testing that they need to perform prior to issue.

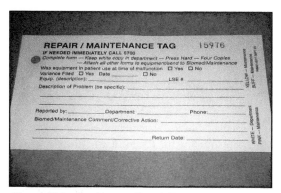

Figure 18.5 – Equipment Repair Tag

Storing Patient Care Equipment

After patient care equipment has been cleaned, inspected, and assembled, it should be placed in storage until needed. In most cases, storage is confined to the Central Service department or a secure location close to it. Sometimes, however, it may be stored in user units. This makes it more accessible for nursing and other patient care staff, and reduces waiting time when the equipment is needed immediately.

All equipment should be stored in a clean, secure location, away from high traffic areas such as visitor hallways. To do otherwise impedes traffic flow, and may provide an opportunity for unauthorized (often curious) people to tamper with it. Then infection control breaches, inadvertent disconnection of critical components, and/or damage can occur.

Some types of patient care equipment require that battery back-up systems be electronically charged. The required number of electrical outlets are needed in all applicable storage areas to enable these items to be plugged in at all times for battery recharge. (See the photo in **Figure 18.6.**) While this equipment is designed to run using wall power, there may be times, including during patient transport when patients are moved while still connected to IV pumps, and during power outages, when the equipment must rely on pre-charged batteries to function.

Tracking Patient Care Equipment

Tracking patient care equipment is a challenge for any Central Service department. The

Legislation and Equipment Safety

The Federal Safe Medical Devices Act of 1990 requires that the healthcare facility report malfunctions of medical devices that have contributed to patient injury, illness, and/or death[2] to the manufacturer and the Food and Drug Administration. Although the act broadly defines a "device," movable patient care equipment is included within this legislation. A proactive equipment management system should accurately record the specific data (for example, pump number, associated serial number, and other information pertinent to the incident) to comply with this legislation.

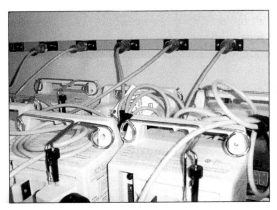

Figure 18.6

equipment is mobile and, in many cases, small, and it can easily be placed in an incorrect location, set aside on a user unit, or otherwise misplaced. Then it becomes very difficult to locate, and this can yield equipment shortages which may delay treatment, necessitate short-term rental of replacement equipment, and increase the hospital's operating costs.

There are several ways to track patient care equipment. It can be done manually using a paper system that tracks each equipment item's specific identifying number. Alternatively, it can be done using computerized programs that automate the tracking process by using bar code stickers that are applied to the device. In some hospitals, equipment is tracked with radio frequency computer chips applied to each device that send signals to a locator system. Note: equipment tracking is discussed in detail in Chapter 19.

Regardless of the type of tracking system used, the main purposes are to provide information:

- About the current location of the equipment.

- To charge using patients (if applicable).

- For equipment usage and trends.

- To track usage.

Tracking patient care equipment allows Central Service personnel to monitor needs, and insures that equipment is available when needed. That

information can also be used to justify additional equipment or for usage information when determining an equipment budget plan.

PROCURING NEW AND ADDITIONAL EQUIPMENT

Learning Objective 4. Describe the differences and explain advantages and disadvantages of purchase, lease, rent, and loan options for patient care equipment.

New technologies and increased need (patient volume) often require healthcare facilities to procure additional patient care equipment. New equipment may be purchased, leased or rented, or it can even be loaned to the healthcare facility by a manufacturer. The decisions to add equipment and its method of acquisition must consider several factors. There are advantages and disadvantages to each alternative, and the facility should make a decision based upon its specific needs.

Equipment Purchase

This method of equipment acquisition has been used by healthcare facilities for decades. Facility personnel identify the need for specific equipment, determine the type (model, style, or brand) that is required, budget for its purchase, and incorporate it into the system. The equipment is then owned by the healthcare facility.

Equipment Lease — long periods of time

As with purchasing, healthcare facility personnel must determine equipment needs. They then contract with a manufacturer or leasing company to lease (use) the equipment for a specific time period. At the end of the contract, the healthcare facility can usually return the equipment (and acquire a newer technology) or purchase it.

Equipment Rental — short time

Equipment rental differs from leasing because it is usually done on a short-term basis. For example, leasing contracts may be for months or years, but rental contracts may be as short as a single day. When renting, the healthcare facility identifies an immediate need, usually because high patient volume has created a demand for existing equipment that has caused a shortage, or because of the unique needs of a specific patient. In either case, the healthcare facility then contracts for a short term rental with an equipment rental company.

Manufacturer's Loan

Occasionally, manufacturers provide equipment to healthcare facilities as part of an agreement in which the facility will use its disposable products such as pads, tubing, and sleeves.

Decisions about the type of equipment acquisition process that will be most beneficial to the healthcare facility should be made by facility administrators. Whatever method is used to acquire equipment, the Central Service Technician's responsibilities remain the same: to provide clean, safe, and complete equipment, and to maintain the availability of that equipment by coordinating workflow.

OTHER PATIENT CARE EQUIPMENT CONCERNS

Learning Objective 5. Review other basic patient care equipment concerns: maintenance and repair and outsourcing.

Equipment Maintenance and Repair

All mechanical equipment must be properly maintained and unfortunately, it sometimes requires repair.

Preventive maintenance (PM) is designed to identify potential problems before they occur. It consists of a safety and function check as specified by the specific equipment manufacturer. PM is conducted on a routine, scheduled basis, and is designed to insure that equipment is in top operating condition. **Equipment repair** is performed as needed when equipment fails to function as it should, and when it appears to be damaged.

Both preventive maintenance and equipment repair should only be performed by trained biomedical equipment technicians.

Outsourcing Equipment Systems

Outsourcing of a hospital's equipment system, people, and resources has become more popular in recent years. Most typically, outsourcing relates to maintenance and repair rather than to maintaining inventory on a daily basis which is a Central Service responsibility. Since non-clinical hospital functions must, increasingly, be cost-justified, many hospital-based equipment management systems will likely be compared against the outsourcing alternative to assess the most cost-beneficial option.

There are several outsourcing options available. The most simple is to transfer management to the outside organization, but to retain all hospital employees and resources involved in the system. A more involved option is to transfer management of the hospital's equipment system, and to require that the external entity recruit and employ staff members to perform the function. Another option involves removing all hospital employees and resources involved in the equipment system, and requiring the outside entity to supply both employees and the equipment. The most radical option involves selling all hospital equipment to the outside entity, and then leasing it back. The outside entity would then own the hospital's equipment, and manage all necessary services.

Preventive maintenance (equipment) – Service provided to equipment to maintain it in proper operating condition by providing planned inspection, and by detecting and correcting failures before they occur; often abbreviated, "PM."

Repair (equipment) – Procedures used to return equipment to proper operating condition after it has become inoperative.

Outsourcing (equipment) – The transfer of control of a hospital equipment management system to an external entity.

Maintenance insurance allows a hospital to retain control of its own equipment. Facilities contract with an external insurance group to manage and insure the costs involved in maintaining the equipment. Some options with this plan include (a) paying the insurance group a flat fee, (b) risk-sharing agreements in which the hospital and the insurance group share the financial risks/rewards of maintaining the equipment, and (c) management contracts in which the hospital incurs most of the financial risk, but the insurance group manages the equipment system.

IN CONCLUSION

Patient care equipment is a vital component of modern healthcare. Central Service Technicians must assure that equipment is clean, assembled, and ready for use. They are also responsible to track the equipment, and insure that patient needs are met. Patient care equipment systems will evolve in healthcare facilities as new technologies emerge, and as different patient support processes are developed. It is important to keep current about these changes, and to remain alert about challenges that may impact patient safety.

ENDNOTES

1. *Joint Commission Accreditation Manual, IC.4.10, The Joint Commission*

2. *Code of Federal Regulations, Title 21, Part 813 – Medical Device Reporting. Subparts A, B, and C. U.S. Government Printing Office. Washington, DC, 2000.*

CENTRAL SERVICE TERMS

Patient care equipment

Preventive maintenance (PM)

Repair

Outsourcing (equipment)

Maintenance insurance

Maintenance insurance – An equipment outsourcing alternative in which a hospital retains control of its equipment, but contracts with an insurance organization to manage and insure the costs involved in maintaining the equipment.

Chapter 19

Tracking Systems

Chapter Learning Objectives:

As a result of successfully completing this chapter, readers will be able to:

1. List the primary reasons for tracking equipment, instruments, and supplies.

2. Discuss the use of computers and information systems to support applications within the facility and Central Service department.

3. Recognize that tracking systems enhance Central Service operations.

4. Explain that tracking systems must address the specific needs of the healthcare facility and Central Service department.

5. Review the features of available instrument and equipment tracking systems.

NEED TO TRACK EQUIPMENT

Learning Objective 1. List the primary reasons for tracking equipment, instruments, and supplies.

Central Service personnel must responsibly manage the equipment, instruments, and supplies owned by their facility that are entrusted to them. These items are in constant movement between departments as they are dispensed, used, and replaced or reprocessed. To maintain order and insure the availability of items for patient care, Central Service staff must track each item to:

- Insure that they can be quickly located.

- Determine when consumable supplies should be replaced.

- Measure item usage.

- Maintain accurate records of processes such as sterilization, distribution, etc.

- Assist with quality processes.

- Obtain information for financial analysis.

Historically, all recordkeeping (tracking) performed by the Central Service Department was done manually. Now most departments use some form of automated information management system to track products and processes. Some departments use a combination of manual and computerized tracking, while others have integrated automated information management throughout the entire department.

Some common types of automated (computer-based) information systems used in the Central Service Department include those for instrument tracking, sterilization logging information, case cart preference lists, patient care equipment tracking, and inventory management.

ROLE OF COMPUTER-BASED INFORMATION SYSTEMS

Learning Objective 2. Discuss the use of computers and information systems to support applications within the facility and Central Service department.

Central Service personnel must maintain and manage a significant amount of data as supplies, instruments, and equipment are stocked and issued to the Operating Room (OR) and various other user and patient care areas. Computers can promote basic and numerous advanced capabilities to support operational activities for healthcare Materiel Management and Central Service processing. Therefore, Central Service Technicians require a solid understanding of how computers are currently and might in the future be used to serve the department's constituencies. Computers and information systems continue to evolve rapidly. When Central Service personnel are involved in evaluating and/or selecting a new computer or system, they must know about the latest advances/technologies.

Basic Functions

Healthcare facilities are in a dynamic state of evolution. Rising materiel costs, concerns about inventories, and the need to improve production and processing functions have resulted in grouping these activities together in an integrated organization. This enables a facility to make more effective use of hospital personnel, and to centralize control and information flows to help decision-making.

Automated information systems have been used since the 1970's to help achieve greater productivity and operational efficiency. Today, automated information systems provide major opportunities for achieving significant improvements in Central Service and related patient care support systems.

To best support clinical needs and financial administration, systems must be joined to other parts (modules) of a comprehensive information system. Hospital information systems comprised of various modules support the diverse needs of the facility by providing the necessary information to those making decisions regarding the management

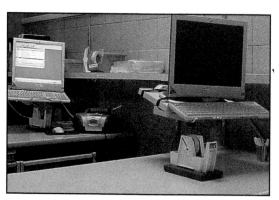

Figure 19.1

of information and materials needed to support patient care.

Much data about the supplies and equipment stocked and issued to all areas of the hospital must be gathered, processed, maintained, and managed. The most important activities include purchasing, receiving, management of inventory and tracking supply and patient charge items (if applicable). Other key areas and customers include the patient care units, the OR (case carts and preference lists), Central Service (instrument sets / trays and equipment), laboratories, radiology, and administrative support areas.

Increasingly, today's emphasis is on point-of-care and point-of-use computing with computer use moving to the bedside, into the physicians' and nurses' hands, and into the Central Service Technicians' work areas (See **Figure 19.1**). This has become possible with the development of electronic patient records and wireless capabilities that provide realtime data and historical record keeping. These systems can be supported with use of hand-held, palm top, and tablet-based computing terminals and wireless communications.

Selection of Department Systems

Many factors must be considered when selecting an information system to support activities for use by a specific department or facility. Key issues and requirements must first be evaluated and defined. These include addressing questions such as: Why do I need it? What do I want it to do? Is it capable of doing these things? Is it compatible with existing systems? Issues about appropriate and acceptable

costs and the projected volume of transactions that the system will process are also important. Other concerns include the types of hardware and operating systems available, the functional needs of the department including the number of users and, if financial or patient-related information is involved, security capabilities.[1]

After a system is selected, hardware and software must be installed. Vendor application software can either be purchased or leased, and application software typically requires implementation support and payment of annual maintenance fees. If software and implementation costs are bundled, their costs may be prorated over many years with a monthly payment. Significant costs are involved, and this purchase is usually treated as a capital expenditure.

TRACKING SYSTEMS FOR CENTRAL SERVICE

Learning Objective 3. Recognize that tracking systems enhance Central Service operations.

The processes and needs of the Central Service department have changed over the years. Advances in sterilization and instrument technologies, durable medical equipment, supply inventory, and costs for instrumentation purchase, instrument repair and replacement have increased the need for better usage and location tracking of these items.

Overview

Central Service personnel represent a key component in achieving the financial goals of reasonable instrument and equipment budgets. The tracking systems available for their use can forecast needs and yield processing costs for trays and single instruments. These tracking systems can also help maximize equipment and inventory usage to yield information as future budgets are developed.

Many healthcare environments use procedures that, while popular for many years, should be re-examined for continued relevance. Central Service personnel must also move out of their safety zones as they improve systems to maintain patient care equipment for nursing units, and to track supplies, instrument sets, and trays used throughout the facility.

Manual methods using hand-written tags, log books, wall-mounted bulletin boards or other methods to track equipment are now computerized. The decision to buy or design the appropriate software is crucial to the system's operation. Many facilities purchase turnkey products with limited support that generates less-than-ideal information. A better tactic involves use of a reputable product that provides updates to best assure that the facility receives necessary support and upgrades.

Tracking Methods

There are several types of tracking systems and methods available. Examples include use of bar codes (laser etched/label printed) to scan an item's last known location, and radio frequency identification (RFID) tracking in real-time. System simplicity, cost, and compatibility with other software systems in use are among the factors affecting the purchase decision.

The tracking system chosen typically involves a stand-alone hospital-based network utilized by both the Central Service department and OR. However, there are also systems available on a monthly subscription basis that provide the same features. This is often an effective way for the facility to control purchase costs and still have the features and abilities that will be important as the facility's and department's needs change. The appropriate software system also depends on the interfaces available to upload and/or download data files to facilitate information about instruments, sets, equipment (and their locations), and for productivity reporting, set/tray list builds, instrument inventory costs, and repair / purchase histories. Some systems even provide for case cart and preference card development and OR Scheduling.

TRACKING SYSTEMS MEET SPECIFIC NEEDS

Learning Objective 4. Explain that tracking systems must address the specific needs of the healthcare facility and Central Service department.

A tracking system must meet the specific needs of the facility that uses it. In some independent healthcare networks for example, there may be special needs of the system utilized by personnel in one site that are never implemented or used at another location. This can involve different locations, types or kinds of procedures used, equipment maintained, facility size, inventory support requirements, and other issues.

Computerized Systems in Use

Today's computerized methods facilitate more effective data tracking for quick report generating and are, respectively, much more comprehensive in scope and faster than yesterday's manual systems. Computerized back-up data is consistently more reliable than that available with a manual system. Computerized standards are accepted by the Healthcare Information Management Systems Society (HIMSS), and are used by applicable facility departments to securely store back-up data.

More About Tracking Systems

The continuing need to update information is critical to the success of any tracking system regardless of its use in a stand-alone or networked system, and regardless of its use for case cart picks, preference cards, inventory control, or other purposes.

Tracking systems perform many functions in Central Service departments. Single instruments can be located within a set/tray using laser-etched dot-type applications. Small bandage-sized RFID transponders provide real-time location when they are affixed to instruments or trays, and bar code labels can be used to assess the last location of sets and trays.

Documenting and scanning for these systems can be done with many different types of devices. These include wireless hand-held devices, devices wired directly to the computer terminal, fixed radio receivers that read the RFID transponder signals throughout the facility, and manual entry keying of information into the computer by keyboard or other human input device.

Decisions about system utilization should consider the specific environment to which the item(s) will be exposed. For example, one must examine the cleaning and sterilization processes for instruments including sets and trays. Chemicals designed for the metals of which instruments are constructed may destroy laser etchings, fade bar code labels, and make them unreadable to the scanner. Heat generated during steam sterilization may melt RFID transponders, and may destroy or cause their power source (usually a battery) located on an instrument set to malfunction. Water, chemicals, and drying temperatures used to clean case carts and other equipment may cause the adhesives utilized to affix the RFID transponders to dissolve causing them to fall off or become damaged from water leakage.

While there are many choices in software applications for tracking, let's take a look at what they can do.

FEATURES OF INSTRUMENT AND EQUIPMENT TRACKING SYSTEMS

Learning Objective 5. Review the features of available instrument and equipment tracking systems.

Instrument and equipment tracking systems can provide many different features to assist Central Service Technicians and personnel in the facility's Operating Rooms and Finance, Nursing, and Administrative departments. All tracking systems include some basic operating features. However, more advanced systems include additional features to enhance their usefulness.

Basic Systems

Basic instrument and equipment tracking systems typically can track (account for):

- Complete instruments and trays.

- Specific equipment items.

- Last known location of a specific instrument set, tray, or equipment item.

- Cost and value of specific equipment and instruments, and the total cost of instrument sets and tray.

- Number of complete processing and use cycles through which instruments and instrument sets have moved.

- Usage of specific equipment.

- Preventive maintenance schedules and repairs made to specific equipment and instrument sets and trays.

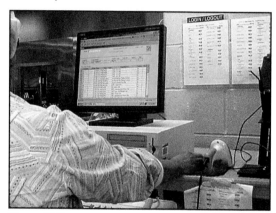

Figure 19.2

Basic instrument and equipment tracking systems also provide other information including:

- Complete Tray List Recipes for accurate tray assembly (See **Figure 19.2**) and equipment set-up procedures such as:
  - Name of Central Service Technician that assembled and inspected the set or equipment.
  - Date set or equipment was processed.
  - Sterilization and cleaning modality (process), if required.
  - Catalog number and manufacturer's name to identify instruments and associated equipment supplies.

- Quantity (individual and total) of instruments included within the set or tray.
- Lists grouped by category or instrument placement order within set.
- Identification of instruments missing from set. (These can be identified on the recipe, and can then be affixed to the outside of the set for identification and tracking.)

- Productivity reporting information:
  - Sets and instruments processed and completed during a specific work shift.
  - Sets and instruments completed by specific employees. Note: this information is helpful for educational and training purposes.
  - Equipment distributed and processed.

- Quality Assurance information for specific facility-based information such as:
  - Sterilization load quarantines.
  - Educational and in-service documentation.
  - Biological monitoring standards and regulations.

- Ability to interface with advanced sterilization and washer/decontamination equipment.

- Financial data for:
  - Instrument replacement and repair.
  - Equipment replacement and repair.
  - Preventive maintenance notification.
  - Preventive maintenance records.
  - Utilization of instrument sets, trays and equipment.
  - Productivity data and staffing requirements for peak operational workflow.

- An interface to the facility's Clinical Systems for associating (linking) the instrument sets and trays and equipment used to each patient's medical records.

Advanced Systems

Instrument and equipment tracking systems may include some advanced features helpful in some healthcare facility applications:

- Radio Frequency Identification (RFID) The real time location of an instrument or equipment item is tracked as it moves through the facility and the processing cycle. The real time location of a complete instrument set or tray can also be assessed.

- Standard Bar Code Label This system allows staff members to know the last location of an instrument set or tray.

- Laser Etched Bar Code This system enables the tracking of a single instrument within a set or tray. It can also identify the set into which a specific instrument was placed.

Note: The information just presented represents a generalized list of features that software and manufacturers typically provide in their instrument and equipment tracking systems. A complete review of a facility's specific needs is required to select the tracking system that best meets its needs.

IN CONCLUSION

Advancements in the technologies available to improve instrumentation processing procedures and techniques and the services Central Service Technicians provide to their customers is on-going. As well, the need to control product and supply costs is critical in today's healthcare environment. A facility's instrument and equipment tracking system will, hopefully, keep up with these improvements and, as they do, significant benefits to a facility will accrue.

As computerization and information systems evolve, additional capabilities will become available to help hospitals better address administrative tasks and to facilitate quality patient care. However, computers are only one part of a total information system. While computers and tracking systems provide numerous benefits, Central Service personnel are the key to providing efficient and effective services to help their department meet the facility's needs.

ENDNOTES

1. Austin, C. Information Systems for Health Services Administration. Ann Arbor, Michigan. AUPHA Press. 1992. (p. 144).

Chapter Outline

Chapter 20
Quality Assurance

Chapter Learning Objectives:

As a result of successfully completing this chapter, readers will be able to:

1. Define "quality" in the context of Central Service operations, and tell how to identify it.

2. Describe components in a quality Central Service program.

3. Discuss quality control indicators:
   - Administrative indicators
   - Customer satisfaction indicators
   - Technical indicators

4. Explain the basics of Failure Mode and Effects Analysis and Root Cause Analysis.

5. Discuss common quality programs:
   - Quality assurance and process improvement
   - Continuous quality improvement
   - Total quality management
   - Other quality programs and standards

6. Review quality procedures in the Central Service Department

Healthcare consumers demand quality in the products and services they receive. They expect nothing less than the best for themselves and their loved ones while using inpatient and outpatient healthcare services. Central Service personnel must establish appropriate quality levels for the products and services they produce, and assure that these levels are consistently attained.

Central Service Technicians directly serve **internal customers** (physicians, nurses, and other professionals working in the facility). The success of Central Service depends upon satisfying the needs of these internal customers so they can best serve the patients. Quality (or lack of it!) can have dramatic consequences on the health and safety of both patients and faculty personnel. How well quality products and services are provided impacts the operation of the department, and significantly impacts the hospital's success.

Central Service Technicians are an integral part of quality service throughout the healthcare industry. Patient care equipment and medical and surgical instrumentation is now processed in many healthcare sectors not serviced by Central Service Technicians including surgi-centers, physician's offices, off-site clinics, nursing rehabilitation facilities, and dental offices. With emerging medication-resistant bacteria and the ever-increasing complexity of surgical instrumentation, it has never been more challenging or rewarding for Central Service personnel to consistently provide quality products and services.

This chapter discusses several established quality programs to assist in monitoring quality within Central Service departments. The ultimate goal is high

> **Customer (internal)** – the physicians, nurses, and other professional personnel served by Central Service staff members.

> **Quality** – The consistent delivery of products and services according to established standards. Quality "integrates" the concerns for the customers (including patients and user department personnel) with those of the department and facility.

quality patient care, and this can best be assured when one or a combination of these programs is selected, implemented, and monitored.

QUALITY IN CENTRAL SERVICE OPERATIONS

Learning Objective 1. Define "quality" in the context of Central Service operations, and tell how to identify it.

Quality requires Central Service Technicians to look at what they do from their customers' perspectives. In many respects, Central Service production is only as good as the last device processed or the most recent service provided. One hundred error-free items can be processed, but one imperfect tray or service will be noticed, and considered as the department's quality outputs are evaluated. While this might objectively seem to be unreasonable, it is very understandable because of the harm to patients and employees that can be caused by the defect.

What Is Quality?

The concept of quality relates to the degree or grade of excellence of a product or service. For example, Emergency Room personnel may feel that an emergency crash cart was delivered efficiently (on a timely basis), but the cart might not provide a needed item that was requested on the pick list (supply listing). This indicates excellent service quality but poor product quality. By contrast, assume a surgical instrument set is needed quickly in the surgical suite, and is delivered with all necessary components. However, if the surgical staff is not informed that the delivery was made, product quality was appropriate, but service quality was unacceptable. In short, quality is measured through the eyes of the customers, and their concerns relate to both products and service.

The patient must be at the center of every quality concern. To help them the most, Central Service personnel must provide properly processed products when they are needed. Just being "good" is not good enough! A surgical tray delivered to the operating room on time that is incomplete or with the wrong instruments does not represent quality service. The patient may have a less than desirable outcome due to instrumentation problems. Patients do not know nor should they have to worry about whether the correct instruments are delivered on time to the Operating Room. Central Service Technicians accept this responsibility and the challenge to consistently meet the facility's product and service standards.

Looking at functions from the customers' perspectives allows the Central Service team to critically review its processes to determine where improvements can be made. However, remember that:

- Quality is not the only way to improve.

- Some things critical to quality cannot be delegated.

- Quality takes time, effort, and participation from everyone in the healthcare facility.

- The quality plan should be the department's business plan.

How is Quality Identified?

Quality (or, at least, aspects of it) can be identified in several ways:

- Products and services might be considered "excellent" if they meet one's needs (they do what they are supposed to do). If a new washer-decontaminator is properly used, but instruments are still dirty after a complete cycle, the equipment will be judged inferior. However, if the equipment meets expectations (it produces clean decontaminated instruments), it is easier to think that "This is a great manufacturer, and I would purchase from this company again."

Case cart – *An inventory control system for products and equipment that is typically used in the operating room. An enclosed cart is prepared for one special surgical case, and is not used for general surgical replenishment.*

This feeling provides a subjective view of quality that provides no basis for measurement, and does not consider the customers' service levels.

- Branding is also a subjective form of quality identification. As suggested above, if one has a great experience with specific equipment, a future purchase from that manufacturer is more likely than if negative experiences occur.

Sometimes professional quality concerns within the Central Service Department establish standards that exceed customers' expectations. Consider an instrument that is missing from an instrument set. If it was not needed, the customer may (or may not) be concerned. The important point is that a "quality" set should contain specific instruments and, if they are not present in the set, it (the set) is not of appropriate quality.

Note: In this example, the definition of "a quality" instrument set may change if customers determine that a specific instrument is no longer needed in a set. Perhaps, for example, a newly available device is judged "better," and will now be a required component in the set. Its availability will then be considered as the quality of future instrument sets is judged.

Sometimes quality can be determined by identifying which Central Service Technician assembled the tray or **case cart**. Knowing that an item is always right when it is processed by a specific person (name) is a type of "branding." However, all staff must be able to perform work within their areas of responsibility to the appropriate quality level.

Products processed by Central Service personnel should always be complete and properly assembled with no defects. Departments attaining this quality standard will be highly regarded throughout the facility. Central Service quality should not be subjective; instead, each item processed or delivered should be documented with valid statistics. An internal-department system should be implemented to identify inferior products before they leave the area. External-department information can be obtained from customers surveyed by using the count sheets in trays, pick tickets on case carts and requested items, and/or by formal surveys

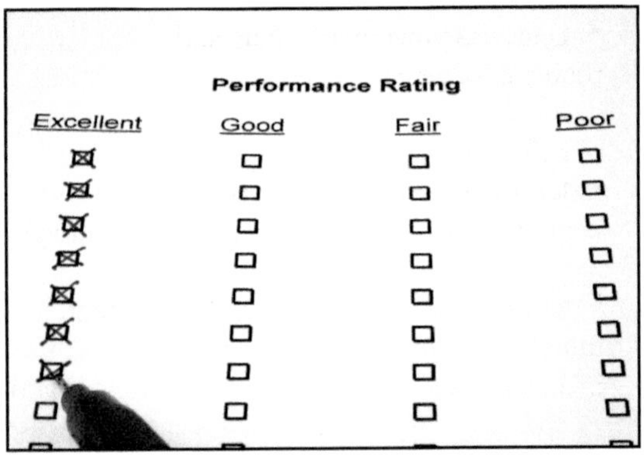

Figure 20.1

designed to learn about quality dimensions from the customers' perspectives. (See **Figure 20.1**) Statistics from both internal and external sources should be analyzed, inferior areas should be studied, and corrective actions should be implemented to best assure quality improvement.

COMPONENTS OF QUALITY

Learning Objective 2. Describe components in a quality Central Service program.

Quality is not a "quick-fix" for healthcare facilities. Achieving world-class (best in the industry) quality requires a multi-year plan to move a facility from its current quality level to the ideal (highest achievable) quality. For example, the Ritz-Carlton hotel chain, the only U.S. lodging organization to win the prestigious Malcolm Baldrige award for quality, began its journey to quality with a benchmark of 60,000 defects per million transactions. It planned a six year process to move to .60 (less than one!) defect per million transactions. The Ritz-Carlton's definition of world-class quality also required a fifty percent reduction in cycle time (the time that passes between an order being placed and being completed). This planned approach to move toward an ideal quality goal is just as relevant to healthcare as it is to hospitality. Quality is the business plan!

Top level administrators must emphasize quality because their support is critical for success. Most problems affecting the employees' ability to accomplish work are caused by systems and procedures that have, in some way, been required or implemented by top-level leaders. Quality requires the efforts and participation from everyone in the facility, and time is required to develop, implement, and monitor any quality program.

Departmental quality should be multi-disciplinary as well as intradepartmental. A true quality program utilizes all Central Service personnel and a cross-section of its customers. (See **Figure 20.2**)

Several concerns are integral to the implementation of a quality program in a healthcare facility. This will now be discussed.

Empowerment

Empowerment is the process of "driving" the process of decision-making and implementation down the facility's chain of command. In other words, some decisions that, in the past, would have been made by managers or higher-level departmental or other administrators are made by supervisors or front line staff members. Empowerment is typically limited to well-defined areas such as **process improvement** changes within the employee's defined areas of responsibility.

Managers must provide training to all personnel about the concept of empowerment who must know how to properly perform all work tasks before they can be empowered.

Leadership

Quality requires committed leaders to help manage the data, plan opportunities, establish priorities, and empower people to implement improved processes.

Empowerment – The act of granting authority (power) to employees to make decisions within their areas of responsibility.

Process improvement – Activity to identify and resolve work task-related problems that yield poor quality; the strategy of finding solutions to eliminate the root causes of process performance problems.

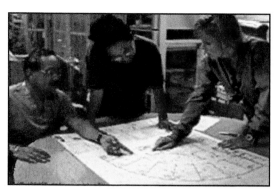

Figure 20.2

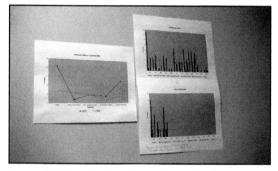

Figure 20.3 Quality Data Posted in a Central Service Work Area.

Effective leaders define standards to be attained in quality products/services, and these will drive the development of strategies that address customer satisfaction and the attainment of the facility's goals.

Senior department leaders should serve as the facility's quality committee. Their responsibilities should include the following:

• Help create and instill standards, and ensure that coaching about standards occurs daily for all employees. Before-shift meetings can focus on facility and departmental quality issues. A daily quality message should be conveyed to every employee in every department.

• Set process priorities. Managers can evaluate suggested projects relative to patient satisfaction or other goals. What are their costs? How difficult will it be to implement recommendations? What is the expected level of savings, and is this level worth the efforts and expenditures required?

• Undertake quality planning and problem-solving activities.

• Be responsible for "error-proofing" (addressing the people aspects of quality through human resources and other functions).

• Address three types of error (inadvertent, intentional and that resulting from incompetence) to reduce their impact on quality.

Department leaders including Shift Supervisors and Lead Technicians should be the first line "guardians" of the quality program to ensure that all department personnel adhere to the standards and priorities set by senior managers. Employees should help their teammates to follow established guidelines. This can be accomplished by interacting with new or less qualified staff members, assisting in on-going training, and participating in daily quality control checks.

Standard Data

Senior leaders must select the data that must be quantified to implement and monitor the department's quality processes. Many managers routinely study financial data; fewer look at organizational data such as turnover costs. Still fewer facilities study patient and employee satisfaction levels, the number of defects, and cycle times. Senior leaders can help to benchmark defects and set quality goals (such as a 50 percent cycle-time reduction, and a 100 percent improvement in patient/customer satisfaction levels as expressed on comment cards). Department leaders should be responsible for implementing and monitoring the above and other specific data while front line staff members assist in data collection and analysis. Figure 20.3 provides an example of data that has been collected and compiled for analysis.

Planning Tools and Procedures

Quality planning can reduce existing and prevent potential problems. It involves:

• Identifying factors which are important to patients and customers. What do they like?

What do they dislike? What's important to them? How do they compare us to the competition? What do patients/customers want from us (for example, no billing errors, no missing instruments, and timely deliveries)?

• Studying the competition. How do other facilities deliver each product and service that their patients/customers want?

• Doing everything better (or at least equal to) the competition.

• Remembering that the process (not people) is the cause of most problems.

• Thinking about how to improve. All levels of staff and customers should be queried to help identify improvement areas and techniques.

One quality planning goal is to design features that customers and employees prefer into the processes used to complete work assignments. A second goal is to design customer and employee dislikes out of the processes.

Steps of quality planning include the following:

• Step One: Identify the needs and requests of the department's customers.

• Step Two: Identify an ideal process to consistently address each need/request.

• Step Three: Compare actual steps and outcomes of each process to the ideal outcome. (for example, 100% error free trays)

• Step Four: Plan process control activities to improve the system.

• Step Five: Measure the defects that result. With a good quality system in place, the number of nonconformities (**defects**) should decrease, and, with continuous quality improvement, defects should continue to decrease.

Defect – A variance from expected standards.

Principles of Quality Management

Several principles of quality management form the foundation of a quality process:

• Patient focus – Assuring that the needs and wants of the patients are the driving force in decision-making, problem-solving and other activities.

• Process management – Placing the emphasis on managing the process rather than upon managing the employees.

• Continuous quality improvement – Believing that things can always be done better, and then undertaking improvement efforts.

• Fact-based decisions – Basing decisions on fact(s) rather than upon assumptions.

Staff Members

How can staff members be developed to support a facility's quality goals? First, define traits that are consistent with those of successful employees. Then provide employees with the knowledge, skills, and tools to do assigned work according to expected standards.

Employees must be empowered to address solutions to immediate problems. For example, they should be allowed to stop what they are doing to help a patient or another employee. Perhaps they can be given some financial discretion. They should be able to enlist the assistance of other workers in problem-solving tasks, when necessary. Further, employees who desire additional responsibilities should be allowed to work on longer term problem-solving projects. This may be done with the use of cross-functional teams who select a process problem, analyze it, develop alternatives, offer solutions, and make implementation suggestions. Senior leaders must recognize superior persons and teams.

Process Management

The only consistent way to achieve goals is with a capable process. Employees may, for example, address ways to shorten cycle times in

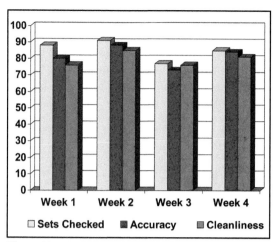

Figure 20.4

decontamination, reduce errors in assembling surgical trays, or increase accuracy while reducing cycle times during inventory replenishment.

Senior leaders must be involved in process management. They can develop and improve some quality processes, and they can recognize basic self-control mechanisms. (Every employee should be a quality engineer!) They can personally ensure that breakthrough improvements become part of the process. Remember that processes always get stronger or weaker; they never stay the same!

Studying processes is critical because process problems cause defects. If defects are identified and resolved, patients and customers will experience fewer problems. (See **Figure 20.4**) Also, employees will have greater success in consistently delivering products and services that meet quality standards. Operating costs will decrease, and financial goals will be better met. Some processes to study for improvement potential are:

- Instrument set turn-around times.

- Instrument set accuracy.

- Surgical case cart accuracy.

- Inventory fill rates.

All employees have a significant role to play in a facility's total quality efforts, including those who directly interact with patients, and those who interact only with other employees. All

staff members at all organizational levels have an integral and important role to play in helping the healthcare facility achieve quality goals. They must consistently attain quality standards designed to meet (and, hopefully, to exceed) the needs and desires of the healthcare facility and the patients it serves. Those who successfully achieve consistently high quality standards should be recognized by the senior management team. Recognition may take place through awards, promotions, and/or bonuses or compensation increases.

The highest levels of quality are difficult to attain and maintain. However, what happens when quality is not emphasized? Inconsistent products, service delays, conflicts between patients and employees, and conflicts among employees are among the results. These problems contribute to higher costs and lower facility revenues.

Quality is a Sequential Process

Quality is a sequential process. Inputs to the process are the facility's resources (for example, people, material, and time). These resources must be used efficiently in a well-defined process or series of processes to produce the products and services desired or required by patients and other customers. This, in turn, yields satisfaction.

What processes should be used to produce the products and services which are needed? The answer can often be best determined by cross-functional teams. One example: a team might consist of staff members from Central Service, Purchasing, Laundry, and other departments interacting with representatives from Nursing, Pharmacy, and Accounting. The perspectives of each of these units can help the team arrive at the best solutions to production process problems. Cross-functional teams can be effective because they address problems which arise from systems and procedures designed (or required) by managers who are not on the day-to-day "firing line."

Administrators spend much money on quality regardless of whether they emphasize quality management. For example, they pay for prevention (the cost of doing things correctly the first time), appraisal (the cost of ensuring that things are done correctly the first time), and failure (the cost of not doing something correctly the first time). Clearly, significant labor costs are devoted to quality assurance. An effective quality process can help to ensure that these costs are minimized and that consistency and effectiveness—from the perspectives of both the facility and the patients—are addressed.

QUALITY CONTROL INDICATORS

Learning Objective 3. Discuss quality control indicators:
- Administrative indicators
- Customer satisfaction indicators
- Technical indicators

Purpose of Quality Control Indicators

Central Service **quality control** indicators are often used to determine how well the department is meeting its objectives of producing the proper quality of goods and services. Several **indicators** of quality should be monitored periodically.

Several threshold variables can be determined which must be met or exceeded to provide the expected quality of performance.

Some examples of Central Service quality indicators are:

- Customer departments receive STAT or urgent medical supplies within five minutes of request.

- Only sterile supplies with current dates are available on unit supply carts.

- Sterilization procedures are acceptable based upon results of mechanical, chemical, and biological indicators.

- Instruments sets contain correct contents.

- Central Service customers are satisfied with departmental services based on a score of 90 or greater on customer survey questionnaires.

- Patient care equipment and supplies are available in proper working condition.

- Results of technical sterilization indicators are properly logged and reported for all sterilizers. (See **Figure 20.5**)

- "Flashing" of instrumentation is done following appropriate protocols and is documented.

- Biological indicators accompany every load requiring biological monitoring.

- Case carts contain correct contents.

Consider instrument set pick lists: an error rate might be established at not more than .60%. When the departmental instrument picking average falls below 99.40% (100.0% - .60%), this indicates unacceptable quality. Then further analysis is needed to correct the problem. Some quality control indicators must be measured and monitored closely; others can be spot-checked occasionally.

There are three categories of quality control indicators: administrative, customer satisfaction, and technical. Each of these will now be discussed.

Administrative Quality Control Monitors

Administrative quality controls are activities regulated by policies, procedures, and other administrative actions to assure safe and efficient departmental performance. They are of three basic types.

Management Control Monitors

The most important quality control in Central Service begins with the management of the department. All directors, managers, supervisors, and lead technicians must be thoroughly trained in modern Central Service principles. They must

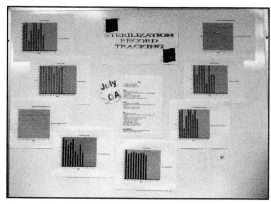

Figure 20.5 Quality Information Posted in a Central Service Work Area.

realize that human resources are their most important resource.

Policies, procedures and standard work assignment lists with times and outcomes are necessary for quality control. The first steps in controlling Central Service work tasks are written procedures and work assignment lists. All tasks require written procedures available to every Central Service Technician. This provides for consistency of on-going operations when new personnel are on duty, and/or when the supervisor is unavailable. Employees must carefully review how to perform all necessary tasks. Communication is necessary for quality assurance. Written procedures help to provide consistent communication.

Quality control checks measure how well products or services meet production standards. For instance, some manufacturers of medical

---

Quality control – A technical, statistical sampling method that measures the quality of production.

Indicator – A measurable variable which relates to the outcome of patient care or employee safety.

Acceptance sampling – Inspection of a sample from a larger lot to decide whether the lot should be accepted.

Random numbers (Table) – A table of numbers generated in an unpredictable, haphazardous sequence that is used to create a random sample.

---

products utilize **acceptance sampling** methods to assess the quality of lots that have already been manufactured. A predetermined number of defective samples from a particular lot size will require rejection of the total lot. If, for example, a lot size of fifty items reveals that two are defective, and if that is the predetermined defect limit, the whole lot is rejected. This approach is difficult when the process is part of an on-going routine such as picking surgical instrumentation for specific cases. Healthcare facilities usually do not have the resources to use this method.

Quality control checks should be performed regularly to determine the levels of Central Service workmanship and service. It is inefficient to constantly check everything that occurs, so a representative and unbiased sample of checks can be made at random.

A Quality Control Grid Table should be developed for each category of items to be checked, and handling sub-systems must be included. For example, the category of items will likely include instruments and case carts, while the sub-systems to be checked will include proper cleaning, set-up, packaging and labeling. To be unbiased, a table of **random numbers** should be used to determine which items to check as well as what aspects of each item are to be checked.

Inspection Control Monitors

Inspection quality controls cross-check other quality control monitors. For example, the Infection Control Coordinator must stay current with modern infection prevention principles and aseptic techniques. He/she can then review patient infections, and keep staff informed about the latest technologies including those relating to disinfectants, isolation precautions, and hospital-acquired infections. The chain of infection from contaminated medical instruments and equipment stops in the decontamination process.

Safety inspections promote quality in the Central Service area. Knowledgeable safety professionals must assist every individual in the facility to remain healthy and to avoid accidents. Safety inspection reports can provide information that may prevent accidents, and they should be encouraged because they help prevent loss of productive working time. Additionally, it is better to keep trained staff on the job than to use new, unskilled employees who require more training.

Regulatory agency inspections involve in-depth inspections concerning all aspects of patient care to assess whether individual departments' policies and procedures are being followed. The Joint Commission is an example of a voluntary/regulatory agency. It is committed to continuous quality improvement, and is patient outcome-oriented. Many agencies provide a detailed summation conference at the end of a several-day inspection to offer recommendations for improving the quality of care. Central Service professionals use these recommendations as indicators of the quality of service being performed.

Facility Meeting Information

Committee minutes provide information about other areas of the healthcare facility that is useful to Central Service personnel. For example, Utilization Management Committee minutes might indicate that supply usage for physicians who perform specific procedures has not been standardized. If so, this is a good time to discuss cost savings from supply standardization with this group, because patients as well as the facility could benefit from this cost containment measure. Also, assume that Safety or Infection Control Committee minutes indicate an increase in needle sticks by the IV therapy team. Distribution personnel within the Central Service Department might suggest a new product that attaches to the IV poles to hold needles, and decrease the probability of needle sticks.

Staff meeting minutes allow for ideas that enhance excellent service by identifying problems before they happen. Trained Central Service Technicians have great practical knowledge, especially in daily operations, and they are an excellent resource. Their ideas and suggestions should be documented in departmental minutes and shared with others.

Customer Satisfaction Quality Control Indicators

Anyone with an expectation about Central Service products or services is a customer. They include patients, medical personnel, diagnostic imaging technicians, physicians, surgical service personnel, and motor pool drivers. Remember, it is in the eyes of the customer that quality is measured.

Customer Surveys

Customer survey results can indicate potential problems that may not be apparent to Central Service personnel. For example, staff nurses may be inconvenienced with the storage of IV solutions and administration sets. Perhaps they are stored too far from each other, or too low on the shelf, and it is difficult for the nurse to obtain these supplies from the cart with efficient body mechanics. Central Service Technicians may also be having difficulty stocking heavy solutions on higher shelves. Surveys provide opportunities for developing excellent customer relations because they facilitate open communication. Physicians and nurses communicate with individual Central Service Technicians, and their input is important to provide quality patient care.

Incident Reports

Incident reports can be useful in determining trends. Assume there is an incident report about the omission of some important pieces which are part of a loaner orthopedic instrument set. As a follow-up to this report, perhaps the company representative was unaware that these pieces were needed for the surgical case. Documentation of communication with the company representative prior to delivery may prevent similar problems. An incident report may be the only document that warns of possible poor quality service.

It is our goal to always provide the highest possible quality of products and service. Your comments about the quality of this tray would be greatly appreciated.

_____

_____

_____

_____

Tray Name: _____

This tray was assembled by: _____

Please send all comments to the Central Processing Department (Quality Control) or call ext. xxxx and ask for Bill Smith.

Figure 20.6

Tray Cards

Tray cards that accompany trays or surgical instrument sets are valuable in obtaining feedback about the department and individual technicians. **Figure 20.6** shows a sample tray card.

Effectively used, tray cards can generate user comments about quality, and they can also express the Central Service department's philosophy about service excellence. Include the department's telephone number and the type of tray or set. In addition, leave some space for comments. Positive comments from users can be provided to the Central Service Technician whose name is on the tray card to reinforce his/her morale and excellent service. Tray cards need not be limited to trays or instrument sets. They can be used with anything manufactured and distributed by the department including patient care equipment and case carts. Even direct shipments from outside vendors that are assembled in the receiving area can include these cards.

Customer Complaints

Customer complaints express dissatisfaction with Central Service quality efforts. It takes courage to tell someone that the department is performing inadequately on a particular project or shift.

Take all complaints seriously even if most are isolated events and not systemic problems, and assure that they are promptly addressed to avoid becoming widespread. The credibility of the department is enhanced when these issues are resolved quickly in a professional manner.

Staff Complaints

Staff complaints are one of the first indications of a problem. Professional Central Service Technicians want to provide excellent service to all units. They often know how to improve operations, and their input should be used to enhance the department's services and products.

Technical Quality Control Indicators

Technical quality control indicators are utilized in the more intricate and precise areas of Central Service including sterile processing which is considered a manufacturing area because medical items are reprocessed for re-use. These process

Technical quality control indicators – *Process control measures utilized to assure that planned technical conditions within sterilizers and aerators are met.*

control measures help assure that planned technical conditions within sterilizers and aerators are met, and that sterility (the absence of all microorganisms on an inanimate item) results. Many processes can be measured to assure quality beginning with the decontamination area and continuing with the cleaning, assembling and packaging areas and, finally, to the terminal sterilization process.

Technical quality control indicators should be used in all areas/departments that perform sterile processing. This includes sterile processing activities which occur outside of the Central Service department including in surgery, clinics, endoscopy, and cardiac catheterization areas.

The sterilization process is often the final step before an item will be used in a patient procedure. This step is of premier importance because the product may be used in a patient invasive procedure. It is difficult to prove that an item is sterile without contaminating it, so the conditions that lead to sterility must be shown to be present. Medical items that have been sterilized must have proof that they met conditions for sterility. The following is a list of technical control indicators which have been discussed at length in earlier chapters:

- Mechanical Indicators: pressure gauges and temperature and pressure graphs and charts.

- Chemical indicators/integrators.

- Biological indicators.

ANALYSIS OF QUALITY CONCERNS

Learning Objective 4. Explain the basics of Failure Mode and Effects Analysis and Root Cause Analysis.

Failure Mode and Effects Analysis (FMEA) and Root Cause Analysis (RCA) are two widely-used methods to analyze issues discovered within quality systems. Although these methods are not always recognized or practiced in their original form, their popularity has continued to grow. Both concepts are important tools that can be used in a quality program.

Failure Mode and Effects Analysis

Failure mode and effects analysis (FMEA) has its origins in the military and industrial fields. It is a proactive process aimed at predicting the adverse outcomes of various human and machine failures. FMEA looks forward to prevent future adverse outcomes. It addresses questions such as "If the sump pump fails on a washer decontaminator, what malfunction would follow?" If the malfunction is unacceptable, the sump pump might be redesigned, or a new pump might be installed. FMEA deals with hypothetical events and, since it requires analysts to imagine the unthinkable, is not widely used in the medical field.

The Institute for Safe Medication Practices (ISMP) uses a healthcare version of FMEA to analyze potential medical errors. It examines the use of new products and the design of new services and processes to determine points of potential failure and what their effect would be before any error actually happens. A proactive process looks more carefully and systematically at vulnerable areas or processes before purchase and implementation of new services, processes, or products to identify potential failure modes. Then steps can be taken to avoid errors before they occur if FMEA shows that a specific error could cause a specific injury.

Root Cause Analysis

Root cause analysis (RCA) is a reactive process used after an unwanted event has occurred to analyze what may have led to the event. RCA uses historical analysis of an adverse outcome to help prevent its recurrence. Assume a washer

Failure mode and effect analysis (FMEA) – A process designed to predict the adverse outcomes of various human and machine failures to prevent future adverse outcomes.

Root cause analysis (RCA) – A process that "looks backwards" at an event to help prevent its future occurrence.

Sentinal Event - An unexpected occurrence involving death, serious physical or psychological injury, or the risk thereof.

decontaminator sump pump malfunctioned and caused instruments to be improperly cleaned. Each event after the pump failure would be examined to determine what could have occurred, and what can be done to resolve this issue in the future. RCA is widely utilized in the medical field to examine contributing factors to adverse events.

Note: Joint Commission standard LD.5.2 requires facilities to select at least one high risk process for proactive (FMEA) risk assessment each year. This standard also requires facilities to conduct root cause analysis on any **sentinel event** that has occurred.[1]

QUALITY PROGRAM ALTERNATIVES

Learning Objective 5. Discuss common quality and process improvement:
- Quality assurance and process improvement
- Continuous quality improvement
- Total quality management
- Other quality programs and standards

Total Quality Improvement

Many Central Service departments utilize a **quality assurance** program because it is comprehensive. It requires the gathering of data to assure that a quality product is regularly produced. The numbers of items not meeting quality requirements is compared to the total number of items produced. Although this process requires quality checks, it does not help to identify reasons for the defects.

Process improvement is another strategy of finding solutions to eliminate the root causes of process performance problems. It determines the number of errors produced and strives to reduce the error rate.

Total quality improvement (TQI) involves measuring the current output of a process or procedure, and then modifying it to increase the output, increase efficiency, and/or increase effectiveness. TQI can be applied to organizational and individual performance. Assume Central Service staff can produce fifty trays daily that meet quality requirements. Then, by changing the method of wrapping, personnel can now produce fifty-five trays daily without sacrificing quality requirements. As well, Judy can answer ten phone calls in an hour, but use of a headset allows her to answer fifteen phone calls per hour. TQI usually focuses on four areas of improvement:

- Input – Reduce working material or the reorder time for that material.

- Throughput – Increase process efficiency or time while reducing waste and resource utilization.

- Output – Decrease costs or increase quantities while not increasing costs.

- Outcome – Determine whether the improvement makes a difference.

TQI recognizes that improvement can occur with an individual, a team, an organizational unit such as the Central Service department, or the organization itself. This process is often seen as a cycle in which goals and objectives are established, coaching is used to provide feedback, performance is adjusted, and appraisal is used to formally document individual performance.

Quality assurance – A comprehensive and measured effort to provide total quality. Also, a technical, statistical sampling method that measures production quality.

Total quality improvement (TQI) – The concept of measuring the current output of a process or procedure, and then modifying it to increase the output, increase efficiency, and/or increase effectiveness.

Continuous Quality Improvement (CQI)

Continuous quality improvement (CQI) is a statistical method to improve **work processes.** Consider a current instrument set pick list signed by a Central Service Technician which accompanies the tray to the point of use. This is an example of a work process that helps assure the quality of instrument sets. When the instrument set pick lists are returned, they can be tallied to quantitatively assess the amount of quality delivered to the customer. A computerized database can assist in determining departmental performance by case, service, physician, set, date and Technician. CQI methods can be used for numerous purposes within the Central Service department. Perhaps none is more important than to assure that consistent processes are used to sterilize instruments while using optimal patient safety procedures.

Four concerns integral to quality control at time of instrument sterilization are:

- Integrity checking and careful cleaning before sterilization.

- Use of the correct sterilizing procedures.

- Routine (random) checking of difficult-to-sterilize instruments to assure that sterilization is adequate.

- Feedback to staff when inspections indicate problems.

Planning and implementing a CQI program for instrument processing involves the receipt and use of input from decontamination staff, reprocessing employees, nursing and physician personnel, and all others involved in equipment use. Sterilization procedures also depend, in part, upon the materials used to construct the instrument to be sterilized. Therefore, manufacturers' recommendations for sterilization of the instrument(s) must also be included in the planning process.

Quality control measures to reprocess items that have contacted patient secretions and fluids are absolutely critical. The risk of infection from exposure to blood and body fluids of infected patients due to improper reprocessing is difficult to determine. However, the greatest risk involves critical items which enter sterile body sites.

Audits should be an integral part of the CQI process because they can:

- Assist in assessing instruments being returned from all hospital units for sterilization. Manufacturers typically provide instructions about utilization of sterilizer equipment and cleaning compounds. With this exception, there are relatively few guidelines available to Central Service personnel about how to ensure continuous quality improvement. In the past, the proper use of biological and chemical indicators has provided adequate indicators of appropriate sterilization for many items. However, it is apparent that these controls are less sufficient for difficult-to-sterilize critical items. While one cannot test every difficult-to-sterilize instrument being processed, spot checks using predefined factors as part of a CQI process will help to ensure process validation.

- Assist in assessing the most appropriate sterilization methods. Even if the correct sterilization procedures are in place, instruments may not be sterilized properly if adequate cleaning procedures are inconsistently used. Central Service employees should not believe that use of technology means no mistakes are possible.

- Assist in identifying areas where additional staff training and education are needed.

- Promote communication between Central Service staff and personnel in other

Continuous quality improvement (CQI) – A scientific approach which applies statistical methods to improve work processes.

Processes (work) A series of work activities which produce a product or service.

---

departments. Audits provide feedback, and input from users of Central Service products and services helps to identify problems and improve processes. Likewise, feedback from Central Service personnel received from user department personnel serves the same purpose.

- Quality standards should be available for, and CQI should address, the reprocessing and re-sterilization of single-use items.

Total Quality Management (TQM) and Six Sigma

Total quality management (TQM) is an organization-wide quality approach based on participation of all members that aims at long-term success through customer satisfaction and benefits to all members of the organization and society. TQM requires that the facility maintain its quality standards in all aspects of its business, that it ensures work tasks are performed correctly the first time, and that defects and waste are eliminated from operations.

TQM starts with a random sampling of the product or service which can than be tested for the concerns that most matter to end users. Causes of failures are isolated and corrected. Variances in measurement ranges and what failures caused them to be chosen are monitored and recorded.

The objective of **Six Sigma** is to deliver high performance, reliability, and value to the end customer. It is a highly-disciplined and complex process that focuses on developing and delivering near-perfect products and services in an on-going quality effort.

Total quality management (TQM) – A quality management approach based on participation of all members aimed at long-term success through customer satisfaction and benefits to all members of the organization and society.

Six Sigma – A quality process that focuses on developing and delivering near-perfect products and services.

Six Sigma is a disciplined, data-driven approach for eliminating defects that measures how far a given process deviates from perfection. The premise: if one can measure how many defects exist in a process, he/she can determine how to eliminate them and move as close to zero defects as possible. A Six Sigma process produces no more than 3.4 defects per one million opportunities. Note: a defect in this program is defined as anything outside of customer specifications. It focuses on process improvement and variation reduction by use of Six Sigma improvement projects.

The DMADV process (define, measure, analyze, design, and verify) is used to develop new processes. As well, DMAIC procedures (define, measure, analyze, improve, control) monitor and improve existing processes.

Roles required for Six Sigma implementation include:

- Executive Leadership - (includes all top-level administrators) Responsible for establishing a vision. They must empower their team with the freedom and resources to explore new ideas and improvements.

- Champions - These persons, drawn from upper administrative levels, are responsible for implementation across the organization. They act as mentors to Master Black Belts, also known as quality leaders.

- Master Black Belts - These champions act as in-house expert coaches for the organization, and devote all of their time to Six Sigma efforts as they guide black and green belts.

- Black Belts - apply Six Sigma methodology to specific projects, and focus on project execution.

- Green Belts - incorporate Six Sigma responsibilities with other job obligations.

- Orange Belts - receive training that enables them to understand Six Sigma methodology. They are prepared to be good team members and support Black Belts and Green Belts.

- Experts - work across company boundaries to improve services, processes, and products for their suppliers, and they work across multiple sites and departments to incorporate lessons learned throughout the facility.

Other Quality Programs and Standards

The Joint Commission

The Joint Commission is an industry-driven organization that ensures quality standards are set, monitored and maintained by member healthcare facilities. It has established many health and safety program requirements for patients and staff using recommended practices and guidelines from national and federal organizations including AAMI and OSHA. Routine and unannounced inspections are used to monitor standards, and each member facility is graded on its performance.

Magnet Status

Magnet Status is an award given by the American Nurses Credentialing Center to hospitals that satisfy factors that measure the strength and quality of their nursing care. Qualifying facilities are surveyed to determine the extent to which:

- Nurses deliver excellent patient outcomes.

- Nurses have a high level of job satisfaction with a resulting low nurse turnover rate.

- The facility has an appropriate grievance resolution process.

- Nurses are involved in data collection about and decision-making in patient care. Note: this emphasis reinforces positive collaborative relationships.

Magnet status – An award given by the American Nurses Credentialing Center to hospitals that satisfy factors that measure the strength and quality of nursing care.

ISO 9000 – An international standard used by participating organizations to help assure that they consistently deliver quality services and products.

- Managers value nurses, and improve their core values through empowerment, pride, mentoring, nurturing, respect, integrity, and teamwork.

- There is open communication between nurses and other healthcare team members to improve patient quality outcomes.

Magnet designation recognizes facilities with quality nursing programs which demonstrate the importance of nursing to the entire organization. It is viewed as one of the highest achievements a hospital can attain. Central Service personnel are involved with Magnet surveys in much the same way with Joint Commission surveys: critical areas impacting positive nursing and patient outcomes are surveyed to assess compliance with core goals.

International Standards Organization (ISO)

ISO 9000 is an international standard that companies use to ensure that their quality system is effective. This process is believed to guarantee that a company consistently delivers quality services and products. A company formally documents policies and procedures used to implement quality standards designed to ensure repeatable products or processes. Variables to this process (mistakes) are documented and analyzed to yield plans to modify the process to yield desired standards. Once these documents are in place and the process has been implemented, an outside agency examines the process and the documents to verify compliance. Note: while many healthcare organizations have subscribed to ISO standards, few Central Service departments have applied or qualified for ISO status.

QUALITY CENTRAL SERVICE PROCEDURES

Learning Objective 6. Review quality procedures in the Central Service Department

Focus on Central Service Technicians

Central Service personnel are expected to consistently attain desired quality standards as they undertake their normal responsibilities. While this is a difficult goal to attain, it is a necessary one. Central Service Technicians have a significant role to play in implementing quality within their facilities. They can, for example, consistently follow all of the instrument processing procedures discussed throughout this manual. They do not, however, work by themselves, and they are an integral part of the entire healthcare team. To assure the highest quality of patient care, all staff members must work together, and the sum of all contributions by all personnel in all departments represents the facility's accomplishments. All employees not just some employees must emphasize quality in all work assignments.

Quality in Central Service Processing Areas

There are many quality processes that all Central Service Technicians must consistently practice in their daily routine. Let's review some of these on a by-area basis within the department.

Decontamination Area

• Always wear personal protective equipment when working in this area to protect yourself and other staff and patients when you leave the area.

• Disassemble all items meant to be disassembled to assure that all instrument parts are accessible for cleaning.

• Measure chemicals properly. Improperly measured chemicals are not effective cleaners or disinfectants.

• Load and operate washers properly. Improperly loaded or operated washers cannot properly clean instruments.

• Follow all written procedures for cleaning and disinfecting items. Ensure that items are cleaned according to the manufacturer's recommendations.

• Clean as you were trained to do so. Do not take shortcuts or use items such as abrasives to best assure that items are cleaned without damage to the instrument.

• Check processing equipment before using to ensure that it is in proper working order. Equipment which is not working properly can cause harm to staff and patients.

Preparation and Packing Areas

• When using linen, always check for holes and lint even if linen is pre-delinted, because lint can cause infections in surgical patients.

• Check for holes in all wrappers and disposable filters to ensure that they are intact before sterilization. Normal handling can cause a small percentage of wrappers and filters to become damaged prior to use.

• Never use a wrapper, filter, or instrument that has fallen on the floor. If this occurs, instruments should be re-cleaned, and wrappers and filters should be discarded.

• Always follow count sheets. Even if you have extensive experience performing the assigned task, changes may have occurred to a par, case cart, or instrument count sheet. Remember that patient care personnel require the right supplies when they are needed.

• Check instruments for functionality, cleanliness, alignment, proper assembly, and sharpness. Failure to do so could result in patient harm.

Sterilization Area

• Always load sterilizer carts as trained. Improperly loaded carts can result in wet or non-sterile loads.

• Always verify mechanical and chemical indicators after a sterilization cycle to ensure that the process was properly completed.

• Do not touch sterilized items until cool.

• Properly complete all documentation including load and biological and implant logs.

Storage and Distribution Areas

- Always follow established pick sheets to ensure that all items are picked and delivered.

- Check product packaging for holes, expiration dating, and appropriate color changes.

- Carefully load items on carts, shelves and other storage units to ensure they stay intact.

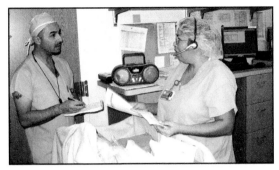

Figure 20.7

All Central Service/Distribution Areas

- Pay attention to what you are doing; do not talk and work at the same time. Excessive visiting or other distractions like a loud radio, can take your mind away from the task at hand and items could easily be missed or the wrong items could be placed on the tray or cart. (See **Figure 20.7**)

- Do not do anything that you have not been trained to do. Always inform someone when you have not been trained for a procedure that you have been requested to do.

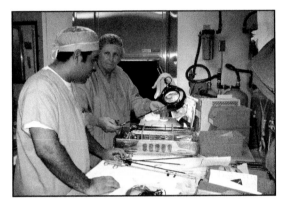

Figure 20.8

- If you are unsure about a completed project, ask someone to check your work. This is much better than to have an incomplete or wrong item leave the department. (See **Figure 20.8**)

- If distracted, check the entire project to ensure that it is done correctly.

- If you can't perform to a 100% level, don't do the project. Do not start a project if you know someone else will need to finish it.

- Re-check all work. The short time required to do so can eliminate an incident in a patient care area.

- Remember that neatness counts.

- Always help other staff members even if they don't think they need help.

- If you think something is wrong, speak-up.

- Report inoperative or damaged equipment.

- Attend all educational in-services, seminars, infection control, service technician, and vendor-sponsored programs that you can. The more education you can obtain, the better Central Service Technician you will become.

- Always follow the rules. They are in place for a reason (which usually is to protect you and other staff and the patients).

- Question anything about which you are unsure.

Remember that quality is the responsibility of every employee, and every employee must be involved, motivated, and knowledgeable if the Central Service Department is to consistently produce and deliver quality products and services.

ENDNOTES

1 . *The Joint Commission, Accreditation Manual for Hospitals, Oakbrook Terrace, IL, The Joint Commission, 2006*

REFERENCES

What is Quality Assurance: A definition. http:// whatis.com

Six Sigma: What is Six Sigma? http://isixsigma.com

Making Customers Feel Six Sigma Quality www.ge.com/sixsigma

Key Elements of Quality: Customer, Process and Employee www. ge.com/sixsigma

Senders, J. FMEA and RCA: The Mantras of Modern Risk Management. Magnet Status Fletcher Allen Health Care.

Benefits of Becoming a Magnet-Designated Facility. American Nurses Credentialing Center. Silver Spring, MD.

What is Magnet Status, and How's That Whole Thing Going? The Center for Nursing Advocacy. http://www.nursingadvocacy.org

CENTRAL SERVICE TERMS

Customer (internal)

Quality

Case cart

Empowerment

Process improvement

Defect

Quality control

Indicator

Acceptance sampling

Random numbers (table)

Technical quality control indicators

Failure mode and effects analysis (FMEA)

Root cause analysis (RCA)

Quality assurance

Process improvement

Total quality improvement (TQI)

Continuous quality improvement (CQI)

Processes (work)

Total quality management (TQM)

Six Sigma

Magnet Status

ISO 9000

Chapter 21

Safety

Chapter Outline

CHAPTER LEARNING OBJECTIVES:

As a result of successfully completing this chapter, readers will be able to:

1. Discuss common safety hazards applicable to Central Service functions and work areas, and explain how employee injuries can be prevented.

2. Describe special safety precautions for handling Ethylene Oxide.

3. Review procedures to report employee accidents and injuries.

4. Explain the importance of ergonomics and health awareness for Central Service Technicians.

5. Discuss procedures to prevent patient accidents and injuries and to report them if they occur.

6. Explain basic procedures which address three occupational hazards: fire, hazardous substances, and bloodborne pathogens.

7. Discuss the basics of internal and external disaster plans for a healthcare facility.

The concept of "safety" relates to freedom from danger, risk, or injury. Safety is something that most of us take for granted most of the time. In our personal lives, wise homeowners change the batteries in their smoke detectors, and concerned parents tell their children why they should not play with fire. It also makes sense to assure that our work areas are free from potential harm. Employee health and safety can never be compromised, and they are the responsibility of every healthcare employee, including all Central Service staff members and managers.

COMMON WORKPLACE SAFETY HAZARDS

Learning Objective 1. Discuss common safety hazards applicable to Central Service functions and work areas, and explain how employee injuries can be prevented.

The safety of healthcare employees continues to receive attention from administrators, unions and trade associations, insurance carriers, and state and federal agencies. Maintaining health and safety issues at the forefront of decision-making processes helps ensure that these concerns are integrated into day-to-day operations.

Central Service Technicians must be responsible for working safely after they are made aware of the hazards. Knowing about and paying close attention to existing and potential hazards in work areas within and outside of their immediate department can prevent most accidents. The belief that "it will never happen to me" is a false security that results in many injuries and exposures each year. Central Service personnel are among those considered at high risk and, therefore, they must be aware of potential hazards and work practices necessary to prevent injuries and accidents. In this section, we'll review hazards and safety precautions in each major area of the Central Service department.

Soiled Receiving and Decontamination Areas

Exposure to blood and other body fluids and harsh chemicals can cause injury, disease, and even death. These can be prevented by wearing personal protective equipment (PPE) including gloves,

head and foot covers, fluid resistant gowns or suits, masks, and eye goggles or face shields. (See **Figure 21.1**) It is the employer's responsibility to provide these items, but it is the employees' responsibility to protect themselves by consistently and correctly using them.

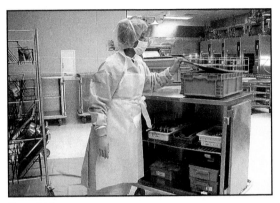

Figure 21.1

Mishandling contaminated **sharps** such as knife blades, needles, pins, and other sharp devices can break the skin's surface and produce puncture wounds, lacerations, and abrasions. These injuries can result in exposure to disease when pathogenic organisms such as those causing Hepatitis B enter the body through these skin breaks. Also, contact with sharp edges on storage units or shelves, workstations, tables or equipment can cause injuries.

If you are exposed to body fluids or chemicals or hurt by a sharp, immediately notify your supervisor, and obtain appropriate care as outlined in your department's or facility's policies.

Safety tips when working in soiled receiving and decontamination areas include:

- Never put your hands into a basin or container holding contaminated objects unless you can clearly see the objects in the basin or container. Instead, use a sponge stick to grasp the object or pour out any solution that prohibits visual examination, and then

Sharps – Cutting instruments including knives, scalpels, blades, needles, and scissors of all types.

remove objects from basins or containers one at a time. Do not grasp several objects at the same time. (See **Figure 21.2**) Ensure that sharp ends are away from any part of your or anyone else's body while transporting objects.

- Dispose of all disposable sharps such as needles and blades in the appropriate sharps container. (See **Figures 21.3** and **21.4**).

- Never put your hands into a trash container; instead, remove the inner bag, and pour its contents onto a surface, or use an instrument to sort through the contents. Be sure to wear the appropriate PPE.

- Use extreme caution when disarming scalpel blades. Never use your hands. Instead, use a needleholder or another tool to remove it, and wear eye protection glasses and appropriate PPE.

- When processing reusable sharps, separate them from other instruments, and position them in a way which avoids injury to anyone else who holds them correctly.

- Follow the manufacturer's recommendations for safe use of chemicals. Always wear recommended personal protective equipment to protect all skin surfaces and mucous membranes from chemical burns.

- Follow the manufacturer's recommendations for safe operation of cleaning and testing equipment.

- Use caution when approaching or walking in areas where water is used; inspect the floor for slippery surfaces. Utilize mats or non-skid footwear, where appropriate. (See **Figure 21.5**)

- When loading and unloading carts from dumbwaiters or elevators, check the weight on the cart. Ensure that the wheels are aligned straight, and that they will roll over door spaces or uneven edges. Unload some items to lighten the cart if it is too heavy to move easily.

- Sinks and other working surfaces should be at levels to afford easy access, and to reduce back and arm strain.

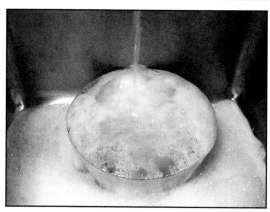

Figure 21.2

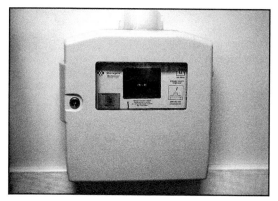

Figure 21.3

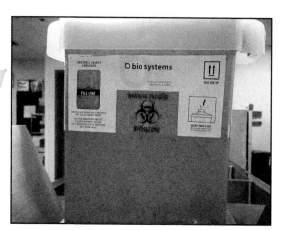

Figure 21.4

- When cleaning instruments in a sink, always scrub below the surface of the water to avoid the formation of **aerosols**. (See **Figure 21.6**)

- Use the concentration of detergents and water recommended by the manufacturer.

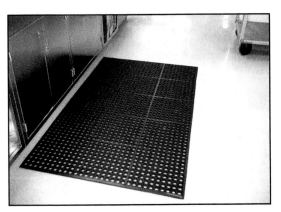

Figure 21.5

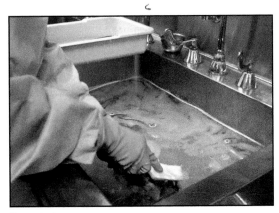

Figure 21.6

Sterile Preparation and Sterilization Areas

The Association for the Advancement of Medical Instrumentation states: "It is recommended that all personnel performing sterile processing activities be certified as a condition of employment."[1] This supports the concern that only those employees who are thoroughly trained in sterilization principles and the care and operation of the sterilization equipment should work in these areas. A well-monitored preventive maintenance program, along with an effective employee education and orientation process, is required to help ensure a safe working environment. Safe and efficient sterile preparation and sterilization areas also benefit patients by ensuring that medical devices are properly sterilized.

Injuries that can occur in sterile preparation and sterilization areas include burns to the skin and mucous membranes caused by misusing chemicals or from being too close to a heat source such as a steam sterilizer or a hot cart. Electrical burns from electric equipment can also result if safe handling precautions are not observed. Splashing chemicals is a common cause of eye injuries, so use of eye protection equipment is required.

Safety tips when working in sterile preparation and sterilization areas include:

• Use thermal insulated gloves when handling sterilizer carts, washer baskets, and other objects subjected to high temperatures.

• Move sterilizer carts to low/no traffic or other designated areas so co-workers will be less likely to come in contact with hot carts.

• Inspect all equipment for frayed electrical cords when servicing or placing them into storage or service. Immediately remove "problem" cords and/or equipment from service until required repairs are made.

• Use caution when using heat sealers. Do not put your fingers inside a sealer to free packaging materials. Ask for assistance and be sure to follow manufacturer's instructions.

• Be cautious when using a cutting edge to prepare paper-plastic packs.

• When lifting instrument sets, size up the load, and use the larger muscles in your legs and arms. Hold the item as close to your body as possible. Remember that one end may weigh more then the other and create a balance problem.

• Procedures for using, reading, recording, and disposing of biological sterilization indicators must be developed and consistently followed by all employees.

• Continuously check sterilizers for obvious damage to doors, door seals, hinges, and other

Aerosol – *A suspension of ultramicroscopic solid or liquid particles in air or gas; a spray.*

parts. If a damaged unit is observed, don't use it, and contact your supervisor about repair.

• Only authorized, experienced service personnel should access the control panels and inner parts of sterilization equipment to perform mechanical alterations and/or adjustments. If a question arises, the credentials of the person involved should be verified.

• Those who operate sterilizers should be trained and authorized to do so.

• Unauthorized hospital personnel, patients, or visitors should not enter a room or area containing sterilization equipment.

• Ensure that proper signs and labels are posted to warn of hot surfaces or other hazards.

Supply Receiving, Breakout, and Storage Areas

To ensure a safe and efficient supply receiving area, adequate storage space and traffic access must be available. Supply storage and shelving units must be secure and steady. Shelves should be arranged to facilitate maximum space efficiency, and to allow employees easy access to supplies. Heavy and bulky materials and cases of glass containers should be stored on lower shelves. Lighter, less frequently used items should be placed on higher shelves. Items used most frequently should be placed on middle shelves to enable them to be easily and safely accessed by employees.

Personnel should use appropriate equipment (for example steps, stands, and ladders) to safely reach upper shelves. Climbing on shelves is not acceptable. Procedures for the safe operation of dollies, hand trucks, and fork lifts or carts to handle bulk materials must be available, and employees must be trained to consistently comply with them. Staff must be provided with and taught how to use safe tools for opening and sealing cases and crates.

Closed trash containers should be available to properly dispose of unwanted materials. Containers for the appropriate storage of hazardous or

flammable materials must be readily available to avoid exposure to hazardous substances. For example, 100% Ethylene Oxide (EtO) canisters should be stored in a storage cabinet that is designed specifically for chemical storage. (See **Figure 21.7**) Employees working in this area must also follow proper procedures when disposing of and removing hazardous materials. Material safety data sheets (MSDSs) must be available for reference where these substances are used.

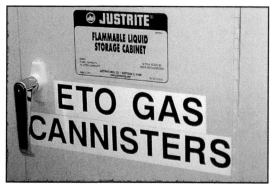

Figure 21.7

There are several types of hazards commonly found in the supply receiving and breakout areas. Employees must be aware of activities in loading docks at all times. For example, when supply trucks enter the loading dock area, the dock must be clear. Do not climb on or off trucks until they are secured. Climbing up and down or swinging from the dock area can result in strains, sprains, and broken bones. The use of proper body mechanics is always important. There are also hazards applicable to chemicals and solutions loaded onto and unloaded from trucks and from fumes generated by trucks and fork lifts.

Safety tips for supply receiving, breakout, and storage include:

• Use caution when removing items from storage units or shelves with sharp corners. Examine the workspace; allow time to perform the task, and assure that adequate space is available to maneuver the items being retrieved.

• When using a box-cutting tool, ensure that fingers and other body parts are not in the path of the blade; always cut away from the body or to the side. Retract the blade into the handle, or cover the blade with a sheath when the device is not in use.

• Open scalpel blades should not be used to open supply boxes or containers.

• Handle paper products with care; tiny skin lacerations can result from repetitive handling.

• Do not handle broken glass. Use a utensil to retrieve large pieces, and containerize them before placing the glass fragments in the appropriate container. Do not touch smaller pieces with your hands.

• Avoid twisting and jerking movements when picking up or removing objects from tight spaces.

• Inspect work areas for objects left in pathways or equipment with parts that protrude into a traffic path. Aisles and doorways must be kept clear at all times.

• When working in small areas, be aware of traffic patterns and the entrances where doors could be a hazard. Be sure doors are in view, or secure them while working in these areas.

Using signs to inform individuals to use caution when opening doors may also reduce injuries.

• Perform appropriate stretching exercises prior to work to avoid injuries to the back and other areas affected by lifting, pushing, and pulling motions.

Equipment Distribution and Central Transport Areas

Areas where supplies and equipment are stored awaiting requests from patient care areas can also be dangerous. There may be storage carts, cabinets, and equipment such as gurneys or wheel chairs used to transport patients in this area with substantial activity and often limited space to move about freely. Many items of patient care equipment require electrical charging, so multiple electrical outlets must be available. All portable electrical equipment including items used in Central Service and patient care areas must comply with applicable electrical codes. All plugs on all electrical equipment (installed or portable) must be three-wire and grounded, and all electrical outlets must accommodate these plugs. Inspecting electrical cords for frayed ends or bent prongs is a responsibility of Central Service Technicians who must be familiar with electrical safety practices to avoid burns or shocks.

Preventive Maintenance For Equipment

The Joint Commission and some State and local regulatory agencies require a preventive maintenance program to ensure optimal operation and function of equipment used for sterile processing functions. This equipment includes autoclaves, washer-decontaminators, and heat sealers which should be routinely inspected and serviced by certified, experienced service personnel with credentials to verify their expertise. Inspection records should be maintained with copies available in the Central Service department. They should be verified by the department head to ensure that the equipment used by Central Service employees is safe for use.

The federal Safe Medical Devices Act states that it is the healthcare facility's responsibility to report

malfunctions of medical devices causing injury and/or death to a patient. Each piece of patient care equipment must be tested prior to issuing. While the testing will not be detailed, it should, at least, indicate that, for example, a battery is fully charged. Verification that the equipment was processed by Central Service personnel should be part of routine record keeping.

Patient care equipment should be inspected by the Biomedical Engineering Department as specified by the manufacturer or internal risk management committee. Records of this inspection must be available and accessible. It is also necessary to use an equipment management system to verify and track equipment issued to each patient.

Adequate storage space should be provided, and shelving should be of adequate capacity and strength. Rugged, easily controlled carts should be provided for transferring supplies to the dispensing counter or mechanical conveyor. Rotation of supplies and recognition of manufacturers' expiration dates should be part of operating procedures in this station. Also, continuous inspection for imperfections in the condition and packaging of sterile supplies is necessary.

Safety tips when working in supply areas or when involved in equipment distribution and central transport activities include:

• When transporting supply carts, patients, or equipment ensure that the path in front and on each side of the transport equipment is visible.

• Ensure clearance on each side of the object being transported to avoid injury to arms or hands.

• Inspect floors for uneven surfaces or defective tiles or edges to ensure that equipment being transported will not be thrown off balance.

• Use caution when approaching automatic doors or elevators. Be aware of how the doors open and at what interval.

• Use caution when approaching corners or intersections of hallways; use safety mirrors whenever available.

• Use caution when pushing objects up or down hallway inclines. Push from behind when going up an incline (object goes first), and pull from in front of an object being transported down an incline (person goes first).

• Do not ride or step on wheeled supply carts or other vehicles.

• Consider the acquisition and use of powered carts for moving heavy or awkward loads.

Handling Compressed Gas Cylinders

Central Service Technicians are often involved in the handling, transport, and storage of medical gas cylinders dispensed for direct patient care and treatment or for use as equipment components. These cylinders may contain oxygen, nitrous oxide, helium, nitrogen, EtO, or other gasses. Specific safety protocols should be used for each specific gas, and should be in compliance with the product's handling instructions in the applicable MSDS.

Medical gas cylinder safety precautions include:

• No gas cylinder should be dispensed for use without a label.

• Gas cylinders should be secured at all times to prevent tipping by placing them in a secured holder for this purpose, or by securely strapping or chaining them in an upright position.

• Cylinders should be handled carefully during transport, and they should never be rolled, dragged, or dropped.

• A cover cap should be used to protect the cylinder's valve during transport.

• Cylinder regulators are gas-specific and not necessarily interchangeable, so an appropriate regulator for the cylinder's contents is required.

• Threads on cylinder valves, regulators, and other fittings should be inspected for damage before connection.

• All cylinders should be clearly labeled as full, in use, or empty.

• Empty cylinders should not be stored with full ones.

• Gas cylinder regulators are equipped with either a hand wheel or stem valve. Stem valves require a key that should remain with the regulator at all times. (See **Figure 21.8**)

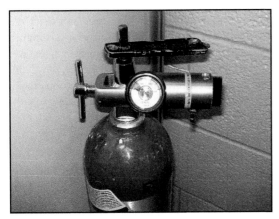

Figure 21.8

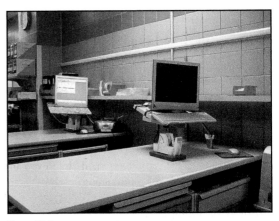

Figure 21.9

Clerical and Other Work Stations

Poor workstation design can create chronic physical conditions for Central Service personnel. Repetitive activities such as bending over sinks, sitting at a computer desk, and standing while assembling instrument sets should be evaluated in efforts to reduce unnecessary stress and strain. The term, "**ergonomics**," means finding ways to change work or working conditions to reduce employee stress, and will be discussed later in this chapter.

Safety tips in clerical or other work stations include:

• Assembly work should be performed at levels that will least fatigue and strain employees. (See **Figure 21.9**)

• Floors in work areas where employees must stand should have fatigue mats to relieve leg strain.

• Appropriate chairs should be used at computer, clerical, and instrument work stations to properly support the employees' backs.

• Computer glare screens should be used to reduce eyestrain.

Ergonomics – The process of changing work or working conditions to reduce employee stress.

• Items used frequently to perform routine tasks should be stored within easy reach to avoid strain to the upper body from repetitive movements to retrieve these items.

• Caution should be exercised when using filing cabinets. When the top drawers are open at the same time, the cabinet can tip over. Also, avoid leaving bottom drawers open when not in use because persons can trip or fall if they open into a walk way.

Surgical Service Areas

Central Service Technicians may have responsibilities that include services in surgery centers or other areas where surgeries are performed. They should become familiar with possible hazards in all areas they visit, and observe applicable safety policies and signage. These spaces have many of the same hazards found in Central Service areas. Additionally, they may have hazards applicable to the use of lasers, x-ray equipment, and chemicals utilized during surgical procedures. Caution is required when entering areas when this equipment is in use. Specific safety precautions provided by the manufacturers should be reviewed and followed by employees.

SPECIAL ETHYLENE OXIDE SAFETY PROCEDURES

Learning Objective 2. Describe special safety precautions for handling Ethylene Oxide.

The ethylene oxide (EtO) sterilization process presents specific hazards for potential EtO exposure in the workplace. In 1984, OSHA established a 1 ppm (in air) permissible exposure limit (PEL), and a 0.5 ppm action level (AL) for EtO. (AL is the concentration level of airborne EtO in or at breathing level.) The PEL and AL limits are expressed as an 8-hour time-weighted average (TWA). They represent the total allowable worker exposure during an 8-hour period, and express it as an average exposure during the period. If the facility can document that employee exposures are below the AL, it need not conduct routine monitoring or periodic medical examinations. If the monitored level is above the AL, the frequency of monitoring is dependent upon whether the measured level is above or below the PEL. The facility may be required to institute a medical surveillance program if specific exposure levels are exceeded. The employer may also be required to develop a written plan to reduce employee exposure to at or below the PEL using engineering and work practice controls. Employers should also have a written emergency plan to address spill response. Figure **21.10** is a sample procedure for an EtO spill response.

In 1988, OSHA amended its rule on occupational exposure to EtO by adding a 5-ppm short-term excursion limit (STEL) over a 15-minute period. The STEL is typically related to tasks such as transferring or handling non-aerated goods, performing sterilizer maintenance, changing gas cylinders, and unloading the EtO sterilizer where there is a potential for exposure to EtO. Monitoring may be discontinued if consecutive measurements taken seven or more days apart indicate exposure levels of less than 5 ppm. When the STEL is exceeded, a written plan must be developed to define actions that will reduce exposure to meet the standard.

To comply with the OSHA standard, employers must determine employee exposure to EtO using breathing zone air samples that are representative of 15-minute short term or the 8-hour TWA exposure levels. OSHA standards do not identify the specific type of monitoring devices required to comply with the standard, but they do define accuracy requirements which the monitoring methods must meet. Both personnel monitoring badges and environmental area monitoring can be employed to comply with the standard.

Let's Review Terms:
OSHA – EtO – PEL – TWA – AL – STEL

[handwritten note: ppm unit of measure]

The Occupational Safety and Health Administration (OSHA) has established several limits on occupational exposure to Ethylene Oxide (EtO). A permissible exposure limit (PEL) is the average concentration of a chemical in the air to which a worker can be legally exposed over a particular period of time (usually eight hours). The PEL for ethylene oxide is 1 part per million (ppm) as an eight-hour time-weighted average (TWA). An action level (AL) is the concentration level of airborne EtO in or at breathing level. Note: it is 0.5 ppm. A short-term excursion limit (STEL) is the maximum concentration of an airborne chemical to which a worker may be exposed over a 15-minute period. OSHA has adopted a STEL of 5 ppm for EtO.

There are several areas where employee exposure to EtO is possible. These include the front of the sterilizer by the door, the rear of the sterilizer by the drains, near emission control devices, and at the tank changing area. Exposure can also result from leakage of an EtO cylinder or connection. Direct contact with this wet, cold liquid or inhalation of the vapor can cause burning of the eyes, a burning sensation in the throat, and skin redness and irritation.

EtO gas sterilizers and aerators must be installed and operated with proper exhaust venting to the building's exterior. Ducts and vents must be directed away from occupied spaces, and they must also be labeled to warn and protect individuals in those areas.

Figure 21.10 Sample Procedure for an EtO Spill Response*

HIGH LEVEL RESPONSE — AUDIBLE HORN AND RED STROBE LIGHT

Upon noticing an audible horn coupled with a visual red strobe light which indicates a HIGH LEVEL exposure of 5.0 ppm or greater:

Proceed to the Ethylene Oxide Monitor's main panel.

Remove clipboard from hook on wall, fill in the appropriate data, and answer all questions.

Identify what color light is flashing on top of main panel (a red light should be flashing), and at what point this is occurring. Point #1 and Point #2 are the EtO sterilization room, and Point #3 is the mechanical access area behind the sterilizers.

Stand in front of the main panel and document the environmental levels for the three monitoring points in the appropriate space provided. Record the levels at the indicated intervals. For example, if the time you first discovered the light was at 13:00, the next reading would be done in 15 minutes (13:15); the next reading would be taken at 13:30, etc. After the first hour, readings are taken every thirty (30) minutes. After the third hour, readings are taken at one hour intervals up to a total of eight hours.

Once the initial time is recorded answer the following questions on the response sheet.

ALL EMPLOYEES ARE TO EVACUATE THE DEPARTMENT IF LEVELS AT POINT #1 AND #2 ARE ABOVE 5.0 PPM AND INITIATE CCF'S CHEMICAL SPILL PROCEDURE AND WAIT FOR FURTHER INSTRUCTIONS. ASSEMBLE IN THE MAIN CORRIDOR.

NO EMPLOYEE IS TO RE-ENTER THE WORK AREA UNTIL LEVELS HAVE BEEN DETERMINED ACCEPTABLE BY THE SPD COORDINATOR, SAFETY MANAGER OR CLEVELAND FIRE DEPARTMENT.

Upon completing the questions, you are to contact your shift coordinator or on-call coordinator. Schedule and pager numbers are posted on back of the clipboard. If the on-call coordinator does not return your call, attempt to call another coordinator or the department head. Continue to document levels. Only at the coordinator's discretion can documentation be stopped.

Evacuate department personnel and close off the area to prevent spread of EtO. All department personnel are to meet in the main corridor outside the department manager's office in the E-building or the ramp outside SPD in the M-building.

Contact the control desk in the Operating Room to advise of potential delays with processing, and that you will keep them posted. THIS WILL NOT INITIALLY INVOLVE CANCELLATION OF SURGERY. THIS WILL BE DECIDED BETWEEN THE DIRECTOR OF SURGERY AND DEPARTMENT MANAGER ONLY.

Call the department shift coordinator/manager and Director of Safety. Have department blueprints available to designate problem area (laminated to back of clipboard).

Only trained personnel with self-contained breathing apparatus will shut off EtO at spill site. Carefully document spill and personnel involved on an Incident Report. Attach a copy of the EtO Spill Response, and turn it into the Safety Director.

Exhaust System Failure (not tied into maintenance system) visual and audible signals are located outside EtO sterilization room.

In the event of failure:

1. Immediately notify Maintenance/Powerhouse at ext. xxxx.
2. Request that someone check EtO exhaust fan: #B-1 in the E-building or #EF-2 in the M-building.
3. When the problem is repaired, notify the shift coordinator or the on-call coordinator.

Courtesy of Cleveland Clinic Foundation, Cleveland, Ohio

Reducing Exposure to EtO

Today, healthcare facilities routinely use passive dosimeter badges (See **Figure 21.11**) to measure employee exposure levels to EtO, and to document compliance with OSHA standards. Efforts continue to further improve worker safety because legal concerns emphasize reducing exposure to levels "as low as reasonably achievable." In fact, one of the driving forces to convert to alternative methods of sterilization such as gas plasma is the desire to minimize safety risks, and to maximize compliance with OSHA standards.

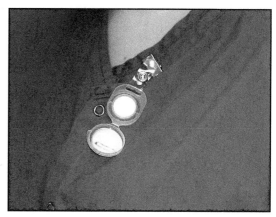

Figure 21.11

Today, most EtO sterilizers perform in-chamber aeration. However, a further reduction in exposure such as during load transfer and from within-device residual EtO levels is desired. These goals continue to encourage the development and validation of faster and more efficient methods of degassing EtO sterilized supplies.

Voluntary or mandated enforcement of low real-time exposure levels encourages the development and installation of more sophisticated environmental monitoring devices and/or real-time personnel monitors.

While environmental and air quality regulations differ between states, most require that EtO exhaust be vented into an emission control device to prevent the gas from entering the atmosphere. These devices are designed to capture the exhaust including that which may go into the drain. Since EtO is recognized as a hazardous chemical, Central Service personnel must comply with all applicable state and local environmental and safety regulations. The employer is required to have environmental surveys performed in the Central Service department to ensure that employees are not being exposed to EtO while working there.

Other safety precautions when working with EtO equipment include:

• When transferring sterilized items to aeration cabinets, employees should wear gloves made of neoprene or another appropriate protective material. They should not hold items close to their bodies nor inhale in the zone close to the items.

• When transporting a cart from the sterilizer to the aerator, pull it instead of pushing it to avoid inhaling EtO fumes.

• Employees should avoid working in areas immediately adjacent to the EtO sterilizer during its cycle. When possible, separate general work areas from those where EtO sterilizers are located. This concept should be incorporated into renovation or new space designs.

• Healthcare facilities using EtO must have an operational, dedicated ventilation system to remove fumes exhausted during the cycle. This exhaust system should be checked regularly to ensure that any fumes in the employees' breathing zone are captured. It is also necessary to have an audible and visual alarm that will sound in case of any malfunction.

• Ensure compliance with all federal, state, and local air quality and worker safety regulations relating to employee safety, discharge, air monitoring, and recordkeeping.

• With some older sterilizers, the door of the chamber must be opened six inches after the cycle is completed, and the sterilizer is turned off. The contents are then allowed to remain in the chamber for fifteen minutes.

During this time, the area close to the sterilizer should be cleared. Note: as older sterilizers are replaced, this step will no longer be required.

- After items have been placed in an aeration cycle or cabinet, the cycle should not be interrupted to retrieve items. It is important to develop and follow a policy that no item will be removed from the aerator until it is thoroughly aerated according to the equipment manufacturer's recommendations. The Safety and Risk Management departments should approve this policy. All procedures should be based on manufacturers' recommendations for specific aeration times for reusable medical devices and patient/employee safety precautions.

- Do not mix loads in the aerator. Don't add newly sterilized items to an aerator that already has items in a current aeration process.

- The exposure of any person to EtO must be reported immediately to the health nurse, emergency department, or employee health service for evaluation.

- Observe "Out of Order" or electrical lock-out signage to prevent injuries or exposures to Central Service or other staff.

REPORTING EMPLOYEE ACCIDENTS AND INJURIES

Learning Objective 3. Review procedures to report employee accidents and injuries.

Even significant efforts to emphasize safety and accident prevention cannot eliminate all employee accidents, and Central Service Technicians can still be injured on the job. If an injury occurs, it must be documented and reported to the appropriate

Work-related musculoskeletal disorder (WMSD) – An injury to or disorder of the musculoskeletal system where exposure to workplace risk factors may have contributed to the disorder's development or aggravated a pre-existing condition.

administrative personnel, in compliance with OSHA regulations for healthcare facilities. An investigation is needed to provide information about the cause, the situation, and/or the behaviors that were involved to identify contributing factors, hazards, or unsafe practices. Then, corrective actions must be implemented to revise the systems or physical conditions, and/or to address the behavior which caused the injury in efforts to prevent future injuries or accidents.

No matter how insignificant an injury seems, the appropriate supervisor, manager, or director should be informed immediately. Details regarding time, place, tasks being performed, and a description of exactly what happened must be properly recorded on the appropriate form. It should then be submitted to the facility's safety officer, personnel department, employee health or other administrators, and risk management personnel must always be informed of potential problems. **Figure 21.12** (Initial Employee's Report of Injury) shows a sample notification form.

All ABOUT ERGONOMICS

Learning Objective 4. Explain the importance of ergonomics and health awareness for Central Service Technicians.

An effective ergonomics program includes a job safety analysis to ensure that the equipment and tools required for a specific job are appropriate for the worker and will not cause or contribute to an ergonomic-related injury. The primary goal is to reduce **work-related musculoskeletal disorders (WMSDs)** by adapting the work to fit the employee rather than by forcing the staff member to adapt to the workstation, equipment, or tools. Persons who perform repetitive or physical work including Central Service Technicians are most at risk for ergonomic injuries.

Ergonomic stressors that employees may encounter include:

- Force – Such as heavy lifting or manipulating equipment or tools.

Please complete this form within 24 hours and send immediately to Safety Director.

EMPLOYEE'S STATEMENT (Every question must be answered fully)

Last Name	First Name	Middle	Employee No.

Date of Accident: Time: ☐ am ☐ pm		Job Title of Employee:
Exact Location Where Injury Occurred Be Specified e.g., 3-W, X-ray, etc.		Supervisor Name and Ext.
Part of Body Injured:		Department of Employee and Ext.

What was Employee doing when injured? Please be specific: identify tools, equipment or material the employee was using, and describe in full the event that caused the injury.

_____

_____

_____

Could You Have Prevented Your Injury?   Yes ☐   No ☐

_____ / _____

                   Employee's Signature   Date

SUPERVISOR'S INVESTIGATION OF CAUSE OF ACCIDENT (To be filled out by immediate supervisor)
What was employee doing when accident occurred? _____

Describe in full how the accident happened _____

_____

What machine, tool, substance, or object was most closely connected with the accident? _____

What does the supervisor recommend for preventing a recurrence of this injury? Be specific; almost every accident can be prevented. To not say "Unavoidable" or "Be more careful." _____

_____

What has the supervisor done to prevent recurrence? _____

Has employee returned to work? _____ If yes, give date _____ If not, was employee paid for date of injury? _____
List names and addresses of witnesses. _____

Was another person responsible? _____ (If yes, give names, address, liability carrier, names and addresses of witnesses, and details on reverse side.)

Nature of injury and part of body affected _____
Did employee go to Employee Health? _____ Emergency Department Physician? _____

_____ / _____

                   Supervisor's Signature   Date

Investigation Warranted/Not Warranted _____
Completed Document _____

_____

_____ / _____

                   Safety Director's Signature   Date

Figure 21.12 Initial Employee's Report of Injury

• Repetition – Using the same motion or series of motions continually or frequently.

• Awkward Positions – Assuming positions that place stress on the body such as reaching or twisting the body while lifting.

• Vibration – Rapid oscillation of the body or a body part.

• Contact Stress – Pressing the body or a body part against a hard or sharp edge.[2]

Exposure to these stressors can cause numerous problems including ligament sprains, joint and tendon inflammation, pinched nerves, herniated spinal discs, and other WMSDs. These problems may develop gradually (such as from word processing), or from a single event (such as from improperly lifting a heavy object), and the injuries can cause pain, loss of work, and disability.

The number and severity of WMSDs can be reduced if the work environment and work practices are effectively adjusted. To do this:

• Management commitment and employee participation are required. This forms the foundation for ergonomic improvements because a sustained effort, allocation of resources, and frequent follow-up is needed. Staff member "buy in" to equipment and work procedure changes is of special importance.

• Training is needed. Training can help employees (a) recognize the signs and symptoms of WMSDs so they can respond to them, (b) report potential problems, (c) recognize jobs/tasks that have ergonomic stressors, and (d) know how to control them.

• Evaluation is necessary. The effectiveness of training programs must be assessed. Appropriate evaluation requires leading indicators (which identify events that prevent accidents and injuries) and trailing indicators (which measure historical results).

Employees should also lead a lifestyle appropriate to and maintain their personal health and fitness

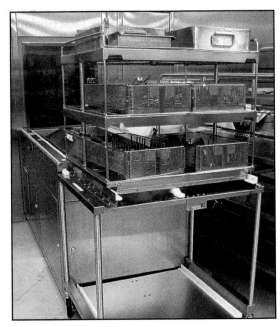

Figure 21.13

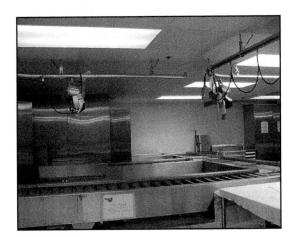

Figure 21.14

in a manner consistent with the physical demands of their work to help minimize the potential for injuries.

A process of work site analysis can help to identify conditions and aspects of work activities that increase risks to employees. It will also help to assure that corrective actions that are implemented will address the problems creating the hazard. Note: **Figures 21.13** and **21.14** show transport carts and overhead lift systems that can be used to move heavy instrument sets.

Loading Washer Racks: Task Description

Carts are brought to surgical processing carrying trays of surgical tools. The trays are on shelves either 9 or 24 inches high. The trays are lifted off the carts, and placed on washer racks with shelves at about 34, 42, and 50 inches. The trays weigh 10 to 16 pounds each; there are 2 to 3 trays per case; about 200 cases are moved each day by 4 people. Therefore, the typical worker in this job will lift about 125 trays per day (an average rate of about 1 tray every 4 minutes).

Evaluation

The following data is used to determine whether the lifting task is likely to lead to injury.

Horizontal reach	18 inches
Pick-up height	9 inches (worst case)
Vertical distance moved	41 inches (placed at shoulder height)
Trunk twist	0 degrees (assume good body mechanics)
Grip	Good
Frequency	1 every 5 minutes
Duration	8 hours

Based on the 1991 National Institute for Occupational Safety and Health (NIOSH) guidelines, 90% of the population can safely lift 17 pounds under these lifting conditions. Since this is greater than the actual lift, this task does not present a significant risk of injury.

Figure 21.15 Sample Ergonomic Evaluation

Work site analysis also examines the duration, frequency, and magnitude of ergonomic stressors to assess whether employees are subject to potential injury. Potential stressors are frequently apparent when the job is observed. Unfortunately, at other times the causes of pain or injury are not easily identified. For example, a Central Service Technician may be observed correctly lifting a rigid container full of sterilized instruments. However, an observer might not realize that this task must be repeated many times during the work shift, and its repetition causes WMSD.

Those conducting work site analyses typically observe the job and discuss job tasks with employees. Employee questionnaires can be used to identify whether there is a pattern of ergonomic-related injuries in selected jobs or with certain work tasks. Information can also be obtained from other facilities to determine the problems being experienced, and to compare them to problems in one's own facility. Note: **Figure 21.15** shows a report developed as a result of work site analysis.

PREVENTING AND REPORTING PATIENT INJURIES

Learning Objective 5. Discuss procedures to prevent patient accidents and injuries and to report them if they occur.

Central Service personnel have responsibilities to help prevent patient injuries, accidents, and infections. They do so as they perform the important tasks of decontaminating, disinfecting, inspecting, testing, assembling, packaging, sterilizing, and aseptic handling of sterile items according to established procedures. When their job is done correctly, the chance of a patient being injured or involved in an accident is greatly reduced. A check and balance system is needed to ensure that these important functions are always done correctly. For example, sterilizers must be inspected while they are in use. They must be monitored by testing with a biological challenge test, and the results must be recorded.

Patient Care Equipment

Patients receiving equipment that has not been tested for proper operation and function before being used can be subjected to complications from malfunctioning equipment or delayed treatment.

Safety tips include:

- Test and document all patient care equipment before it leaves the department according to the manufacturer's guidelines and departmental procedures.

- Ensure that all equipment has been decontaminated, and is free from any soil, damage, defects, or hazards that could affect the use of the equipment (for example, frayed electrical cords, sharp appendages, and bent parts).

- Be sure that the equipment is identified and controlled by a tracking system. A usage history for each piece of equipment is helpful in legal situations where the responsibility of the healthcare facility is being challenged.

- Perform regularly scheduled preventive maintenance on patient equipment. Since the Central Service department can be held accountable for this under Joint Commision standards, records about equipment use and maintenance should be retained, and made available upon request.

- Ensure that the facility's biomedical engineering department assists with equipment acceptance and regular testing programs.

- Assure that safety guards are placed over items such as heat lamps and heat cradles to ensure that parts are not broken during transport.

- Always cover contaminated equipment being transported to Central Service areas to prevent cross-contamination throughout the healthcare facility. Covering cleaned equipment in storage or awaiting transport is recommended to reduce the risk of contamination while the equipment is waiting for distribution.

Contaminated Supplies and Reusable Medical Devices

Contaminated supplies, equipment, and unsterile reusable medical devices are a hazard to patients undergoing surgical procedures or treatment because nosocomial infections can result. Also, complications resulting from delays in surgical procedures can occur when items are not properly reprocessed and must be flash sterilized.

Safety tips include the need to ensure that:

- All items are thoroughly disassembled, cleaned, inspected, reassembled, prepared for sterilization, packaged appropriately, sterilized, and aseptically handled and stored.

- All equipment used to perform any sterile processing function is tested and operates properly.

- All personnel responsible for equipment operation can demonstrate appropriate techniques for its care and operation. (Document applicable training.)

- All instrument components are complete, and all instrument parts are functioning properly. (Document the inspections.)

- All sterilization equipment is visually monitored by inspecting throughout the cycle, and mechanically monitored by review of the mechanical printouts. Also, biological and chemical indicators, and/or air detection tests should be utilized.

Chemical Residues

Patients coming in contact with items having chemical residues can receive chemical burns or other complications from these chemicals.

Safety tips include:

- All items sterilized with EtO must be fully aerated to ensure that no EtO residue or by-products are introduced into patients during surgical procedures.

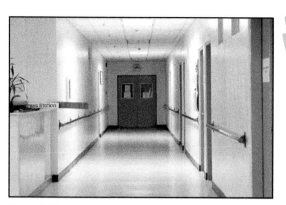

Figure 21.16

- Items to be sterilized in EtO must be dry to avoid ineffective sterilization.

- All items soaked in gluteraldehyde or other chemicals for disinfection must be fully rinsed to ensure that no residues or by-products are transferred to patients during surgical procedures.

Supply and Equipment Transport

Often there is frequent traffic including food service and supply carts and patient transportation devices such as gurneys and wheelchairs in many patient care areas. There may be hallways, corners, and elevators that present hazards if proper techniques are not used by employees transporting patients and other items.

Safety tips include:

- Use caution when approaching doorways, hallways, elevators, and high-traffic areas.

- Do not use a transport vehicle to push or prop open automatic doors.

- Carts and mobile equipment should not be parked in hallways where it may block traffic or door access. Always keep hallways clear for the free flow of traffic. (See **Figure 21.16**)

Patient Accident and Injury Reporting Procedures

Whenever a patient accident or injury occurs, it must be investigated, and a record of the incident is necessary. Any practices or physical conditions within the facility that can cause a patient accident or injury must also be investigated and reported. All healthcare workers must report unsafe practices or hazards that could affect patients or employees to minimize accidents and to prevent their recurrence.

If a sterilization process malfunctions, all items in any loads thought to be unsterile must be recalled, and should be quarantined until biological and chemical indicators are read. Central Service departments must have a procedure to recall sterile items, and basic components should include:

- Obtain a list of all supplies known to be in the load that are suspect.

- Verify the sterilization controls.

- Notify the Central Service supervisor, manager, or director.

- Notify areas throughout the healthcare facility where any supplies known to be unsterile could be stored.

- Retrieve as many items as possible on the list.

- Notify the Infection Control and Operating Room supervisor or coordinator and administrative departments according to policy.

- Notify physicians if items known to be unsterile were used in any surgical procedures they performed.

- Document all steps taken.

- Notify Risk Management personnel about any possibility that unsterile equipment was used on a patient.

- Ensure that qualified service personnel inspect any malfunctioning sterilization equipment, that a comprehensive report is generated, and that a biological run is performed before the next use. Consult AAMI ST79 for guidelines for sterilizer testing.

If the recall is a result of a malfunctioning sterilizer, ensure that it is taken out of service.

CENTRAL SERVICE OCCUPATIONAL HAZARDS

Learning Objective 6. Explain basic procedures which address three occupational hazards: fire, hazardous substances, and bloodborne pathogens.

Occupational hazards relate to the potential for injury caused by something in the workplace environment. The three categories of hazards are physical (including fire), chemical (relating to hazardous substances), and biological (including infectious waste and blood-borne diseases). Each of these important occupational hazards for Central Service Technicians will be discussed in this section. (See **Figure 21.17**)

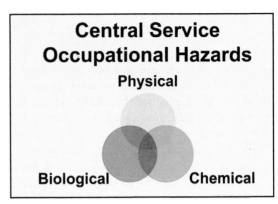

Figure 21.17

Fire Safety Programs

Fire is an oxidation-reduction chemical reaction. Fire requires three elements to be present at the same place and at the same time, and these elements make up the "Fire Triangle" (**Figure 21.18**):

- A **combustible** or flammable substance.

- A source of oxygen.

- A source of ignition.

To prevent fires, at least one of the elements in this triangle must be eliminated.

Risk Management and Central Service

Risk management involves methods used to assess the risks of a specific activity, and to develop a program to reduce losses from exposure to them. It also involves injury prevention and claims management: the settlement, defense, and prevention of claims and lawsuits.

Risk management originated in the insurance industry as the result of the increased number of medical malpractice suits that have cost healthcare facilities billions of dollars over the past quarter century. Healthcare personnel must effectively manage injury prevention and the reporting of accidents that involve patients and employees. Various authorities, including The Joint Commission, have mandated that healthcare facilities develop and implement procedures to ensure that the care which is rendered meets minimal standards.

A risk management program is closely related to and is an integral part of a facility's quality assurance program with one major difference: risk management includes claim management. It relates to the prevention of accidents and/or injuries, and ensures the accurate reporting and follow-up needed to assist in preventing similar incidents.

After a situation is examined and hazards or unsafe practices have been discovered, risk management personnel assure that corrective actions are taken to improve systems, behavior, and/or the physical conditions to help prevent employee and patient accidents and injuries.

Fire and Explosions

A fire occurs when the temperature of a flammable or combustible substance is raised high enough for the individual carbon and hydrogen atoms to combine with oxygen, and the resulting energy is released. If the material is a solid, it will burn only at its surface. In contrast, if the material is a volatile liquid such as alcohol which readily vaporizes or a gas such as ethylene oxide, the burning or flame front passes quickly through the substance. The result is an explosion accompanied by the instantaneous generation of large quantities of heated gases. Their rapid expansion creates a very loud pressure wave that can cause great damage

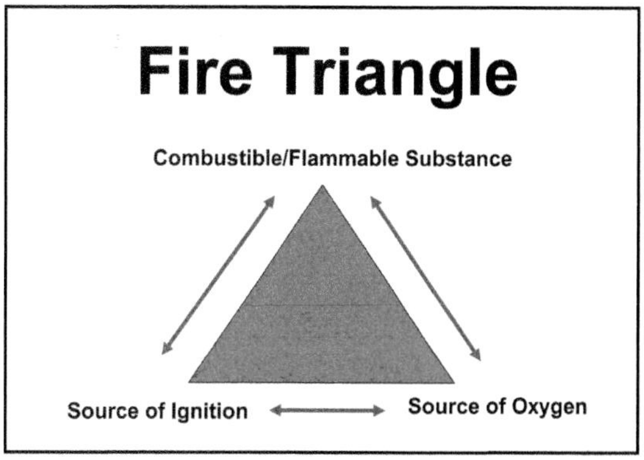

Fire Triangle

Combustible/Flammable Substance

Source of Ignition ←→ Source of Oxygen

Figure 21.18

Combustible loading is the weight of combustible materials per square foot of area in which those materials are located.

Disposable materials including surgical drapes, gowns, caps, masks, shoe covers, tubing, bed pans, syringes, and their packaging contribute to heavy combustible loads in hospitals. This problem occurs principally in central storage areas such as Central Service, operating and delivery suites, nursing units, and trash handling facilities.

The presence of large volumes of combustible materials and flammable substances in close proximity to nonambulatory patients poses unique risks. The large combustible loading created by single-use items and their wrappings in storage and as trash is especially dangerous. When these materials burn, large quantities of highly toxic smoke are produced. Even with hospital compartmentalization features that limit the spread

of smoke and fire, a high-risk situation occurs. Evacuation of bedridden patients is generally impractical or impossible. Therefore, healthcare fire safety programs must include the following:

- Minimization of the combustible load.
- Fire response plans.
- Early detection.
- Removal of persons in danger.
- Containment of the fire and combustible products.
- Extinguishment.
- Evacuation.

Minimize combustible loads

It is important to minimize the volume of combustible substances because a prime rule of fire protection is: "Don't give fire a place to start." Tactics to minimize combustible loads include:

- Minimize use of disposable items. Conduct a cost analysis study before switching to single-use items.

- Assure that single-use items are safely stored by keeping them in areas with the proper temperature and humidity. (The fire-resistant properties of some operating room drapes, gowns, and similar fabrics are reduced by high temperature and low humidity). Use dedicated storage locations which are adequately compartmented from the rest of the building, and equipped with fire detection, alarm and suppression devices.

Risk Management – *The methods used to assess the risks of a specific activity, and to develop a program to reduce losses from exposure to those risks.*

Combustible – *A substance that, if ignited, will react with oxygen and burn.*

Combustible loading – *The weight of combustible materials per square foot of area in which those materials are located.*

• Minimize the volume of combustible substances even when adequate storage facilities are available. Consider purchase systems in which the supplier retains possession of, but not title to, items until actually needed.

• Minimize trash build-up. Each facility must have an adequate trash handling program which includes covered trash containers of noncombustible construction and adequate volume at each site of trash generation. Regular pickup from these containers for transfer to a central trash collection facility is required as is a disposal program which addresses environmental protection concerns.

More About Combustible Materials Storage Areas

Areas where combustible supplies are stored must be separated from other parts of the hospital with fire-rated walls and doors that comply with fire, life safety, and building codes. Openings or penetrations in fire and smoke barriers above the ceiling must be sealed.

Doors should be equipped with automatic closers. If traffic into the storage area is heavy, the door may be equipped with an automatic hold-open device that will release the door, and allow it to close and latch when the fire alarm is activated by a smoke detector. The use of wedges to prop open doors should not be permitted.

Develop Fire Response Plan

Every healthcare facility requires a comprehensive fire response plan, and each staff member in every department must know his/her specific role in these plans. The fire safety emphasis should begin at the time of new employee orientation, and should continue with on-going training. In addition, staff must actively participate in routine fire drills in all areas in which they routinely work. A training program should include at least the topics listed in **Figure 21.19**.

Many facilities use the term, "R-A-C-E" to help staff recall appropriate fire response procedures.

Figure 21.19 Elements in a Comprehensive Program

A. Life Safety Systems Testing

B. Training
- All staff.
- Fire response personnel.
- Department specific responsibilities.
- High hazard areas (storage areas, kitchens, labs, oxygen-enriched environments).

C. Fire Response Activities

D. Drills (per Joint Comission and other regulatory agency requirements)

E. Materials Storage
- Combustible load considerations.
- Non-interference with fire detection, alarm, and suppression systems.
- Trash collecting, handling, disposal.

F. Inspections
- Routine.
- High hazard areas.

G. Construction Safety
- Inspections
- Contractors
- Hot work (welding)

H. Evacuations
- Central Service role to equip and supply alternate care sites.

I. Alarms
- Central Service employees' role in the department.
- Central Service employees' role when in other departments.

J. Suppression

K. High Hazard Areas

L. Regulatory Compliance

M. Minimize Sources of Ignition
- Electricity.
- Equipment.
- Smoking.

R Remove persons in danger.

A Alarm. Call 911 and activate alarms.

C Contain the fire. Close doors in the area.

E Extinguish the fire only if safe or Evacuate the area horizontally or vertically.

Note: even though R-A-C-E is presented in sequential steps, ideally many staff members are implementing these steps simultaneously.

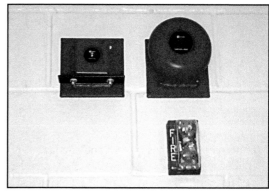

Figure 21.20

Early Detection

Early detection requires use of ionization smoke detectors in areas where combustible materials are stored. These smoke detectors should be connected to the facility's fire alarm system. As an added precaution, sprinkler protection with water flow indicators connected to the same alarm system may be installed. Infrared smoke detectors and sprinklers may, in accordance with fire codes, be required in patient care areas. Staff should be knowledgeable about the fire and life safety systems serving the buildings in which they work.

Notifying persons about fires involves activating alarm stations, calling emergency (911) fire response personnel and facility personnel identified in the fire response plan, and alerting others in the vicinity.

Activating alarm stations will trigger audible and visual alarms that notify occupants that there is a potential fire. (See **Figure 21.20**) In many facilities, alarm activation alerts persons at a central monitoring station who then initiate a fire response team and call the local fire department.

Co-workers in the immediate area should also be notified so they can implement fire response procedures that include securing the safety of patients, possible fire suppression, and identifying the source of the fire, smoke, or smell.

Removal of Persons in Immediate Danger

Everyone must be removed from the immediately dangerous fire or smoke area. This allows employees to help patients, visitors, and co-workers. Note: patients should only be moved if they are at imminent risk from fire or smoke.

Containment

Staff should know whether the buildings where they work are constructed with compartmentalization features that allow a "defend-in-place" strategy for protecting themselves and patients, or whether patients must be evacuated during a fire.

Upon evidence of a confirmed, or notification of a possible fire, doors in the area should be closed to prevent smoke migration and the spread of fire. Special fire doors may close automatically when smoke is detected, or when the alarm is activated; however, it is still necessary to ensure that these doors have closed and latched properly. Responding fire response personnel and the fire department must be informed of the locations of patients still in their rooms.

Extinguishment

Some patients can be evacuated quickly and safely. However, many (for example, those who are immediately post-operative) are difficult to evacuate. Still others such as those in intensive care may not be able to be evacuated without direct threat to their lives. Therefore, fires must be extinguished as quickly as possible.

Fire extinguishers appropriate to the hazard that is present (paper, wood, fabric, electrical, elastic, flammable liquids), must be properly placed

Figure 21.21 Use of Portable Fire Extinguishers

Burning Material	Type of Fire[1]	EXTINGUISING AGENT			
		Water2	Carbon Dioxide	Ammonium Phospate[3]	Halon 1211
Paper, wood, cloth, plastic	A	*	*4	*	*4
Flammable liquid	B		*	*	*
Energized electrical equipment	C		*	*	*
Computer equipment	C				*

1 Each extinguisher listed by Underwriters Laboratories is prominently labeled (has the UL seal) for the type of fire on which it will be effective. Personnel should acquaint themselves with the labeling of extinguishers available in Central Service.

2 Once the electrical equipment is de-energized, water may be used.

3 Ammonium phosphate is the most effective form of dry chemical extinguishing agent currently available.

4 Carbon dioxide and Halon 1211 will suppress, but may not completely extinguish, a fire involving ordinary combustible substances.

throughout the facility to ensure quick and easy access. (See **Figure 21.21**)

Evacuation

Patient evacuations involve the coordinated efforts of many people. Communication is critical to ensure that it is effective and efficient. Staff must be familiar with the different types of evacuations, when each is appropriate, and their specific roles to assist with them.

In most fire situations, horizontal evacuation from a threatened area to a non-threatened area should provide adequate safety for patients and staff. Adequate compartmentalization, use of smoke-stopping doors, and a proper ventilation system should contain fire-generated smoke, and prevent fire from spreading into patient care areas. Unfortunately, these tactics may not keep combustible products out of all patient care areas. Therefore, a fire response strategy should include plans for fire events in numerous areas, and all employees, including Central Service personnel, should be well-versed about these plans. For example, egress corridors and other evacuation routes must be kept clear of equipment, supplies, and other clutter that may impede an evacuation. Central Service staff

are usually important participants in a facility's corridor clearance program.

For buildings without compartments, patients must be moved horizontally beyond a set of fire doors, vertically to another floor, or completely out of the building, according to the facility's fire response plan.

Hospital buildings should only be evacuated when it is unsafe to remain in the structure. Usually all available staff are engaged in moving the patients or preparing the alternate care site to receive patients. Central Service staff would normally transport necessary patient medical supplies, including disaster medical supply caches, to a designated site. In addition, they must help to ensure that critical medical supplies are available for longer-duration evacuations.

Hazardous Substances

Central Service managers must develop a hazardous materials management program to best ensure the health and safety of employees, as is required by state and federal regulations and Joint Commission requirements.

Information about chemicals and substances classified as hazardous must be available to all employees. OSHA "Employee Right to Know" regulations mandate that a comprehensive hazard communication program be in place to help ensure that employees know about hazards around them. Components of an effective departmental hazardous substance management program include container-labeling requirements, use of MSDSs, employee information and training, procedures to manage and handle hazardous substances, employee monitoring, and hazardous waste management.

Container Labeling

No container of hazardous substances should be released for use unless it is clearly labeled to specify contents and appropriate hazard warnings, and it must indicate the name and address of the manufacturer. All secondary containers must be labeled with an extra copy of the original manufacturer's label or with a generic label that identifies hazard warnings and directions.

Material Safety Data Sheets

A **Material Safety Data Sheet (MSDS)** contains important information about hazardous materials that employees must know to work safely with any given material. MSDSs, which are developed and provided by the manufacturer of the material, are specific for each hazardous material. They contain at least the following information:

- Product identification – Product name, manufacturer's name, address and telephone number, product item number (manufacturer's ID), and synonym names.

- List of hazardous ingredients.

- Physical data – Vapor pressure, evaporation rate, solubility in H_2O, freezing and boiling points, specific gravity, acidity (pH), vapor density, appearance, and odor.

- Fire and explosion information – Flash point, flammable units, extinguishing media, special fire fighting procedures, and unusual fire and explosion hazards.

- Reactivity data – Stability, incompatibility, hazardous decomposition products, and conditions contributing to hazardous **polymerization**.

- Health hazard data – Effects of over-exposure.

- Storage recommendations – Incompatible materials and storage temperatures.

- Emergency and first-aid procedures.

- Spill or leak procedures, spill management, and waste disposal methods.

- Protection information and control measures.

- Special precautions.

The employer is responsible to ensure that MSDSs are readily available to employees who may work with or routinely be in the vicinity of hazardous materials. In turn, employees are responsible for becoming familiar with the MSDS information, and to consistently follow the instructions given for the products they handle and use.

Employee Information and Training

All new Central Service employees should attend a health and safety orientation provided by Risk Management or Safety Department personnel to become familiar with hazards and safety practices throughout the facility. They should also attend a department-specific orientation which focuses on, at least, the following:

Material Safety Data Sheet (MSDS) – A written statement providing detailed information about a chemical or toxic substance including potential hazards and appropriate handling methods. An MSDS is provided by the product manufacturer to the product buyer, and it must be posted and/or made available in a place that is easily accessible to those that will use the product.

Polymerization – A molecular reaction that creates an uncontrolled release of energy.

• An overview of the requirements contained in the hazard communication regulations including employees' rights under the regulations.

• Notification of employees about any operations in their work area where hazardous substances are present.

• Location and availability of the written hazard communication program information.

• Physical and health effects of the hazardous substances with which they may encounter.

• Methods and observation techniques used to determine the presence or release of hazardous substances in the work area.

• How to lessen or prevent exposure to these hazardous substances through safe control and work practices, and use of personal protective equipment.

• Steps the department has taken to lessen or prevent exposure to these substances.

• Emergency and first aid procedures to follow if employees are exposed to hazardous substance(s).

• How to read labels and review MSDSs to obtain appropriate hazard information.

• Emergency spill procedures for glutaraldehyde, EtO, hydrogen peroxide, and PA.

Handling Hazardous Substances

Each state acknowledges certain chemicals and substances as hazardous. Each Central Service Department should have an easily accessible, understandable, and current list of all hazardous substances with which employees could come in contact, **Figure 21.22** lists substances commonly classified as hazardous which are found in healthcare facilities.

Periodically, employees may be required to perform hazardous non-routine tasks such as changing EtO cylinders. Prior to performing such tasks,

they must be given information about the hazards to which they may be exposed. This information should include identification of specific hazards, use of personal protective equipment, safety measures to be employed, and emergency response procedures. Employers should take extra measures to minimize hazards to employees. These could include increased area ventilation, respirators, presence of other employees to assist, and rehearsing of emergency procedures.

Employee Monitoring

To prevent potential health hazards to workers, OSHA has established permissible exposure limits (PELs) for many chemicals used in sterilant and disinfectant formulations. These include EtO, hydrogen peroxide, formaldehyde, and others. One exception is glutaraldehyde, a chemical commonly used in Central Service as a high-level disinfectant. The National Institute for Occupational Safety and Health (NIOSH) recommends that exposure to glutaraldehyde be under 0.2 parts per million (ppm) time weighted average over an eight hour work shift. The American Conference of Governmental Industrial Hygienists (ACGIH) recommends a ceiling value of 0.05 ppm which should not be exceeded at any time.

Healthcare facilities are required by OSHA to:

• Institute engineering controls such as ventilation systems.

• Establish safe work operating procedures.

• Provide personal protective equipment.

• Implement other methods to ensure that occupational exposure limits are not exceeded in the workplace.

Figure 21.23 lists regulated chemicals and exposure limits.

Figure 21.22 Common Hazardous Materials by Hospital Department or Location

Central Service
- ethylene oxide
- infectious agents
- soaps, detergents
- flammable gases
- needle sticks

Dialysis Units
- infectious agents
- formaldehyde
- needle sticks

Dental Service
- mercury
- ethylene oxide
- ionizing radiation
- infectious agents
- needle sticks
- anesthetic gases

Engineering
- solvents
- asbestos
- flammable liquids
- sewage
- mercury
- boiler compounds
- PCBs

Food Service
- soaps, detergents
- caustic solutions (oven, drain cleaners)
- solvents
- disinfectants
- pesticides

Housekeeping
- infectious agents
- needle sticks
- disinfectants, cleansers
- solvents

Laboratory
- infectious agents
- toxic chemicals
- (solvents, reagents, formaldehyde, dyes)
- needle sticks
- carcinogens
- flammable liquids and gas

Laundry
- infectious agents
- needle sticks
- detergents, bleaches, soaps

Maintenance
- asbestos
- pesticides
- caustic cleaners
- sewage
- flammable liquids
- ammonia
- carbon monoxide
- paints, solvents
- adhesives
- infectious agents

Nuclear Medicine
- radionuclides
- infectious agents
- ionizing radiation

Nursing (including aides, attendants)
- infectious agents
- needle sticks
- ionizing radiation
- cytotoxic drugs
- anesthetic gases

Occupational Therapy
- chemicals used in arts & crafts
- (paints, fixatives, glazes)

Operating Rooms
- anesthetic gases
- antiseptics
- methacrylate
- compressed gases
- infectious agents
- sharp instruments/ needle sticks
- sterilizing gases
- radiation (ionizing and nonionizing)

Pathology
- infectious agents
- formaldehyde
- freons
- solvents
- phenols
- sharp instruments

Pharmacy
- pharmaceuticals
- cytotoxic agents
- needle sticks
- flammable liquids
- mercury

Physical Therapy
- chlorine and other swimming pool chemicals

Print Shops
- inks
- solvents

Radiology
- radiation
- infectious agents
- chemicals (fixers, developers)
- resins

Radiation Oncology
- alloys
- chemicals (fixers, developers)

Respiratory Therapy
- infectious agents
- disinfectants
- compressed gases
- needle sticks

Note: This list is not all inclusive.

Employees who work in the hospital receiving area and loading dock may handle chemicals from several of these areas.

Figure 21.23 Some Regulated Chemicals and Exposure Limits

CHEMICAL	USE	TWA	STEL	MONITORING METHOD
Ethylene oxide	Sterilant, fumigant	1.0 PPM	5.0 PPM	Infrared analysis Gas chromatography Passive exposure badges Metallic oxide semiconductors Photoionization
Gultaraldehyde	Sterilant, disinfectant	None	0.2 (ceiling)	None
Formaldehyde	Preservative, disinfectant, sterilant	1.0 PPM	2.0 PPM	Infrared analysis Gas chromatography Passive exposure badges Photoionization
Nitrous oxide	Anesthetic	50 PPM* (dental) 25 PPM (hospital)	None	Infrared analysis comp Passive exposure badges Photoionization
Xylene	Solvent cover slips in laboratory	100 PPM	150 PPM	Passive exposure badges Gas chromatography
Toluene	Solvent - thins	100 PPM mounting medium	150 PPM	Passive exposure badges Gas chromatography
Benzene	Solvent	1.0 PPM Occupational Carcinogenic	5.0 PPM	Passive exposure badges Gas chromatography
Mercury (alcohol)	Disinfectant	.01 PPM	.03 PPM	Mercury meter
Mercury (vapor)	Instrument	.05 PPM	None	Mercury meter
Ammonia	Cleaning solvent	25 PPM	35 PPM	Infrared analysis Photoionization
Chlorine	Disinfectant ingredient	.5 PPM	1.0 PPM	Infrared analysis Photoionization
Alcohols: Methyl Ethyl Isopropyl	Disinfectant	200 PPM 1 000 PPM 400 PPM	250 PPM None 500 PPM	Gas chromatography Photoionization
Methyl methacrylate	Glue used in orthopaedics	100 PPM	None photoionization	Infrared analysis

*NIOSH recommended standard for hospitals is 25 ppm.

Hazardous Waste Management

The facility's and Central Service department's **hazardous waste** management program is intended to provide employees with a safe, efficient protocol for disposing of hazardous chemicals while ensuring that the hazardous waste is disposed of properly and in compliance with applicable regulations. Not all hazardous chemicals are classified as hazardous waste; therefore, it is important to review the MSDSs, and refer to specific guidelines under federal, state, and local regulations to ensure proper disposal.

Many facilities contract the services of a waste management company to make routine pickups to remove hazardous waste. Hazardous waste containers must be labeled with the contents and the date with which waste was first disposed of in that container. There are other specific federal, state, and local regulations that pertain to the definition, generation, storage, containers used for, and labeling of hazardous waste. These regulations should be consulted when establishing a chemical waste program.

Bloodborne Pathogens

OSHA's Occupational Exposure to Bloodborne Pathogens standard has established requirements to protect workers from exposure to bloodborne pathogens. The agency summarized the rule as follows:

"Based on a review of the information in the rule making record, OSHA has made a determination that employees face a significant health risk as the result of occupational exposure to blood and other potentially infectious materials because they may contain bloodborne pathogens, including hepatitis B virus which causes Hepatitis B, a serious liver disease, and human immunodeficiency virus, which causes Acquired Immunodeficiency Syndrome (AIDS). The Agency further concludes that this exposure can be minimized or eliminated using a combination of engineering and work practice controls, personal protection clothing and equipment, training, medical surveillance, Hepatitis B vaccination, signs and labels, and other provisions."[3]

Figure 21.24 provides details about the OSHA bloodborne pathogens standard.

Since the early 1990's, OSHA has based compliance and enforcement policies and procedures for inspections involving occupational exposure to TB on guidelines from the Centers for Disease Control and Prevention (CDC). It is recommended that the local OSHA office be contacted for information about regulations applicable to specific Central Service activities.

DISASTER PLANS AND PREPAREDNESS

Learning Objective 7. Discuss the basics of internal and external disaster plans for a healthcare facility.

A third component of the Central Service safety program is a response plan for internal and external disasters. An **internal disaster** is any situation with the potential to cause harm or injury to Central Service Department employees or where the loss of utilities may drastically impact departmental operations. Examples of internal disasters include a hazardous chemical spill or leak, a loss of power, or a failure of a utility such as water, electricity, or steam.

An **external disaster** is a situation in which activities external to the facility affects departmental or facility operations. Examples that may necessitate activation of the external disaster plan include earthquakes, floods, hurricanes, and a large number of seriously injured patients sent to the facility from

Hazardous waste – Substances that cannot be disposed of in the facility's normal trash system.

Disaster (internal) –Any situation with the potential to cause harm or injury to Central Service employees, or where the loss of utilities may drastically impact department operations.

Disaster (external) –A situation in which activities external to the facility affects departmental or facility operations.

Figure 21.24 OHSA Bloodborne Pathogens Standard

Bloodborne Pathogens

OSHA regulations applicable to bloodborne pathogens (Standards, - 29CFR, 1910.1030) provides details about requirements needed to minimize risk. Regulations require that:

- Employers shall provide at no cost to the employee, appropriate personal protective equipment including gloves, gowns, laboratory coats, face shields/masks and eye protection and mouth pieces, resuscitation bags, pocket masks or other ventilation devices. (Personal protective equipment will be considered appropriate only if it does not permit blood or other potentially infectious materials to pass through to or reach the employees work or street clothes, undergarments, skin, eyes, mouth or other mucous membranes under normal conditions of use and for the duration of time which the protective equipment will be used.)

- The employer shall ensure that the employee uses appropriate personal protective equipment.

- The employer shall ensure that the appropriate personal protective equipment in the appropriate sizes is readily acceptable at the work site or is issued to employees.

- If a garment is penetrated by blood or other potentially infected materials the garment shall be removed immediately or as soon as possible. All personal protective equipment shall be removed prior to leaving the work area.

- Employers shall ensure that the work site is maintained in a clean and sanitary condition. The employers shall determine/implement an appropriate written schedule for cleaning and method of decontamination based upon the location within the facility, the type of surface to be cleaned, the type of soil present and tasks/procedures being performed. All equipment, environmental, and working surfaces shall be cleaned and decontaminated after contact with blood or other potentially infectious materials.

- Reusable sharps contaminated with blood or other potentially infectious materials shall not be stored/processed in a manner that requires employees to reach by hand into the containers where these sharps have been placed.

- Contaminated sharps shall be discarded immediately or as soon as feasible in containers that are closeable, puncture-resistant, leak-proof on sides and bottom and appropriately labeled or color-coded.

- Hepatitis B vaccination shall be made available after employees have received appropriate training and within 10 working days of initial assignment to all employees who have occupational exposure unless the employee has previously received the complete Hepatitis B vaccination series, antibody testing has revealed that the employee is immune or the vaccine is contra-indicated for medical reasons. The employer shall not make participation in a pre-screening program a prerequisite for receiving Hepatitis B vaccination.

- If an employee initially declines Hepatitis B vaccination but at a later date decides to accept the vaccination, the employer shall make available Hepatitis B vaccination at that time. The employer shall assure that employees who decline to accept Hepatitis B vaccination offered by the employer sign an appropriate statement.

- Manual training for all employees is required. Applicable topics shall include at a minimum:

    - An accessible copy of applicable OSHA standards/regulations.

- A general explanation of the epidemiology and symptoms of bloodborne diseases.

- An explanation of the modes of transmission of bloodborne pathogens.

- An explanation of the employer's exposure control plan.

- An explanation of the appropriate methods for recognizing tasks/activities that may involve exposure to blood and other potentially infectious materials.

- An explanation of the use and limitations of methods that will prevent or reduce exposure.

- Information on the types, proper use, location, removal, handling, decontamination and disposal of personal protective equipment.

- An explanation of the basis for selection of personal protective equipment.

- Information on the Hepatitis B vaccination.

- Information on the appropriate actions to take and persons to contact in an emergency involving blood/potentially infectious materials.

- An explanation of the procedure to follow if an exposure incident occurs.

- Information on the post-exposure evaluation follow-up that is required for an employee following an exposure incident.

- An explanation of the signs and labels and/or color coding of sharps containers.

- An opportunity for interactive questions/answers with the trainer.

- The employer shall establish/maintain a sharps injury log to record percutaneous injuries from contaminated sharps. The confidentiality of the injured employee must be maintained. The log shall contain:

  - The type/brand of device involved in the incident.

  - The department/work area where the incident occurred.

  - An explanation of how the incident occurred.

a plane crash. When there are external disasters, the entire facility is placed on alert, and personnel from each department are expected to perform tasks based on the type of situations that exist.

Disaster Plans

Central Service department disaster plans, like those of other departments, should be consistent with, and support, the facility's plans. Most hospitals use an incident command system (ICS) to manage their disaster response. Central Service managers must ensure the Central Service disaster response activities and expectations are included in the overall ICS plan.

Elements of a Central Service disaster plan typically include:

- An emergency call list outlining the lines of authority, and the key individuals to be notified in specific types of disasters. (These could differ for each type of disaster.)

- Protocols for inventory, replenishment, and delivery of emergency supplies. Usually supply distribution department personnel are responsible for the maintenance of supplies and, in times of disaster, will deliver to an area for emergency patient care.

- Posted evacuation plans and practice drills for employees to ensure that they know alternative ways to leave the department if their safety is at risk.

- A well-known and understood organizational structure that presents lines of authority.

- Responsibility lists to identify employees responsible for certain tasks during disaster situations.

- Directions for alternative communication and transportation if existing facilities such as elevators and telephone systems cannot be used.

- Directions for locations of utility and power shut-off points.

- Plans for prioritizing sterile processing and supply distribution functions based on failing utilities or internal damage.

- A risk assessment that presents the likelihood, potential severity, and the facility's current level of preparedness, to help guide planning efforts.

- Description of how the institution's disaster planning and response efforts are integrated with other community response organizations.

All potential disaster situations that may either impact hospital operations or to which the facility may respond in support of the community, should be addressed in departmental disaster planning activities.

New Concerns

The United States has experienced the use of anthrax bacteria as a terrorist weapon to intentionally cause death, illness, and panic. The potential use of other biological agents for terrorism purposes including botulism, hemorrhagic fever, plague, smallpox, and tularemia is also possible. Chemicals can also be used in terrorist attacks. These include nerve, blister, blood, and choking agents. As a consequence, disaster plans must include preparedness and response protocols associated with terrorist threats in addition to natural disasters.

Infection control practices for patient management following suspected or confined terrorism events must be well-organized and rehearsed.[4] Factors that should alert healthcare providers to the possibility of a bioterrorism attack include:

- A rapidly increasing disease incidence (for example, within hours or days) in a normally healthy population.

- An epidemic curve that rises and falls during a short period of time.

- An unusual increase in the number of people seeking care, especially with fever, respiratory, or gastrointestinal complaints.

- An **endemic disease** rapidly emerging at an uncharacteristic time or in an unusual pattern.

- Lower attack rates among people who had been indoors, especially in areas with filtered air or closed ventilation systems, compared with people who had been outdoors.

- A cluster of patients arriving from a single locale.

- Large numbers of rapidly fatal cases.

- Any patient presenting a disease that is relatively uncommon and has bioterrorism potential (for example, pulmonary anthrax, tularemia, or plague).

While it is important for the entire facility to quickly react in a coordinated approach, there are special concerns applicable to Central Service:

- Isolation Precautions. Standard Precautions prevent direct contact with body fluids (including blood), secretions, excretions, nonintact skin (including rashes), and mucous membranes. Standard Precautions routinely

Endemic disease – *One that occurs more or less continuously throughout a community.*

practiced by healthcare providers include hand washing and use of gloves, masks/eye protection or face shields, gowns (and shoe covers in suspected or confirmed cases of smallpox).

• Cleaning, disinfection, and sterilization of equipment and environment. Standard Precautions should be generally applied for the management of patient care equipment and environmental control.

• For some biological agents including suspected smallpox, all linen and laundry should be kept in the isolation room until the diagnosis has been established. Linens should be placed in a biohazardous plastic bag, and should then be put in a soiled linen bag that is securely closed. All linen should be treated as infectious and transported to the laundry in a safe manner. It should not be sorted.

• All trash in suspected or confirmed smallpox outbreaks must be placed in bio-hazardous trash boxes and disposed of in the usual manner for infectious waste.

Checklist for Disaster Readiness[5]

A healthcare facility's disaster plan must be reconsidered in terms of the potential for unimaginable activities that can become a reality. Here are some suggestions:

• Focus efforts on a general all hazards plan to yield a framework for crisis situations.

• Upgrade existing disaster plans. Components must now include mass casualty terrorism including chemical and biological situations.

• Integrate the facility's plan with those of the community's emergency response agencies.

• Develop a plan to support the families of staff members.

• Review back-up communication capabilities.

• Assure that essential facility information systems and data storage have effective storage and recovery capabilities.

• Interact with community leaders and lawmakers; let them know what your facility can do.

• Review your supply and inventory strategies; just-in-time systems may not work with a mass casualty event.

• Examine how to protect the physical security of your hospital.

• Know how your facility relates to the National Disaster Medical System or to a Metropolitan Medical Response System.

• Ensure that medical staff report unexpected illness patterns to the Public Health Department and, if appropriate, to the CDC.

• Inventory your staff; key members may be called up if they are members of the Military Reserves or part of an Office of Emergency Preparedness Response Team.

ENDNOTES

1. *ANSI/AAMI. Comprehensive guide to steam sterilization and sterility assurance in health care facilities. American National Standard ST 79. Arlington, Va. 2006. (Section 4.2.2)*

2. *Adapted from: Occupational Safety and Health Administration (OSHA). Ergonomics for the Prevention of Musculoskeletal Disorders: Guidelines for Nursing Homes. www.OSHA.gov/ ergonomics/guidelines/nursinghome/index.html*

3. *Federal Register 56:64004, December 6, 1991.*

4. *This section is adopted from disaster preparedness procedures developed by the Cleveland Clinic Foundation. Cleveland, Ohio. 2001.*

5. *Adapted from: American Hospital Association. Advancing Health in America. Disaster Readiness Advisory. 2001.*

CENTRAL SERVICE TERMS

Sharps

Aerosol

Ergonomics

Work-related musculoskeletal disorder (WMSD)

Risk Management

Combustible

Combustible loading

Material Safety Data Sheet (MSDA)

Polymerization

Hazardous waste

Disaster (internal)

Disaster (external)

Endemic disease

Chapter Outline

Chapter 22

Communication and Human Relations Skills

Chapter Learning Objectives

As a result of successfully completing this chapter, readers will be able to:

1. Explain the need for Central Service Technicians to utilize effective communication and human relations skills.

2. Define the term, "professionalism," list traits of professional Central Service Technicians, and describe their fundamental beliefs and behaviors.

3. Use basic tactics of effective communication in the workplace.

4. Practice procedures to enhance and maintain effective working relationships.

5. Discuss tactics to improve teamwork.

6. Define the term, "diversity," explain why it is important, and review how Central Service Technicians can develop a "diversity mind-set."

7. Practice basic customer service skills, and utilize tactics to appropriately handle customer complaints.

8. Review concerns applicable to handling promotions, relating experience to job success, setting priorities, and committing to patient care during disasters.

The responsibilities of Central Service Technicians relate directly to the health and well-being of the patients, and they must have the knowledge and skills to address the sophisticated concepts addressed in this Technical Manual. However, they must also interact with other persons in their department and in other units within the facility as well as, frequently, patients, vendors, and suppliers. To do so requires the consistent use of the communication and human resources skills that are the topics of this chapter.

NEED FOR EFFECTIVE COMMUNICATION AND HUMAN RELATIONS SKILLS

Learning Objective 1. Explain the need for Central Service Technicians to utilize effective communication and human relations skills.

Central Service Technicians (and all other persons in healthcare facilities) must have effective interpersonal skills. Communication abilities are one dimension of interpersonal skills because they allow a person to understand someone else's needs and interests. Human relations skills then become important as one uses the information gained from communication to interact with other persons.

Let's define terms: **Communication** is the process of transmitting information and understanding from one person to another by use of words and non-verbal expressions such as body language.

The concept of **human relations** involves the development and maintenance of effective interpersonal (between people) relationships that enhance teamwork.

There are many communications and human relations principles applicable to the job, and most can be used off the job as well. While people are unique and different in many respects, they also share many things in common. These include specific needs, wants, and desires that form a framework for developing an approach to human relations, and effective communication is a key element in determining and addressing these common concerns.

The use of appropriate communication and human relations skills is important whenever two persons interact. However, the world of health care is very labor intensive: machines do not replace the need for human judgment and skills as Central Service Technicians undertake their job responsibilities. They must work with their peers (other technicians), and with department supervisors and managers. They also represent their department as they interact formally and informally with staff members in other departments throughout the facility. Central Service Technicians are also likely to come in contact with patients and their families and with visitors to the facility including those conducting business with department managers.

In these days when health care organizations receive scrutiny from society, the need for effective communication and the application of appropriate human relation skills continues off-the-job. What one says (and does not say) and what one does (and does not do) reflects on the individual. However, there is also a carry over effect, and all health care employees, including Central Service Technicians, reflect not only on themselves, but also on their employer in their off-work words and actions.

How often do "communication problems" occur, and what causes them? Interestingly, these problems happen all-too-frequently even when everyone speaks the same language. What is likely to happen when Central Service Technicians

Communication – *The process of transmitting information and understanding from one person to another by use of words and non-verbal expressions such as body language.*

Human relations – *The development and maintenance of effective interpersonal (between people) relationships that enhance teamwork.*

Jargon - *Specialized words or phrases known only by persons working in a position.*

interact with persons who speak a different native language? While use of basic communication principles discussed in this chapter will not resolve all of these problems, it will help to address many of them. Questions that can be interpreted differently such as, "Can you come to work early? (What time is early? Do you just mean earlier than usual?), and the inconsistent meaning of **jargon** hinders communication and the understanding that is supposed to result from it. Inappropriate tactics such as blaming some persons, criticizing others, and ignoring still others are examples of the ineffective use of human relations skills that damage effective interactions in the workplace.

While it may seem strange, some persons can easily understand details of microbiology and apply specialized skills to operate sophisticated sterilization equipment, but have difficulty interacting with others. The proper use of communication and human relations skills is important for the success of all Central Service Technicians in all health care facilities. Fortunately, these principles can be learned and are easy to apply on the job. The ability to do so is a characteristic of professional Central Service Technicians.

CENTRAL SERVICE TECHNICIANS ARE PROFESSIONALS

Learning Objective 2. Define the term, "professionalism," list traits of professional Central Service Technicians, and describe their fundamental beliefs and behaviors.

What is a professional? A professional is a person working in an occupation that requires extensive knowledge and skills to do so. A profession involves membership limited to those with education and experience in a specialized body of knowledge. Membership is usually controlled by licensing, registration, and/or certification, and is governed by a universal code of ethics.

The practice of Central Service technology requires professionalism, and includes the essential elements of a profession. The Central Service discipline will be fully classified as a profession when requirements for formal education, certification, and a universal code of behavior are fulfilled and become requirements for employment.

Figure 22.1 summarizes selected characteristics of professional Central Service Technicians.

More About Professionalism

Professionals are proud of themselves and the work they do. They can do the job correctly, and they always try to do better and improve their profession in the process. A professional "goes the extra mile," is part of the team, tries to put forth the best possible effort to meet the facility's and department's goals, and is truly interested in other employees and the patients.

Professional Central Service Technicians know what their supervisor expects of them and consistently meet these standards. They are effective communicators, and they are courteous and

What Should Central Service Technicians Expect from their Employer?

All staff members have a right to:

- Fair pay for the work which is done

- Safe working conditions

- Training to meet job standards, and then additional training to maintain performance and, possibly, advance to more responsible positions.

- Help to make sure that all employees work well together

- An explanation of all applicable policies, rules, and regulations

- A fair evaluation of their work

Employees who believe that one or more of these considerations are not provided should discuss the situation with their supervisor. Professionals want to help the team become the best it can be. By working toward solutions, an employee helps make the department better.

concerned about the problems encountered by other staff members.

Job success is affected by how well employees get along with their supervisor. Hopefully, this is easy to do because of mutual respect and understanding between both parties. However, sometimes friction

Professional Central Service Technicians:

- Have a positive attitude and pride in themselves, and the important work they do.
- Possess the knowledge and skills required to be proficient.
- Are alert to the need for on-going improvement.
- Contribute "110%" to help their team meet its goals.
- Are genuinely interested in helping others.
- Know and attain (exceed) their facility's quality and quantity standards.
- Are competent communicators.
- Practice appropriate human relations skills.
- Respect their supervisors and their peers.
- Have imagination.
- Are creative.
- Follow high ethical and moral standards.
- Are self-confident.
- Are courteous to their co-workers and all others with whom they have contact.
- Admit mistakes and learn from them.
- Follow appropriate personal hygiene and dress standards.
- Have a sense of humor.

Note: *Many of these characteristics relate to the practice of human relations skills that are discussed later in this chapter.*

Figure 22.1 Characteristics of Professional Central Service Technicians

can occur. Then it may be difficult but even more important to develop, maintain, and improve the relationship. Central Service Technicians should recognize that the boss may not be their friend or "buddy." However, a professional relationship will address job tasks and human relations concerns.

Those who obtain promotions, pay raises, and most quickly attain career goals enjoy the respect of their peers and supervisors. This respect is most likely when an employee cooperates, is dependable, has ambition, and is willing to work hard to be successful.

Technical Competence is Important

Central Service professionals understand their role, and they know the challenges in their day-to-day work are best met with technical competence. The health and safety of others are compromised when employees who work with chemicals, explosive/flammable agents, pathogenic organisms, and hazardous wastes do not know what they are doing. Central Service Technicians must be knowledgeable about every aspect of their work and follow procedures correctly. Appropriate training is absolutely necessary to consistently meet standards.

Safety practices must be understood and followed 100% of the time because carelessness and lack of understanding are not acceptable. Use resources such as the facility's Safety Committee, Infection Control Coordinator, Material Safety Data Sheets (MSDSs), and other resources to increase knowledge. Professionals are prepared to respond to any emergency, and know how to protect themselves and others during daily operations.

Moral, Legal, and Ethical Considerations

Central Service Technicians must follow a professional code of behavior that includes moral, legal, and ethical aspects of responsibility.

Moral behavior relates to basic principles about what is right and wrong. Patients who enter the hospital entrust their lives to the staff. Central Service Technicians must honor this trust as a member of the health care team. They must carry out their duties in compliance with each detail and procedural step. They accept responsibility to follow work schedules, maintain good attendance, and follow established policies and procedures in the best interests of patient care. Central Service Technicians utilize resources wisely. They do not question or ridicule a patient's religious beliefs or personal possessions. They care for and protect the patient's property including valuables, toys, and religious and sentimental items. Occasionally, personal objects may be sent to Central Service for cleaning and sterilization, and these require safeguarding for return to the patient.

Central Service professionals also respect the beliefs and rights of their co-workers. They do not promote gossip or conduct that affects their department's best interests. They recognize their responsibility to preserve personal values and beliefs, and they do not engage in activities that violate personal moral or religious beliefs.

Legal behavior is determined by the authority of laws, and one must never overstep the limitations of these responsibilities. Laws protect staff as well as patients. Central Service Technicians will be held legally responsible for their actions. They are expected to perform job duties as they have been taught, and they do not accept responsibility for or attempt to carry out a job task for which proper instructions or training has not been provided. They do not perform duties that have been designated for or assigned to a licensed or registered professional. Negligence is grounds for legal action. They pay attention to details, follow each step of written procedures, and maintain thorough records and documentation. Short cuts and carelessness may cause patient infections, undue suffering, harm, and even loss of life.

Ethical behavior relating to what is right and wrong relative to the standards of conduct for one's profession is of concern today. There is a perception, for example, that it is no longer just a few "unethical" businesspersons who abuse the system. There is concern that many officials in business and other organizations lack social responsibility and behave unethically. Health care facilities, as they grow larger and become more focused on financial,

political, and other issues, are more likely to become part of the "big business" infrastructure that fosters the public's attitudes of mistrust and suspicion.

Ethical conduct is required of Central Service Technicians at all times. However, the difference between what is "right" and what is "wrong" can be viewed from different perspectives. Consider the following:

• A Central Service Technician knows that another staff member regularly "beats the system" by arriving late and leaving early. A friend takes care of the time clock; both this employee and the friend spend lots of time in unproductive work while "on the clock." This situation represents a case where there is a loser: the facility. However, the attitude of "It's none of my business" seems to prevail.

• A Central Service supervisor consistently emphasizes the need for "quality, quality, and more quality." At the same time, many decisions place a higher priority on cost than on quality. There are inconsistent words and actions; in effect the supervisor is saying, "Do what I say—not what I do!" Are inconsistent words and actions of a role model (the supervisor) acceptable? Do they (or can they) impact the attitudes and behavior of the Central Service Technicians who do not know the supervisor's definition of "what is right?"

Will the situations above be handled without an effort to consider ethical and social responsibility aspects of the situation? The answer lies with the individual(s) confronted by the situation.

How does one decide if a proposed action is ethical? Answers to the following questions may be helpful:

• Is the proposed action legal?

• Does the proposed action hurt anyone?

• Is the proposed action fair?

• Am I being honest as I undertake the proposed action?

- Can I live with myself if I do what I am considering?

- Would I like to publicize my decision?

- What if everyone did it?

Many organizations develop Codes of Ethics to help identify acceptable and unacceptable behavior. **Figure 22.2** reviews popular components in the codes of ethics of many organizations.

A code of ethics identifies how employees of a health care facility should interact with and relate to each other, and the constituencies whom they serve. Today, being "ethical" might give some health care facilities a competitive edge over counterparts whose actions are sometimes less than ethical. However, less-than-consistently ethical organizations will not survive. Therefore, Codes of Ethics and the conduct that they mandate in the future will be a prerequisite for success—not a factor that better assures it.

Figure 22.2 Codes of Ethics

Major components of codes of ethics often include:

- Preamble (purpose, goals, and objectives).

- Member responsibilities to the profession.

- Member responsibilities to the patients (or those served).

- Member responsibilities to the employing organization.

- Member responsibilities to employees/peers.

- Member responsibilities to the community/society.

- Member responsibilities to the oneself (the professional).

- Matters relating to violations of code of ethics.

BASICS OF COMMUNICATION

Learning Objective 3. Use basic tactics of effective communication in the workplace.

Some employees cannot effectively express their thoughts to co-workers, and others think about something else while someone speaks to them. The first concern relates to speaking, and the second involves listening to problems. These are examples of obstacles that create communication breakdowns, and interfere with the successful exchange of information from one person to another.

You've learned that the ability to communicate successfully is important for Central Service Technicians. Fortunately, we can all learn to communicate more effectively. Communication is a skill and, like all skills, to do well requires practice.

Central Service Technicians play an important role in their facility's communication process. For example, they provide feedback including ideas and suggestions to their supervisors who, in turn, communicate information up and down the chain of command. Each person's role in this communication process is vital to its success.

Some employees think communication is easy. (After all, they have been doing it all their lives!) In fact, the process is not difficult, but it does require use of basic principles. Some of these are addressed in **Figure 22.3** (Take the Communications Test). A personal analysis of its results may suggest whether additional efforts to improve one's communication skills could be helpful.

Check It Out!

To view the Code of Ethics of, literally, thousands of associations, non-profit organizations, companies, and business on the world-wide web, just enter "code of ethics" into your favorite search engine.

Figure 22.3 Take the Communications Test

	Correct	Incorrect
1. I do not hold **stereotypes** of people who are not like me.	☐	☐
2. I try to keep personal matters from affecting me on the job.	☐	☐
3. I know that the volume and tone of my voice impacts my message when I talk.	☐	☐
4. I look at the person with whom I'm speaking most of the time.	☐	☐
5. I use my hands, arms, shoulders, and head to emphasize what I'm saying.	☐	☐
6. Generally, my facial expressions suggest the same as my words.	☐	☐
7. I try to think of a single point I want a person to remember before I speak.	☐	☐
8. I ask questions to help me determine if my listener understands what I said.	☐	☐
9. I know that listening is an important part of communicating.	☐	☐
10. I generally don't interrupt a person who is speaking to me.	☐	☐
11. I generally give persons my full attention while they are talking to me.	☐	☐
12. I control myself when someone sets off one of my emotions.	☐	☐
13. I know that my "body language" supplements my communication (and can be the most important aspect of it).	☐	☐
14. I use proper protocols when writing and sending e-mails.	☐	☐
15. I minimize the use of jargon when talking.	☐	☐

Scoring the test: The more times you answer "correct," the more effective are your communication abilities. If some questions were answered "incorrect," try to think about and correct these concerns as you communicate with others.

Stereotype – A preconceived belief or opinion about a group of people that is applied to every person in that group.

Feedback – A step in communication that occurs when the listener asks a question, repeats information or otherwise helps the speaker to know if the message has been correctly received.

Communication Myths

These are some common misunderstandings about communication that, when applied, impact its effectiveness. Here are several communication myths.[1]

- *We only communicate when we want to* – People do not control every aspect of communication. If a Central Service Technician does not respond to a situation, this conveys a message just as clearly as do words that express a low priority or disinterest.

- *Words mean the same to everyone* – In fact, words have special meanings based upon a person's experience. For example, the use of nicknames and abbreviations for common medical instruments can cause "communication" problems when they are not understood by both Central Service Technicians and operating room personnel.

- *Words are the primary way we communicate* – Remember the saying, "Actions speaks louder than words." The way one looks and acts while speaking or listening often communicates a person's feelings about a topic being discussed. As well, the volume and tone of the speaker's voice (loud or soft, harsh, mild-mannered or happy, for example) help to portray a message that may be the same as or different from that which is intended.

- *Communication is a one-way process: the sender "tells" the receiver* – In fact, communication should normally be a two-way activity. Effective communicators talk "with" rather than "at" or "to" others. Effective communicators use feedback from the listener to assess communication effectiveness. If **feedback** is interpreted correctly, the sender knows whether and to what extent the receiver has understood the message. It helps assure that the message one wants to be communicated is the message that is received.

- *A message should contain all possible information* – While too little information is certainly not good, too much information can also be a problem. We sometimes distort messages with unnecessary information. The term information overload is often used when too much information is given. The concern should be with the quality of information rather than the quantity of information that is communicated.

Communication Roadblocks

Communication should be a simple, clear process. Unfortunately, it is often made more difficult than necessary when, for example, roadblocks interfere with the intended message and cause misunderstandings. Six special problems that Central Service Technicians should consider when they communicate include:

- *Unfair comparison* – Do not compare one employee with another. Everyone has unique talents and abilities, and deserves one's best communication efforts.

- *Just-like-me* – People tend to like others who behave or think as they do, and who have similar backgrounds and characteristics. Conversely, less attention may be given to those who are different. Learn to communicate in ways all people will understand. This requires the use of different approaches for different people.

- *Stereotypes* – You've learned that these occur when a person forms general opinions about certain groups, and then applies these opinions to every person in that group. It is incorrect to think that all people who belong to a group are the same. Everyone is an individual. Do not assign a behavioral characteristic such as "low energy" or "untrustworthy" to a person unless that is the actual behavior of that individual.

- *Good day/bad day effect* – Everyone has good and bad days, and personal feelings can affect communication. When experiencing a bad day, one may be more critical of others. Consistent and appropriate communication and interactions with others are necessary on both good days and bad days.

- *Halo effect* – One practices the halo effect when a person is favored because of a quality found to be attractive or valuable. In the process, negative behavior may be overlooked. Favoritism hurts communication.

The best tactic: be a consistently effective communicator with everyone.

• *Pitchfork effect* – The opposite of the halo effect, this occurs when one dislikes another person because of a specific quality or personal characteristic. Don't let the pitchfork effect become a barrier to communication.

All Central Service Technicians must be effective communicators. Myths about and roadblocks to effective communication should be considered as effective speaking and listening are developed.

Basic Speaking Tactics

Here are some principles that should be used when you speak with others.

• Know what you want to say, and keep on target as you speak.

• Identify the main points in the message; organize what you will say, and assure that, while speaking, you address each main point.

• Stay focused; do not ramble, digress, or talk about things that are not critical to your message.

• Concentrate on the listener rather than on yourself. Remember that the main objective of speaking is to communicate – not to make a good impression.

• Speak enthusiastically. Be committed to the purpose of your message and show interest and enthusiasm when speaking.

• Be able to support the information provided. If points are well documented, the listener can concentrate on what you say rather than questioning whether your statements are accurate.

• Think about your listener's background, and speak in a way that will help assure that the message is accurately received. Use feedback methods such as asking open-ended questions ("Why do you think this is a problem?" rather

than "Is this a problem?"), or requesting intermediate comments to assess whether the listener understands the message.

• Use language that the listener will understand.

Basic Listening Tactics

Many Central Service Technicians spend more time listening than they do speaking. Basic techniques to improve your listening ability include:

• Concentrate on the central idea the speaker is trying to convey. (Recall the point made above: a well-organized speaker makes it easier for the listener because the message will be clearly thought out and stated.)

• Focus on what the speaker is saying; do not be become distracted.

• Don't let your emotions influence you. Remember the old saying, "We hear what we want to hear." Avoid an immediate evaluation of the message, and try to think about its content objectively.

• Don't "tune out" the speaker because the message seems familiar, strange, or unimportant.

• Consider the speaker's perceptions as you listen to the message.

• Don't just listen for specific facts. There may be a "hidden agenda" that is a subtle but important part of the message.

• Understand the speaker's basic ideas before objectively criticizing them.

• Don't let an uncomfortable physical environment cause distraction. There may be few places within a busy Central Service Department where the environment is ideally acceptable for effective communication; therefore, try to make the best of it.

• Search for special meaning in the speaker's message. Some elements may be more important than others.

- Note the speaker's non-verbal communication. Sometimes the "real" message can only be understood if you recognize implications of the non-verbal communication that accompanies the message.

- Don't avoid listening to information that is complicated. Use feedback such as "I really don't understand what you are saying," or "Can you please say that in another way" to tell the speaker that the message was not effectively conveyed.

- Concentrate on the message and its content not on its delivery. Problems with the speaker's voice, speed of speech, and/or pronunciation can cause difficulties, but it is important to attempt to learn the real meaning of the message.

- Allow the speaker to finish, and than react fairly and sensibly to the message that was stated.

- If applicable, take notes if the information is detailed or specific, and/or if it will be helpful in the future.

- Don't formulate a response to the message while listening to the speaker.

Types of Communication

Communication flows through formal and informal channels within the Central Services Department. Examples of formal communication include:

- Instructions, advice, and **coaching** undertaken by managers and supervisors.

- Facility and department policies and procedures that help regulate behavior and work practices.

- Discussions in departmental and other meetings.

Coaching – *Positive reinforcement used to encourage Central Service Technicians to follow proper work practices, and negative reinforcement to discourage inappropriate work practices.*

- Individual and group training presentations.

- Facility and departmental bulletins, memos, newsletters, and related communication tools.

- Performance evaluation sessions.

- Employee work schedules.

- Conversations related to delegated project assignments.

- Monitoring of on-going work activities.

The list of formal types of communication within the Central Services Department can continue, and could become very lengthy. The variety, frequency, and importance of formal communication emphasize the need to consistently apply basic principles including those presented in this chapter.

Informal methods of communication also exist within Central Service Departments. These include the "grapevine" (the informal channel of communication throughout the organization), casual conversations between employees before, during, and after work, and while on breaks. Much of this communication is beneficial because it can improve the working relationships of staff members. Unfortunately, informal communication can also be damaging. Consider, for example, rumors: information that is circulated without knowledge of its source or whether it is true.

Useful tactics to address rumors include questioning whether it could be true. Ask questions such as, "Why am I being told?" "Would the person telling me gain something by saying something untrue?" "Does the person have access to the required information?" And, finally, "Can the information be confirmed?" When rumors appear to be gossip, ask the person why you are being told, inform the subject of the rumor about it, and do not repeat the information.

Understanding the Interview Process

Central Service Technicians were involved in interviews as part of their initial selection process, and they participate in performance evaluations that typically include an interview component. While much of the interview process is controlled by the manager or supervisor conducting the interview, the interviewee (Central Service Technician) can still benefit from the use of basic speaking and listening techniques during these sessions. This is especially so since contemporary interview methods emphasize a participative approach in which the person conducting the interview interacts with rather than "lectures to" the interviewee.

There are two types of questions that interviewees can ask:

- Open-ended questions permit the interviewee to respond in an unstructured manner. Examples: "What do you think the role of a Central Service Technician should be?" "What are the main challenges you have encountered since our last discussion?"

- Closed-ended questions call for a brief response. Examples: "Do you like your job?" "Do you understand the correct way to do this task?"

Many interviews include both types of questions. One important step in preparing for any interview is to anticipate the types of questions that are likely to be asked, and to plan a response for them.

There are four basic steps in any type of interview:

- Step 1 – It must be planned. Be sure you know the exact purpose of the interview, and the "mechanics" of it (time, location, and estimated duration).

- Step 2 – Transitional conversation is helpful. Hopefully, there will be an initial discussion of mutual topics of interest to move the discussion away from on-going work considerations to the specific topic. Professional Central Service Technicians will have the confidence, pride, expertise, and positive attitude to reduce tension, and to allow them to be confident during the interview.

- Step 3 – Questions will be asked. This is where the interviewee's anticipation of potential questions and ability to effectively

speak and listen will be most useful. It is also where application of the speaking and listening tactics discussed earlier will be most helpful.

- Step 4 – The interview discussion can be reviewed. Hopefully, the interviewer will provide a summary. The Central Service Technician should provide reactions to this review, so both parties can agree on what was decided and what, if any, follow-up activities should be undertaken.

Telephone and E-Mail Etiquette

The manner in which Central Service Technicians answer and talk on the telephone reflects on their department and on themselves. The need to be professional, courteous, and helpful is obvious, and to do so involves the use of several tactics:

- Try to answer the phone in the fewest possible rings. (Many organizations use the "within three rings" rule.)

- When answering the telephone, state your name and department: "Hello, this is Lani in the Central Services Department." Do so in a professional but friendly tone of voice.

- If you answer someone else's phone, identify the individual for whom you are answering: "Hello, this is Joe in Mrs. Jones's office."

- When answering calls, identify yourself. For an internal call, you might say, "Hello, this is Renee," and this is probably a wise tactic even if the facility's phone system shows the name and number of the caller.

- If calls must be screened, never ask who is calling before you inform the caller about whether the individual is available.

- Ask the caller if he/she wishes to leave a name and telephone number if the person being called is unavailable.

- If a caller must be placed on hold, ask if he/she prefers to be on hold or to be called back. (Avoid the phrase, "Hold please.") Update the caller, if necessary: "I'm very sorry that you're still waiting; do you prefer to hold, or may I take your number so Mr. Jones can return your call?"

• When transferring calls, give the caller the number to which the call is being transferred. Then he/she can call the number if the transfer is unsuccessful, or if he/she wants to call the number later. If possible, stay on the line to assure that transfer is completed.

• When taking messages, be sure to get the caller's name and company affiliation, date and time of the call, complete telephone number, and any additional information the caller provides. Repeat the message to assure that you have taken it correctly.

Remember that good telephone manners are always in order. Be pleasant, be professional, and offer to help the caller. Also, use a pleasant "thank you for calling" rather than a "bye-bye," and allow the caller to hang-up before you do.

Most of today's Central Service Technicians are common users of electronic mail (e-mail). E-mail and traditional (hardcopy) memos share some things in common. For example, both create opportunities for misspelled words (although spell check systems in word processing software reduce the problem during e-mail communication). Also, there is still a need to carefully study the message. Is the content correct? Is it presented as clearly as possible? How is it likely to be interpreted by the reader?

There are, however, some things unique to or, at least different from, common written memos:

• People other than the intended receiver may read the message when it is sent.

• Messages might be sent to the wrong mailbox. (If the message is confidential or contains frank comments, e-mail may not be the best communication medium.)

• E-mail may not be received for numerous reasons. If a timely response is not received, a friendly follow-up query is typically in order.

• Remember that phrases and e-mail symbols used by experienced e-mail writers may confuse rather than communicate.

• If possible, limit the message to one screen (or, hopefully, much less!) to eliminate the need for a reader to scroll up and down through an extensive message. Remember, the purpose of e-mail is to quickly and effectively communicate important information, not to entertain.

• It is typically best to use e-mail for messages that require urgent attention.

• Don't let e-mail become a substitute for personal and telephone conversations.

• All types of communication including "old-fashioned" letters and memos and "new" e-mail techniques can be improved by remembering the human aspects in communication. A personal salutation, a thank-you, and the ever-appropriate "please" are always in order. While technology enables quick and effective communication, empathy, thoughtfulness, and courtesy will always be important in effective communications.

Whose Technology is it?

Healthcare facilities and the Central Service Departments within them have invested significant financial resources in communications technology. It is increasingly difficult for many people to imagine how they could cope in their professional and personal lives without seemingly constant access to the wide variety of computers, copiers, printers, fax machines, telephones, and other electronic communication equipment that is available. With its convenience, however, comes the opportunity for misuse when facility equipment is used for personal purposes (examples: shopping on the internet, sending personal e-mail, and photocopying private materials). Problems include unproductive time away from the job, increased facility expenses for supplies, and the blurring of the distinction between acceptable and unacceptable work practices.

Most facilities have policies that address these and related concerns. They are often addressed in Codes of Ethics, and clearly identified in employee handbooks or other documents. Professional Central Service Technicians know about these policies, understand their importance, and consistently comply with them.

HUMAN RELATIONS

Learning Objective 4. Practice procedures to enhance and maintain effective working relationships.

Earlier in this chapter the term, "human relations," was defined as the development and maintenance of effective interpersonal (between people) relationships that enhance teamwork. Central Service Technicians may have the knowledge and skills required to do their job correctly, but they cannot be successful unless they know how to "get along" with their supervisors, peers, and others.

Professional Central Service employees have the following human relations concerns:

- They try to understand each of their fellow employees as individuals and, when possible, to incorporate this understanding into how they interact with other staff members.

- They help other employees to achieve their highest possible levels of job satisfaction.

- They increase their contributions to their team because this benefits the team, the facility, and their profession.

- They develop a genuine spirit of cooperation and teamwork among themselves, their peers, and those at higher organizational levels.

It is relatively easy to talk about human relations skills and the positive impact they have on the organization. It is, however, much more difficult for Central Service Technicians to consistently apply these skills. The world of work requires staff members to interact with many employees with differing backgrounds, interests, challenges, and job responsibilities. These are among the factors that make it increasingly difficult to practice the "art and science" of human relations.

Fortunately, some techniques of human relations are really "common sense," and are used by many professional Central Service employees because they involve the use of principles that are relatively easy to recall. Other principles may require new philosophies about working and interacting with peers. While these are more difficult to use, they are also necessary.

Many observers of the world of work believe that managers and supervisors cause many of the problems that occur in the workplace. This may be true for problems including resource allocation, scheduling, training (or lack of it), layout, design, and equipment availability in the Central Service Department, and related concerns. However, Central Service Technicians are also integral to the team, and they must accept some responsibility for and share in the issues that affect the success of their department. To do so, they must have the appropriate knowledge and skills (topics of the other chapters in this book), and effective interpersonal skills (the topic of this chapter).

There are numerous ways that Central Service Technicians apply their human relations skills on the job. These include:

- Doing all that is reasonably possible to maintain sound working relationships with supervisors, peers, and others in the health care facility.

- Acting in a professional manner as discussed earlier in the chapter.

- Serving as a contributing member of the department and facility team.

- Accepting the responsibility to continually learn and, when applicable, helping their peers to do so as well.

- Promoting cooperation among their peers. This is done by helping others, by sharing knowledge and experience, and by trying to understand the perspectives of other persons.

CENTRAL SERVICE TECHNICIANS AND TEAMWORK

Learning Objective 5. Discuss tactics to improve teamwork.

Improving Teamwork

To be successful, every Central Service Department requires people working in different positions. Individuals must work as part of a team because the work they do relates directly to that being done by others. Consider, for example, that the main goal of every Central Service Technician, like all other staff members employed by the facility, is to help the patients. Everyone must work together as a team to assure that the patients are best served. If employees do not perform their work correctly, the consequences can be tragic.[2]

Employees cannot do their work without the help of others. This is another reason why teamwork is so important. What one does (or does not do) affects the work of others, and the success (or failure) of the Central Service Department.

Teamwork is beneficial to the facility in other ways as well. For example, it can:

- Increase patient satisfaction levels through increased awareness of employees' roles.

- Improve productivity through increased staff cooperation and reduced interpersonal competition.

- Increase employees' job satisfaction.

- Improve the work environment by creating a common agenda (purpose) for the staff.

- Decrease job-related stress.

> **Attitude** – *A person's emotions or willingness that cause him/her to react in a predetermined way to people or situations.*

Teamwork Factors

Several factors must be present for teamwork to occur:

- Attitude – A proper **attitude** is the most important factor necessary for teamwork. The attitudes of Central Service Technicians about their job, peers, and patients affect their actions. An employee's attitude is often influenced by co-workers. If one is part of a team in which everyone gets along, likes their jobs and the facility, and wants to provide good service, each staff member will probably have a good attitude. This helps to make the team even stronger. By contrast, if a co-worker does not like the job, supervisor, or the facility and does not care about the quality of work, teamwork will suffer.

- Cooperation – To provide good service, one must be willing to help and work with other employees.

- Promptness – When an employee is late to work or does not show up, this affects other employees. The remaining members of the team must work harder, and/or goals related to work quantity and quality standards suffer.

- Loyalty – A good member of a team trusts co-workers and supervisors. At the same time, co-workers and supervisors trust each team member.

Figure 22.4 lists characteristics of successful groups.

Types of Groups

Central Service Technicians are members of two types of work groups: formal groups and informal groups. Teamwork concerns are important for both types.

A health care facility is comprised of a formal group of employees who, at the highest organizational level, have the same

Figure 22.4 Characteristics of Successful Groups
Successful groups generally share the following characteristics:

1. Common goals are defined and accepted by group members.
2. Group members cooperate as a team.
3. Group members have the resources necessary to attain goals.
4. Group members help each other.
5. The atmosphere within which group members work is comfortable.
6. Group members participate in discussions about matters affecting the group.
7. Group members are creative; they contribute ideas without fear of ridicule.
8. There can be 'healthy" disagreement between group members.
9. There is generally group consensus – not just a simple majority – about decisions affecting the entire group.
10. Group members do not subjectively criticize each other's ideas or positions.
11. Group members feel free to express their feelings.
12. Assignments are made and accepted when action must be taken.
13. There is seldom a power struggle between group members.
14. The group leader does not always dominate nor does group attention focus on "who controls." Instead, "what must be done" is the primary concern of group members.
15. Group members know how the group operates.

boss: the Hospital Administrator and Board of Directors. As staffing plans are developed, smaller work groups are established. The facility is divided into several large units and one, Materiel Management, typically becomes responsible for specific functions including Central Service. One formal group, the Central Service Department, provides, among other functions, sterilization and supply services for other departments. Work in the

Central Service Department may be divided into still other formal groups including those relating to specific work units and work shifts.

Each formal work group has a formal leader responsible for coordinating, directing, and controlling the work group.

A task group is another example of a formal group. Members work together to perform essentially non-routine activities. For example a committee might address a specific concern, and a work team can develop a job breakdown for training purposes. After the work of a task group is completed, the group is typically dissolved.

Informal groups develop for several reasons including common interests of members, a desire to be "close" to others in a similar situation, economic reasons, and a desire to satisfy specific but common personal needs. Examples of informal groups may include employees who take lunch or other breaks together, participate in after-work activities, and those who car-pool.

Informal work groups are not necessarily "good" or "bad" because they can assist, harm, or have no impact on the facility's efforts to attain goals. Informal groups frequently develop an informal communication system called the "grapevine." This system can spread rumors or provide helpful information depending on the situation.

You've learned that common interests influence persons to become affiliated with informal groups. It is unlikely, then, that Central Service Technicians with positive attitudes about the facility and work will be drawn to informal groups comprised of members who do not share these concerns.

Teamwork and Decision-Making

Two other aspects of teamwork are important, and both involve decision-making. Hopefully, managers and supervisors recognize the advantages to group decision-making. If they do, Central Service Technicians have great opportunities to generate and evaluate alternatives for decision-making and/ or problem resolution concerns that address their department. As they do so, they bring the benefit of their knowledge, experience, and "common sense" to the process by which patients are better served, and their organizations become more successful.

In some health care facilities, Central Service Technicians enjoy another opportunity to participate in the decision-making process: participation in cross-functional teams: a group of employees from different departments within the health care facility that works together to resolve operating problems. Consider, for example, a problem that involves instruments that are not available when needed in the operating room. A traditional problem solving approach in which operating room personnel address the problem may determine that the majority of concerns relate to those in the Central Service Department. While these observations may be correct, there may be other potential causes of the problem that relate to operating room personnel. Therefore, a **cross-functional team** comprised of Operating Room, Central Service, and staff from other departments may yield creative alternatives that would not be considered when only a group with a more narrow focus addressed the issue.

Special Teamwork Concerns

Central Service Technicians may experience anxiety and tension when they begin their employment and join their new team. Most are seeking affirmation that their decision to work at the facility was a good one and, therefore, new job experiences, both positive and negative, are very meaningful. An evolutionary process beginning with uncertainty and mistrust will, hopefully, evolve into mutual respect and trust. Then, new staff members will begin to communicate candidly with other members of the team. Mutual activities such as group decision-making is the next step in the process and, over time, cooperation rather than competition becomes commonplace. Then group members find satisfaction in and become committed to working towards the group's success because the members have common goals.

The process described above applies to both formal groups and to their informal counterparts. Groups become stronger as each of the above stages evolve. For example, if problems arise during the early stages of group affiliation, it may be difficult to resolve them. By contrast, mature groups confronting the same problems often generate creative and effective solutions. In all instances, successful groups emphasize the development and attainment of mutual goals.

Experienced Central Service Technicians should consider how they felt when they first began work. This can help to provide empathy for their recently-employed peers who probably have the same concerns, and who desire to have the same questions addressed. Facility and department orientation programs should provide much basic information. However, this does not replace the friendly "helping hand" that experienced Central Service Technicians can provide for their recently employed peers.

Teamwork is affected by the ability of the group to adapt to members of different cultural backgrounds, of different ages, and who speak different native languages. These and related concerns along with other diversity-related issues will be discussed next.

CENTRAL SERVICE TECHNICIANS AND DIVERSITY

Learning Objective 6. Define the term, "diversity," explain why it is important, and review how Central Service Technicians can develop a "diversity mind-set."

What is Diversity?

The concept of **diversity** has received a great deal of attention in modern organizations. To some, it means providing equal opportunities to persons of selected characteristics such as age, gender, mental/physical abilities, sexual orientation, race, or ethnic

Cross-functional team – A group of employees from different departments within the healthcare facility that works together to resolve operating problems.

Diversity – The broad range of human characteristics and dimensions that impact the employees' values, opportunities, and perceptions of themselves and others at work.

heritage. To others, the concept implies responses to legal concerns such as for equal employment opportunities. In fact, diversity should be defined in the broadest possible way so that all employees are included, and everyone's diversity is valued.[3]

A reasonable definition of "diversity" might separate the entire population into the six characteristics noted above. Those mentioned do influence how everyone experiences the world. In addition, however, there are numerous secondary dimensions that also shape one's values, expectations, and experiences. These include education, family status, organizational role and level, religion, first language, income, geographical location, and numerous others. As you can see, then, every person is unique, and brings special qualities to the job that influences his or her attitudes about it, and opportunities to contribute to it.

Many persons argue that a diversity effort should be implemented and kept on-going because "it is the right thing to do." However, it is also possible to make a strong business case for a diversity effort. Advantages include:

- A welcoming and rewarding work environment encourages excellent job performance.

- The changing make-up of the U.S. labor force increasingly requires the employment of those with diverse personal dimensions.

- When persons are valued, turnover and absenteeism are minimized, and associated costs are reduced.

- A culture of understanding, respect, and cooperation encourages teamwork with its benefits.

- Diverse backgrounds create more creative alternatives as decisions are made, and as problems are resolved. (Recall our discussion about employee input to decision-making, and the use of cross-functional teams in the previous section.)

Equal Employment Opportunity and Affirmative Action Programs Are Different From Valuing Diversity Efforts.

Equal Employment laws and Affirmative Action address the prevention and/or correction of employment practices that discriminate against individuals based on age, color, disability, Vietnam-era veteran status, national origin, race, religion, and gender. Affirmative Action programs are implemented to address these types of discrimination. Their goal: to close gaps by establishing targets and time frames to modify race and gender profiles in organizations. Many organizations that are exempt from these requirements implement programs to better match their employee profile to that of the external labor pool.

Organizations that implement valuing diversity efforts move beyond race and gender concerns, and attempt to provide an environment that is welcoming and rewarding for every staff member. The goal is to move beyond satisfying legal requirements to address environmental concerns, to improve productivity, and to increase morale. In other words, these organizations attempt to create cultures in which diversity is desired because it yields the full utilization of the diverse talents of every staff member.

How is a valuing diversity effort implemented? It does not happen because top-level officials require it, nor does it occur because the Central Service Director desires it. As well, it is not a "program" in which a committee "decides what to do," and an employee training effort follows. Instead, valuing diversity represents a significant organizational culture change that must have the on-going commitment from those mentioned. However, it must also have buy-in from employees in every department throughout the facility.

Implementing Diversity Efforts

Basic change management strategies are required to successfully implement a valuing diversity effort. People typically respond to new ideas in predictable ways based on the extent to which they tolerate perceived risk. Those who perceive little or no risk in valuing diversity view it as a creative opportunity, and will endorse the concept first. Those who are more cautious about exploring new ideas will view diversity as desirable after it has been proven useful in the facility. Other staff members with the highest level of perceived risk see diversity as changing the "status quo" (how things have always been). They will mistrust it, and will be interested in keeping things as they are.

Strategies to implement a valuing diversity effort should begin by involving those to see its value, and should recognize that those employees who are anxious about and/or fearful of it are not likely to change their attitudes quickly. There are no "quick fix" implementation plans to "convince" employees that a valuing diversity mind-set is useful. Instead, it involves life-long learning, personal commitment, and on-going self-improvement. In other words, it involves a change in attitude.

Central Service Technicians who value diversity have some basic beliefs that form the framework for their mind-set:

- Valuing diversity requires a change in the organizational culture, and these change efforts never end.

- When diversity is valued, benefits accrue to employees and to their health care facility.

- Efforts to implement diversity efforts should include everyone, because every staff member brings diverse attitudes, backgrounds, and experiences to the job.

- Everyone benefits when the organization values the diversity of all of its staff members.

It typically takes longer than leaders initially believe to change an organizational culture. Attitudes that have built-up over many years and that have passed down through many generations must be changed. Even when it becomes an accepted organizational goal, it will take a long time for many employees to value diversity, and some staff members are unlikely to ever accept it.

Central Service Technicians working for facilities with diversity goals should maintain a long-term vision of their purpose and desired results. They can do their part by respecting all staff members, by cooperating and participating in efforts to implement a valuing diversity emphasis, and by recognizing that it is an effort that will never end. They should also recognize that all employees want to be recognized for who they are and appreciated for what they do. As well, all staff members want to feel comfortable with whom they work. They want to believe that their input is valued, and that they have some impact on the decisions that affect them. As the importance of diversity is better recognized and addressed in the workplace, the basic human needs of all staff members will be better recognized.

CUSTOMER SERVICE SKILLS FOR CENTRAL SERVICE TECHNICIANS

Learning Objective 7. Practice basic customer service skills, and utilize tactics to appropriately handle customer complaints.

Basics of Customer Service

Customer service relates to the relationship between the Central Service team and its customers. These customers include anyone who utilizes its services including doctors, nurses, clinicians, and patients. The communication and human relations skills being discussed in this chapter are very important for all Central Service Technicians. One brief positive (hopefully) or negative (unfortunately) encounter with a customer can leave a lasting impression about the entire department that will be passed on to other customers.

Providing a service is not always easy. Some customers of the Central Service Department are the direct patient caregivers who, themselves, have customers (the patients). Central Service personnel must be committed to provide excellent support service so their counterparts throughout the facility can provide excellent service and care to the ultimate customer: the patient.

Providing top-quality service requires the consistent dietary of products and services that meet standards of departmental performance. Each employee must possess shared values, beliefs, and work ethics that support the facility's and department's goals.

Each functional area and work shift in Central Service depends on others. The quality of each step in the reprocessing cycle is affected by previous and subsequent steps. If decontamination and cleaning procedures are not done effectively or in a timely manner, the sterilization process may not be effective, and/or products may not be available when needed. Just as the quality of a finely crafted watch is dependent upon the detailed working mechanisms of each tiny part, Central Service is dependent on the performance and contribution of each team member. Central Service Technicians must function as a team to achieve quality customer service.

With practice, one can improve customer relations skills. Self-discipline and control are very important, especially in difficult encounters. Keep focused on real issues, maintain composure, and don't allow emotions or personalities to influence performance goals. Be objective when it is necessary to say no to a request. Explain the reasons and offer alternatives. Honesty is always the best policy; never make excuses. If an error occurs, admit it, and work toward a resolution. Credibility and trust are essential, and the customers trust must never be betrayed.

It helps to personalize services, to get to know customers, and to use their names. This will make them feel important and good. Provide your full attention and find ways to handle special requests. Cheerful, courteous, and friendly behavior projects the proper image, and is great for promoting customer service. The provision of good service requires Central Service Technicians to constantly assess the quality of their services. Follow-up on commitments and solicit feedback. Quality service is a reflection of professionalism, and it requires maturity, self-esteem, competence, confidence, and a positive attitude.

Emergencies and crisis situations are a reality in the health care environment, and then stress and tension can mount. Even then emotional stability must prevail because anxiety cannot be transmitted to the customer at a time when prompt service is most required.

Cooperation with Operating Room Personnel[4]

No two departments in a typical health care facility work more closely than do personnel in Surgery and Central Service. The outcome of every patient procedure depends on effective communication and cooperation between personnel in these two departments. They work within a fast-paced, ever-changing environment and, therefore, communication can break down, and relationships can become strained.

Much of the relationship between Surgery and Central Service staff relies on mutual trust. Trust, however, is earned, and the actions and responses to issues of employees in both departments build or erode the trust necessary to reduce communication roadblocks.

Differences between systems used by both departments can create communication challenges. Slang terms, jargon, and nicknames used to describe medical instruments and supplies may not be familiar to all staff working in both departments. Also, instrument and supply needs change (often several times a day) and, if information doesn't travel smoothly, frustrations can increase, and relationships can be damaged.

There are several ways to enhance communication between the Surgery and Central Service departments. Sometimes, for example, a specific issue should first be addressed. At other times, a broader tactic such as a survey to identify and prioritize communication roadblocks may be best. After a specific issue is selected, it should be addressed without assigning blame to individuals or work groups. Instead, the focus should be on identifying and correcting problems. A questioning process can be used:

- Is adequate training provided for the task?

- Does everyone involved in the process under stand their role?

- Is there adequate equipment and are expectations realistic?

- Do other factors interfere with the process?

Hopefully, Central Service Technicians are involved in the process used to define and address these and related questions.

After problems are identified, staff from both departments can work together to resolve them. By taking the personal element out of the process, staff can focus on the issues without allowing personal frustrations and feelings to impact the problem solving process.

Communication between staff in the Surgery and Central Service departments should not just occur when an incident has occurred, or after the issue has been identified. Instead, it should be on-going. Joint projects can be completed, or a solution that addresses mutual concerns can be identified and implemented. Also, simple actions such as showing appreciation for the efforts and assistance of personnel in the other department can help establish a bond between both groups.

Central Service Technicians Interact With Patients

Patients are very special customers of the Central Service department. They are the reason health care employees have a job! The satisfaction of their needs must be at the top of the list of a Central Service Technician's professional responsibilities and priorities. Here are some tips for improving patient relations:

- Always look professional: neat and well-groomed.

- Perform your job well, and have pride in the work and facility. Staff performance has a significant impact upon the patients' health and well-being, and their attitudes about the facility.

- Follow applicable service strategies that focus on patients.

- Solicit ideas about ways to be more patient friendly from customers.

There is an old saying that the customer is always right. A slight modification (the patient is always right) suggests a philosophy that should guide service standards used to provide a high quality of products and services to patients. In today's competitive health care environment, the patients' perceptions about the facility and the word of mouth impact that their experiences have on the community become additional reasons why Central Service Technicians must consistently practice effective patient relations.

Handling Customer Complaints

In spite of the best procedures and protocols, and staff members who are trained to follow them, customer complaints can arise. Hopefully, the facility endorses the concept of **empowerment.** Then Central Service Technicians can more easily resolve customer complaints than other staff members without the authority to suggest resolution alternatives. Modern business text books use a new term, **"service recovery"**, to explain the procedures by which customer complaints can be handled, and empowered employees are integral to this approach.

Figure 22.5 reviews tactics in a service recovery model. Use of these tactics can typically help to satisfactorily address customer complaints.

Empowerment –The act of granting authority to employees to make key decisions within the employees' areas of responsibility.

Service recovery –The sequence of steps used to address customer complaints and problems in a manner that yields a win-win situation for the customer and the department.

Figure 22.5 Steps in Service Recovery Process

Tactic	Tactic in Action
1. Acknowledge the customer.	This service recovery example involves an operating room nurse who is alleging that an improper instrument set has been delivered.
2. Carefully listen to the customer's problem.	The nurse explains that the proper instrument set must be delivered immediately.
3. Remain calm and give undivided attention.	The Central Service Technician who is speaking with the operating room nurse gives her complete attention, and is not distracted by anything in the area.
4. Ask questions.	"Farrah, I'm sorry about the mix-up. What instrument set do you need?"
5. Empathize with the customer.	"It must be very frustrating when this problem occurs. I know this is a serious problem, and I know it must be taken care of immediately."
6. Apologize for the problem, and accept responsibility to resolve it.	I'm very sorry, Farrah, I'll be right there with the instruments you need.
7. Do not justify or place blame.	The Central Service Technician does not tell the nurse that the instrument set delivered is that which was ordered. He does, however, know that this information must be relayed to the Central Service Director who can initiate discussions to help assure that problems with instrument set descriptions do not continue.
8. Provide time frame for remedial action.	I can return within five minutes with the instruments you need
9. Monitor problem resolution progress.	The Central Service Technician cannot be distracted as he returns to the department, and returns with the correct instrumentation.
10. Follow-up with the customer.	The Central Service Technician (or his supervisor who has been notified) later contacts the operating room nurse to confirm that the problem was resolved.
11. Learn from the experience.	This customer complaint has identified a problem. Since it has been brought to the attention of the Central Service Director, corrective action can be taken to reduce the possibility that improper instrument sets are delivered in the future.

SPECIAL HUMAN RELATIONS CONCERNS

Learning Objective 8. Review concerns applicable to handling promotions, relating experience to job success, setting priorities, and committing to patient care during disasters.

There are, seemingly, innumerable human relations concerns and issues that are confronted by Central Service Technicians. This chapter has presented detailed information about several important concepts, and will conclude with a brief review of several others.

Handling Promotions

Many Central Service Technicians who perform their jobs well have opportunities for promotion to positions with additional responsibilities and higher compensation levels. Those that accept these positions will likely find many differences in tasks, especially if they assume supervisory duties. Challenges arise when a staff member who has been a peer (co-equal) to other employees then becomes their supervisor. Relationships change, and friendships on the job and, probably, off the job as well, must reflect the new supervisor-**subordinate** relationship.

Supervisors must consider the broader needs of the department and the health care facility before the specific needs of individual staff members. However, this is difficult to do when they have personal (friendship) relationships with some of those whom they supervise.

Central Service Technicians considering promotions should also recognize that some tasks will be different. One with the knowledge and skills to perform cleaning, decontamination, and related tasks may not be as comfortable performing supervisory activities such as planning, coordinating, directing, controlling, and evaluating. As well, even if these and related responsibilities appear interesting, one should recognize the need

> **Subordinate** – *An employee who is supervised by someone in a higher organizational position.*

for, probably, extensive training and experience to become proficient.

Long-term planning leading to promotion decisions should be an integral part of career management considerations of interested Central Service Technicians. Details about this process go beyond the scope of this chapter.[5]

Relating Experience to Job Success

Experience should, but does not always, impact job success. For example, a Central Service Technician may note that he or she has 20 years of experience in the profession. In effect, however, this staff member may really have one year of experience that was repeated 20 times! The usefulness that experience brings to the work situation is not the same as time on the job. In the fast-paced world of Central Service, on-going professional development and continuing education is absolutely critical for one to make a full contribution. Unfortunately, experience can encourage some persons to find shortcuts, to inform newly-employed staff members about how things should really be done, and to develop an attitude of entitlement. (I've been here so long, and I've done so much; I am owed for it!)

By contrast, experience can be invaluable because it provides insight about what has and has not been successful in the past. This type of input is important when experienced staff members are encouraged to be part of the participative decision-making process, or when individuals serve on cross-functional teams.

Experience can improve the knowledge, skills, and common sense that helps Central Service Technicians to be successful. However, it is interesting to note (and most Central Service Managers will agree) that problem employees are frequently not those with the inability to effectively perform physical aspects of their job. Instead, unsuccessful staff members are most typically those with attitudinal problems and/or an inability (unwillingness) to appropriately interact with others. Experience can improve one's human relations skills. However, these skills are also affected by one's attitudes about people. Unfortunately, attitudes are more difficult to change and, in many instances, this is increasingly true as years on the job increase.

Setting Priorities

Basic work tasks for Central Service Technicians are determined in job descriptions, and others may be specified as employee schedules are developed. Experienced Central Service staff members realize that numerous unexpected challenges occur frequently, and can have a significant impact on the work to be done. Professional Central Service Technicians are willing to do whatever reasonable work tasks are assigned when the task is assigned, because managers have a "big picture" overview of what needs to be done that is unavailable to others.

The most significant priority is anything that can be done to assist with a patient or other emergency. This is the time when careful compliance with instructions and providing assistance is most needed.

Teamwork has been emphasized throughout this chapter. It provides another example of setting priorities. When peers need help, and when one's supervisors or managers request assistance, these instances should receive a priority over other activities that can be postponed.

There may be times when Central Service Technicians have some freedom to decide what they wish to do. How should priorities be established in these instances? The most important things should be done first, and these might be identified by asking questions such as:

* What is the most important part of my job?

* What few things make the biggest difference in how I perform my job?

* What task would I want done if I were the supervisor?

* What is the best use of my time right now?

* What can I do to help my team?

* What are things I've been waiting to do until I get around to it? (That time might be available now.)

Central Service Technicians who work smarter not harder may be able to enjoy the opportunity to better manage their work and, in the process, will be able to make more contributions to their department.

Committing to Patient Care During Disasters

No one can forecast when disasters will occur. However, each health care facility including Central Service departments within it should anticipate the most likely crises that may arise. Then plans that incorporate the most appropriate responses to these crises can be developed. Training staff members who will implement the disaster plans is an important next step after their roles have been identified.

What are appropriate actions of Central Service Technicians in the event that their facility must respond to disasters? Here are several:

* Study your department's and hospital's disaster plans, and ask questions, if necessary. Make sure you thoroughly understand your role and that of your department if a disaster occurs.

* Take disaster drills seriously. When you have practiced your department's response tactics, you will be able to react more quickly, efficiently, and confidently if there is a need to implement emergency plans.

* Keep your department informed of your current telephone number so an accurate call back roster will be available if it is needed.

* Think about what you would do in the event of an actual disaster. Make personal plans that will allow you to support patient care. For example, have a back-up arrangement for child care and family communications if you must remain at the hospital for an extended time.

• Remember to keep calm and positive during a disaster. The stress level will be high, and making a conscious effort not to add to the stressful environment will help everyone.

• Focus on your job, and what is needed to meet the patients' needs.

• Recognize that your knowledge, skills and experience are an integral part of your facility's emergency response, and your efforts as part of the Central Service team are critical to save lives.

• Do not share patient information with anyone outside of the hospital including your family and friends. If you are asked for general information about the emergency and your facility's response, know and refer those who inquire to the appropriate spokesperson identified in the facility's disaster plan.

IN CONCLUSION

The work of Central Service Technicians is very challenging because of the vast amount of knowledge and skill that is necessary to perform their job. Their work is, at the same time, critical to patient care. In the course of their work, these professionals must utilize a wide array of communication and human relations skills. There are a few, if any, positions in a health care environment where more science (technical knowledge) and art (interpersonal skills) is needed. Professional Central Service Technicians have the people skills necessary to effectively interact with internal customers (their peers in the Central Service department) and their external customers (all other persons with whom they must interact while on the job).

ENDNOTES

1. This and the following section are adapted from: Ninemeier, J. Supervision Principles: Leadership Strategies for Healthcare Facilities. Second Edition. Chicago, Il., International Association of Health care Central Service Materiel Management, 1997. (Chapter 14).

2. For detailed information about teamwork see: Ninemeier, J. Supervision Principles: Leadership Strategies for Healthcare Facilities. Second Edition. Chicago, Il, International Association of Health care Central Service Materiel Management, 1997. (Chapter 12). Some of the information in this section is adopted from this reference.

3. This section is loosely adopted from: Marilyn Loden. Implementing Diversity. Boston, Ma. McGraw- Hill. 1996.

4. This section is adapted from: Enhancing Cooperation between the Central Service and Operating Room Departments. International Association of Healthcare Central Service Materiel Management. Self-Study Lesson Series. Lesson #88. May, 2006.

5. Readers interested in additional information about career management are referred to: Ninemeier, J. Supervision Principles: Leadership Strategies for Healthcare Facilities. Second Edition. Chicago, Il, International Association of Healthcare Central Service Materiel Management, 1997. (See Chapter 16)

CENTRAL SERVICE TERMS

Communication

Human relations

Jargon

Stereotype

Feedback

Coaching

Attitude

Cross-functional team

Diversity

Empowerment

Service recovery

Subordinate

Chapter Outline

Chapter 23

Sterile Processing for Ambulatory Surgery and Other Practices

Chapter Learning Objectives

As a result of successfully completing this chapter, readers will be able to:

1. Review basic similarities and some differences between sterile processing in hospitals and other healthcare facilities.

2. Explain basic standards and practices used for sterile processing in ambulatory surgical centers:
   - Overview and History
   - Ownership and Regulatory Standards
   - Accreditation Standards
   - ASC Processing Personnel
   - Processing Environment

3. Explain basic standards and practices used for sterile processing in dental facilities:
   - Environmental Issues
   - Instrument Processing Procedures

4. Provide an overview of Veterans Administration (VA) facilities, and list sterile processing differences between VA and other healthcare facilities.

STERILE PROCESSING SCIENCE IS UNIVERSAL

Learning Objective 1. Review basic similarities and some differences between sterile processing in hospitals and other healthcare support facilities.

Most Central Service Technicians serve patients in for-profit and not-for-profit hospitals. However, the profession also extends to other types of healthcare and healthcare support facilities. Surgical instruments and equipment are prepared or used for patient care and treatment in ambulatory surgical centers, dental facilities, Veterans' Administration (VA) institutions, and clinics. Veterinary hospitals, third party reprocessing operations, and some manufacturers also require sterile processing skills for some of their operations. Someone in these facilities must insure that the items are safely processed between uses and/or that the items, along with disposable supplies, are ready when needed. While titles differ, persons with these responsibilities perform the duties of Central Service Technicians.

Even though the type of facility may vary, the science behind cleaning, disinfection, and sterilization does not change, nor does the need for knowledge of medical terms and skills related to human relations, quality, and customer service. Information presented in this Technical Manual is important regardless of where Central Service duties are performed.

However, the processes by which some types of facilities are regulated, their structure, and the types of services performed, may differ from traditional hospital settings, and this chapter provides an overview of some of these operations that require Central Service skills. For example, while all facilities have the same goal of providing quality patient care, different regulations and standards have, in some cases, led to modifications of some standards and practices detailed earlier. This chapter will create an awareness of other systems and related practices that may be encountered as one explores the broad dimensions of the Central Service discipline. However, certification from the International Association of Healthcare Central Service Materiel Management is driven by the Association for the Advancement of Medical Instrumentation (AAMI) standards, and by the recommended practices, standards, and regulations outlined in previous chapters of this text.

AMBULATORY SURGERY CENTERS

Learning Objective 2. Explain basic standards and practices used for sterile processing in ambulatory surgical centers:
- Overview and History
- Ownership Regulatory Standards
- Accreditation Standards
- ASC Processing Personnel
- Processing Environment

Ambulatory Surgery Centers (ASCs) provide selected surgical and procedural services that do not require hospital admission.

Overview and History

Ambulatory surgery centers are not urgent care facilities, rural health care centers, or physicians' offices. All surgery centers must have at least one dedicated operating room and the equipment necessary to perform safe surgical procedures to ensure quality patient care.

Before the mid-1970s, virtually all surgery was performed in hospitals. Over time, selected surgical procedures began to be performed in physicians' offices. As they proved to be a successful and growing alternative to hospital inpatient services, surgeons began to develop surgical facilities outside of traditional hospital environments.

Although many hospitals have outpatient departments that provide surgical services, these are typically part of the facility itself, and not a stand-alone facility. Hospital outpatient departments (HOPDs) offer the benefit of overnight services for patients requiring extended recovery times,

Ambulatory surgery center – A healthcare facility that allows patients to have selected surgical and procedural services performed that do not require hospital admission.

and/or in single- or multi-specialty stand-alone facilities. Some specialize in gastroenterology (GI), and provide services for diagnostic and/or minor minimally invasive surgical procedures done endoscopically including colonoscopies and proctoscopies. Others provide services for minimally invasive opthalomological (eye) procedures including those for cataract removal, to treat glaucoma, and for laser services that do not require hospitalization. Sports medicine has become an avenue for specialty ASCs providing surgical procedures including arthroscopies, ACL reconstruction, and minor fracture repairs.

Multi-specialty ASCs can provide all procedures within one facility. In addition, surgical procedures provided by ambulatory surgery centers may include the following:

- Cosmetic
- Facial Plastic & Reconstructive
- Gastroenterology
- General Plastic
- General
- OB/GYN
- Opthalomological
- Oral/Maxillofacial
- Orthopedic
- Podiatry
- Urology
- Cardiovascular /Vascular

The first ASC was organized in 1970 by physicians in efforts to provide patients with high quality, cost-effective surgical services as an alternative to inpatient hospital care. Their subsequent development has allowed physicians to find a better way of dealing with Operating Room (OR) scheduling delays, limited OR room availability,

and the challenges of obtaining new equipment due to hospital budget constraints.

Ownership and Regulatory Standards

Physicians are involved in the ownership of approximately 90% of all ASCs. Many are jointly-owned by local hospitals and physicians as hospitals have become increasingly aware of their value. Approximately 20% of existing ASCs have hospital ownership interest, and 3% are owned entirely by hospitals.[1]

Healthcare facilities, including ASCs, are highly regulated by federal and state agencies. Most states require ASCs to be licensed, and each state determines licensure requirements which include initial and on-going reporting and on-site inspections.

Medicare has reimbursed ASCs for applicable patient services since 1982, and those serving Medicare patients must be certified by the Medicare program to comply with federal government standards. The scope of surgical procedures reimbursed by Medicare is tightly controlled by federal regulations. They generally limit services to elective procedures with short anesthesia and operating times that do not require an overnight stay. The number of Medicare-certified ASCs has grown from 2786 in 1999 to 4506 in 2005, an annual growth rate of 8.3%.[2]

Growth Will Continue

The number of ambulatory surgical centers is likely to continue to grow for three primary reasons: advances in technology that will create additional minimally invasive procedures, faster acting and more effective anesthetics, and an aging population that will continue to place greater demands on the need for increased numbers of surgical procedures.

***Accreditation** – A voluntary process by which an organization measures the quality of its services and performance against nationally recognized standards.*

Accreditation Standards

Accreditation is a voluntary process by which an organization measures the quality of its services and performance against nationally recognized standards. It is usually accomplished through a comprehensive review of a facility's compliance with recognized standards and on-site inspection surveys undertaken by an independent accrediting organization. The concept of accreditation began in hospitals, but it is now achievable and sought after by stand-alone healthcare facilities as well.

Accreditation is viewed as a distinction of quality and excellence, and ASCs seek accreditation from one of four organizations:

- Joint Commission

- Accreditation Association of Ambulatory Health Care (AAAHC)

- American Association of Accreditation of Ambulatory Surgery Facilities (AAAASF)

Sterility Assurance Guidelines

The ANSI/AAMI ST79:2006 Comprehensive Guide to Steam Sterilization and Sterility Assurance in Healthcare Facilities includes sterility assurance guidelines for ambulatory surgery settings in its recommended practices. Additionally, AORN includes ambulatory surgery facilities in its recommended practices. Note: this organization references ST 79 in the development of its guidelines and recommended practice statements.

- American Osteopathic Association (AOA)

ASC Processing Personnel

Infection control plays an important role in the continuous effort to provide education for best practices in the ambulatory setting. Many facilities do not have a dedicated sterile processing practitioner. Instead, an RN staff member, RN manager, or Surgical Technologist is often appointed and educated about the role of infection control, referencing guidelines and best practices provided by the Association for Professionals in Infection Control and Epidemiology (APIC). The standards and best practices of ambulatory surgery facilities for decontamination and sterilization should be no different than those applicable to a hospital setting.

The surgery environment in an ASC is fast-paced, and turnover of instrumentation must be done quickly and efficiently. Those responsible for terminally cleaning and sterilizing instrumentation do so at the end of each day, picking cases for the following day's OR schedule, stocking disposable inventory, and maintaining sterile storage areas.

ASCs with multiple OR suites may employ trained Central Service Technicians, and may additionally require certification as an employment prerequisite. Placing sterility assurance in the hands of persons trained and experienced in decontamination and sterilization practice allows OR staff to focus on the needs of the patients and directly assist the surgeons.

As ASCs thrive and expand, and as surgical instrumentation continues to evolve, and as procedures become less invasive, the demand for certified Central Processing Technicians in the ASC setting will grow.

Processing Environment

You've learned that Central Service professionals in ASCs must work in a fast-paced environment. Demands of the OR require moving between processing areas throughout the day, and flexibility, patience, and a sound knowledge of infection control protocols are necessary.

The instrument processing area is typically in close proximity to the OR suites, and is often centered around them to provide easy access. Central Service Technicians do not typically work within an OR setting and, at first, the need to work directly with OR staff may seem very different from the more traditional relationship between these professionals. In most ASC facilities, Central Service Technicians work along side OR staff to accomplish the day's tasks, and they must consistently use best practices and professional know-how as they do so.

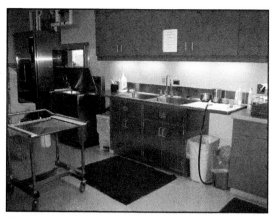

Figure 23.1

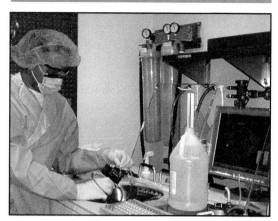

Figure 23.2

The configuration of the decontamination and sterilization areas varies greatly between facilities depending on the size and the type of specialty services provided. However, the work flow from "dirty" to "clean" is necessary regardless of the facility's layout.

Most facilities have a decontamination area with a sink for sorting and manual cleaning, and automated cleaning equipment that may include ultrasonic cleaners and automatic washer/decontaminators. (See **Figure 23.1**) These areas may also contain automated endoscope reprocessors, (See **Figure 23.2**) high level disinfection set-ups, and/or low temperature sterilizing units.

The need to use the equipment manufacturers' recommendations for cleaning and sterilizing surgical instrumentation is applicable to any facility that reprocesses reusable surgical instrumentation. Careful attention must be paid to the reprocessing of single- or limited-use surgical instrumentation.

As in any decontamination area, the best practices of proper personal protective equipment (PPE) and adherence to Standard Precautions are always important. The need for quick or rapid turnover of instrumentation never negates the use of best practices for patients or staff members. Policies and procedures should be established to provide consistent and accountable practice.

Proper monitoring of low temperature automated and non-automated disinfection/ sterilization units is critical in facilities where non-dedicated staff

perform cleaning/decontamination procedures. The more people involved in a process the more likely errors may occur. Accurate record keeping for disinfection/sterilization processes is necessary, and this provides a method of tracking any possible lapses in best practice policies and procedures.

The area dedicated to instrument assembly and sterilization can also vary greatly in configuration between facilities. Typically this area houses the unsterile instrument inventory, and wrapping, packaging, and labeling equipment much as in a hospital's Central Service setting. Sterilizers used for wrapped and peel pouch packaged instrumentation are also usually located in this area. Sterilization methods may include use of steam sterilizers, gas plasma units, and/or ozone sterilization units. Smaller facilities may use table top sterilizers.

The volume of surgical procedures that can be done less invasively and, therefore, more quickly, means there is usually a limited number of sets for each case. This may result in the need for flash sterilization of sets after sterile sets have been used. Central Service professionals may need to prepare instruments for flash sterilization and, in some situations, initiate the sterilization process.

Ethylene oxide gas sterilization is not generally used in ASCs, in part because of the need for a more efficient turnover of instrumentation, installation constraints, and environmental concerns.

The role of Central Service professionals in

ambulatory surgical settings enables them to contribute best practices in all reprocessing areas from decontamination to sterile storage. Their employment represents another area of growth for IAHCSMM members, and their continued dedication to education and professionalism will provide many future opportunities.

DENTAL FACILITIES

Learning Objective 3. Explain basic standards and practices used for sterile processing in dental facilities.
- Environmental Issues
- Instrument Processing Procedures

Dental facilities commonly require decontamination, sterilization, and inventory management activities. The range of instruments processed by dental facilities includes items from basic instrumentation to complex instruments such as powered hand pieces. (See **Figure 23.3**) Dental professionals must insure that their practices provide a safe environment and experience for their patients.

The Centers for Disease Control (CDC) has outlined guidelines for the sterilization and disinfection of patient care items in dental facilities.[3] This resource addresses environmental issues and instrument processing procedures which are summarized below.

Environmental Issues

The instrument processing area in a dental facility should be divided into four sections:

- Receiving, cleaning, and decontamination.

- Preparation and packaging.

- Sterilization.

- Storage.

Ideally, these areas should be separated by walls or partitions. If not possible, they should be separated by adequate space. The goal: to minimize the risk of cross-contamination between soiled and clean areas.

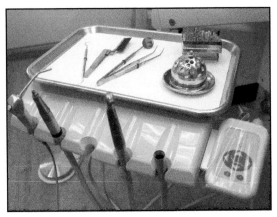

Figure 23.3

Environmental infection control concentrates on **environmental surfaces** which are surfaces or equipment that do not contact the patient directly, but may become contaminated during patient care. Examples of environmental surfaces include light switches, power unit switches, and drawer knobs. Environmental surfaces are separated into two categories: clinical contact surfaces and housekeeping surfaces.

Clinical contact surfaces are environmental surfaces that can be directly contaminated during patient care. This usually results from sprays, spatter, or direct contact with a dental healthcare professional's gloved hand. Examples of clinical contact surfaces include light handles, switches, chair side computers, drawer and faucet handles, and countertops. Clinical contact surface

Environmental surfaces (infection control) – *Surfaces or equipment that do not contact the patient directly, but may become contaminated during patient care; examples: light and power unit switches and drawer knobs.*

Clinical contact surfaces (infection control) – *Environmental surfaces that can be directly contaminated during patient care; examples: from sprays, spatter, or direct contact with a dental professional's gloved hand.*

Housekeeping surfaces (infection control) – *Environmental surfaces such as floors, walls, and sinks that pose a risk of disease transmission.*

contamination is minimized and controlled by the use of specialized barrier products, and by routine cleaning and disinfection between patients.

Housekeeping surfaces are environmental surfaces such as floors, walls, and sinks. These areas also pose a risk of disease transmission, and should be cleaned on a regularly scheduled basis, and whenever they are visibly soiled.

In addition to environmental guidelines, there are guidelines for dental instrument processing.

Instrument Processing Procedures

Contaminated instruments should be transported in an enclosed container from the point of use to the receiving, cleaning, and decontamination area. Items should be processed as soon as possible after use and, if they cannot be processed in a timely manner, they must be kept moist to prevent soil from drying on them.

Dental healthcare professionals must select the cleaning option (manual or automatic) that best fits the instrument's cleaning specifications. (See **Figure 23.4**) Regardless of the option chosen, items must be thoroughly cleaned. Inadequate cleaning can result in a failed disinfection or sterilization process which can endanger patients and staff.

While working in the receiving, cleaning, and decontamination area, the risk of exposure to blood borne pathogens is high, and all workers must wear PPE to insure their safety.

Preparation and Packaging

Before sterilization, all items must be inspected and prepared for sterilization. (See **Figure 23.5**) General guidelines for sterilization preparation include inspecting instruments for soil and functionality, unlocking hinged instruments, and any other tests or inspections that are required by the instruments' manufacturers.

After inspection and assembly, items should be prepared for sterilization. For unwrapped loads, a chemical indicator should be placed in each tray. For wrapped loads, a chemical indicator should be

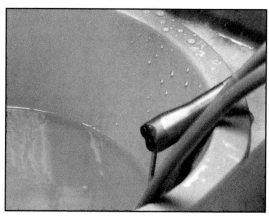

Figure 23.4

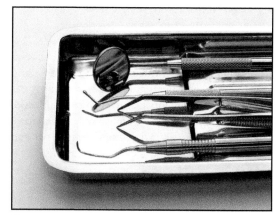

Figure 23.5

placed inside each tray or package and, since that indicator will not be visible after the sterilization process, an external chemical indicator must also be used. For example, chemical indicators are usually visible after sterilization processes in paper-plastic peel pouches, but they may not be visible in cassettes or wrapped trays. Only approved sterilization packaging materials should be used.

Sterilization

Sterilization in dental facilities is most often performed using steam under pressure, dry heat sterilization, or unsaturated chemical vapor. In addition to these primary methods, liquid chemical sterilization and ethylene oxide gas sterilization are sometimes used. It is important to follow the sterilizer manufacturer's recommendations for all sterilization methods.

Steam under pressure is the most common form of sterilization performed in dental facilities because it is dependable and economical. Dental facilities typically use tabletop steam sterilizers. Most are gravity displacement sterilizers; however pre-vacuum sterilizers are becoming more common.

Dry heat sterilizers are used in dental facilities to sterilize items such as burrs and certain orthodontic instruments that may be damaged by moist heat. Dry heat sterilization is economical and non-corrosive, but it requires high exposure temperatures and long cycle times so it is generally not suitable for all sterilization needs.

Two basic types of dry heat sterilizers are used in dental facilities. Oven-type sterilizers are constructed with heating coils on the bottom and sides of the chamber, and they heat the load contents through natural convection. Rapid heat transfer sterilizers circulate heated air throughout the chamber at a high speed to quicken heat transfer and reduce sterilization times.

Unsaturated chemical-vapor sterilizers heat a chemical solution (usually a mix of alcohol and formaldehyde) in a pressurized chamber. This process is less corrosive than steam sterilization on carbon steel instruments such as dental burrs, and cycle times are less than with dry heat sterilization.

Liquid chemical germicides such as glutaraldehyde, peracetic acid, and hydrogen peroxide are also used in dental facilities as sterilants or high level disinfectants. With all chemical sterilization and disinfection processes, care must be taken to handle each chemical in compliance with manufacturer's instructions.

Dental facilities employ sterilization quality assurance methods such as cycle monitoring, biological testing, and chemical indicators to measure sterilization process parameters.

Storage

Dental facilities should store sterile items in enclosed cabinets, if possible. Care should be taken

to protect the integrity of each package, and each sterile package should be inspected before use for signs of contamination.

Dental facilities should have clearly written procedures for all decontamination, inspection, packaging, sterilization and storage processes, and all employees who work within those processes should receive training.

VETERANS ADMINISTRATION (VA) FACILITIES

Learning Objective 4. Provide an overview of Veterans Administration (VA) facilities, and list differences between VA and other healthcare facilities.

"To care for him who shall have borne the battle and for his widow, and his orphan." This is the motto for the U.S. Department of Veterans Affairs, and President Abraham Lincoln first used the phrase in his second inaugural address in 1865. It is inscribed on most (if not all) VA cemeteries, hospitals, and office buildings, and is a grand charter the VA strives to achieve.

Overview

VA hospitals are located throughout the United States, and a Supply, Processing and Distribution (SPD) department performs Central Service functions for each facility.

The Department of Veteran's Affairs has its own certification program that is only offered to current SPD employees in VA operations. All SPD employees are expected to complete the program.

Annual continuing education units (CEUs) to maintain VA Certification differ by position:

- Chiefs of SPD - 20 CEUs.

- Supervisory personnel - 17 CEUs.

- SPD Technicians - 5 CEUs.

SPD employees in VA facilities must comply with regulations called Directives which are contained in VA Directives 7176.[4] This document outlines the requirements of SPD operations relating to organizational structure, employee development, infection control, inventory management, safety standards, decontamination, preparation area, loading/operating sterilizers, distribution, inventory, equipment tracking, and quality control.

Practice Differences

Some differences between VA processing requirements and those of other healthcare facilities include:

- VA facilities do not permit an indefinite shelf life for reprocessed products. Items in inventory for more than one year must be reprocessed, if applicable.

- Third party reprocessors are not used. VA facilities must use the services of other VA sites if additional sterilization activities must be performed.

- No single use disposable products are reprocessed.

- Two wrappers sequentially wrapped must be used for wrapped items or trays to provide aseptic opening and maintain a sterile field.

- SPD Technicians must use heat-seal peel pouches because of concerns about the consistent proper sealing of self-seal peel pouches.

- Requirements prohibit writing on packaging material because of concerns that the integrity of the packaging material will be compromised. One must write on sterilization tape that is then placed on the package.

- All items must undergo a sterilization process before moving to the preparation area for further processing.

- Biological tests must be incubated and read at 48 hours. Three hour enzyme tests can be used; however, 48 hour readings are still required and must be documented.

- Validation of reprocessed products is not performed by VA personnel. Only those recommendations used on the manufacturer's approved 510K application are allowed.

- Use of internal chemical indicators is at the discretion of SPD personnel.

- Sterilization of solutions is not permitted.

There are other different requirements; however the ones listed above are some of the main differences. The thought behind some of the differences is to assure that the practices used in the VA are proven practices for providing the best care available to the veteran.

Additional Related Practices

Types of Central Service functions are also performed in clinics, veterinary hospitals, third party reprocessing facilities, and some manufacturers. As mentioned at the beginning of this chapter, it is safe to say that wherever instruments, equipment and supplies are needed for patient care, there is a need for Central Service skills.

ENDNOTES

1. *Foundation for Ambulatory Surgery in America, Physician Ownership of Ambulatory Surgery Centers, Alexandria, VA, 2006. (www.fasa.org)*

2. *American Association of Ambulatory Surgery Centers, Ambulatory Surgery Centers; A Positive Trend in Healthcare, Johnson City, TN, 2006. (www.aaasc.org)*

3. *Centers for Disease Control. Guidelines for Infection Control in Dental Health-Care Settings. Washington, D.C. 2003.*

4. *Department of Veterans Affairs, VA Directive 7176, Washington D.C. 2006.*

CENTRAL SERVICE TERMS

Ambulatory surgical centers

Accreditation

Environmental surfaces (infection control)

Clinical contact surfaces (infection control)

Housekeeping surfaces (infection control)

Glossary

A

AAMI Short for Association for the Advancement of Medical Instrumentation.

ABC analysis Inventory management strategy that indicates storeroom controls should first address the relatively few items with the greatest value (A items), and should lastly consider the many items with the lowest value (C items).

abdomen Part of the body between the chest and the pelvis.

abduction Movement away from the midline; turning outward.

abort Failed or incomplete machine cycle caused by a malfunction.

abrasive Any of a wide variety of natural or manufactured gritty substances used to grind, wear down, rub away, smooth or scour.

abscess Area of tissue breakdown; a localized space in the body containing pus and liquefied tissue.

absolute pressure (steam sterilizer) Gauge pressure (machine produced) + atmospheric pressure (14.7 pounds per square inch at sea level).

absorbent towel All-cotton towel having a plain weave with only the warp yarns tightly twisted.

acceptance sampling Inspection of a sample from a larger lot to decide whether the lot should be accepted.

ACGIH Short for American Conference of Governmental Industrial Hygienists.

acid Compound with a pH of less than 7.0 with a sour, sharp, or biting taste; a compound with a water solution that contains positive hydrogen ions (for example, HCl).

acid detergent Organic, acid-based cleaning agent, best used for removing mineral deposits.

acid-fast bacteria Bacteria that do not de-colorize when acid is added to the stained smear.

acidity Measurement of the amount of acid present.

acidosis Condition that results from a decrease in the pH of body fluids.

acid scrubber Type of EtO emission control device.

acquired immune deficiency syndrome Viral disease that attacks the immune system; commonly abbreviated "AIDS."

acquired immunity Immunity acquired by a person after birth.

action level For certain chemicals, the airborne concentration of an air contaminant, calculated as an 8-hour time-weighted average, above which particular monitoring, medical surveillance, or other stated Occupational Safety and Health Administration requirements apply.

acute Short in time; relatively severe in degree.

acute disease Disease that runs a rapid course with more or less severe symptoms.

adhesion Holding together of two surfaces or parts; a band of connective tissue between parts that are normally separate; the molecular attraction between contacting bodies.

adipose Referring to fatty tissue.

adrenal Endocrine gland located above the kidney; suprarenal gland.

aerate To expose gas-sterilized items to warm, circulating air.

aeration Process in which a device is actively subjected to moving air; example: items being sterilized with ethylene oxide gas.

aerator (ethylene oxide) Machine designed to speed up removal of ethylene oxide residuals from sterilized items by subjecting them to warm, circulating air.

aerobe Microorganism that requires the presence of air or oxygen for growth.

aerobic (bacteria) Those capable of growing in the presence of free oxygen; requiring oxygen.

aerosol Suspension of ultramicroscopic solid or liquid particles in air or gas; a spray.

affinity Attraction.

agar Extract of red seaweed used as a solidifying agent in culture media.

AIDS Short for Acquired Immune Deficiency Syndrome; the advanced symptomatic and ultimately fatal disease in the progression of an HIV infection.

airborne Suspended or carried in a gas or air stream.

air count Method of estimating the number of bacteria or microbes in a specific quantity of air.

albumin Protein in blood plasma and other body fluids that helps to maintain the osmotic pressure of the blood.

alimentary canal Pathway that food takes through the body's digestive system.

alkalies Chemicals which release an excess of hydroxyl ions (OH) in a solution to yield a pH of more than 7.

alkaline In solution; having a pH greater than 7.

alkalosis Condition that results from an increase in the pH of body fluids.

alkylation Process by which Ethylene Oxide destroys microorganisms resulting in the inability of the cell to normally metabolize and/or reproduce.

allergen Substance that causes hypersensitivity; substance that induces allergy.

allergic Caused by allergy.

allergy Tendency to react unfavorably to a certain substance that is normally harmless to most people; hypersensitivity.

alveolus (pl. alveoli) One of millions of tiny air sacs in the lungs through which gases are exchanged between the outside air and the blood; tooth socket.

ambient condition Environmental conditions such as pressure, temperature, and humidity which are normal for a specific location.

ameba (pl. amebas) Protozoon that moves by extruding finger-like elements (pseudopods); also spelled amoeba (pl.amoebae).

amebiasis Infection with pathogenic amebas; acute amebiasis is called amebic dysentery.

amino acid Building block of protein; organic chemical compounds containing an amino group and a carboxyl group, which form the chief structure of proteins.

amitosis Direct cell division.

amniocentesis Removal of fluid and cells from the amniotic sac for prenatal diagnostic tests.

amniotic sac Fluid-filled sac that surrounds and cushions the developing fetus.

amoeboid movement Crawling movement of cells that occurs as the cell successively becomes longer and then retracts.

anaerobe Microorganism that grows only or best in the absence of oxygen.

anaerobic (bacteria) Capable of growing in the absence of free oxygen; not requiring oxygen.

analgesic Relieving pain; a pain-relieving agent that does not cause loss of consciousness.

anaphylaxis State of hypersensitivity to a protein resulting from a previous introduction of the protein into the body; can result in death without treatment.

anastomosis Surgical or pathological formation of a passage between two normally distinct structures such as tubular organs.

anatomy Study of body structure.

anemia Reduction in the amount of red cells or hemoglobin in the blood resulting in inadequate delivery of oxygen to the tissues.

anesthesia Loss of sensation (particularly of pain).

aneurysm Bulging sac in the wall of a vessel.

angina Severe choking pain; disease or condition producing such pain.

angina pectoris Suffocating pain in the chest usually caused by lack ofoxygen supply to the heart.

angstrom Unit of measure for visible light.

animate Having life.

anion Negatively charged particle (ion).

anionic Compounds with a negative electrical charge on the large organic portion of the molecule which are relatively hydrophobic and lipophilic; used as synthetic detergents.

anorexia Loss of appetite.

anoxia Lack of oxygen.

ANSI Short for American National Standards Institute.

antagonist Muscle with an action opposite that of a given movement; substance that opposes the action of another substance.

anterior Toward the front or belly surface; ventral.

anthrax Infectious disease of cattle and sheep caused by a spore-forming bacterium (Bacillus anthracis) which may be transmitted to man through handling of infected products.

antibacterial serum Antiserum that destroys or prevents the growth of bacteria.

antibiotic Substance produced by one microorganism that will kill or inhibit another microorganism.

antibody Protein produced in the body which reacts against a specific foreign molecule (antigen).

antigen Substance which causes the body to produce antibodies.

antiseptic Solution which inhibits the growth of bacteria; usually used topically and only on animate objects.

antiserum Serum containing antibodies given to provide passive immunity.

antitoxin Immune serum which neutralizes the action of a toxin.

anus Lower opening of the alimentary canal.

anvil One of the three middle ear bones; attaches to the hammer and stirrup.

AORN Short for Association of Operating Room Nurses; also known as The Association of peri-Operative Registered Nurses.

aorta Largest blood vessel in the body.

APIC Short for Association of Practitioners in Infection Control.

aqueous humor Watery-like fluid between the cornea and the eye lens.

aqueous solution Liquid in which a chemical substance is dissolved in water.

areriole Vessel between a small artery and a capillary.

arrhythmia Abnormal rhythm of the heartbeat.

arteries Vessels that carry blood away from the heart.

arteriosclerosis Hardening of the arteries.

arthritis Inflammation of the joints.

asepsis Absence of microorganisms that cause disease.

asepsis (medical) Procedures performed to reduce the number of microorganisms to minimize their spread.

asepsis (surgical) Procedures to eliminate the presence of all microorganisms, and/or to prevent the introduction of microorganisms to an area.

aseptic Free from pathogenic organisms; a means of preventing infection.

aseptic technique Activity or procedure that prevents infection or breaks the chain of infection.

ASHCSP Short for American Society of Healthcare Central Service Personnel.

asphyxia Condition caused by lack of oxygen in inspired air.

aspirate To draw by suction; examples: when fluid is removed with a syringe and material is drawn into the lungs during inspiration.

asset Something of value owned by an organization or person.

asset (current) Asset that is expected to be used within one year.

atherosclerosis Hardening of the arteries caused by deposits of yellowish, fat-like material on blood vessel linings.

atom Fundamental unit of a chemical element.

atria The two upper chambers of the heart.

atrium One of the two upper chambers of the heart.

atrophy Wasting or decrease in size of a part.

attenuated Weakened. attitude A person's emotions or willingness that cause him/her to react in a predetermined way to people or situations.

austenitic (stainless steel) Non-magnetic stainless steel that cannot be heat-hardened, and which is more corrosion-resistant than martensitic stainless steel; also called 300 series stainless steel..

autoclave Equipment that uses steam under pressure to sterilize, usually at temperatures of 250° or 270°F (121°C or 132°C).

automated supply replenishment system Replenishment system in which items removed from inventory are automatically identified and tracked. When a reorder point is reached, item information is generated on a supply pick list in the central storeroom. Items are then issued, and transferred to the appropriate user area.

automatic endoscope reprocessor (AER) Automated equipment designed to clean, disinfect, and rinse flexible endoscopes.

autonomic nervous system Part of the nervous system that controls smooth muscle, cardiac muscle, and glands; motor portion of the visceral or involuntary nervous system.

autopsy Examination of the internal organs of a dead body.

axilla Hollow beneath the arm where it joins the body; armpit.

B

bacillus (pl., bacilli) Rod-shaped bacteria; a genus of the family Bacillaceae.

bacillus atrophaeus Resistant microorganism used to challenge Ethylene Oxide sterilizers.

bacillus stearothermophilus See geobacillus stearothermophilus.

bacillus subtilis See bacillus atrophaeus.

bacteremia Condition in which bacteria are in the bloodstream.

bacteria (sing. bacterium) Single-celled, plantlike microbes that reproduce by splitting; some cause diseases; also called "germs."

bacterial count Method of estimating the number of bacteria in a sample unit.

bactericidal Relating to the destruction of bacteria.

bactericide Substance that kills bacteria.

bacteriology Science of the study of bacteria.

bacteriophage Virus that parasitizes and multiplies exclusively in bacteria.

bacteriostasis Condition in which bacterial growth is inhibited, but the organisms are not killed.

bacteriostat Substance that inhibits the growth of bacteria.

bacteriostatic Inhibition of bacterial growth without their destruction.

balance sheet Financial summary of what a healthcare facility owns (assets), owes (liabilities), and is worth (equity) at a specific point in time (example: the last day of every month).

bar code Numerous machine-readable rectangular bars and spaces arranged in a specific way to represent letters, numbers, and other symbols.

barrier cloth Fabrics made of blends or cotton/polyester.

barrier properties Ability of a material to resist the penetration of liquids and/or microorganisms.

basal ganglia Gray masses in the lower part of the forebrain that assist with muscle coordination.

base Compound with a pH above 7.0, a compound whose water solution yields negative hydroxyl ions (example: NaOH), and combines with an acid to form a salt and water; turns red litmus paper blue.

basophil Granular white blood cell that shows large, dark blue cytoplasmic granules when stained with basic stain.

BCG (Bacillus of Calmette-Guerin) Vaccine against tuberculosis made from a bovine strain of tubercle bacilli attenuated through long culturing.

benign Tumor that does not spread, is not recurrent or becoming worse; not malignant.

bevel Angle at which the point of a needle is ground.

bile Substance produced in the liver that emulsifies fats.

binary fission Typical method of bacterial reproduction in which a cell divides into two equal parts.

bioburden Number of microorganisms on a contaminated object; also called bioload or microbial load.

biodegradable Readily decomposed by bacteria or enzymatic actions.

biofilm Matrix that contains living and dead cells and a polysaccharide that is exuded by microorganisms when they grow in water or water solutions or in vivo (example: the bloodstream). Biofilm prevents antimicrobial agents such as sterilants, disinfectants, and antibiotics from reaching microorganisms.

biohazard signage Notices in easily-seen locations that alert persons about the presence of harmful bacteria, viruses, or other dangerous biohazardous agents or organisms.

biohazardous Relating to infectious agents that present a risk or potential risk to human health either directly through infections or indirectly through the environment.

biological Relating to biology.

biological indicator (BI) Sterilization process monitoring device consisting of a standardized, viable population of microorganisms (usually bacterial spores) known to be resistant to the mode of sterilization being monitored.

biological transfer of infection Mode of transfer of infection from host to host by an animal or insect in which the disease-causing agent goes through a development cycle.

biology Science which studies living things, both animals and plants.

biomedical engineering department Hospital department that performs safety inspections and function tests on medical equipment; frequently abbreviated "Biomed Department."

biopsy Removal of tissue or other material from the living body for examination, usually under the microscope.

blood Connective tissue fluid that transports many substances throughout the circulatory system.

borosilicate Alkaline-free silicate glass having at least 5% boric oxide and used especially in heat resistant glassware; a very hard glass (Pyrex).

botulism Food poisoning caused by the toxin of an anaerobic, spore-forming bacterium, (clostridium botulinum) in contaminated canned or smoked foods.

Bowie Dick Test Test run daily to validate the vacuum function of the sterilizer. The test should be run in an empty load, and at the same time of the day each day.

box locks Point where the two jaws or blades of an instrument connect and pivot.

bradycardia Heart rate of less than 60 beats per minute.

brain Main control unit of the central nervous system.

brain stem Controls many automatic body functions such as heartbeat and breathing.

broad-spectrum Term indicating that an antibiotic is effective against a large array of microorganisms.

bronchi Tubes extending from the trachea into both sides of the lungs.

bronchiole One of the small bronchial subdivisions that branch throughout the lungs.

brownian motion Dancing motion of finely divided particles in suspension.

buffer Substance that prevents sharp changes in the pH of a solution.

bursa Small, fluid-filled sac in an area subject to stress around bones and joints.

C

calibration Comparison of a measurement system or device of unknown accuracy to a national standard of known accuracy to detect, correlate, report, or adjust any variation from the required performance limits of the unverified measurement system or device.

cancer Uncontrolled growth of a tumor that spreads to other tissue; a malignant neoplasm.

cannulas Surgical instruments with a hollow barrel (or lumen) through their center; often inserted for drainage.

capillaries Vessels that connect veins and arteries.

capillary action Attraction or repulsion force caused by the surface tension of liquids in hair-like tubes.

capital equipment Item of major importance; usually defined by a set dollar amount and which is depreciated over the useful life of the equipment rather than being expensed at purchase.

capsule Gelatinous, colorless envelope or slime layer surrounding the cell wall of certain microorganisms; a membrane or sack containing a body part.

carbohydrate Simple sugar or compound made from simple sugars linked together.

carbon dioxide Gaseous waste product of cellular metabolism; CO_2.

carcinogen Cancer-causing substance.

carcinoma Malignant growth of epithelial cells; a form of cancer.

cardiopulmonary resuscitation Method to restore heartbeat and breathing by mouth-to-mouth resuscitation and closed chest cardiac massage; also called "CPR."

carditis Inflammation of the heart; myocarditis .

career ladder Plan projecting progressively more responsible professional positions that serves as a foundation for a professional development program.

caries Tooth decay.

carpals Wrist bones.

carrier Individual who harbors and disseminates specific pathogenic microorganisms without manifesting clinical symptoms, and who serves as an intermediary in the transfer of diseases to a susceptible person.

cartilage Type of flexible connective tissue.

case cart pull sheet (pick list) List of specific supplies, utensils, and instruments used to assemble the items needed for individual surgical procedures.

case cart system Inventory control system for products/ equipment typically used in operating room. An enclosed cart is generally prepared for one special surgical case and is not used for general supply replenishment.

CAT Scan See computed tomography.

catalyst Substance which influences the speed of a chemical reaction without being consumed.

catalytic converter Type of Ethylene Oxide emission control device.

cataract Opacity of the eye lens or lens capsule.

catheter Slender, flexible tube of rubber, plastic, or metal used for draining a body cavity or injecting fluids through a body passage.

cation Positively charged particle (ion).

cation resin tank Tank into which untreated hard water flows, and in which sodium ions are exchanged for calcium and magnesium ions to produce soft water.

cationic Compounds containing a positive electrical charge on the large organic hydrophobic molecule which exhibit germicidal properties.

causative agent (chain of infection) – Microorganism that causes an infectious disease.

caustic Corrosive and burning; agent, particularly an alkali, that will destroy living tissue.

cautery Burner; a means of destroying tissue by electricity, heat, or corrosive chemicals. Thermocautery consists of a red hot or white hot object, usually a wire or pointed metallic instrument, heated in a flame or with electricity.

cavitation Process used by an ultrasonic cleaner in which low-pressure bubbles in a cleaning solution burst inward to dislodge soil from instruments.

CDC Short for Centers for Disease Control (part of the The Department of Health and Human Services) whose primary function is to investigate outbreaks of and control various diseases.

cecum Small pouch at the beginning of the large intestine.

ceiling limit According to OSHA: "the employee's exposure (to an air contaminant which shall not be exceeded during any part of the work day. If instantaneous monitoring is not feasible, then the ceiling shall be assessed as a 15-minute time-weighted average exposure which shall not be exceeded at any time over a working day;" see also threshold limit value.

cell Basic unit of life; the smallest structural unit of living organisms capable of performing all basic life functions.

cell membrane Outer covering of a cell; regulates what enters and leaves cell.

cellulitis Diffuse inflammation of connective tissues.

centigrade Thermometer temperature scale with 100° between the melting point of ice at 0° and the boiling point of water at 100°.

central nervous system Part of the nervous system that includes the brain and spinal cord; abbreviated CNS."

centrifuge Device used to spin test tubes; used in the laboratory.

cerebellum Second largest part of the brain that controls muscle coordination, body balance, and posture.

cerebrospinal fluid Fluid that circulates in and around the brain and spinal cord; a bbreviated "CSF."

cerebrovascular accident Condition involving bleeding from the brain or obstruction of blood flow to brain tissue, usually resulting from hypertension or atherosclerosis; abbreviated "CVA;" also called stroke.

cerebrum Largest part of the brain that controls mental activities and movement.

cervix Constricted portion of an organ or part; neck.

CFC (chlorofluorocarbon) Inert (inflammable) gas often mixed with a flammable gas to create an inflammable solution; has been used with Ethylene Oxide to create an inert gas..

challenge test pack Used in qualification, installation, and on-going quality assurance testing of hospital sterilizers.

chamber Enclosed area that holds products to be sterilized.

chelating agents Chemicals that hold hard water minerals in solution, and prevent soaps or detergents from reacting with the minerals.

chemical indicators (CIs) Systems that reveal a change in one or more predefined process parameters based on a chemical or physical change resulting from exposure to a process.

chemical sterilization Process using a chemical agent to render a product free of viable microorganisms.

chemotherapy Treatment of disease without injury to patient with chemicals having a specific effect on microorganisms.

chickenpox Varicella; a rather mild, highly contagious virus disease characterized by fever and the appearance of vesicles.

chisels Wedge-shaped instruments used to cut or shape bone.

CHL Short for Certification in Healthcare Leadership(International Association of Healthcare Central Service Materiel Management)

CHMMC Short for Certification in Healthcare Materiel Management Concepts (International Association of Healthcare Central Service Materiel Management)

chloride Compound commonly found in water created when chlorine is combined with another element or radical; examples: salt and hydrochloric acid.)

chlorophyll Molecule in plants that absorbs sunlight, and converts it to energy in process called photosynthesis.

cholesterol Organic, fat-like compound found in animal fat, bile blood, myelin, liver, and other parts of the body.

chromium Blue-white metallic element found naturally only in combination and used in alloys and electroplating.

chromogenic Producing a pigment.

chromosome Rod-shaped masses of chromatin appearing in the cell nucleus during mitosis which play an important part in cell division and transmit the cell's hereditary characteristics..

chronic Referring to a disease (illness) that is not severe but is continuous, recurring, protracted, and prolonged.

cilia (sing. cilium) Hairlike elements that spring from certain cells and, by their action, create currents in liquids; if the cells are fixed, the liquid is made to flow, if the cells are unicellular organisms suspended in the liquid, the cells move.

circumduction Circular movement at a joint.

cirrhosis Chronic disease (usually of the liver) in which active cells are replaced by inactive scar tissue.

CIS Short for Certified Instrument Specialist (International Association of Healthcare Central Service Materiel Management)

CJD (Creutzfeld-Jakob Disease) Brain debilitating fatal disease; see prions.

class 5 (chemical integrators) Integrating indicators designed to react to all critical parameters over a specified range of sterilization cycles.

cleaning Removal of all visible and non-visible soil, and any other foreign material from medical devices being reprocessed.

clostridium Genus of cylindrical-shaped bacteria which are anaerobic, gram-positive, and spore-forming.

coaching Positive reinforcement used to encourage Central Service Technicians to follow proper work practices, and negative reinforcement to discourage inappropriate work practices.

coagulase Enzyme that causes coagulation or clotting of blood serum.

coagulation Clotting (as of blood).

coccus Round-shaped (spherical) bacterium.

coccyx Tail bone.

cochlea Coiled portion of the inner ear that contains the organs of hearing.

cold boil Cavitation which is not dependent upon heat for its bubbling action.

coliform bacteria Group of intestinal microorganisms of which Escherichia coli is a member.

collagen Flexible white protein that gives strength and resilience to connective tissue including bone and cartilage.

colon Main portion of the large intestine.

colony Visible growth of microorganisms seen in culture medium; usually obtained from a single organism.

colony count Determination of the number of visible clumps of bacteria derived from the multiplication of specific microorganisms on or in a culture medium.

combining vowel Letter, usually an "o," sometimes used to ease the pronunciation of a medical term.

combustible Substance that, if ignited, will react with oxygen and burn.

combustible loading Weight of combustible materials per square foot of area in which the materials are located.

combustion Chemical process accompanied by the rapid production of heat and light.

commissioning (installation qualification) Obtaining and documenting evidence that equipment has been provided and installed in accordance with its specifications, and that it functions within predetermined limits when operated in accordance with operational instructions.

communicable Disease whose causative agent is easily transmitted from person to person by direct or indirect contact.

communication Process of transmitting information and understanding from one person to another by use of words and non-verbal expressions including body language.

complication Secondary illness imposed upon a person with a primary illness.

compound Substance composed of two or more chemical elements.

computed tomography Imaging method in which multiple x-ray views taken from different angles are analyzed by computer to show a cross section of an area; used to detect tumors and other abnormalities; abbreviated "CT" or "CAT" (computed axial tomography).

conditioning Treatment of products within the sterilization cycle but before sterilant admission to attain a predetermined temperature and relative humidity; may be carried out at atmospheric pressure or under vacuum.

conduction Heat transfer method in which heat is absorbed by an item's exterior surface, and passed inward to the next layer.

conduction heating Process in which heat is transmitted in a solid substance from molecule to molecule by molecular impact or agitation.

conductivity (of water) A measurement of the ability of water to carry an electrical current.

congenital Present at birth.

conjunctiva Membrane that lines the eyelid, and covers the anterior part of the sclera.

conjunctivitis Inflammation of the conjunctiva of the eye.

contagious Highly communicable; easily transmitted.

contaminate To render unfit for use through introduction of a substance which is harmful or injurious.

contamination State of being soiled or infected by contact with infectious organisms or other material.

continuous quality improvement (CQI) Scientific approach which applies statistical methods to improve work processes.

contraception Prevention of fertilization of an ovum or implantation of a fertilized ovum; birth control.

convalescence Period during which recovery takes place following illness.

convection Process of heat transfer by the circulation of currents from one area to another.

convection heating Transfer of heat in a fluid or gas from one place to another by the motion of the fluid or gas.

copious Present in a large amount (such as large volume of rinsing water).

cornea Clear portion of sclera that covers the front of the eye.

coronary Referring to the heart or to the arteries supplying blood to the heart.

corrosion Act of wearing away gradually by a chemical reaction.

corrosive Having the power to corrode or wear away.

cortex Outer layer of an organ such as the brain, kidney, or adrenal gland.

counterstain Second stain of a contrasting kind applied to a smear for the purpose of making the microorganisms treated with a primary stain more distinct.

CPR Short for cardiopulmonary resuscitation.

CPU Short for central processing unit.

craze Spider web cracking of plastics under chemical stress.

CRCST Short for Certified Registered Central Service Technician. (International Association of Healthcare Central Service Materiel Management)

crisis Change in a disease which indicates whether the result will be recovery or death.

critical devices (Spaulding medical device classification system) Instruments or objects introduced directly into the bloodstream or other normally sterile body areas.

critical parameters Parameters that are essential to the sterilization process and that require monitoring.

cross-contamination Migration of contaminants from one person, object, or work location to another.

cross-functional team Group of employees from different departments within the healthcare facility that work together to resolve problems.

cross-infection Infection acquired from an animate or inanimate contaminated environment, usually accidentally.

culture Growth of microorganisms on a nutrient medium; to grow microorganisms on such medium.

culture medium Substance or preparation used for the growth and cultivation of microorganisms.

customer (internal) Physicians, nurses, and other professional personnel served by Central Service personnel.

cutaneous Referring to the skin.

cyanosis Bluish color of the skin and mucous membranes resulting from insufficient oxygen in the blood.

cycle buying Purchasing method in which an order is placed at a scheduled interval.

cycle (gravitation-displacement type; steam sterilization) Sterilization cycle in which incoming steam displaces residual air through a port or drain in or near the bottom of the sterilizer chamber.

cycle (sterilization) Defined sequence of operational steps designed to achieve sterilization; carried out in a sealed chamber.

cycle time Total elapsed time of a sterilization cycle from when the sterilizer door is closed and the cycle is activated until the cycle is completed and the door is opened.

cystitis Inflammation of the urinary bladder.

cytology Study of cells.

cytoplasm Living matter of a cell between its membrane and nucleus.

D

D-value Amount of time required to kill 90% of the microorganisms present.

debridement Surgical removal of dead or unhealthy tissue.

decontamination Removing or reducing contamination by infectious organisms or other harmful substances.

decontamination area Location within a health care facility designated for collection, retention, and cleaning of soiled and/or contaminated items.

defecation Act of eliminating undigested waste from the digestive tract.

defect Variance from expected standards.

deflocculate To reduce or break up into very fine particles.

degeneration Breaking down (as from age, injury, or disease).

degerm To remove bacteria and other microbes by mechanical cleaning and applying antiseptics or disinfectants.

dehydration Excessive loss of body fluid.

deionization Process by which ions with an electrical charge are removed from water.

deionize To remove ions from (as water by ion exchange); demineralize.

denatured alcohol Alcohol that has been rendered unfit for use as a beverage by the addition of substances which impart an unpleasant odor and taste (examples: wood alcohol and benzene).

density Degree of compactness; closely set or thickness.

deoxyribonucleic acid (DNA) One of two nucleic acids; essential for biological inheritance.

dermatitis Inflammation of the skin.

dermis True skin; deeper part of the skin.

detergent Cleaning agent composed of a "surface wetting agent" which reduces surface tension, a "builder" which is the principle cleaning agent, and a "sequestering" or "chelating agent" to suspend the soil; detergents may also have additional additives such as blood solvents or rust inhibitors; any chemical which causes oil or grease to dissolve in water and cleans the item on which it is used. Unlike soap, does not contain fats and lye.

detergent/germicide Combination of a cleaning agent and a disinfectant.

detergent/sanitizer Combination of chemicals which possesses antibacterial and cleaning properties.

dextrose Glucose; simple sugar

diabetes mellitus Disease in which glucose is not oxidized in body tissues for energy because of insufficient insulin.

diagnosis Identification of an illness.

dialysis Method to separate molecules in solution based on differences in their rates of diffusion through a semi-permeable membrane; method for removing nitrogen waste products from the body by hemodialysis or peritoneal dialysis.

diaphragm Dome-shaped muscle under the lungs that flattens during inhalation; a separating membrane or structure.

diarrhea Loose and frequent bowel movements.

differential staining Staining techniques to distinguish between different bacteria.

diffusion Movement of molecules from a region of higher concentration to a region of lower concentration.

digestion Process of breaking down food into absorbable particles.

dilation Widening of a part (examples: pupil of the eye, blood vessel, or uterine cervix); dilatation.

diphtheria Acute, infectious disease of the mucous membranes of the upper respiratory tract; characterized by patches of pseudomembrane and caused by Corynebacterium diphtheriae.

diplococci Pairs of cocci.

direct contact Spread of disease directly from person-to-person.

disaster (external) Situation in which activities external to the facility affects departmental or facility operations.

disaster (internal) Situation with the potential to cause harm or injury to Central Service or other employees, or where the loss of utilities may drastically impact department operations.

disease State of illness characterized by marked symptoms caused by an infectious agent producing a definite pathological pattern.

disinfectant Chemical which kills most pathogenic organisms but not spores; is not a sterilant.

disinfectant/detergent Chemical compound that contains both detergent and disinfectant. Usually the action of both is compromised because of the combination.

disinfection Destruction of nearly all pathogenic microorganisms on an inanimate surface.

disinfestation Destruction of insects, rodents, or other animals which transmit infections to other animals, humans, or their surroundings.

displacement Ionic change in which one element exchanges with another element by oxidation or reduction; a chemical change in which one element, molecule, or radical is removed by another.

dissociation Physical breaking apart of a molecule.

distal Farther from the origin of a structure or from a given reference point.

distill To vaporize by heat, and condensing and collecting the volatilized product.

distillation Changes from liquid to vapor to liquid; a process for removing impurities from liquids.

distilled water Water that has been heated to boiling point, vaporized, cooled, and condensed into liquid form; a condensate with no minerals and a pH of 7.0.

distribution Movement of supplies throughout the facility; primarily consumable supplies from storeroom to clinical units and reprocessed supplies from Central Service to operating room.

diversity Broad range of human characteristics and dimensions that impact the employees' values, opportunities, and perceptions of themselves and others at work.

DNA See deoxyribonucleic acid.

Doctor's (Physician's) preference card Document that identifies a specific physician's needs (requests and preferences) for the instruments, equipment, supplies, and utensils for a specific procedure.

dominant Referring to a gene that is always expressed if present.

dorsal Toward the back; posterior.

down time rate (equipment) Number of down days/Number of devices (x) 365.

droplet infection Infection transmitted by small drops (particles) of sputum or nasal discharges expelled into the air while talking, coughing, or sneezing.

duct Tube or vessel.

duodenum First portion of the small intestine.

dust cover Protective plastic bag used to maintain the sterility of an item by protecting it from the environment; also known as a sterility maintenance cover.

dye Coloring material used for staining or coloring bacteria for microscopic examination.

dyspnea Difficult or labored breathing.

E

ebonize Exposure of an instrument to a chemical dip which blackens the metal.

ECG Short for electrocardiogram; a picture of the electrical activity of the heart used to determine if heart disease is present.

economic order quantity (EOQ) Specific mathematical formula used to determine the most appropriate order quantity based upon usage and other variables.

ectoplasm Outer clear zone of the cytoplasm of a one-celled organism.

edema Presence of abnormally large amounts of fluid in intercellular tissue spaces of the body.

EDI Short for electronic data interchange. Orders, invoices, and other transactions are transferred electronically between the customer and the vendor to create a "paperless" and more efficient system.

EEG Short for electroencephalogram; a picture of the electrical activity of the brain.

effusion Escape of fluid into a space or part; the fluid itself.

ejaculation Expulsion of semen through the urethra.

ejaculatory duct Duct formed by the joining of the seminal vesicles with the vas deferens, through which semen moves during ejaculation.

electrocardiograph Instrument to study the electric activity of the heart; record made is an electrocardiogram; abbreviated "EKG" and "ECG."

electroencephalograph Instrument used to study electric activity of the brain; record made is an electroencephalogram; abbreviated EEG."

electrolyte Compound that forms ions in solution; substance that conducts an electric current in solution.

electron Negatively-charged particle that moves around the nucleus (central core) of an atom.

electroplating To plate with an adherent continuous coating by electrodeposition.

electrostatic Pertaining to the attractions and repulsions of electrical charges.

element One substance from which all matter is made; a substance that cannot be decomposed into a simpler substance.

embolus Blood clot or other obstruction in the circulation system; the condition is an embolism.

embryo Developing offspring during the first two months of pregnancy.

emesis Vomiting.

emphysema Pulmonary disease characterized by dilation and alveoli destruction.

empowerment Granting authority (power) to employees to make decisions within their areas of responsibility.

empyema Accumulation of pus in a body cavity, especially the chest.

emulsification Dispersion of two mutually immiscible (unable to be mixed) liquids.

emulsify To break down large volumes of fats oils, and greases into small globules which are held in suspension.

encephalitis Inflammation of the brain.

encephalomyelitis Inflammation of the brain and spinal cord.

endemic disease One that occurs more or less continuously throughout a community.

endocarditis Inflammation of the endocardium (lining membrane) of the heart including heart valves.

endocardium Membrane that lines the heart chambers and covers the valves.

endocrine Gland that secretes directly into the bloodstream.

endogenous Originating within the organism.

endometrium Lining of the uterus.

endoscope Flexible tube with an attached viewing system used to view the inside of organs and cavities. The tube is passed through a body opening or a small slit made through the skin.

endothelium Epithelium that lines the heart, blood vessels, and lymphatic vessels.

engineering controls Controls (examples: sharps disposal containers and self-sheathing needles) that isolate or remove bloodborne pathogen hazards from the workplace.

enteric Pertaining to the intestines.

enteric bacteria Bacteria living in or isolated from the intestinal tract.

entrained Trapped in the stream. Example: water can be trapped in the stream of steam.

environment Space that surrounds or encompasses a person or an object.

enzymatic solution Solution containing special enzymes that dissolves proteinaceous materials.

enzyme Substance that initiates chemical changes such as fermentation without participating in them; a catalyst, usually protein, produced by a living cell with a specific action and optimum activity at a definite pH value.

EPA Short for Environmental Protection Agency.

epicardium Membrane that forms the outermost layer of the heart wall, and is continuous with the lining of the pericardium; visceral pericardium.

epidemic Occurrence of a disease among many people in a given region at the same time.

epidemiology Study of the occurrence and distribution of disease; usually refers to epidemics.

epidermis Outermost layer of the skin.

epididymus Tube that carries sperm cells from the testes to the vas deferens.

epiglottis Leaf-shaped cartilage that covers the larynx during swallowing

equipment (capital) Relatively expensive assets such as sterilizers or washers that require significant advance planning for their purchase.

equipment utilization rate Days used/Number of devices (x) 365.

ergonomics Process of changing work or working conditions to reduce employee stress.

erythema Redness of the skin.

erythrocyte Red blood cell (corpuscle).

esophagus Tube that carries food from the throat to the stomach.

estrogen Group of female sex hormones that promote development of the uterine lining, and maintains secondary sex characteristics.

ethylene oxide Chemical (gas) used in low temperature sterilization; performs as a very effective general purpose sterilant for items that are heat or moisture-sensitive; also used as a fumigant; abbreviated "EO" or "EtO."

etiology Study of the cause of a disease or the theory of its origin.

EtO See ethylene oxide.

eustachian tube Tube that connects the middle ear cavity to the throat; auditory tube.

exacerbation Increase in the severity of a disease.

exchange cart system Inventory system in which desired inventory items are placed on a cart assigned a specific location. A second, duplicate cart is maintained in another location, and the two carts are exchanged once daily to ensure that sufficient supplies are always available.

excretion To eliminate or give off waste products (examples: feces, perspiration, or urine).

exfoliate To come off in strips or sheets; particularly the stripping of the skin after certain exanthematous diseases.

exotoxin Soluble poisonous substance excreted by a living microorganism; can be obtained in bacteria-free filtrates without death or disintegration of the microorganism.

expiration date Date calculated by adding a specific period of time to the date of manufacture or sterilization of a medical device or component that defines its estimated useful life.

expiration statement Statement indicating that the contents of a package are sterile indefinitely unless the integrity of the package is compromised.

exposure time Time for which the sterilizer's chamber is maintained within the specified range for temperature, sterilant concentration, pressure, and humidity.

external solutions Solutions normally used for irrigating, topical application, and surgical use given orally or by inhalation.

extracellular Outside the cell.

extraction Use of physical force (usually centrifugal or strike/impact) to remove excess water from a wash load prior to drying.

extraneous Outside the organism; and not belonging to it.

extrinsic From without.

exudate Accumulation of a fluid in a cavity or matter that penetrates through the vessel walls into adjoining tissue.

F

facultative Having the power to do something but not ordinarily doing it. Capable of adapting to different conditions. (Example: a facultative anaerobe can live in the presence of oxygen but does not ordinarily do so.)

fahrenheit Thermometer scale in which the space between the freezing point and the boiling point of water is 180°; 32° is the freezing point and 212° is the boiling point. To convert from Fahrenheit to Centigrade scales: 5/9 (°F - 32) = °C.

failure mode and effect analysis (FMEA) Process to predict the adverse outcomes of various human and machine failures to prevent future adverse outcomes.

fallopian tubes Slender tubes that convey the ova (eggs) from the ovaries to the uterus.

families (chemicals) Groups of chemicals that have similar characteristics.

fascia Band or sheet of fibrous connective tissue.

FCS Short for Fellowship in Central Service. (International Association of Healthcare Central Service Materiel Management)

FDA Short for Food and Drug Administration.

febrile Characterized by or pertaining to fever.

feces Waste material discharged from the large intestine; excrement; stool.

feedback Step in communication that occurs when the listener asks a question, repeats information, or otherwise helps the speaker to know if the message has been correctly received.

femur Upper leg bone.

fenestrated Having openings.

fermentation Decomposition of complex organic molecules under the influence of ferments or enzymes; usually associated with living microorganisms.

fertilization Union of an ovum and a spermatozoon.

fetus Developing offspring from the third month of pregnancy until birth.

fever Abnormally high body temperature.

fibrin Blood protein that forms a blood clot.

fibula Smaller bone of the lower leg.

filter Device secured to a rigid sterilization container's lid and/or bottom that allows passage of air and sterilants, but provides a microbial barrier.

filter retention system Mechanism on a rigid sterilization container that secures disposable filters in place.

filtrate Liquid that has passed through a filter.

fimbriae Finger-like projections extending from the fallopian tubes that draw ova (eggs) into the fallopian tube.

first In, first Out Stock rotation system in which the oldest product (that which has been in storage the longest) is used first; abbreviated "FIFO."

fissure Deep groove.

flagella Long, hair-like processes extending from the cell wall of a microorganism that helps an organism to move (especially in liquids).

flammable Combustible substance that ignites very easily, burns intensely, or has a rapid rate of flame spread.

flash sterilization Process by which unwrapped instruments are sterilized for immediate use when an emergency situation arises; process of sterilizing an item that is not packaged.

flash sterilizer Sterilizer that uses higher temperatures for shorter exposure times for emergency sterilization of dropped instruments.

flatus Gas in the digestive tract.

flexion Bending motion that decreases the angle between bones at a joint.

fluid invasion Damage to powered surgical instruments when water or solution enters the instrument's internal components.

focal infection Localized site of more or less chronic infection from which bacteria or their by-products are spread to other parts of the body.

fomite Inanimate object that can transmit bacteria.

foot candle Amount of light equivalent to that produced by one standard candle at a distance of one foot.

forceps Instrument for grasping, holding firmly, or exerting traction upon objects.

forging To form by heating and hammering.

formaldehyde Class of disinfectants most often used to disinfect hemodialysis equipment; also used as a preservative and fumigant. Use with caution because of its potential carcinogenic effect and irritating fumes.

fractional sterilization Sterilization performed at separate intervals, usually for 15 minute periods over three to four days, so spores will develop into bacteria that can then be destroyed.

fumigation Disinfection by exposure to the **fumes** of a gaseous or vaporized disinfectant.

fungicide Substance that kills fungi.

fungus (pl. fungi) Type of plant-like microorganism; unicellular and multi-cellular vegetable organisms that feed on organic matter; examples: molds, mushrooms, and toadstools.

G

gamma globulin Protein component of blood plasma that contains antibodies.

ganglion Collection of nerve cell bodies located outside the central nervous system.

gangrene Death of tissue due to loss of blood supply; accompanied by bacterial invasion and putrefaction.

gas State of matter in which molecules are practically unrestricted by cohesive forces. A gas has neither shape or volume, nor is it liquid nor solid.

gas cylinder safety relief device Device installed in a gas cylinder or container to prevent rupture of a cylinder by overpressures resulting from certain conditions of exposure; device may be a frangible (breakable) disc, fusible plug, or relief valve.

gasket Pliable strip on sterilization containers that seals the lid and the container to prevent entry of microorganisms.

gas pressure regulator Device that may be connected to the cylinder valve outlet to regulate the gas pressure delivered to a system.

gastroenteritis Inflammation of the stomach and intestines with symptoms similar to enteritis and dysentery; often caused by enteric group of bacteria (examples: Salmonella paratypih and Salmonella schottmuller).

gastrointestinal Pertaining to the stomach and intestine or the digestive tract as a whole; abbreviated "GI."

gauge pressure (steam sterilizer) Absolute pressure (-) atmospheric pressure (14.7 pounds per square inch at sea level); also called "overpressure."

gene Biological unit of heredity, self-reproducing and located in a definite position (locus) on a specific chromosome.

generalized infection One involving the whole body.

genetic Pertaining to genes or heredity.

genus Group of one or more related species.

geobacillus stearothermophilus Highly resistant but relative harmless nonpathogenic microorganism used to challenge steam and dry heat sterilizers.

germ Microorganism that causes disease.

germicidal Related to destroying germs.

germicide Agent that kills germs.

glaucoma Disorder involving increased fluid pressure within the eye.

glucagon Hormone that can increase the blood sugar level.

glucose Simple sugar; main energy source for the cells; dextrose.

gonad Sex gland; ovary or testis.

gonorrhea Contagious venereal disease of the genital mucous membranes; caused by Neisseria gonorrhoeae.

gram Basic unit of weight in the metric system.

gram-negative Losing the purple stain or decolorized by alcohol in Gram's method of staining; a primary identification characteristic of certain microorganisms

gram-positive Retaining the purple stain or resisting decolorization by alcohol in Gram's method of staining.

gram stain Differential stain used to classify bacteria as gram-positive or gram-negative depending upon whether they retain or lose the primary stain (crystal violet) when subjected to a decolorizing agent.

gravity Pull toward the center of the earth.

greenhouse gases Gases such as carbon dioxide (CO2,) methane (CH4), halogenated fluorocarbons (HCFCs), and ozone (O3) which contribute to potential climate change.

gross soil Tissue, body fat, blood, and other body substances.

H

halogen Any of the four very active non-metallic chemical elements: chlorine, iodine, bromine, and fluorine.

hammer One of the three middle ear bones; attaches to the tympanic membrane.

hand bacterial count Method of estimating the number of bacteria present on one's hand.

hand hygiene Act of washing one's hands with soap and water or using an alcohol-based hand rub.

hardness Amount of dissolved minerals in water which alters the effectiveness of many disinfectants, detergents, and soaps.

hazardous waste Substances that cannot be disposed of in the facility's normal trash system.

HCFC Short for hydrochlorofluorocarbon gas; when mixed with other gases, it yields an inflammable gas.

health care products Medical devices, medicinal products (pharmaceuticals and biologics), and in vitro diagnostics.

heart Muscular organ that pumps blood throughout the body.

heat sink Heat-absorbent material; a mass that readily absorbs heat.

heat-up time Time required for entire load to reach a pre-selected sterilizing temperature after the chamber has reached that temperature.

hematocrit Volume percentage of red blood cells in whole blood; packed cell volume; abbreviated "Hct."

hematoma Swelling filled with blood.

hematuria Blood in the urine.

hemodialysis Removal of impurities from the blood by passage through a semi permeable membrane.

hemodialyzer Equipment used to remove impurities and waste products from blood before returning it to the patient's body.

hemoglobin Iron-containing protein in red blood cells that transports oxygen; abbreviated "Hb."

hemolysis The destruction of red blood cells which leads to the release of hemoglobin from within the red blood cells into the blood plasma.

hemolytic Destruction of red blood cells with the liberation of hemoglobin.

hemorrhage Loss of blood.

hemostasis Stoppage of bleeding.

hemostatic forceps Surgical instrument used to control flow of blood.

heparin Substance that prevents blood clotting; anticoagulant.

hepatitis Inflammation of the liver; usually caused by the hepatitis virus.

heredity Transmission of characteristics from parent to offspring by genes.

hernia Protrusion of an organ or tissue through the wall of the cavity in which it is normally enclosed.

herpes simplex Mild, acute, eruptive, vesicular virus disease of the skin and mucous membrane.

herpes zoster Shingles; an acute virus disease characterized by a vesicular dermatitis which follows a nerve trunk.

high efficiency particulate air filter Special filters with minimum efficiency of 99.97%; commonly called " HEPA filter."

high-level disinfection Process that utilizes a sterilant for a shorter contact time than that used for sterilization, and that kills all microbial organisms but not necessarily large numbers of bacterial spores.

histology Study of tissues.

HIV Short for human immunodeficiency virus; an HIV infection is a chronic viral infection characterized by progressive destruction of the T-cell, which impairs the body's immune system; disease severity is relates to degree of immune suppression.

HMO Short for health maintenance organization.

homeostasis State of balance within the body; maintenance of body conditions within set limits.

hormones Chemical messengers that travel through the blood and act on target organs.

host Animal, plant, or human that supports the growth of microorganisms.

huck towel All-cotton surgical towel with a honeycomb- effect weave.

human immunodeficiency virus Virus that causes AIDS.

human relations Development and maintenance of effective interpersonal (between people) relationships that enhance teamwork.

humerus Upper arm bone.

hydration Act of combining with water.

hydrocarbon Chemically identifiable compound of carbon and hydrogen.

hydrogen ion concentration Degree of concentration of hydrogen ions in a solution used to indicate the reaction of that solution; expressed as pH (the logarithm of the reciprocal of the hydrogen ion concentration).

hydrologic cycle Continual movement of water from the atmosphere to the earth and back to the atmosphere.

hydrolysis Splitting of large molecules by the addition of water (as in digestion).

hydrophilic Describing a substance that absorbs or adsorbs water.

hydrophobic Describing a substance that does not absorb or adsorb water.

hyperglycemia Abnormal increase in the amount of glucose in the blood.

hypertension High blood pressure.

hypertonic Solution with a higher osmotic pressure than that of a reference solution.

hypoglycemia Abnormal decrease in the amount of glucose in the blood.

hypotension Low blood pressure.

hypothermia Abnormally low body temperature.

hypotonic Solution which is of less than isotonic concentration.

hypoxia Reduced oxygen supply to the tissues.

I

IAHCSMM Short for International Association of Healthcare Central Service Materiel Management.

icteric Yellow pigmentation of the tissues, membranes, and secretions caused by the deposit of bile pigment; usually a sign of liver or gall bladder disease.

idiopathic Of unknown cause.

idiosyncrasy Individual and peculiar susceptibility or sensitivity to a drug, protein, or other matter.

ileum Last portion of the small intestine.

immune Exempt from a given infection.

immunity Power of an individual to resist or overcome the effects of a particular disease or other harmful agent.

immunization Process of conferring immunity on an individual.

impact marker Tool which engraves with a forceful impact that indents and "breaks" the polished metal surface leaving an inscribed marking.

impingement Spray-force action of pressurized water against instruments being processed to physically remove bioburden.

implosion Bursting inward; the opposite of an explosion; occurs when cavitations in an energized solution collapse.

inactivation To stop or destroy activity.

inanimate Not endowed with life or spirit; not alive.

incipient Just beginning.

incompatible Not capable of being mixed without undergoing destructive chemical changes or antagonism.

incubate To maintain under optimum environmental conditions favorable for growth.

incubation period Period between when infection occurs and appearance of first symptoms.

incubator Apparatus for maintaining a constant and suitable temperature for the growth and cultivation of microorganisms.

indefinite shelf life Shelf life of hospital-sterilized items without a definite expiration date; based on premise that shelf life is event- not time-related. User must assure the integrity of the packaging is intact, clean, and properly identified.

indicator (quality) Measurable variable which relates to the outcome of patient care or employee safety.

indirect contact Transfer of infection by means including inanimate objects, contaminated fingers, water, and food.

infarct Area of tissue damaged from lack of blood supply caused by blockage of a vessel.

infection Invasion of body tissue by microorganisms which multiply and produce a reaction.

infection control Control of active infectious disease; requires (a) working knowledge of the usefulness and applications of physical and chemical agents that suppress or kill microorganisms and (b) familiarity with the sources of potentially dangerous microorganisms, routes by which they spread, and their portals of entry into the body.

infectious Having the ability to transmit disease.

inferior Below or lower.

infestation Lodgment, development, and reproduction of arthropods on a body or clothing.

inflammation Reaction of the tissues to an injury; a protective mechanism to an irritant on tissues.

inhibition Act of checking or restraining.

inoculate To implant or introduce causative agents of disease into an animal or plant or microbes onto culture media.

inoculated carrier Carrier on which a defined number of test organisms has been deposited.

inorganic Composed of matter other than plant or animal: minerals.

installation qualification (IQ) Obtaining and documenting evidence that equipment has been provided and installed in accordance with its specifications.

instrument Utensil or implement.

instrument washer sterilizer (IWS) Combination units that wash and sterilize instruments to insure the safety of processing personnel.

issue Act of withdrawing supplies from storage for transfer to areas for use

insulin Hormone that reduces the level of sugar in the blood.

integrated delivery network (IDN) System of healthcare providers and organizations which provide (or arrange to provide) a coordinated range of services to a specific population. .

integrating indicator Chemical indicator designed to react to all critical parameters over a specified range of sterilization cycles, and whose performance has been correlated to the performance of the relevant biological indicator (BI) under the labeled conditions of use.

intercellular Between cells.

intermediate-level disinfection Process that utilizes an agent that kills viruses, mycobacteria, fungi, and vegetative bacteria, but not bacterial spores.

intermittent (fractional) sterilization Destruction of microorganisms by moist heat for given periods of time on several successive days to allow spores during the rest periods to germinate into vegetative forms (which are most easily destroyed).

interstitial Between; pertaining to spaces or structures in an organ between active tissues.

intracellular Within a cell or cells.

intravenous Within or into the veins.

in-use testing Evaluation of infection-control chemicals, aseptic techniques, and sanitary and sterilization procedures under actual working conditions.

inventory Reusable equipment and consumable items used to provide healthcare services for patients.

inventory (consumable) Assets such as wrapping supplies, processing chemicals, and other items which are consumed as healthcare services are provided to patients.

inventory (official) Consumable products found in Central Service and other storerooms, warehouses, and satellite storage areas. Official inventory is included as an asset on a healthcare facility's balance sheet.

inventory (reusable) Relatively inexpensive assets such as medical devices and sterilization containers that can be reused as healthcare services are provided to patients.

inventory service level Percentage of items filled (available) when an order is placed.

inventory stock out rate Percentage of items that cannot be filled (are not available) when an order is placed.

inventory turnover rate Number of times per year (or other time period) that inventory is purchased, consumed, and replaced.

inventory (unofficial) Consumable products found in user areas such as surgical locations and labs. Unofficial inventory has usually been expensed to user units and is stored in various locations on the units.

in vitro Referring to a process or reaction carried out in a culture test tube or Petri dish.

in vivo In the living body.

iodophor Disinfectant that is a combination of iodine and a solubilizing agent (or a carrier) which slowly liberates or releases free iodine when diluted with water.

ion Electronically-charged particle formed by the loss or gain of one or more electrons.

ionize To dissociate into ions or to become electrically charged.

iris Circular colored region of the eye around the pupil.

ischemia Lack of blood supply to an area.

islets Groups of cells in the pancreas that produce hormones; islets of Langerhans.

ISO 9000 International standards used by participating organizations to help assure that they consistently deliver quality services and products.

isolate To place by itself; to separate from others.

isotonic Solution having the same osmotic pressure as that of another solution taken as a standard reference.

isotope Form of an element with the same atomic number as another but with a different atomic weight.

J

jargon Specialized words or phrases known only by persons working in a position.

jaundice Excess of bile pigments in blood, skin, and mucous membranes with a resulting yellow appearance of the individual.

jaw Either of two or more opposable parts that open and close for holding or crushing something between them.

jejunum Second portion of the small intestine.

JIT Short for "just in time," a method of inventory distribution where a vendor holds inventory for an organization, and delivers items on a regular basis which go directly to supply carts.

job description Human resources tool that identifies the major tasks performed by persons in specific positions.

joint Any place where two bones meet

Julian date - The Julian day or Julian day number is the number of days that have elapsed since January 1 of a specific year.

K

kidneys Organs that remove excess water and waste substances from the blood in a process that yields urine.

killing power Ability of a chemical to kill bacteria under laboratory conditions and during in-use testing.

L

labeling Legend, work, or mark attached to, included in, belonging to, or accompanying any medical device.

lacrimal Referring to tears or the tear glands.

lactation Secretion of milk.

lactic acid Organic acid that accumulates in muscle cells functioning without oxygen.

laminar airflow Filtered air moving along separate parallel flow planes to surgical suites, nurseries, bacteriology work areas, and pharmacies; prevents collection of bacterial contamination or hazardous chemical fumes in work areas.

large intestine (colon) Digestive organ that dehydrates digestive residues (feces).

larynx Voice box.

laser Device that produces a very intense beam of light.

latching mechanism Mechanical device that secures a rigid sterilization container's lid to the container's bottom.

latent heat Additional heat required to change the state of a substance from solid to liquid at its melting point, or from liquid to gas at its boiling point after the temperature of the substance has reached either of these points.

lateral Farther from the midline; toward the side.

latex Common form of rubber used in the manufacture of hospital and medical supplies.

latex sensitivity Sensitivity (allergic reaction) of some persons to latex caused by exposure to latex that is improperly processed; symptoms range from skin rash, primarily on the hands, to anaphylactic reaction.

leak test (endoscope) Endoscope processing procedure that ensures the device's flexible covering and internal channels are watertight.

lens Biconvex structure of the eye that changes in thickness to accommodate near and far vision; crystalline lens.

lesion Wound or local injury; a specific change or morphological alteration by disease or injury.

lethal Pertaining to death.

leukemia Malignant blood disease characterized by abnormal development of white blood cells.

leukocyte White blood cell.

ligament Band of connective tissue that connects a bone to another bone.

lipids Group of fats or fatty substances characterized by insolubility in water.

lipid virus A virus whose core is surrounded by a coat of lipoprotein. Viruses included in this structural category are generally easily inactivated by many types of disinfectants, including low level disinfectants.

liquid-proof Material that prevents the penetration of liquids and microorganisms.

liquid-resistant Material that inhibits the penetration of liquids.

liter Basic unit of volume in metric system.

liver Organ that filters the blood to remove amino acids and neutralize some harmful toxins.

load configuration All attributes defining the presentation of products to sterilization process including (a) orientation of products within the primary package (b) quantity and orientation of primary packages(s) within secondary and tertiary packages (c)quantity, orientation, and placement of tertiary packages on sterilizer pallets or within carriers and (d) quantity and placement of the pallets (or carriers) within the vessel or area.

load control number Label information on sterilization packages, trays, or containers that identifies the sterilizer, cycle run, and date of sterilization.

loaner instrumentation Instruments or sets borrowed from a vendor for emergency or scheduled surgical procedures that will be returned following use.

local exhaust hood System that captures contaminated air and conducts it into an exhaust duct; also called venting hood.

local infection One confined to a restricted area.

logarithm Exponent indicating the power to which a fixed number (the base) must be raised to produce a given number.

lot (load)control number Numbers and/or letters by which a specific group of products can be traced to a particular manufacturing or sterilization operation.

low-level disinfection Process that utilizes an agent to kill vegetative forms of bacteria, some fungi, and lipid viruses.

lumen Interior path through a needle, tube, or surgical instrument.

lungs Organs of respiration.

lux One-tenth of a foot candle.

lymph Fluid in the lymphatic system.

lymphatic system Series of tiny vessels throughout the body that carry lymph fluid to protect the body against disease.

lymphocyte White blood cell involved in antibody production.

M

macromolecules Large molecules (proteins, carbohydrates, lipids, and nucleic acids) within a microorganism

macroscopic Visible to the naked eye.

magnet status Award given by the American Nurses Credentialing Center to hospitals that satisfy factors measuring the strength and quality of nursing care.

magnetic resonance imaging (MRI) Method for studying tissue based on nuclear movement following exposure to radio waves in a powerful magnetic field.

maintenance insurance Equipment outsourcing alternative in which a hospital retains control of its equipment, but contracts with an insurance organization to manage and insure the costs involved in maintaining it.

malaise Indisposition, discomfort, or feeling of ill health.

malignant Describing a tumor that spreads or a disorder that becomes worse and causes death.

malnutrition State resulting from lack of food, lack of an essential component of the diet, or faulty use of food in the diet.

mandible Lower jaw bone.

Mantoux test Tuberculin skin test.

manufacturer Maker or producer of items or equipment.

martensic (stainless steel) Metal also known as 400 series stainless steel, that is magnetic and may be heat-hardened.

Materiel Management Department Healthcare department responsible for researching, ordering, receiving, and managing inventory (consumable supplies).

mastectomy Removal of the breast; mammectomy.

mastication Act of chewing.

measles Rubeola; acute, infectious virus disease characterized by fever, catarrh, coryza, Koplik spots on buccal mucous membrane, and a papular rash.

medial Nearer the midline of the body.

mediastinum Region between the lungs and the organs and the vessels it contains.

Medicaid Federal and state assistance program paying covered medical expenses for low-income persons.

medical device Any instrument, apparatus, appliance, material or other article, used alone or in combination, including software necessary for its proper application intended by the manufacturer to be used for human beings for (a) diagnosis, prevention, monitoring, treatment, or alleviation of disease (b) diagnosis, monitoring, treatment, alleviation of, or compensation for an injury or handicap (c) investigation, replacement, or modification of the anatomy or of a physiological process or (d) control of conception.

Medicare Federal medical insurance program that primarily serves those over 65 years of age regardless of income, and younger disabled persons and dialysis patients; medical bills are paid from trust funds into which covered persons have paid.

MedWatch Program Safety information and adverse event reporting system that serves healthcare professionals and the public by reporting serious problems suspected to be associated with the drugs and medical devices they prescribe, dispense, or use.

meiosis Process of cell division that halves the chromosome number in the formation of the reproductive cells.

membrane Thin sheet of tissue.

memory Inherent ability of a substance to return to its original shape and contours.

meningitis Inflammation of the meninges.

menopause Time at which menstruation ceases.

menses Monthly flow of blood from the female reproductive tract.

mesentery Membranous peritoneal ligament that attaches the small intestine to the dorsal abdominal wall.

mesophiles Bacteria that grow best at moderate temperatures: 68°F-113°F (20°C-45°C).

metabolic rate Rate at which energy is released from nutrients in the cells.

metabolism Total chemical changes by which the nutritional and functional activities of an organism are maintained.

metacarpals Hand bones.

metallurgy Science and technology of metals.

metastasis Spread of tumor cells.

metatarsals Bones of the foot.

meter Basic unit of length in the metric system.

methicillin-resistant staphylococcus aureus (MRSA) Staphylococcus aureus bacteria that have developed a resistance to methicillin, the drug of choice; usually occurs with patients who have had antibiotic therapy for a long time.

microaerophilic Microorganisms which require free oxygen for their growth, but in an amount less than that of the oxygen in the atmosphere.

microbes Organisms of microscopic or submicroscopic size generally including viruses, rickettsiae, bacteria, algae, yeasts, and molds.

microbiology Study of microorganisms; science which treats the nature, life, and action of microorganisms.

micron Unit of measurement; 1/1000 of a millimeter or 1/25,000 of an inch or one millionth of a meter. (Note: meter equals 39.37 inches.)

microorganisms Forms of life which are too small to see with the naked eye. Bacteria, viruses, and fungi are types of microorganisms; also called "germs" and "microbes.")

midbrain Upper portion of the brain stem.

mil Unit of length or thickness equal to .001 of an inch.

mineral Inorganic substance; diet element needed in small amounts for health.

min/max (minimum/maximum) System in which orders are placed to reach a predetermined maximum when a predetermined minimum level is reached.

minimum effective concentration (MEC) Percentage concentration of the active ingredient in a disinfectant or chemical sterilant that is the minimum concentration at which the chemical meets all label claims for activity against specific microorganisms.

mitosis Cell division that produces two daughter cells exactly like the parent cell.

mitral valve Valve between the left atrium and left ventricle of the heart; bicuspid valve.

mixed culture Growth of two or more microorganisms in the same medium.

mixed infection Simultaneous process of two or more microorganisms causing an infection.

mixture Blend of two or more substances.

mode of transmission (chain of infection) Method of transfer of an infectious agent from the reservoir to a susceptible host.

molds See fungus.

molecular attraction Adhesive forces exerted between the surface molecules of two bodies in contact.

molecule Smallest quantity of matter that can exist in a free state and retain all of its properties.

monel A trademark used for an alloy of nickel, copper, iron, and manganese.

monitor To systematically check or test to control the concentration of a specific ingredient or the execution of a process; may include qualitative and/or quantitative measurements.

mouth Opening through which air, food, and beverages enter the body; beginning of the alimentary canal.

MRC Short for minimum recommended concentration; minimum concentration at which the manufacturer tested the product and validated its performance.

MRI See magnetic resonance imaging.

MRSA See methicillin resistant staphyloccus aureus.

MSDS Short for material safety data sheets; Manufacturers' information about workplace chemicals and hazardous materials required by the Occupational Safety and Health Administration. Required information includes manufacturer's name, address, telephone number, hazardous Ingredients, health hazard data, and precautions for safe handling and use.

mucosa Lining membrane that produces mucus; mucous membrane.

mucous Thick protective fluid secreted by mucous membranes and glands.

mucous membrane Membrane lining all body cavities that open externally including mouth, nose, and intestines that secretes mucous.

multiparameter indicator Indicator designed for two or more critical parameters that indicates exposure to a sterilization cycle at stated values of the parameters.

murmur Abnormal heart sound.

muslin Broad term describing wide variety of plain-weave cotton or cotton/polyester fabrics with approximately 140 threads per square inch.

mutation Change or alteration in the gradual evolution of a microorganism.

mycology Study of molds, yeasts, and fungi.

myocardium Middle layer of the heart wall; heart muscle.

N

nasopharynx Portion of the pharynx above the palate.

natural immunity Immunity with which a person or animal is born.

necropsy Postmortem examination or autopsy.

necrosis Death of a mass of tissue while part of the living body.

needleholders Surgical instruments to drive suture needles to close or rejoin a wound or surgical site

negative air pressure Situation that occurs when air flows into a room or area because the pressure in the area is less than that of surrounding areas.

neoplasm Abnormal growth of cells; tumor.

nephron Microscopic functional unit of the kidney.

nerve Nerve fibers outside the central nervous system.

neuritis Inflammation of a nerve.

neuron Nerve cell.

neutral Neither acid nor base.

neutralizer Substance added to a medium which stops the action of a antimicrobial agent.

NFPA Short for National Fire Protection Association.

node Small mass of tissue such as a lymph node; space between cells in the myelin sheath.

nomenclature System of names used to identify parts of a mechanism or device.

non-critical devices (Spaulding medical device classification system) Those that contact intact skin.

noncritical zone Area of a gown or drape where direct contact with blood, body fluids, and other potentially infectious materials is unlikely to occur.

nonionic Atoms with no electrical charges; compounds containing a nondissociated hydrophilic group which forms a bond with water.

nonlipid virus A virus whose nucleic acid core is not surrounded by a lipid envelope. These viruses are generally more resistant to inactivation by disinfectants.

nonpathogenic Not capable of producing disease.

nonpyrogenic Free from fever-causing substances.

nontoxic Not poisonous; not capable of producing injury or disease.

nonwoven Fabric made by bonding (as opposed to weaving) fibers together

normal flora Normal bacterial population of a given area.

nose Nasal cavity.

nosocomial Hospital-acquired infection (HAI); pertaining to a hospital; applied to a disease caused in the course of being treated in a hospital.

noxious Physically harmful or destructive to living beings.

nucleotide Building block of deoxyribonucleic acid (DNA) and ribonucleic acid (RNA).

nucleus Functional center of a cell that governs activity and heredity.

O

occluded Closure of an opening.

ohm Unit of measurement that expresses the amount of resistance to the flow of an electric current.

olfactory Pertaining to the sense of smell.

oncology Study of tumors.

ophthalmic Pertaining to the eye.

opportunists Microbes that produce infection only under especially favorable conditions.

optimum temperature Applied to bacterial growth, the temperature at which bacteria grow best.

order point (order quantity system) Method of reordering a predetermined quantity of products when a predetermined on-hand level is reached.

organ Part of the body containing two or more tissues that function together for a specific purpose.

organic Describing compounds containing oxygen, carbon and hydrogen; characteristic of, pertaining to, or derived from living organisms.

organism Living thing, plant or animal; may be unicellular or multicellular.

origin Source; beginning; end of a muscle attached to a nonmoving part.

OSHA Short for Occupational Safety and Health Administration; concerned with safe work environment and employee safety.

osmosis Net movement of solvent molecules across a selectively permeable membrane from areas of higher to lower concentrations.

osmotic pressure Tendency of a solution to draw water into it; directly related to the concentration of the solution.

ossification Process by which cartilage is replaced by bone.

osteoblast Bone-forming cell.

osteomyelitis Inflammation of bone marrow.

osteoporosis Abnormal loss of bone tissue with tendency to fracture.

osteotomes Chisel-like instruments used to cut or shave bone.

otitis media Inflammation of the middle ear.

outsourcing (equipment) Transfer of control of a hospital's equipment management system to an external entity.

ovaries Female reproductive glands.

ovulation Release of a mature ovum from a follicle in the ovary.

ovum Female sex cell.

oxidation Process by which a molecule, atom, or ion loses an electron; act or process of oxidizing: chemical breakdown of nutrients for energy.

oxidative chemistries Class of compounds containing an additional atom of oxygen bound to oxygen that uses oxidation to interrupt cell function.

oxidize To change by increasing the proportion of the electronegative part or change (an element or ion) from a lower to higher positive valence.

oxidizing agent Material that removes electrons from another substance.

oxygen Gas needed to completely break down nutrients for energy within the cell.

ozone A reactive and unstable oxygen molecule.

P

packaging Application or use of appropriate closures, wrappings, cushioning, containers, and complete identification up to, but not including, the shipping container and associated packing.

pandemic Very widespread epidemic (even of worldwide extent).

papers (kraft-type) Medical grade paper packaging material used for numerous sterilization applications.

PAR Short for periodic automatic replenishment; inventory system in which the desired amount of products which should be on hand is established, and inventory replenishment returns the quantity of products to this level; often abbreviated "par system."

paracentesis Puncture through the wall of a cavity (usually to remove fluid or promote drainage).

parametric release Declaring product to be sterile on the basis of physical and/or chemical process data, rather than on the basis of sample testing or biological indicator results.

parasite Plant or animal that lives upon or within another living organism (host) from which it obtains nourishment and at whose expense it grows without giving anything in return.

par cart Distribution method in which a supply cart remains in a given location is inventoried and replenished on a regular basis.

parenteral solutions Solutions administered to patients intravenously.

parietal Pertaining to the wall of a space or cavity.

par level (inventory) Desired amount of inventory which should be on hand.

particle Piece of matter with observable length, width, and thickness; usually measured in microns.

particulate matter General term applied to matter of miniature size with observable length, width, and thickness (contrasted to nonparticulate matter without definite dimension).

parturition Childbirth; labor.

patient care equipment Portable (mobile) equipment used to assist in the care and treatment of patients; examples: suction units and heat therapy units.

passivation Chemical process applied during instrument manufacture that provides a corrosion-resistant finish by forming a thin transparent oxide film.

passive carrier Carrier who harbors the causative agent of a disease without having had the disease.

passive immunity Immunity produced without the body of the person or animal that becomes immune participating in its production; example: production of immunity to diphtheria by injection of diphtheria antitoxin.

pasteurization Process of heating a fluid to a moderate temperature for a definite period of time to destroy undesirable bacteria without changing its chemical composition.

patella Kneecap.

pathogen Capable of causing disease; disease-producing microorganism.

pathogenic Capable of producing disease.

pathology Study of disease.

pawl Pivoted tongue or sliding bolt on one part of an instrument adapted to fall into notches or interdental space on another part to permit motion in only one direction.

PEL Short for permissible exposure limit.

pelvis Basin-like structure; lower portion of the abdomen; large bone of the hip.

penicillin Antibiotic produced by the mold, Penicillium notatum.

penis Male organ of urination and intercourse.

peracetic acid (PA) Liquid oxidizing agent that is an effective biocide at low temperatures; used in a sterilization system that processes immersible diagnostic and surgical instruments (primarily flexible and rigid scopes); items must be used immediately after sterilization because they are wet and cannot be stored.

performance qualification (PQ) Obtaining and documenting evidence that equipment, as installed and operated in accordance with operational procedures, consistently performs according to predetermined factors and meets specifications.

perineum Pelvic floor; external region between the anus and genital organs.

periosteum Membrane of connective tissue that closely invests all bones except at the articular surface.

peripheral Located away from a center or central structure.

peripheral nervous system All nerves and nerve tissue outside the central nervous system.

peristalsis Wavelike movements in the wall of an organ or duct that propel its contents forward.

peritoneum Serous membrane that lines the abdominal cavity, and forms the outer layer of abdominal organs; forms supporting ligaments for some organs.

peritonitis Inflammation of the peritoneum.

permissible exposure limits (PEL) Limits developed by the Occupational Safety and Health Administration to indicate the maximum airborne concentration of a contaminant to which an employee may be exposed over the duration specified by the type of PEL assigned to that contaminant.

perpetual inventory system System which tracks all incoming and issued supplies to determine, on an on-going basis, the quantity of supplies in storage.

personal protective equipment (PPE) Specialized clothing or equipment worn by an employee for protection against a hazard.

pertussis Whopping cough.

petri dish Shallow, covered cylindrical glass or plastic dish, used to culture bacteria and in which bacterial colonies may be observed without removing the cover.

pH Measure of alkalinity or acidity on a scale of 0-14; pH of 7 is neutral (neither acid or alkaline); pH below 7 is acid because of an excess of hydrogen ions; pH above 7 indicates an excess of hydroxyl ions making it alkaline; see hydrogen ion concentration)

phagocyte Cell capable of ingesting bacteria or other foreign particles.

phagotization Process by which some cells can ingest bacteria or other foreign particles.

phalanges Bones that comprise the fingers and toes.

pharynx Throat.

phenol Carbolic acid (phenyl alcohol); a colorless crystalline compound (C_6H_5OH) with strong disinfectant properties.

phenol coefficient Method of designating the disinfecting properties of a chemical by comparing its activity to that of phenol.

phlebitis Inflammation of a vein.

physiology Study of the function of living organisms.

PI Short for performance improvement; a process to continually improve patient care that identifies performance functions and associated costs which affect patient outcomes, and the perception of patients and families about the quality and value of services provided..

pick and pack Inventory control system for forms and office supplies. Items are shipped/charged to the customer as ordered in minimal quantities, and the customer is financially responsible for the vendor's agreed-upon inventory.

placenta Structure that nourishes and maintains the developing individual during pregnancy.

plague Acute, often fatal epidemic disease, caused by Pasteurella pestis and transmitted to man by fleas from rats and other rodents.

plasma Liquid portion of blood.

plasmolysis Shrinkage of a cell or its contents due to withdrawal of water by osmosis.

plasmoptysis Escape of protoplasm from a cell due to rupture of the cell wall.

platelet Cell fragment that forms a plug to stop bleeding and acts in blood clotting; thrombocyte.

pleura Serous membrane that lines the chest cavity and covers the lungs.

pneumonia Inflammatory consolidation or solidification of lung tissue due to presence of an exudate blotting out the air-containing spaces; see exudate.

pneumothorax Accumulation of air in the pleural space.

point of use processing That which occurs when a medical device is processed immediately before use, and/or close to the patient care area.

poliomyelitis Virus disease in which there is inflammation of the gray substance of the spinal cord; commonly called infantile paralysis.

pollution State of rendering unclean or impure by adding harmful substances.

pounds per square inch gauge (psig) Measure of ambient air pressure; the pressure that a gas would exert on the walls of a one-cubic foot container.

polycarbonate Type of plastic.

polyethylene Thermoplastic polymer capable of being produced in thin sheets; exhibits good moisture-vapor barrier qualities, but has a high sloughing tendency.

polymerize Process of joining many simple molecules into long chains of more complex molecules whose molecular weight is a multiple of the original and whose physical properties are different.

polyp Protruding growth (often grape-like) from a mucous membrane.

polypropylene Type of plastic.

polystyrene Type of plastic.

polyurethane Type of plastic.

polyvinyl chloride (PVC) Type of plastic.

porous Possessing or full of pores (minute openings).

portability Not fixed; can be transported.

portal of entry (chain of infection) Path used by an infectious agent to enter a susceptible host.

portal of exit (chain of infection) Path by which an infectious agent leaves the reservoir.

positive air pressure Situation in which air flows out of a room or area because the pressure in the area is greater than that of surrounding areas.

posterior Toward the back; dorsal.

ppm Short for parts per million.

preconditioning Treatment of product prior to the sterilization cycle in a room or chamber to attain specified limits for temperature and relative humidity; see conditioning.

preconditioning area Chamber or room in which preconditioning occurs. .

prefix (word element) Word element that comes before the root word element.

preservative Substance that prevents biologic decomposition of materials when added to them.

preventive maintenance (equipment) Service provided to equipment to maintain it in proper operating condition by providing planned inspection, and by detecting and correcting failures before they occur; often abbreviated "PM."

primary infection First of two or more infections.

prions A disease-causing agent that is neither bacterial nor fungal nor viral and contains no genetic material. A prion is a protein that occurs normally in a harmless form. By folding into an aberrant shape, the normal prion turns into a rogue agent. It then co-opts other normal prions to become rogue prions. Prions have been held responsible for a number of degenerative brain diseases, including scrapie (a fatal disease of sheep and goats), mad cow disease, Creutzfeldt-Jacob disease and others.

process challenge device (PCD) Object that simulates a predetermined set of conditions when used to test sterilizing agent(s)

process equivalency Documented evaluation that the same sterilization process can be delivered by two or more pieces of sterilization equipment.

process improvement Activity to identify and resolve work task-related problems that yield poor quality; the strategy of finding solutions to eliminate the root causes of process performance problems.

process indicators Devices used with individual units (examples: packs or containers) to demonstrate that the unit has been exposed to the sterilization process, and to distinguish between processed and unprocessed units.

processes (work) Series of work activities which produce a product or service.

processing area Area in which decontaminated, clean instruments and other medical and surgical supplies are inspected, assembled into sets and trays, and wrapped, packaged, or placed into container systems for sterilization; commonly called "preparation and packaging area" if part of Central Service and "pack room" if textile packs are assembled there.

processing group Collection of products or product families that can be sterilized in the same EO sterilization process. All products within the group have been determined to present an equal or lesser challenge to the sterilization process.

product adoption Process of formally including a candidate product into an existing validated sterlization process.

product family Collection of products determined to be similar or equivalent for validation purposes.

progesterone Hormone produced by the corpus luteum and placenta; maintains the lining of the uterus for pregnancy.

prognosis Prediction of the probable outcome of a disease based on the patient's condition.

prophylactic Agent used to prevent infection or disease.

prophylaxis Prevention of disease.

prostate gland Organ that produces a fluid element in semen that stimulates the motility of sperm.

prosthesis Artificial replacement of a body part such as an arm or leg.

protein Complex combinations of amino acids containing hydrogen, nitrogen, carbon, oxygen and, usually sulfur and sometimes other elements; essential constituents of all living cells.

prothrombin Clotting factor; converted to thrombin during blood clotting.

proton Positively-charged particle in the nucleus of an atom.

protoplasm Thick mucous-like substance that is colorless and translucent that forms the biochemical basis of life found within the cell nucleus.

protozoan One-celled animal-like microorganism of the sub-kingdom, protozoa.

proximal Nearer to point of origin or to a reference point.

prudent Marked by wisdom or judiciousness; wise.

pseudopodia "False feet;" temporary protrusions of ectoplasm to provide locomotion.

psia Pounds per square inch absolute.

psychrophiles (bacteria) Cold-loving bacteria whose optimum temperature for growth is 59°F-68°F (15°C-20°C) or below.

pulse Wave of increased pressure in blood vessels produced by contraction of the heart.

pupil Opening in the center of the eye through which light enters.

pure culture Specific bacterial growth of only one species of microorganism.

purulent Containing pus.

pus Semifluid creamy product of inflammation consisting of blood cells (mainly white), bacteria, dead tissue cells, and serum.

pyogenic Pus-producing.

pyrex Type of hard glass made from borosilicate which is alkaline free.

pyrexia Fever.

pyrogen Fever-producing substance.

pyrogenic Fever-producing; by-products of bacterial growth or metabolism.

Q

quadrant One part of four; to be divided into four equal parts.

qualified personnel Prepared by training and experience to perform a specified task.

quality Consistent delivery of products and services according to established standards.

quality assurance Comprehensive and measured efforts to provide total quality.

quality control Technical, statistical sampling method that measures production quality

quarantine Isolation of infected persons and contacts who have been exposed to communicable diseases for the time equal to the longest incubation period of the disease to which they have been exposed.

quaternary compound Group of disinfectants having derivatives of benzalkonium chloride as the active ingredient.

quiescent Not active.

R

radiation heat Transmission of heat from one object to another without heating the space in between; process of emitting radiant energy in the form of waves or particles.

radical Group of atoms that behaves as a single atom in a chemical reaction.

radio frequency identification (RFID) Term used to describe a system in which the identity (serial number) of an item is wirelessly transmitted with radio waves.

radius One of the two bones in the forearm

random numbers (table) Compilation of numbers generated in an unpredictable, hap-hazardous sequence used to create a random sample..

ratchet (or rachet) Part of a surgical instrument that "locks" the handles in place.

rationale Underlying reason; basis.

recessive Gene that is not expressed if a dominant gene for the same trait is present

Recommended Practices and Standards (AAMI) Voluntary guidelines representing a consensus of AAMI members intended for use by healthcare facilities to help ensure the safety of medical instrumentation for patient use.

rectum Last several inches of the large intestine.

reflex Involuntary response to a stimulus.

refraction Bending of light rays as they pass from one medium to another of a different density.

regulation Mandatory law or rule issued by a governing body.

relative humidity Amount of water vapor in the atmosphere; expressed as a percentage of the total amount of vapor the atmosphere could hold without condensation.

remission Diminution or abatement of disease symptoms.

reorder point (ROP) Inventory level available when an order is placed to replenish inventory.

repair (equipment) Procedures used to return equipment to proper operating condition after it becomes inoperative.

requisition system Method of inventory distribution in which product needs are requested (requisitioned), and removed from a central storage location for transport to the user department.

reservoir Carrier of an infectious microorganism; generally refers to a human carrier.

reservoir of agent (chain of infection) Place where an infectious agent (microorganisms) can survive.

resident bacteria Bacteria normally occurring at a given anatomical site.

residual Pertaining to or constituting what is remaining; leftover.

residual (EtO) Amount of EtO that remains inside materials after they are sterilized.

residual property Capacity of an antiseptic or disinfectant to kill microorganisms over a long period of time after initial application.

resistance Ability of an individual to ward off infection.

resorption Loss of substance (such as bone).

respiration Exchange of oxygen and carbon dioxide between outside air and body cells.

retina Innermost layer of the eye; contains light sensitive cells (rods and cones).

retractors Surgical instruments primarily used to move tissues and organs to keep them exposed throughout surgery.

retroperitoneal Behind the peritoneum (kidneys, pancreas, and abdominal aorta).

reusable medical device Devices intended for repeated use on different patients, with appropriate decontamination and other processing between uses.

reusable surgical textile Drape, gown, towel, or sterilization wrapper intended to be used during in or assist in preparing for surgery; made from a fabric (usually woven or knitted), fabric/film laminate, or non-woven material intended to be used more than once with appropriate reprocessing between uses.

reverse osmosis Diffusion (flowing) of water through a semi-permeable membrane to eliminate impurities; water treatment process in which dissolved impurities are separated from water by forcing the water through a semi-permeable membrane under pressure.

rhinitis Inflammation of the mucous membrane of the nose.

rib spreaders Retractor used to expose the chest.

ribonucleic acid (RNA) One of two types of nucleic acids; found in nucleus and cytoplasm and involved in protein synthesis.

risk management Methods to assess risks of a specific activity, and to develop a program to reduce losses from exposure to those risks.

rod Straight, slim mass of substance related to microorganisms; example: rod-shaped bacteria.

roentgenogram Film produced with of x-rays.

rongeurs Surgical instruments to cut or bite away at bone and tissue.

root cause analysis (RCA) Process that "looks backwards" at an event to help prevent its future occurrence.

root (word element) Tells the primary meaning of a word; also called base word element.

rubeola Measles.

S
sacrum Lower portion of vertebral column.

safety stock Minimum amount of inventory that must be on hand.

saline Containing or pertaining to salt; an isotonic aqueous solution of sodium chloride for temporarily maintaining living cells.

saliva Secretion of salivary glands; moistens food and contains an enzyme that digests starch.

sanitary Relating to health; characterized by, or readily kept in, cleanness.

sanitize To reduce the microbial flora in materials or on articles such as eating utensils to levels judged safe by public health standards.

saponification Action of detergent alkalies on an item's fat or soil contents to form soaps.

sarcoma Malignant tumor of connective tissue; a form of cancer.

saturated steam Steam that contains the maximum amount of water vapor; steam that exerts the maximum pressure for water vapor at a given temperature and pressure.

scapula Shoulder blade.

schizomycetes Plant class to which all bacteria belong.

scissors Surgical instruments used to cut, incise, and/or dissect tissue.

sclera Outermost layer of the eye; "white" of the eye.

scrotum Sac in which testes are suspended.

seals (tamper-evident) Sealing method for sterile packaging that allows users to determine if packaging has been opened contaminated) and helps them identify packages unsafe for patient use.

sebaceous Secreting or pertaining to sebum.

sebum Oily secretion of sebaceous gland that lubricates the skin.

secondary infection Superimposed infection occurring in a host who is already suffering from an earlier infection.

selective action Ability to inhibit or kill one group of microbes and not another.

semen Mixture of sperm cells and secretions from several male reproductive glands.

semi-critical devices (Spaulding medical device classification system) Those which come in contact with non-intact skin or mucous membranes.

seminal vesicle Gland that produces semen.

sensitivity State of being susceptible.

sensitization Process of sensitizing or making susceptible.

sepsis Condition, usually with fever, that results from the presence of microorganisms or their poisons in the blood stream or other tissues.

septic Relating to the presence of pathogens or their toxins.

septicemia Presence of pathogenic microorganisms or their toxins in the bloodstream; blood poisoning.

septum Dividing wall; examples: between heart chambers or sides of the nose.

sequestering agents Chemicals that remove or inactivate hard water minerals.

sequestration Removal or inactivation of water hardness elements by formation of a soluble complex or chelate.

serology Science that deals with serum.

serrations Parallel grooves in the jaws of surgical instruments.

serum Clear fluid exuded when blood coagulates.

service Activity that helps one or more persons or groups.

service recovery Sequence of steps to address customer complaints and problems to yield a win-win situation for the customer and the department.

sex-linked Gene carried on a sex (usually X) chromosome.

sharps Cutting instruments including knives, scalpels, blades, needles, scissors, chisels, osteotomes, some curettes, dissectors, elevators, rongeurs and cutting forceps, punches, saws and trocars.

shelf life Period of time during which product sterility is assumed to be maintained.

shelf life (disinfectants) Length of time a disinfectant can be properly stored after which it must be discarded.

shock Pertaining to circulation: inadequate output of blood by the heart.

short-term exposure limit (STEL) An employee's 15-minute time weighted average exposure which shall not be exceeded at any time during a work day unless another time period is specified (by OSHA). If another time period is specified, the time weighted average exposure over that time period shall not be exceeded at any time during the working day;" see threshold limit value.

sigmoid colon Last portion of large intestine.

sign Manifestation of a disease noted by an observer.

silicate Mineral commonly in water derived from silca in quartz and other components.

simple stain Staining technique using only one dye.

single-parameter indicator Designed for one critical parameter that indicates exposure to a sterilization cycle at a stated value of the chosen parameter.

six sigma Quality process that focuses on developing and delivering near-perfect products and services.

skin Organ containing sweat glands that, through perspiration, produces and eliminates sweat.

sloughing To cast off one's skin; to separate dead tissue from living tissue.

small intestine Digestive organ where the greatest amount of digestion and nutrient absorption into body cells occurs.

smear Thin layer of material spread on a glass slide for microscopic examination.

SMS (spunbond-meltblown-spunbond) Non-woven packaging material which is the most popular flat wrap.

soap Compound of one or more fatty acids or their equivalent with an alkaline substance.

softening (sequestering) Process of removing selected substances from hard water.

soft glass Glass made from alkaline materials which cannot be subjected to high temperatures without causing chemical reactions and possible shredding of the glass.

soluble Able to be dissolved.

solution Mixture with components evenly distributed.

solvent Liquid capable of dissolving another substance.

species One kind of organism; the subdivision of a genus.

sperm Male sex cell.

spermatozoon Male reproductive cell; gamete.

sphincter Muscular ring that regulates the size of an opening.

sphygmomanometer Device used to measure blood pressure.

spirillum Spiral-shaped bacterium of the genus spirillum; chief pathogens causing rat bite fever and Asiatic cholera.

spirochete Slender, corkscrew-like or spiral-shaped bacteria found on man, animals, plants and in soil and water; moves in a waving and twisting motion, and some cause disease.

spleen Lymphoid organ in the upper left region of the abdomen.

sporadic disease Disease that occurs in neither an endemic nor epidemic.

spore Microorganisms capable of forming a thick wall around themselves to enable survival in adverse conditions; a resistant form of bacterium.

spore strip Paper strip impregnated with a known population of microorganisms and that meets the definition of biological indicator.

sporicide Agent which destroys spores.

stain Substance used to color cells or tissues to differentiate them for microscopic examination and study; see gram stain.

standard Uniform method of defining basic parameters for processes, products, services, and measurements.

standards (AAMI) Recommendations representing a consensus of AAMI members that provide guidance to device manufacturers about design, performance, labeling, and other factors applicable to instruments they manufacture.

standards (regulatory) Comparison benchmarks mandated by a governing agency and, if not complied with, may cause a facility to be in violation and liable for legal penalty.

standards (voluntary) Comparison benchmarks strongly recommended by a governing agency or professional organization that provide recommendations and guidelines for patient care.

standardization Being made uniform.

standard precautions – Using appropriate barriers to prevent transmission of infectious organisms from contact with blood and all other body fluids, non-intact skin, and mucous membranes; applies to all patients, regardless of diagnosis or presumed infectious status.

staphylococci Gram-positive bacteria which grow in grape-like clusters.

stasis Stoppage in the normal flow of fluids such as blood, lymph, urine, or contents of the digestive tract.

stat. Abbreviation for the Latin "statim" meaning immediately or at once.

statute Written and enforceable law enacted by a governing body.

steam Water vapor at 212°F (100°C) or above.

steam purity Degree to which steam is free of dissolved and suspended particles, water treatment chemicals, and other contaminants.

steam quality Weight of dry steam present in a mixture of dry saturated steam and entrained water.

STEL Short for short term excursion limit.

stenosis Narrowing of a duct or canal.

stereotype Preconceived belief or opinion about a group of people applied to every person in that group.

sterilant/sterilization agent Physical or chemical entity, or combination of entities, that has sufficient microbicidal activity to achieve sterility under defined conditions.

sterile Completely devoid of all living microorganisms.

sterile field Immediate environment around trauma site or surgical incision; includes all materials in contact with the wound, gowns worn by the surgical team (front panel from chest to the level of the operative field and sleeve from the cuff to two inches above the elbow), patient drapes (area adjacent to the wound, and table covers (top surface).

sterile storage area Area of healthcare facility designed to store clean and sterile supplies and to protect them from contamination.

sterility assurance level (SAL) Probability of a viable microorganism being present on a product unit after sterilization.

sterility (event-related) Concept that items are considered sterile unless the integrity of the packaging is compromised (damaged) or suspected of being compromised (damaged) regardless of the sterilization date; sometimes referred to as ERS (event-related sterility).

sterility (time-related) Concept that a package is considered sterile until a specific expiration date is reached.

sterilization Process by which all forms of microbial life including bacteria, viruses, spores, and fungi are completely destroyed.

sterilization area Location of steam sterilizers, including the space for loading, queuing carts, cool-down, and unloading carts.

sterilization process monitor Physical/chemical device used to monitor one or more parameters to detect failures due to packaging, loading and/or sterilizer functioning. These devices cannot guarantee, assure, or prove sterilization; they measure physical conditions.

sterilization wrap Device intended to enclose another medical device to be sterilized by a healthcare provider, and to maintain sterility of the enclosed device until used.

sterilizer Equipment to sterilize medical devices, equipment, and supplies by direct exposure to sterilizing agent.

sterilizer (ethylene oxide) Sterilizing equipment that utilizes ethylene oxide under defined conditions of gas concentration, temperature, and percent relative humidity.

sterilizer (steam) Sterilizing equipment that uses saturated steam under pressure as the sterilant.

sterilizer (steam, dynamic-air-removal type) Steam sterilizer in which air is removed from the chamber and the load by means of pressure and vacuum excursions, or by means of steam flushes and pressure pulses.

sternum Breast bone.

stethoscope Instrument that conveys sounds from the patient's body to the examiner's ears.

stilet (or stylet) Small, sharp, pointed instrument used to probe, stabilize needles or catheters for insertion, and to remove obstructions from lumens of needles and tubes.

stockless inventory Distribution method in which supplies are stored by an outside vendor and delivered to the hospital on a regular basis in case lot quantities. Advantage: minimum inventory is held and paid for by the facility.

stock outs (inventory) Condition that occurs when reusable or consumable inventory items required to provide healthcare services to patients are not available.

stomach Pouch that serves as a reservoir for food that has been consumed.

strain Specific specimen or "culture" of a given species.

streptococci Bacteria which divide to form chains; members of the genus streptococcus which are Gram-positive, chain-forming bacteria.

strike-through Penetration of liquid or microorganism through a fabric.

subcutaneous Under the skin.

subordinate Employee who is supervised by someone in a higher organizational position.

suction devices Surgical instruments used to extract blood from a surgical site.

surfactant Surface-acting agent that lowers the surface tension of a liquid so it can penetrate deeper; prevents debris from being re-deposited on the item to which the soil was attached.

suffix (word element) Word element that comes after the root word element.

superheated steam Steam at a temperature which exceeds that of saturated steam at the same pressure; "dry" steam; the condition of steam when its temperature is too high relative to its pressure in a steam table.

superheating Condition that arises when steam is at a temperature which exceeds that of saturated steam at the same pressure.

superior Above; in a higher position.

surface tension Contractile surface force of a liquid which makes it tend to assume a spherical form (example:, to form a meniscus); also exists at the junction of two liquids.

surfactant Surface-active substance; alters (usually lowers) the surface tension of water; used in, wetting agents, and detergents; three types: nonionic, anionic and cationic.

surgical drape Device made of natural or synthetic materials used as a protective patient covering; purpose: to isolate a site of surgical incision from microbial and other contamination.

surgical gown Devices worn by operating room personnel during surgical procedures to protect the patient and operating room personnel from transfer of microorganisms, body fluids, and particulate matter.

surgical towel Absorbent product, typically made of cotton, intended to be used in a patient-care procedure.

susceptible host (chain of infection) Person or animal that lacks the ability to resist infection by an infectious agent.

suspension Mixture that will separate unless shaken.

suture Joint in which bone surfaces are closely united (example: skull); stitch used in surgery to bring parts together.

symbiosis Living together or close association of two dissimilar organisms with mutual benefit.

symptom Subjective disturbance due to disease.

synapse Junction between two neurons. or between a neuron and an effecter.

syndrome Group of symptoms characteristic of a disorder.

synergism Action of an inactive material that improves or increases the action of an active material; case in which the sum of the actions of two or more active materials mixed together is greater than the sum of their individual actions.

synovial Pertaining to a thick lubricating fluid found in joints, bursae, and tendon sheaths; pertaining to freely movable (diarthrotic) joint.

synthetic Produced by chemical synthesis rather than of natural origin.

system Group of organs that work together to carry out a specific activity.

systole Contraction phase of cardiac cycle.

T

table-top sterilizer Compact steam sterilizer with a chamber volume of not more than two cubic feet that generates its own steam with distilled or deionized water added by the user.

tachycardia Heart rate over 100 beats per minute.

tap water Treated water that is acceptable for drinking.

tarsals Ankle bones.

t cell Lymphocyte active in immunity that matures in the thymus gland; destroys foreign cells directly; T lymphocyte.

technical quality control indicators Process control measures utilized to assure that planned technical conditions within sterilizers and aerators are met.

tendinitis Inflammation of tendon.

tendon Cord of fibrous tissue that attaches a muscle to a bone.

terminal disinfection Disinfection of room after it has been vacated by a patient.

terminal infection Infection with streptococci or other pathogenic bacteria that occurs during the course of a chronic disease which causes death.

terminal sterilization Process of sterilizing a packaged item.

testes Male reproductive gland that forms and secretes sperm and several fluid elements in semen.

testosterone Male sex hormone produced in the testes; promotes the development of sperm cells and maintains secondary sex characteristics.

tetanus Constant contraction of a muscle; infectious disease caused by a bacterium (Clostridium tetani); lockjaw.

tetany Muscle spasms due to abnormal calcium metabolism as in parathyroid deficiency.

therapy Treatment of disease.

thermal disinfection Use of heat to kill all organisms except spores.

thermal equilibrium Condition in which all parts of a system have reached the same temperature; in a steam autoclave or hot-air oven, when the temperature throughout the entire load is the same.

thermocouple Device composed of two lengths of wire, each of which is made of a different homogenous metal; used to measure temperature changes by connecting a potentiometer or pyrometer into the thermocouple circuit.

thermolabile Easily altered or decomposed by heat.

thermophiles (bacteria) Bacteria which grow best at a temperature of 122°F – 158°F (50°C – 70°C).

thermostable Not easily affected by moderate heat.

thermostatic Controlled by temperature.

thorax Chest; thoracic.

threshold limit value (TLV) According to ACGIH: TLVs refer to airborne concentrations of substances, and represent conditions under which it is believed that nearly all workers may be repeatedly exposed day after day without adverse health effects (ACGIH, 1999).

thrombocyte Blood platelet; participates in clotting.

thrombus Blood clot within a vessel.

thumb forceps Tweezer-like instrument with smooth tip; used to grasp objects.

thyroid Endocrine gland in the neck.

tibia Large bone in lower leg.

time-weighted average (TWA) The employee's average airborne exposure in any 8-hour work shift of a 40-hour work week which shall not be exceeded; see also threshold limit value.

tincture Liquid in which a chemical is dissolved in alcohol.

tissue Group of similar cells that performs a specialized function.

tissue culture Cultivation of tissue cells in vitro.

tissue forceps Tweezer-like instrument with teeth to grasp tissue.

titer Concentration of infective microbes in a medium; amount of one substance to correspond with given amount of another substance.

titration Volumetric determination against standard solutions of known strength.

TLV-C The concentration that should not be exceeded during any part of the working exposure. If instantaneous monitoring is not feasible, the TLV-C can be assessed by sampling over a 15-minute period except for substances that may cause immediate irritation when exposures are short"

TLV-TWA The time weighted average concentration for a normal 8-hour workday and a 40-hour work week, to which nearly all workers may be repeatedly exposed, day after day, without adverse effect

TLV-STEL A 15-minute TWA exposure which should not be exceeded at any time during a workday even if the 8-hour TWA is within the TLV-TWA Exposure above the TLV-TWA up to the STEL should not be longer than 15 minutes, and should not occur more than four times per day. There should be at least 60 minutes between successive exposures in this range.

tolerance Ability to withstand or endure without ill effects.

tonsil Mass of lymphoid tissue in the pharynx region.

total acquisition costs All costs incurred by a facility to purchase a specific supply or equipment item from the point of authorization through its disposal.

total quality improvement (TQI) Concept of measuring the current output of a process or procedure, and then modifying it to increase the output, increase efficiency, and/or increase effectiveness.

total quality management (TQM) Quality management approach based on participation of all members aimed at long-term success through customer satisfaction and benefits to all members of the organization and society.

toxemia General intoxication caused by absorption of bacterial products, usually toxins, formed at a local source of infection.

toxic Poisonous.

toxin Poison; poisonous substance produced by and during the growth of certain pathogenic bacteria.

toxoid Detoxified toxin that produces specific antibodies; neutralized specific toxins used to immunize against bacteria that produce specific toxins.

TQM Short for total quality management.

trachea Windpipe.

tracheostomy Surgical opening into the trachea to introduce a tube through which the patient may breathe.

trait Characteristic.

transducer Device that converts energy from one form to another; ultrasonic transducer changes high-frequency electrical energy into high-frequency sound waves.

transmission Transfer of anything (such as a disease).

transplant Portion of a bacterial culture which has been transferred from an old pure culture to a fresh new medium.

triage System designed to sort out or classify emergency room patients according to severity of injury or disease.

tricuspid valve Valve between the right atrium and right ventricle of the heart.

tuberculin Filterable substance produced in the growth of mycobacterium tuberculosis in culture media; when injected intracutaneously in persons exposed to the tuberculosis bacillus or its products, a reaction is produced in 24 to 48 hours consisting of infiltration and hyperemia.

tuberculocidal Having the ability to kill tubercle bacilli.

tuberculosis Highly variable and communicable disease of man and some animals caused by the tubercle bacillus (Mycobacterium tuberculosis) and characterized by the formation of tubercles in the lungs or elsewhere.

turbidity Occurs when water contains sediments or solids that, when stirred, make the water appear cloudy.

TWA Short for time weighted average.

tympanic membrane Membrane between the external and middle ear that transmits sound waves to the bones of the middle ear; eardrum.

U

ubiquitous Present everywhere or in many places.

ulcer Area of the skin or mucous membrane in which the tissues are gradually destroyed.

ulna One of the two bones in the forearm.

ultrasonics Physical science of acoustic waves that oscillate in approximate range of 18 to 80 KHz.

ultraviolet radiation (UV) Invisible component of sun's radiation; used infrequently to degerm air and inanimate objects.

umbilical cord Structure that connects the fetus with the placenta; contains vessels that carry blood between the fetus and placenta.

umbilicus Small scar on the abdomen that marks the former attachment of the umbilical cord to the fetus; navel.

unicellular Composed of a single cell.

universal precautions See standard precautions.

unsanitary Deficient in sanitation; unclean to such a degree as to be injurious to health.

UPC Short for universal product code.

ureters Tube-like structures extending from the kidneys to the urinary bladder that move urine between these organs.

urethra Tube that discharges urine and semen.

urinary bladder Reservoir for urine.

urine Liquid waste excreted by kidneys.

use life (disinfectants) Length of time (or number of times) used after which the efficiency of a disinfectant is diminished.

utensil Instrument or container for domestic use; in hospitals, an item used for basic patient care such as a bedpan or washbasin..

uterus Female organ within which the fetus develops during pregnancy.

uvula Soft, fleshy, V-shaped mass that hangs from the soft palate.

V

vaccination Introduction of vaccine into the body.

vaccine Substance used to produce active immunity; usually a suspension of attenuated or killed pathogens given by inoculation to prevent a specific disease.

vagina Muscular canal in a female that extends from an external opening to the neck of the uterus.

validation Decontamination procedures used by equipment manufacturers to obtain, record, and interpret test results required to establish that a process consistently produces a sterile product.

value analysis Study of the relationship of design, function and cost of a product, material, or service.

valve Structure that prevents fluid from flowing backward (as in the heart, veins, and lymphatic vessels).

vancomycin-resistant enterococcus (VRE) Enterococcus bacteria that are no longer sensitive to vancomycin; transmission can occur either by direct contract or indirectly by hands.

vapor Substance in the gaseous state that is usually a liquid or solid.

variance Difference between the amount of a supply that should be available (from records), and the amount that is available (from physical count) when a perpetual inventory system is used.

varicella Chickenpox.

varicose Pertaining to an unnatural swelling; example: varicose vein.

variola Smallpox.

vas deferens Duct that transfers sperm from the epididymus to the seminal vesicle.

vasoconstriction Decrease in the diameter of a blood vessel.

vasodillation Increase in the diameter of a blood vessel.

VD Short for venereal disease.

vector Carrier of pathogenic microorganisms from one host to another (examples: flies and fleas, mosquitoes.

vegetative bacteria Nonsporeforming bacteria or sporeforming bacteria in a nonsporulating state.

vegetative stage State of active growth of microorganisms (as opposed to resting or spore stages.)

veins Vessels that carry blood back to the heart.

vena cava One of two large veins that carry blood into the right atrium of the heart.

venereal disease Disease acquired through sexual activity; VD; sexually transmitted disease.

venous Relating to vein or veins.

ventilation Movement of air into and out of the lungs.

ventral Toward the front or belly surface; anterior.

ventricles The two lower chambers of the heart.

venule Very small vein that collects blood from the capillaries.

verification Decontamination procedures used to confirm that the validation undertaken by the equipment manufacturer is applicable to the specific setting.

vertebra One of the bones of the spinal column.

vesicle Small sac or blister filled with fluid.

viable Living; having the ability to multiply.

virology Study of virus and viral diseases.

virucide Agent that destroys or inactivates viruses.

virulence Capacity of microorganisms to produce disease; power of an organism to overcome defenses of the host.

virus One of a group of minute infectious agents that grow only in living tissues or cells

viscera Organs in the ventral body cavities (especially the abdominal organs).

vital Characteristic of life; necessary for life; pertaining to life.

vitreous humor Fluid-filled compartment that gives shape to the eye.

VRE Short for vancomycin resistant enterococcus. When enterococcus bacteria are no longer sensitive to vancomycin, treatment is a challenge. Transmission occurs by direct contract or indirectly by hands.

W

warranty Guarantee or an assurance from a seller to the buyer that the goods or property is or shall be as represented.

washers Automated equipment used to clean, decontaminate, or disinfect (low, intermediate, or low-level) and dry medical devices.

wet pack Containers with moisture after the sterilization process is completed.

wetting agent Substance that reduces the surface tension of a liquid, and allows the liquid to penetrate or spread more easily across the surface of a solid.

wetting power Reduction of the water surface tension which allows the water to run or spread evenly over the surface.

wicking material Approved absorbent material that allows for air removal, steam penetration, and that facilitates drying.

word elements Parts of a word.

work practice controls Controls that reduce the likelihood of exposure by altering the manner in which a task is performed; example: prohibiting recapping needles with a two-handed technique.

work-related musculoskeletal disorder (WMSD) Injury to or disorder of the musculoskeletal system where exposure to workplace risk factors may have contributed to the disorder's development or aggravated a pre-existing condition.

X

x-ray Radiation of extremely short wave length that can penetrate opaque substances and affects photographic plates and fluorescent screens.

Y

yeasts Any of several unicellular fungi of the genus, Saccharomyces, which reproduce by budding.

Index

pH level for 137

for ultrasonic cleaners 138

Digestive system 52-54

Disaster

external 423

internal 423

plans 425-427

Disease, endemic 426

Disinfectants

activity levels of 158-159

chemical action of 159-160

effectiveness of 159-160

environmental evaluation of 172

in healthcare 160-171

risk levels 157-158

safety requirements 171-172

Disinfection

definition of 156

factors influencing effectiveness 156-157

selection of 160

Disposable packaging materials 245-246

Distillation, of water 117-118

Diversity 444-446

Doctor's (physician's) preference card 12-13

Dressing forceps 182

Dry heat sterilization 311-322

advantages 312

disadvantages 312

packaging 314

process challenge devices for 319

procedures 313-314

uses of 311-312

D-Values 322-323

E

Ear (sense organ) 44-45

Education and training, for safety 135

E-mail etiquette 439-440

Employee accidents 408-409

Endocrine system 46-47

Endoscopes

accessories for 225-226

rigid 226-229

semi-rigid 226-229

and Spaulding classification system 207-209

Endoscopic instruments

association guidelines 208

background 206-207

and glutaraldehyde 212

high-level disinfection 211

infection control issues 209-211

and OPA 212

and peracetic acid 212-213

regulations and guidelines 207-208

reprocessing chemicals for 211-213

special processing concerns 207

and staff education 215-216

Environmental Protection Agency (EPA) 90

Enzymatic

detergents 138

products for cleaning 119-120

Enzymes, for cleaning 138

Equal Employment Opportunity 445

Equipment acquisition

lease 368

manufacturer's loan 368-369

purchase 368

rental 368

Skin (organ) 45, 50, 51

Society of Gastroenterology Nurses and Associates (SGNA) 94

Softeners, water 117

Soil, gross 125

Soiled item transport 124-128

Solutions 326-328

Spaulding classification system 157, 276

Speaking, basic tactics 437

Spores 318

Stainless steel, types of 176-177

Standard precautions 16, 103, 134-135

Standards, definition of 78

STAT orders 353

Steam sterilization

absolute pressure 298-299

advantages of 288-289

assembling sets 309

conditions for effective 297-301

contract 297-298

gauge pressure 298-299

moisture 298-301

preparing devices and packs 301-305

temperature 298

time 298

work practices 301-311

wrapping sets 309-310

Steam sterilizers

anatomy of 289-292

cleaning 310-311

conditioning 295-296

cycle phases 295-297

drying 297

dynamic air removal 293

exhaust 296-297

exposure 296

flash 293-294

gravity air displacement 293

instrument washer-sterilizer 294

loading 305-307

steam-flush pressure-pulse 293

table top 292-293, 319

time/temperature relationship 298-301

types of 292-294

unloading 307-308

wet packs 308-309

Steam table 300-301

Sterile packages, transport of 263

Sterile packaging

flat wrapping 255-258

objectives of 239

overview of 238-239

storage of 260-262

universal principles 454

Sterile stock, arrangement of 262-263

Sterile storage, skills for 12-13

Sterility

event-related 260

time-related 260

Sterility assurance level 330

Sterility maintenance 259-260

Sterility maintenance covers 259

Sterilization

basic requirements 330-331

biological indicators 318-322

chemical indicators 315

definition of 156

Verification
of cleaning 152
of sterilization process 321-322
Veterans' administration facilities, overview 460
Viruses 68-69,158

W

Washing, automated 144-146

Waste
categories of 152
infectious 152-153

Water
chemicals in 115-116
deionized 327
distilled 327
filters for 116-117
for cleaning 136-137
pH 115
purification systems 116-117
purified 327
quality 114-116
reverse osmosis 327
softened 327
tap 326-327

Wet packs 244

Word elements (medical technology) 28-32

Work area, cleanliness of 108-109

Workplace hazards
clerical areas 404
decontamination area 398-399
equipment, distribution,
transport areas 402-403
receiving, breakout, storage areas 401-402
soiled receiving area 398

sterile preparation area 400-401
sterilization area 400-401
surgical service areas 404
World Health Organization (WHO) 94

Z

Ziehl-Neilson stain 65